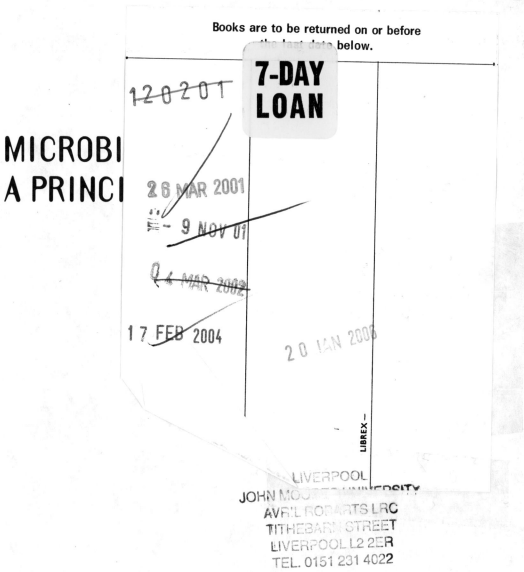

Microbial Pathogenesis: A Principles-Oriented Approach

Bruce A. McClane, Ph.D.
Associate Professor
Department of Molecular Genetics and Biochemistry
University of Pittsburgh School of Medicine
Pittsburgh, Pennsylvania

Timothy A. Mietzner, Ph.D.
Associate Professor
Department of Molecular Genetics and Biochemistry
University of Pittsburgh School of Medicine
Pittsburgh, Pennsylvania

Fence Creek Publishing

Madison, Connecticut

Typesetter: Pagesetters, Brattleboro, VT
Printer: Port City Press, Baltimore, MD
Illustrations by Visible Productions, Fort Collins, CO
Distributors:

United States and Canada
Blackwell Science, Inc.
Commerce Place
350 Main Street
Malden, MA 02148
Telephone orders: 800-215-1000 or 781-388-8250
Fax orders: 781-388-8270

Australia
Blackwell Science, PTY LTD.
54 University Street
Carlton, Victoria 3053
Telephone orders: 61-39-347-0300
Fax orders: 61-39-347-5001

Outside North America and Australia
Blackwell Science, LTD.
c/o Marston Book Service, LTD.
P.O. Box 269
Abingdon Oxon, OX 14 4XN England
Telephone orders: 44-1-235-465500
Fax orders: 44-1-235-465555

1 2 3 4 5 6 7 8 9 10

TABLE OF CONTENTS

Contributors vii

Preface ix

Introduction xi

Part I: Introduction to the Infectious Diseases 1
Overview

Chapter 1 7
Biology of Microbial Pathogens

Chapter 2 27
Bacterial Growth and Physiology

Chapter 3 45
Growth of Viruses

Chapter 4 61
Antimicrobial Therapy

Chapter 5 81
Resistance to Antimicrobial Agents, *Saleem A. Khan, Ph.D.*

Part II: Establishment of Infectious Diseases: Transmission and Colonization 97
Overview

Chapter 6 101
Infectious Diseases Acquired by Ingestion

Chapter 7 119
Pathogens Acquired by Inhalation

Chapter 8 135
Zoonotic Infections

Chapter 9 153
Sexually Transmitted Diseases, *William F. Goins, Ph.D.*

Chapter 10 167
Bloodborne and Transplant-Associated Infections

Chapter 11 179
Normal Microbial Flora Inhibition of Colonization

Chapter 12 189
Colonization I: Adherence

Chapter 13 205
Colonization II: Invasion

Part III: Microbial Subversion of Host Defenses 219
Overview

Chapter 14 223
Overcoming the Physical and Chemical Defenses of the Human Body

Chapter 15 233
   Immune Survival Strategies of Intracellular Prokaryotic and Eukaryotic Pathogens
Chapter 16 251
   Immune Evasion Strategies: Molecular Mimicry
Chapter 17 265
   Immune Evasion Strategies: Antigenic Variation
Chapter 18 281
   Immune Evasion Strategies: Capsules
Chapter 19 295
   Immune Evasion Strategies of Bacteria: Noncapsular Surface Factors and Secreted Factors

Part IV: Mechanisms By Which Pathogens Damage the Host 307
   Overview
Chapter 20 311
   Bacterial Exotoxins
Chapter 21 327
   Sepsis, *Karen A. Norris, Ph.D.*
Chapter 22 335
   Immunopathologic Consequences of Inflammation, *Joanne L. Flynn, Ph.D.*

Part V: Genetics of Microbial Virulence 347
   Overview
Chapter 23 349
   Role of Mobile Genetic Elements in Bacterial Virulence
Chapter 24 363
   Regulation of Bacterial Virulence Factor Expression

Part VI: Host Factors and the Outcome of Infection 377
   Overview
Chapter 25 379
   Consequences of Failure to Clear Pathogens: Persistence, Latency, and the Carrier State,
   William F. Goins, Ph.D.
Chapter 26 391
   Role of Bacteria and Viruses in Tumorigenesis
Chapter 27 403
   Acquired Immunodeficiency Syndrome
Chapter 28 413
   Opportunistic Infections

Part VII: Vaccine Principles 427
   Overview
Chapter 29 431
   Bacterial and Viral Vaccines

Appendixes 451
   1   Diagnostic Medical Microbiology
   2   Control of Pathogens by Sterilization, Pasteurization, and Disinfection
   3   Table: Review of Medically Important Pathogens
Index 473

CONTRIBUTORS

John N. Dowling, M.D.
Professor
Department of Medicine
University of Pittsburgh School of Medicine
Pittsburgh, Pennsylvania

Joanne L. Flynn, Ph.D.
Assistant Professor
Department of Molecular Genetics and Biochemistry
University of Pittsburgh School of Medicine
Pittsburgh, Pennsylvania

William F. Goins, Ph.D.
Associate Professor
Department of Molecular Genetics and Biochemistry
University of Pittsburgh School of Medicine
Pittsburgh, Pennsylvania

Saleem A. Khan, Ph.D.
Professor
Department of Molecular Genetics and Biochemistry
University of Pittsburgh School of Medicine
Pittsburgh, Pennsylvania

Bruce A. McClane, Ph.D.
Associate Professor
Department of Molecular Genetics and Biochemistry
University of Pittsburgh School of Medicine
Pittsburgh, Pennsylvania

Timothy A. Mietzner, Ph.D.
Associate Professor
Department of Molecular Genetics and Biochemistry
University of Pittsburgh School of Medicine
Pittsburgh, Pennsylvania

Karen A. Norris, Ph.D.
Associate Professor
Department of Molecular Genetics and Biochemistry
University of Pittsburgh School of Medicine
Pittsburgh, Pennsylvania

Bruce A. Phillips, Ph.D.
Professor
Department of Molecular Genetics and Biochemistry
University of Pittsburgh School of Medicine
Pittsburgh, Pennsylvania

PREFACE

Infectious diseases are a major medical concern today, claiming over 17 million victims worldwide each year. This fact, coupled with the emergence of new microbial pathogens and the increasing problems with resistance to existing antimicrobial therapies, signals that infectious diseases will continue to be a daily concern of the physician into the future. This reality dictates that today's medical students develop a solid foundation in medical microbiology. The ability of a student to obtain this foundation is increasingly challenged because the field of medical microbiology is undergoing unprecedented changes in its understanding, particularly as molecular tools shed new light on how infectious diseases cause their diverse pathologies (a process that is referred to as "pathogenesis"). The result is a form of knowledge overload that can overwhelm even the most astute medical student seeking to integrate this information in a useful way.

In response, our medical microbiology course moved away from a traditional taxonomy-oriented course (i.e., the infamous "bug parade") to a principles-oriented course that emphasizes common themes in infectious disease. The rationale for this change was our belief that an appreciation for the common principles of infection will foster better long-term retention of relevant material, minimizing the short-term memorization of specific "factoids," many of which may become outdated in a short time.

We have developed this principles-oriented approach over the past six years, and it has been increasingly well received by our students. However, we have struggled to find a textbook appropriate for our course. To meet this perceived need, we have produced *Microbial Pathogenesis: A Principles-Oriented Approach*. This book is organized into seven parts, each of which addresses a particular theme (e.g., Part IV: Mechanisms By Which Pathogens Damage the Host) important for understanding, treating, or preventing infectious diseases. Each chapter within a part addresses one aspect of the theme (e.g., Chapter 20, Bacterial Exotoxins). To reinforce the relevance of medical microbiology to modern medicine, each chapter begins with the introduction of a clinical case that involves the pathogenic principle. The principle is discussed in general terms and then its importance to pathogenesis is illustrated using a medically important microbial pathogen as a paradigm. The clinical case is resolved at the end of the chapter. Following each chapter are review questions (and answers with explanations) that allow the student to self-assess whether they have learned the important information presented.

All of the authors have been involved with this course from its inception. It is our hope that this book reflects our enthusiasm for teaching microbiology in a principles-oriented approach.

Finally, the authors wish to thank the staff at Fence Creek Publishing for their patience and assistance in bringing this book to completion, especially Matt Harris, publisher, for his commitment to this project, and Nancy G. Lucas, production editor. Nancy's enthusiasm, diligence, and careful attention to detail truly facilitated bringing this project to completion.

Bruce A. McClane, Ph.D., and Timothy A. Mietzner, Ph.D.

INTRODUCTION

Microbial Pathogenesis: A Principles-Oriented Approach is one of ten titles in the *Integrated Medical Sciences (IMS) Series* from Fence Creek Publishing. These books have been designed as course supplements and aids for board review for first- and second-year medical students. Rather than focusing on the individual basic science disciplines, the books in the *IMS Series* have been designed to highlight the points of integration between the sciences, including clinical correlation where appropriate. Each chapter begins with a clinical case, the resolution of which requires the application of basic science concepts to clinical problems. Extensive use of margin notes, figures, tables, and questions illuminates core biomedical concepts with which medical students often have difficulty.

Each book in the *IMS Series* shares common features and formats. Attempts have been made to present difficult concepts in a brief and focused format and to provide a pedagogical aid that facilitates both knowledge acquisition and also review.

Given the long period of gestation necessary to publish a book, it is often impossible for publishers to keep pace with the changes and advances that occur so rapidly. However, the authors and the publisher recognize the need to have access to the most current information and are committed to keeping *Microbial Pathogenesis: A Principles-Oriented Approach* as up to date as possible between editions. As the field of medical microbiology evolves, updates to this text may be posted periodically on our web site at http://www.fencecreek.com.

We hope that the student finds the format and the text material relevant, interesting, and challenging. The authors, as well as the Fence Creek staff, welcome your comments and suggestions for use in future editions.

PART I: INTRODUCTION TO THE INFECTIOUS DISEASES

OVERVIEW

NATURE AND MEDICAL IMPORTANCE OF THE INFECTIOUS DISEASES

The infectious diseases are illnesses caused by microbial pathogens or their products. The pathogens most commonly responsible for infectious diseases include bacteria, viruses, fungi, and parasites (a few more exotic microbial pathogens are introduced later in this book). The biologic differences among these groups of pathogens have extremely important consequences for antimicrobial therapy and, thus, are the major focus for Chapters 1–3 of this book.

The infectious diseases have held considerable importance for medicine, being the primary cause of morbidity and mortality in the human population throughout history. For example, single epidemics of bubonic plague are believed to have resulted in the deaths of more than one-third of the population in medieval Europe. However, during much of the 20th century, dramatic progress has been achieved in limiting morbidity and mortality from human infectious diseases, particularly in developed countries. For example, public health measures (e.g., rodent and insect control programs) have significantly reduced the occurrence of diseases involving vectorborne pathogens. Further, the development of several effective vaccines (see Chapter 29) and the introduction of antimicrobial therapy (see Chapter 4) also contributed significantly to this reduction in infectious disease morbidity and mortality. In fact, by the 1970s, these successes had given rise to a commonly held but short-sighted perception that infectious diseases were under control in industrialized countries and were likely to remain so permanently. (Note that infectious diseases were never considered to be controlled in Third World countries.)

Despite this optimism of the 1970s, it has become increasingly clear that the infectious diseases have not been controlled, even in industrialized countries. For example, recent statistics indicate that infectious diseases once again rank as the third leading cause of death in the United States, trailing only heart disease (first) and cancer (second). Several factors are contributing to our renewed problems with infectious diseases. First, a number of newly discovered pathogens (e.g., human immunodeficiency virus [HIV], which causes acquired immunodeficiency syndrome [AIDS]; *Borrelia burgdorferi*, which causes Lyme disease) only recently emerged as major public health problems. Second, pathogens such as *Mycobacterium tuberculosis* (the cause of tuberculosis [TB]) that were among those microbes once considered controlled (at least in developed countries) have now returned as major health concerns in the United States and other developed countries. The re-emergence of these pathogens often appears to be related to societal changes (e.g., increased homelessness, poverty) that contribute to the spread of TB in the United States (see Chapter 22). Third, changes in medical practice are increasingly predisposing patients to infectious diseases. For example, immunosuppression of transplant recipients and chemotherapy of cancer patients often result in lowered host defenses, rendering these patients much more susceptible to infections by opportunistic pathogens (see Chapter 27). A fourth contributing factor to the renewed concern about infectious diseases is the increasing difficulty in treating many of these illnesses. Bacteria that were once sensitive to several different antimicrobials are often now highly resistant to antibiotics, which limits therapeutic options (see Chapters 4 and 5). The bottom line is that infectious diseases are important contemporary medical concerns and will likely remain so for the foreseeable future.

KOCH'S POSTULATES

Throughout this book, statements indicate that a particular pathogen is responsible for a specific infectious disease. How have these relationships been established? Traditionally, one of the most accepted ways of establishing a causal relationship between a pathogen and an infectious disease has been to fulfill a set of rules referred to as Koch's postulates. Fulfilling Koch's postulates involves:

1. Showing that a particular microbe is always found in a diseased host (e.g., humans) but not in a healthy host.
2. Isolating this microbe from the diseased host and growing it in pure cultures away from the host.
3. Showing that the isolated microbe can cause a similar disease when it is inoculated into susceptible experimental animal models.
4. Re-isolating from the diseased experimental animals the same microbe that had been injected into these animals.

Koch's postulates have provided an invaluable framework for establishing the cause of many but not all infectious diseases. Problems are sometimes encountered when trying to fulfill Koch's postulates experimentally. For example, some pathogens (e.g., *Mycobacterium leprae*, the cause of leprosy) cannot be grown away from an animal host, whereas other pathogens (e.g., *Neisseria gonorrhoeae*, the cause of gonorrhea) are so highly specialized for infecting humans that there simply are no adequate experimental animal models. Furthermore, it is increasingly appreciated that many infections involve opportunistic pathogens that cause disease only in immunocompromised individuals (see Chapter 27). Attempting to fulfill Koch's postulates by inoculating opportunistic pathogens into healthy experimental animals can yield false-negative conclusions about the ability of these microbes to cause infectious diseases in immunocompromised humans.

What happens when such problems are encountered in fulfilling Koch's postulates? In this situation, a causal relationship between a pathogen and an infectious disease is usually indirectly inferred from epidemiologic studies aimed at demonstrating a specific statistical association between a microbe and an infectious disease.

MOLECULAR KOCH'S POSTULATES

*A **commensal organism** is a microbe that exists in the healthy body as part of the normal flora without causing detectable damage to the host.*

__Virulence__ is a word with many meanings. In this book (unless otherwise noted), virulence refers to the number of microbes that must be administered to an animal to cause the development of disease (i.e., fewer "high virulence" than "low virulence" microbes are required to cause equivalent disease).

Virulence

Although a particular bacterial species may be identified as the cause of an infectious disease, this does not necessarily mean that all members of that species are able to cause that illness. For example, some strains of *Escherichia coli* can cause human gastrointestinal (GI) infections (see Chapter 12), while other *E. coli* strains are commensal organisms that comprise part of the normal GI flora of healthy humans (see Chapter 11). Continuing with this example, it is now appreciated that the variable ability of different *E. coli* isolates to cause GI disease reflects differences in their virulence, with the virulence of an individual *E. coli* cell (or any microbe) being a function of the virulence factors that a particular microbial cell can produce. Examples of some well-established bacterial virulence factors include toxins, adhesins, and capsules (each of these virulence factors are explored in detail in Chapters 12, 18, and 20–22).

Steps in Fulfilling Molecular Koch's Postulates

How can one evaluate whether a specific microbial product is a virulence factor for a pathogen? The following set of rules, termed molecular Koch's postulates, are commonly used to establish this relationship:

1. The phenotype or property encoded should be associated with pathogenic strains of that species.
2. Specifically inactivating the virulence genes associated with this virulence trait should cause a measurable loss of virulence (i.e., it now takes more of these microbes to cause equivalent disease).
3. Adding a cloned copy of the wild-type gene back to the mutant should restore virulence.

For example, using these rules, one can prove that cholera toxin is a virulence factor for *Vibrio cholerae*:

1. Clinical isolates of *V. cholerae* are colera-toxin positive.
2. Specific inactivation of the *V. cholerae* genes that encode for cholera toxin sharply decreases the ability of the mutant to cause diarrhea in animal models (or human volunteers).
3. Adding a wild-type toxin gene back to the cholera toxin mutant created in step 2 restores virulence (i.e., restores the ability of the mutant to cause diarrhea).

Therefore, it can be concluded that cholera toxin is a virulence factor for *V. cholerae*.

INTRODUCTION TO PRINCIPLES OF MICROBIAL PATHOGENESIS

Microbial Entry, Colonization, and Disease

Before causing disease symptoms, a pathogen faces considerable challenges. This microbe must first compete with normal flora microbes already present at many mucosal surfaces in the body (see Chapter 11). If successful in this competition, the pathogen then usually confronts the necessity of evading, at least temporarily, host defenses. To overcome these challenges, successful pathogens have devised some fascinating strategies; these pathogenic strategies are the focus of a major portion of this book (see Parts II and III).

Before discussing selected paradigm pathogenic strategies in Parts II and III, a few basic pathogenic principles common to most infectious diseases need to be briefly introduced. First, it is important to appreciate that disease does not necessarily occur every time a pathogen enters the human body. It is usually necessary for some minimum number of microbes to enter the body for infection to be initiated (with this number being lower for more virulent microbes). Further, it is even possible for some pathogens to colonize the body successfully in significant numbers without causing illness. For example, *Streptococcus pneumoniae*, which causes pneumococcal pneumonia (see Chapter 18), can be routinely found in the upper respiratory tract of 10%–30% of healthy people. Pneumococcal pneumonia, which is one of the most common types of pneumonia, usually develops following some impairment of a person's respiratory host defenses (see Chapter 18), thus allowing *S. pneumoniae* to proliferate in the lower respiratory tract. Note that pneumococcal pneumonia illustrates the importance of host defense status in determining whether many infectious diseases will develop.

Infection Versus Intoxication

A second basic pathogenic principle is that infection refers to a disease in which viable pathogens are (or were) present in the human body. Most but not all infectious diseases involve infections. The exceptions are the few infectious diseases that involve intoxications, in which the entrance of a microbial toxin alone (i.e., no viable microbes are in the body) is sufficient to induce illness. An obvious example of an intoxication is foodborne botulism, in which all symptoms of this very serious illness (see Chapter 20) are caused by botulinum toxin alone. Foodborne botulism often results from ingestion of foods contaminated with botulinum toxin (i.e., it is not necessary to ingest viable *Clostridium botulinum* cells to become ill with foodborne botulism).

Pathogenic Cycle

Another important principle is referred to as the pathogenic cycle. With the exception of infectious diseases that involve intoxications, most infectious diseases result from microbes that complete most or all of the steps in the following cycle:

1. Entrance of the pathogen into the body (see Chapters 6–11)
2. Colonization and adherence of the pathogen in the human body (see Chapters 11 and 12)
3. Invasion of the pathogen from the epithelium into deeper tissues (see Chapter 13)
4. Production of cell and tissue damage (see Chapters 20–22)
5. Dissemination of the pathogen to initiate infection in a new host (see Chapters 6–11)

As indicated above, each step of the pathogenic cycle is explored in detail in this book. The rationale for this emphasis is that understanding how a pathogen completes its pathogenic cycle often provides important insights into the infectious diseases caused by that microbe. For example, a relationship often exists between how a pathogen enters the body and the type of initial symptoms the pathogen elicits (e.g., pathogens acquired by inhalation often cause, at least initially, respiratory tract disease, involving symptoms such as coughing). Before leaving this introduction to the pathogenic cycle, it is necessary to note that although most pathogens complete this entire cycle, there are some exceptions. For example, although *V. cholerae* enters the body (via ingestion), colonizes the GI tract (by adhering to intestinal epithelial cells), produces physiologic damage to the host (through a toxin-induced voluminous diarrhea that causes severe fluid and electrolyte loss), and disseminates from the infected host to others (by fecal contamination of water supplies), this bacterium does not invade the intestinal epithelium and typically does not utilize an elaborate immune evasion strategy.

Intracellular Versus Extracellular Pathogens

The final pathogenic principle to be introduced in this overview is the importance of determining whether a pathogen is present intracellularly or extracellularly during disease (Table I-1). The extracellular pathogens are unable to grow inside mammalian cells and, therefore, as implied by their name, must exist extracellularly during disease. The obligate intracellular pathogens absolutely require mammalian cells for their growth. Unlike the extracellular and facultative intracellular pathogens described below, the obligate intracellular pathogens cannot grow on artificial media. A final group, the facultative intracellular pathogens, are capable of growing inside or outside mammalian cells, although they are often found inside appropriate host cells in vivo.

Inspection of Table I-1 clearly confirms that either an intracellular or extracellular life style can be used successfully to cause infectious disease. In fact, adopting either of these life styles holds both advantages and disadvantages for a pathogen. For example, pathogens residing inside mammalian cells have the advantage of being shielded (at least initially) from the immune system. An intracellular location also provides some pathogens, such as *Chlamydia* species (see Chapter 9), with access to energy generated

TABLE I-1
Major Intracellular Versus Extracellular Pathogens

Intracellular		Extracellular
Obligate	**Facultative**	
All viruses		
Bacteria		
Mycobacterium leprae (af)[a]	*Brucella* species (−)[a]	*Bacillus* species (+)
Chlamydia species (−)[b]	Some *Escherichia coli* (−)[b]	*Clostridium* species (+)
Rickettsia species ("- like")[b]	*Legionella* species (−)[a]	*Corynebacterium diphtheriae* (+)
	Campylobacter species (−)[b]	Most strains *E. coli* (−)
	Other *Mycobacteria* species (af)[a]	*Haemophilus* species (−)
	Salmonella species (−)[a]	*Klebsiella* species (−)
	Shigella species (−)[b]	*Helicobacter* species (−)
	Yersinia species (−)[a]	*Proteus* species (−)
	Neisseria gonorrhoeae (−)[b]	*Pseudomonas* species (−)
	Neisseria meningitidis (−)[c]	*Vibrio cholerae* (−)
	Bordetella pertussis (−)[c]	*Borrelia* species (−)
	Group B streptococcus (+)[c]	*Treponema* species (−)
	Listeria monocytogenes (+)[a]	*Staphylococcus* species (+)
		Group A streptococcus (+)
		Bacteroides-like group (−)
Fungi		
None	*Histoplasma capsulatum*[a]	*Cryptococcus neoformans*
	Blastomyces dermatitidis[b]	
	Candida albicans[b]	
	Coccidioides immitis[a]	
Parasites		
None	*Plasmodium* species[b]	*Giardia lamblia*
	Leishmania species[a]	*Trypanosoma brucei*
	Trypanosoma cruzi[b]	
	Cryptosporidium species[b]	
Others		
None	None	*Pneumocystis carinii*

Note. af = acid fast; (+) = gram positive; (−) = gram negative.
[a] Intracellular growth in professional phagocytes.
[b] Intracellular growth in other cells.
[c] May be found intracellularly but thought to exist primarily as extracellular organisms in the human body.

by the host cell or some pathogens, such as viruses (see Chapter 3), with access to the host cell's protein and nucleic acid synthesis machinery. A final advantage for an intracellular life style is that the pathogen is afforded protection from certain antimicrobial agents that do not easily penetrate mammalian cells (see Chapter 4). However, an intracellular life style has a major (and obvious) disadvantage: the pathogen must survive and grow inside mammalian cells, particularly professional phagocytes, which have developed defense mechanisms specifically aimed at killing (or limiting the growth of) intracellular invaders. Therefore, to succeed as an intracellular pathogen, particularly in professional phagocytes, a microbe must devise a strategy to overcome the natural defenses of the mammalian cell. Even if a pathogen succeeds in devising such a strategy, it is then usually necessary for the pathogen to devote a considerable portion of its efforts toward implementation of its survival strategy.

1

BIOLOGY OF MICROBIAL PATHOGENS

CHAPTER OUTLINE

Introduction of Clinical Case
Biology of Microbial Pathogens
• Taxonomic Definitions and Their Medical Utility
Viral Pathogens
Prokaryotic Pathogens
• Similarities among Prokaryotic Pathogens
• Structural Differences among Bacteria
Gram Stain
• Bacterial Anatomy and the Basis for the Gram Stain
• Medically Important Pathogens Unreactive to Gram Stain
Eukaryotic Pathogens
• Fungi
• Parasites
• Difficult-to-Categorize Eukaryotic Pathogens
Resolution of Clinical Case
Review Questions

INTRODUCTION OF CLINICAL CASE

A working mother brought her 14-month-old son from a day care facility to the pediatrician's office, complaining that the child had a slight fever, an intermittent cough, and a runny nose. The mother also described the child within the past week as generally irritable and lacking his normal appetite. Physical examination of the toddler revealed left ear tenderness, and inspection of the inner ear showed signs of inflammation. The pediatrician suggested that the child be observed for the next couple of days to see if the symptoms resolved. The mother, at her wits' end with the child's irritability and under extreme pressure at work, demanded that the pediatrician prescribe something to alleviate the child's affliction.

Several obvious questions arise with regard to this clinical case:

• Why is the child experiencing these symptoms?
• If this is an infectious disease, what is the biologic agent responsible for the child's symptomology and where is he likely to have "caught" it?
• How should the pediatrician respond to the mother's demand to prescribe something to alleviate the child's symptoms?

This clinical scenario is experienced nearly every day by practicing pediatricians. Many of the answers to these questions rely on a basic understanding of the biology of microbial pathogens that cause disease.

BIOLOGY OF MICROBIAL PATHOGENS

Understanding the biology of microbial pathogens is fundamental to understanding the diseases that they cause and to designing appropriate management regimens, whether these regimens are antibiotics or vaccines. The major divisions of pathogens causing infectious diseases have traditionally been the viruses, bacteria, and eukaryotic pathogens. A virus consists of a core of genetic material (either DNA or RNA) enclosed in a protein shell, and it depends on host cells to supply necessary functions such as protein synthesis and energy metabolism. Bacteria represent the next level of biologic complexity. These unicellular microbes usually do not depend on a host cell for proliferation, but there are some exceptions (see Part I, Overview). Bacteria lack internal membrane organelle organization, including the complete absence of a nuclear membrane, and so are described as *prokaryotic* ("before" a nucleus). This cellular organization is in contrast to pathogens described as *eukaryotic* ("true" nucleus), including fungi and parasites, which have a biologic architecture resembling the mammalian host that they infect. The similarities between the host cell and eukaryotic pathogens present a particularly difficult challenge to the host defenses (see Part IV) as well as for antimicrobial therapy (see Chapter 4). The basic biologic differences between viral, bacterial, and eukaryotic pathogens are summarized in Table 1-1.

Major Divisions of Pathogens
- *Viruses*
- *Prokaryotic pathogens (bacteria)*
- *Eukaryotic pathogens (fungi, parasites)*

TABLE 1-1 ▶

Characteristics of the Major Microbial Pathogens

Characteristic	Viruses	Bacteria	Fungi	Parasites
Size (μm)	0.02–0.2	0.1–10.0	3.0–10.0	15–100
Presence of a cytosol	No	Yes	Yes	Yes
Presence of a nucleus	No	No	Yes	Yes
Presence of ribosomes	No	70S	80S	80S
Presence of mitochondria	No	No	Yes	Yes
Cell wall composition	None	Peptidoglycan	Chitin, mannin, glucan	None
Germ-line nucleic acid	RNA or DNA	DNA	DNA	DNA
Reproduction	Asexual	Asexual	Sexual	Sexual

Taxonomic Definitions and Their Medical Utility

Because of the diversity of pathogens that can parasitize humans, the formal classification of pathogens (i.e., taxonomy) is often a source of frustration for the student attempting to appreciate the complexity of infectious disease. Although frustrating, a basic vocabulary describing microbial pathogens associated with certain etiologic outcomes must be established to link the cause-and-effect relationships of infectious diseases, as well as to design effective disease management measures (e.g., public health intervention, antimicrobial therapy, vaccination). By convention, classification is accomplished by organizing pathogens into kingdom, family, genus, and species relationships. This scheme is used for bacteria and the eukaryotic pathogens, but because of their unique biology, it is not used for the viruses. The specific rationale for the classification of viruses, bacteria, and parasites is described further in the sections that pertain to their biology.

As introduced above, one distinguishing feature of microbial pathogens is the presence or absence of a nucleus. A second distinguishing characteristic of pathogens is their size, as depicted in Figure 1-1. Viruses cannot be observed by conventional microscopy; they typically require visualization by electron microscopy. By contrast, prokaryotic pathogens are generally larger than viruses, with dimensions ranging between 0.1 and 10.0 μm. These dimensions allow them to be visually observed by high-power light microscopy using 1000X magnification (achieved using a 10X ocular lens in conjunction with a 100X objective lens and oil immersion). Although prokaryotic pathogens (with exceptions) are larger than viruses, they are roughly one-fifth to one-tenth the size of eukaryotic pathogens. Most eukaryotic pathogens can be visualized by light microscopy using relatively low-power magnification (achieved using a 10X ocular lens, a 40X objective lens, and no oil immersion).

Taxonomic ranks using Escherichia coli *as a specific example. The most practical organization includes the ranks of* **family,** **genus,** *and* **species.**

Formal Ranks	**Example**
Kingdom	*Procaryotae*
Division	*Gracilicutes*
Class	*Scotobacteria*
Order	*Eubacteriales*
Family	*Enterobacteriaceae*
Genus	*Escherichia*
Species	coli

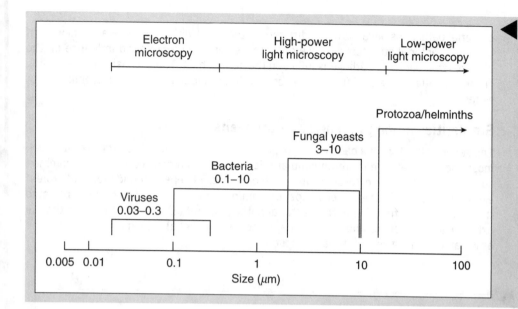

FIGURE 1-1
Microbial Pathogens on the Molecular Ruler. The representation of microbial pathogens on the scale of the molecular ruler is a useful means to organize the three major groups of microbial pathogens—viruses, prokaryotes, and eukaryotes.

VIRAL PATHOGENS

Because viruses require a host cell for replication, they lack the autonomy of most prokaryotic and eukaryotic pathogens. Thus, they are not taxonomically organized in a scheme involving kingdom, family, genus, and species. Rather, viruses are categorized based upon the mechanisms by which they maintain their infectivity. This correlates with the general status of their infectious genetic material (e.g., DNA, RNA, segmented, linear, double stranded, single stranded). These aspects of viral classification are described in detail in Chapter 3, and an understanding of this scheme should not be viewed as an exercise in rote memorization. For example, a clinician prescribes the drug azidothymidine (AZT) to a patient with acquired immunodeficiency syndrome (AIDS) specifically because this drug inhibits the human immunodeficiency virus (HIV) enzyme, reverse transcriptase. AZT is effective against HIV because reverse transcriptase is critical for the conversion of viral RNA to DNA, a step that is essential for the proliferation of this virus (see Chapters 3 and 27). A similar antiviral therapy would not be appropriate for herpesvirus, because this DNA virus does not employ reverse transcriptase as part of its infectious process (see Chapters 3 and 9). This is but one of many examples that underscore the importance of understanding the biologic classification of viruses.

Viruses are ubiquitous to the environment in which humans live. They can occur as inconspicuous proviruses that are integrated into the human genome, allowing them to be maintained within the host from generation to generation (vertical transmission). More frequently, viruses are transmitted between people (horizontal transmission). Regardless of how they are transmitted, viruses cause a variety of human diseases by essentially "hijacking" normal host-cell processes and exerting their pathology either by causing host-cell dysregulation or by eliciting an immune response that results in the destruction of host tissues (immunopathology). The basic biology of viruses, their medical significance, and their ubiquity are more thoroughly described in Chapter 3.

Vertical transmission refers to the transmission of the insulting agent from germ line to germ line. In this context, viruses are unique among the microbial pathogens because they can integrate into chromosomal DNA as proviruses; a property that allows them to be passed from parent to progeny during sexual recombination.
Horizontal transmission of infectious disease refers to the transfer of disease between individuals.

PROKARYOTIC PATHOGENS

Within the kingdom Procaryotae, there exists the order Eubacteriales, referring to the "true bacteria" (eubacteria), which includes the most common bacterial pathogens. Bacterial pathogens are classified as eubacteria based on their size and the similarities of their biologic structures. Despite these similarities, there is tremendous diversity among bacterial pathogens because of the differences that exist within the general framework of common bacterial structures. These differences can have a profound influence on the diseases that bacterial pathogens inflict on the human host. Thus, a basic understanding of these similarities and differences is critical to an understanding of microbial pathogenesis.

Similarities among Prokaryotic Pathogens

The general structure of a bacterial pathogen is depicted in Figure 1-2. At the basal level, most bacterial pathogens are unicellular microorganisms organized into three common compartments: (1) the cytosol, in which the processes of genetic replication and protein expression occur; (2) the cell envelope, containing a cell wall and membranes critical to the structure and function of the bacterial pathogen; and (3) surface structures that lie external to the cell envelope (e.g., capsules, pili, flagella) and may or may not be associated with a given bacterial pathogen.

FIGURE 1-2 ▶

General Organization of a Bacterium. The basic structure of a bacterial cell includes a cytoplasm, a plasma or cytoplasmic membrane, a cell wall, and structures that lie beyond the cell wall.

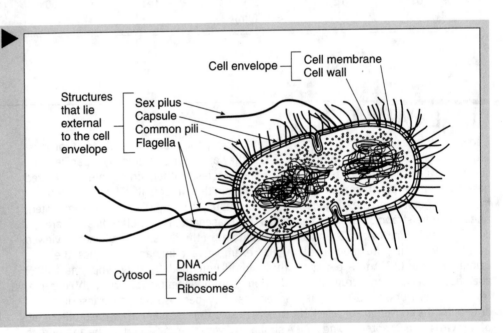

COMMON BACTERIAL BIOLOGY

Nucleic Acid Replication and Genetic Exchange. A key feature that distinguishes prokaryotic pathogens from eukaryotic pathogens is that bacteria have a single *haploid* circular chromosome containing a single origin of replication. This is in contrast to the complex, multiple *diploid* chromosomal arrangement typical of eukaryotes. The implication of having a single haploid chromosome is quite profound; it requires that a prokaryote divide asexually by the process of binary fission, in contrast to the sexual reproduction exhibited by many eukaryotes. The genetic differences between prokaryotes and eukaryotes are beyond the scope of this text, and the interested student is advised to consult a basic genetics textbook for a complete discussion of these differences. What is important to appreciate is that eukaryotes and prokaryotes use unique enzymes for DNA replication (e.g., polymerases, topoisomerases, helicases), which can be targets of the selective strategy of antimicrobial therapy (see Chapter 4).

A theoretical restriction of binary fission is clonal proliferation. If all organisms developed as clones using an identical DNA blueprint, as implied by strict binary fission, then the host immune system would have little trouble eliminating all progeny derived from the parental clone. In fact, this does not occur. Instead, antigenic and phenotypic diversity is the norm rather than the exception for bacterial pathogens (see Chapter 17). Faced with environmental pressures, such as those imposed in a host–pathogen relationship, bacteria are able to overcome specific and nonspecific immune mechanisms using a variety of strategies, as described in Table 1-2.

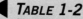

Mechanism	Example
Environmental sensing	Expression of *Pseudomonas aeruginosa* exotoxin A in response to the iron-limiting conditions of the human host (see Chapter 5)
Episomal transfer (conjugation)	Plasmid-mediated antibiotic resistance (see Chapter 5)
Phage transfer (transduction)	Phage-encoded diphtheria toxin expression (see Chapter 23)
Uptake of naked DNA (transformation)	Gonococcal pilus diversity (see Chapter 17)
Somatic mutation	Flagellar immune modulation (see Chapter 24)
Genomic rearrangement	Duplication of the cholera toxin gene in virulent strains of *Vibrio cholerae* (see Chapter 20)

TABLE 1-2
Mechanisms of Bacterial Antigenic/Phenotypic Diversity

One biologic strategy that prokaryotic pathogens employ to exercise their diversity is the differential expression of genes in response to changes in their environment. A classic example of this is the overexpression of *Pseudomonas aeruginosa* exotoxin A in response to the iron-limiting environment of the human host (see Chapter 5). Other environmental cues, such as oxygen, phosphate, or carbohydrate limitation, may also alter the molecular composition of bacterial pathogens (see Chapter 24).

Another common means of spreading genetic diversity among prokaryotes is by autonomously replicating extrachromosomal nucleic acids, commonly referred to as plasmids. The resistance plasmids (R-plasmids) are of great significance in contemporary medicine because they confer resistance to commonly used antibiotics (see Chapter 5). Plasmids may also encode virulence genes (e.g., encoding attachment factors or toxins) that can confer a selective advantage to a bacterial pathogen within the context of the host environment and can be spread from bacteria to bacteria. This spread can be accomplished by conjugation, which requires intimate contact (mediated by sex pili) between bacterial cells or by the exchange of naked DNA in a manner that is independent of cell-to-cell contact (see Transformation, Chapter 5). Another mechanism of genetic exchange between bacteria is transduction, which uses bacteriophages (i.e., viruses that specifically infect bacteria). Finally, genetic diversity can also be accomplished through somatic mutations or chromosomal rearrangements that occur during the process of bacterial replication. The mechanisms by which prokaryotic pathogens control the differential expression of genes contribute significantly to the course of disease.

Protein Expression. One more feature that distinguishes prokaryotes as a group of organisms is how they carry out the process of protein expression. Prokaryotes can transcribe their messenger RNA (mRNA) in a polycistronic fashion, which means that each mRNA contains the information for the translation of multiple polypeptides. Further, bacterial mRNA species are not extensively modified, spliced, or capped with a polyadenosine sequence. It is also notable that the half-lives of prokaryotic mRNAs are generally on the order of minutes, compared to hours for eukaryotic mRNAs. This affords bacteria the capacity to respond quickly to changes within their environment. Contributing to this rapid response time is the fact that translation of mRNA in prokaryotes is closely coupled with transcription. This is possible because no nuclear barrier separating ribosomes from nucleic acid processes exists. Bacterial RNA polymerase can produce mRNA at approximately 55 nucleotides per second, and bacterial ribosomes can produce polypeptide chains at approximately 18 amino acids per second, meaning that prokaryotic pathogens can produce proteins as fast as they receive the information from the mRNA. This allows bacteria to respond quickly to the diverse environments that they encounter during the course of infection.

Translation of bacterial mRNA is accomplished with ribosomes that are smaller and simpler in structure than eukaryotic ribosomes. The ribosomal complex of prokaryotes is termed a 70S ribosome, as compared with the 80S ribosome of eukaryotes. The designation of 70S or 80S refers to the sedimentation properties (expressed in Svedberg [S] units) of the ribosomes and reflects important differences in their composition. These differences are of medical significance and are exploited as targets of antimicrobial therapy (see Chapter 4).

COMMON BACTERIAL STRUCTURES

The cell envelope is the portion of the bacterial cell immediately beyond the cytosol (see Figure 1-2). The cell envelope is important for determining the morphology (e.g., rods, spheres) and arrangement (e.g., pairs, chains, clusters) of bacteria. Two structural components of the cell envelope found in all bacteria are the cytoplasmic membrane and the cell wall.

Cytoplasmic Membrane. The cytoplasmic membrane of most prokaryotes is distinguished from the cytoplasmic membrane of eukaryotes by its lipid composition. The prokaryotic cytoplasmic membrane lacks sterols, the only exception being *Mycoplasma* (see Chapter 4), which incorporates complex lipids (e.g., cholesterol) into their membranes if grown in the presence of these compounds. The bacterial cytoplasmic membrane has the following functions:

- The selective permeability and transport of solutes
- Electron transport and oxidative phosphorylation processes
- Excretion of hydrolytic exoenzymes
- Biosynthesis of DNA, cell wall polymers, and membrane lipids
- Chemotactic and sensory processes that allow pathogenic bacteria to respond to the complex environments that they encounter during the course of infection

Cell Wall. Except for *Mycoplasma*, a feature that distinguishes bacterial pathogens from eukaryotic pathogens is that prokaryotes contain a chemically homogeneous cell wall composed of murein. *Murein* is derived from the Greek root *sacculus* meaning "sack." This describes the primary function of the cell wall, which is to supply rigidity to bacterial cells so that they can withstand osmotic stress. (This is an essential function because bacteria commonly find themselves in both hypotonic and hypertonic environments.) The terms mucopeptide and peptidoglycan accurately describe the biochemical composition of the cell wall, which is composed of a repeating polymer of *N*-acetylglucosamine (GlcNAc) and *N*-acetylmuramic acid (MurNAc) and cross-linked by short peptide units. The general structure of bacterial cell walls is demonstrated in Figure 1-3. The chemical composition of the cell wall is similar among all bacteria except for some variations in the biochemical nature of the peptide cross-links that tie together the individual sheets of peptidoglycan. One constituent of the peptidoglycan peptide unit that is unique to

FIGURE 1-3 ▶

Peptidoglycan Structure. *The basic structure of a bacterial cell wall is common to both gram-negative and gram-positive organisms. It is comprised of a repeating polymer of the disaccharides N-acetylglucosamine and N-acetylmuramic acid (GlcNAc–MurNAc), forming a sheet that surrounds the bacterial cell. Cross-linking these sheets are peptides, as described in the text. The exact composition of each peptide cross-link is unique to each gram-positive and gram-negative species. How these peptide cross-links are biochemically organized define both the Gram-stain reaction of these organisms as well as the morphology of these organisms.*

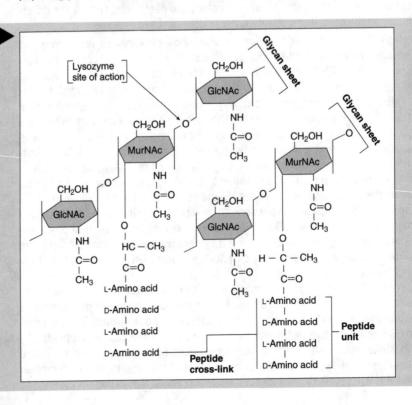

prokaryotic cell walls (especially those associated with gram-negative pathogens) is diaminopimelic acid (DAP). Finally, it should be emphasized that differences in the cross-linking of the cell wall give rise to the characteristic morphologic architecture (e.g., cocci versus bacilli) of different families of bacteria.

Although the general structure of the prokaryotic cell wall is similar, not all bacterial cell walls are equal, as demonstrated by the Gram-stain reaction. The Gram-stain reaction separates most bacteria as gram-positive or gram-negative. This differential staining reaction occurs as a result of the differences associated with the bacterial cell envelope. Figure 1-4 contrasts the basic anatomy of a gram-negative and gram-positive bacterial cell envelope; the former being defined by a thin peptidoglycan layer and an outer membrane, whereas the latter is characterized by no outer membrane and a thick

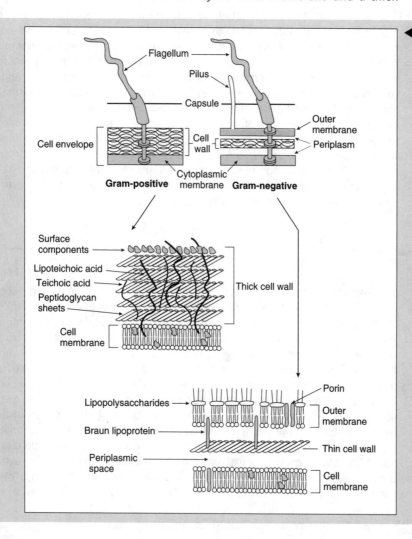

FIGURE 1-4
Comparison of the Gram-positive Cell Envelope with the Gram-negative Cell Envelope Demonstrating Similarities and Differences. *Both types of envelopes have a cytoplasmic membrane, a cell wall, and structures that lie external to the cell wall (as detailed in the upper figure). However, gram-negative bacteria differ from gram-positive bacteria by possessing a characteristically thin cell wall, the presence of a periplasm, and an outer membrane that contains lipopolysaccharide (as detailed in the lower figure). In contrast, gram-positive bacteria have a thick, teichoic acid–containing cell wall and lack an outer membrane (as detailed in the middle figure).*

peptidoglycan layer. For gram-positive bacteria, the cell wall contains as many as 40 sheets of peptidoglycan and can comprise up to 50% by weight of the entire cell envelope. By contrast, gram-negative bacteria cross-link only a few sheets of peptidoglycan. Consequently, this structure is much thinner in nature and represents only a minor component (5%–10%) of the overall cell envelope. These differences in bacterial structure are the focus of a later section of this chapter.

Structures Lying External to the Cell Envelope. Pathogenic bacteria, whether gram-positive or gram-negative, commonly produce hydrophilic polysaccharide polymers that coat the exterior of the cell envelope. When these structures form a condensed layer surrounding the bacteria, they are referred to as a bacterial capsule. When these structures form a loose mesh-like framework around the bacteria, they are referred to as a glycocalyx. In contrast to the typical carbohydrate nature of the capsule or glycocalyx,

*Bacterial capsules are important virulence factors. While most bacterial capsules are composed of repeating **carbohydrate polymers** (polysaccharide), one notable exception is the polypeptide capsule of Bacillus anthracis, which is a **polypeptide capsule** comprised of a repeating polymer of D-glutamic acid.*

flagella and pili (fimbriae) are proteinaceous, oligomeric structures that are also organized external to the cell envelope of many pathogenic bacteria. These structures extend from the bacterial cell surface and can be visualized by electron microscopy as electron-dense, thread-like structures. Flagella function in the process of motility for those bacteria that possess them. Pili are generally shorter and thinner than flagella and function in genetic conjugation, attachment, and antiphagocytic properties of bacteria. The contribution of capsules, the glycocalyx, flagella, and pili (all structures that lie external to the cell envelope) to the pathogenesis of infectious disease is reiterated throughout this text, so these terms should be well understood by the student.

Structural Differences among Bacteria

Shared aspects of DNA replication, mRNA synthesis, protein translation, and cell envelope synthesis generally separate the prokaryotic pathogens from the viral and eukaryotic pathogens. The estimated number of genes expressed by a typical prokaryote is on the order of 3000. Of these 3000 genes, most must be dedicated to essential functions like energy metabolism, macromolecule synthesis, and cellular replication, and these genes (referred to as *housekeeping genes*) are conserved among all bacteria. A smaller subset of the bacterial genome encodes genes allowing a particular organism to specifically cause disease. These genes are often referred to as *virulence genes* and encode virulence factors. The complex environments that are encountered by bacterial pathogens infecting the human host are reflected by the broad array of bacterial pathogens causing human infection and require some taxonomic framework for appreciating their medical significance. Historically, the single most important criterion used to provide this taxonomic framework has been the Gram stain.

GRAM STAIN

The Gram-stain reaction involves fixing bacterial specimens to a glass microscope slide followed by the exposure of the specimen to a basic dye, crystal violet. A solution of iodine is then applied to the specimen to help fix the crystal violet dye in the bacteria. At this point, all bacteria are stained purple. The specimen is then treated with alcohol, which acts as a decolorizing agent and is used to extract the crystal violet dye from bacteria. Gram-positive bacteria retain the crystal violet dye and remain purple, whereas the alcohol treatment extracts the crystal violet dye from gram-negative bacteria. In the last step of the Gram-stain procedure, a counterstain (e.g., the pink dye safranin) is applied to the specimen. This allows any decolorized gram-negative bacteria to stain pink, in contrast to the gram-positive bacteria, which remain a purple color.

Microscopic examination of the Gram-stain reaction provides important information about bacterial morphology that is useful for the taxonomic classification of bacterial pathogens. As demonstrated in Figure 1-5, bacteria can exist with a variety of morphologies, ranging from spheres (referred to as cocci), to rods (referred to as bacilli), to

FIGURE 1-5 ▶
Bacterial Morphologies and Arrangements. The Gram-stain reaction differentiates most bacterial pathogens on the basis of whether or not these organisms stain pink (gram-negative) or purple (gram-positive). This assessment must be made by microscopic examination of bacterial preparations using high-power magnification with oil immersion. In addition to the Gram-stain reaction, a morphologic description of the organisms can be obtained upon microscopic examination of the Gram-stain reaction. This figure summarizes the basic bacterial morphologies and arrangements.

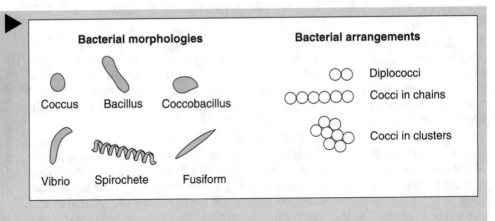

Bacterial morphologies

Coccus   Bacillus   Coccobacillus

Vibrio   Spirochete   Fusiform

Bacterial arrangements

Diplococci
Cocci in chains

Cocci in clusters

something in-between (referred to as coccobacilli). Variations of these common morphologies can also occur. For example, bacteria that exist as very short rods with tapered ends (club-shaped) are referred to as *fusiform*, whereas short rods that are curved are designated as *vibrios*. Bacteria grouped together taxonomically share similar morphologic properties that can be discerned by the Gram stain (e.g., all members of the Enterobacteriaceae are gram-negative rods, and all streptococci and staphylococci are gram-positive cocci). The importance of knowing the Gram-stain characteristics of major pathogens becomes apparent throughout this text, as bacterial pathogens are repeatedly referred to by their Gram-stain reaction and morphology.

In addition to morphologic information, microscopic examination of Gram-stained specimens can provide information on the arrangement of bacteria, which also can be a taxonomically distinguishing property. For example, the gram-positive staphylococci are characteristically organized in grape-like clusters. Streptococci are morphologically similar to staphylococci but are commonly arranged in chains or as pairs (diplococci). These characteristic arrangements provide useful information for the identification and taxonomic organization of bacterial pathogens.

The importance of the Gram stain cannot be overemphasized in microbiology. It is the single most powerful technique used in the clinical microbiology laboratory to identify bacteria, and each student will be expected to perform and interpret this procedure reliably during their medical training.

Bacterial Anatomy and the Basis for the Gram Stain

The explanation for why some bacteria stain as either gram-positive or gram-negative is relatively simple. The single membrane, thick cell wall of gram-positive bacteria favors the retention of the initial crystal violet dye after iodine fixation, despite alcohol extraction. The dual membrane, thin cell wall of gram-negative bacteria does not protect against alcohol extraction of this dye.

Gram-Positive Cell Envelope. As shown in Figure 1-4, distinctive aspects of the gram-positive cell envelope include the presence of a thick cell wall, along with the presence of cell wall–associated teichoic acids. The importance of the cell wall for the maintenance and structure of the gram-positive bacterial cell can be demonstrated in a simple experiment employing lysozyme, which is an enzyme that specifically cleaves the β-1,4 glycosidic linkages between the GlcNAc and MurNAc sugars that comprise the glycan backbone of all bacterial cell walls (see Figure 1-3). Lysozyme is found in large quantities in the granules of human polymorphonuclear cells and secretions (e.g., tears, saliva, vaginal mucus), and it contributes to nonspecific (innate) immunity. When gram-positive bacilli are treated with lysozyme in hypotonic media, they immediately lyse. However, if the osmotic strength of the medium is raised to balance the internal osmotic pressure of the cell (i.e., it becomes isotonic), protoplasts are formed, and the bacilli almost immediately convert to a rounded morphology (Figure 1-6). This experi-

Protoplasts refer to gram-positive bacteria that have lost their cell wall but which retain an intact cytoplasmic membrane. Spheroplasts refer to gram-negative bacterial structures that have an outer membrane and an inner membrane but lack an intact cell wall.

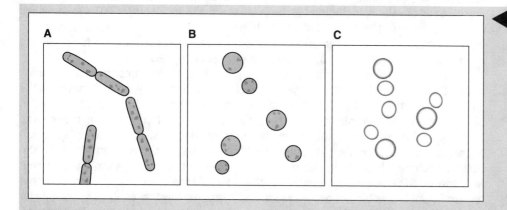

A   **B**   **C**

◀ *FIGURE 1-6*
Susceptibility of Gram-positive Bacteria to Lysozyme. *In this three-panel figure, Bacillus megaterium, a gram-positive rod, is viewed by 1000X phase-contrast microscopy under the following conditions: (A) no treatment; (B) after treatment with lysozyme (protoplasts) under isotonic conditions; and (C) after treatment with lysozyme under hypotonic conditions. The empty structures in panel C are disrupted cytoplasmic membranes that could not sustain their structural integrity in the face of the osmotic differential. The ability to resist osmotic lysis is typically provided by the bacterial cell wall. (Adapted with permission from Brooks GF, Butel JS, Ornston LN, et al: Medical Microbiology, 12th ed. Norwalk, CT: Appleton & Lange, 1995, p 23.)*

ment demonstrates the susceptibility of gram-positive organisms to this enzyme because of the surface exposure of their cell wall. It also demonstrates the structural contribution of the cell wall to bacterial morphology.

Associated with the thick cell wall of gram-positive bacteria are molecules referred to as teichoic acids or lipoteichoic acids. These are polymers of ribitol (teichoic acids) or glycerol (lipoteichoic acids) that are covalently polymerized by phosphodiester linkages. Extending from this backbone are one or more sugar, amino sugar, or amino acid substituents. The general structure of teichoic and lipoteichoic acids are depicted in Figure 1-7. The teichoic acids constitute major surface antigens for many gram-positive bacteria because they are surface localized and therefore are commonly encountered by

> *Teichoic acids and lipoteichoic acids are unique to the cell envelope of gram-positive bacteria.*

FIGURE 1-7 ▶

Basic Structure of Teichoic (Glycerol-containing) and Lipoteichoic Acids (Ribitol-containing)

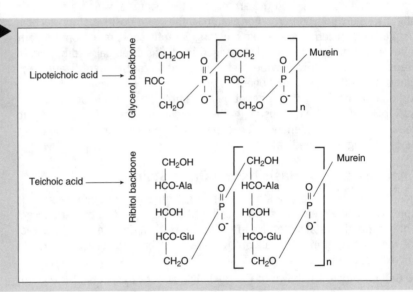

the host immune system. For example, the teichoic acids of *Streptococcus pneumoniae* bear the antigenic determinants referred to as Forssman antigens, which, in part, provide a basis for the grouping of these organisms. Among gram-positive bacteria, teichoic acids may contribute as much as 50% to the weight of the gram-positive cell envelope. They can be associated with the cell wall (in the form of teichoic acids) or anchored to the cytoplasmic membrane (in the form of lipoteichoic acids). The lengths (extent of polymerization), chemical nature (whether lipidated or free), and location (buried within the thick cell wall or surface exposed) of the teichoic acid polymers vary from species to species and sometimes between strains within a given species.

Gram-Negative Cell Envelope. Figure 1-4 contrasts the basic structure of gram-negative and gram-positive bacteria. Three features are uniquely associated with the gram-negative cell envelope, including (1) the presence of a thin cell wall, (2) the existence of an outer membrane that lies external to both the cell wall and the cytoplasmic membrane (inner membrane), and (3) the presence of an intervening space between the outer and inner membranes, referred to as the periplasmic space, or periplasm.

The thin nature of the gram-negative peptidoglycan layer in contrast to the thick gram-positive cell wall is both a consequence of the low peptidoglycan content within the gram-negative cell envelope and the limited number of cross-links that occur between peptidoglycan sheets in gram-negative bacteria. Despite its thin composition, the cell wall of gram-negative bacteria is still responsible for the osmotic resistance and cell morphology of these bacteria, similar to the identical function that the cell wall provides for gram-positive bacteria. However, in contrast to gram-positive bacteria, if lysozyme treatment were applied to a gram-negative bacilli (e.g., *Escherichia coli*), an outcome similar to that seen in Figure 1-6 would not occur even though lysozyme has the identical specificity for the peptidoglycan derived from either gram-positive or gram-negative cell walls. However, in the case of gram-negative organisms, the outer membrane effectively shields this enzyme from the cell wall. This example illustrates the ability of the outer membrane to exclude large molecules, which is a function that underscores its importance as a principal permeability barrier, restricting access of harmful substances to the bacterial cell wall and cytoplasmic membrane.

The outer membrane of gram-negative bacteria is biologically unique because of the asymmetric organization of its lipid bilayer, with lipopolysaccharide (LPS) predominating on the outer bilayer leaflet (see Figure 1-4) and simple phospholipids (e.g., phosphotidylserine, phosphotidylethanolamine) predominating on the inner bilayer leaflet. The gram-negative outer membrane is also unique in that it is not energetically active. This is largely because of the presence of integral membrane proteins, referred to as *porins*, which allow the free diffusion of aqueous solutes with molecular weights of less than 1000 kD (e.g., amino acids, sugars) across this lipid bilayer.

Like the relationship between teichoic acids and gram-positive bacteria, LPS is associated only with gram-negative organisms. LPS is synonymous with endotoxin and is extremely toxic to humans; even minute quantities (e.g., those released into circulation during gram-negative infection) can cause fever and endotoxic shock (see Chapter 21). The general structure of LPS as shown in Figure 1-8 includes three basic chemical

> *LPS* is associated with the outer membrane of all gram-negative bacteria.

> **Classic Gram-negative Bacterial Antigens**
> - *K antigen* is defined by the bacterial capsule.
> - *H antigen* is defined by bacterial flagella.
> - *O antigen* is defined by the repeating polysaccharide of LPS.

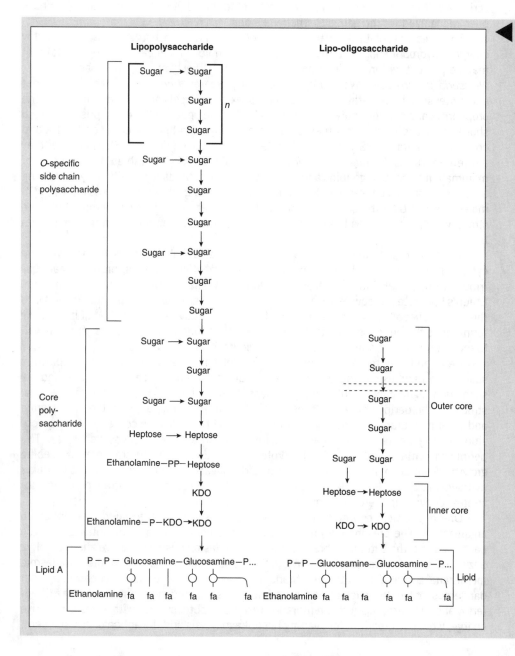

◀ **FIGURE 1-8**
Generalized Structures of the Gram-negative Lipopolysaccharide and Lipo-oligosaccharide Associated with the Outer Leaflet of the Outer Membrane. fa = fully acid; KDO = ketodeoxyoctalonate; P = phosphate.

domains: (1) a surface-exposed carbohydrate O antigen connected to (2) a core antigen, which in turn is connected to (3) lipid A, a chemical moiety buried within the bacterial outer membrane.

Lipid A is the component of the LPS molecule that has endotoxic activity for humans and is organized as units of phosphorylated glucosamine disaccharides to which are attached a number of long-chain fatty acids. One of these attached fatty acids is β-hydroxymyristic acid, a fatty acid which is only found associated with LPS in nature. The presence of other fatty acids, along with substituent groups associated with the lipid A phosphates, varies among bacterial species. The core polysaccharide of LPS is similar in all gram-negative bacteria. This region is notable because it bears two copies of keto-deoxyoctulonate (KDO), a sugar found only in LPS. These KDO residues link lipid A to the rest of the LPS core (which is generally composed of no more than four saccharide moieties, in addition to the two KDO saccharides). Attached to the LPS core is a variable repeat region that is unique to each species and often to particular strains within a given species. This variable region is composed of repeated linear trisaccharides or branched tetra- or pentasaccharides, with these structures repeated as often as 25 times. This repeated saccharide is the structure referred to as the O antigen, and it can be highly variable within a given genus. For example, more than 1000 different O antigens have been recognized for the genus *Salmonella* alone.

The presence of LPS on the surface of gram-negative bacteria creates a highly charged, hydrophilic surface that retards hydrophobic substances (e.g., bile salts) that may be present within the intestinal environment. Other gram-negative bacteria (e.g., *Neisseria gonorrhoeae, Neisseria meningitidis, Haemophilus influenzae*) that do not encounter such bile-containing environments (existing largely on mucosal surfaces of the oropharnyx and genitourinary tract) express LPS homologues that are comprised of much shorter polysaccharide constituents. These homologues retain the common lipid A and core components of LPS yet lack a repeated O antigen (see Figure 1-8). Therefore, they are referred to as *lipooligosaccharides (LOS)*. LOS closely resembles the structure of mammalian glycosphingolipids and, as a result, it contributes to the difficulty in clearing these organisms by conventional immune mechanisms. Like the O antigens of LPS, LOS molecules exhibit extensive antigenic and structural diversity even within the same strain, which complicates the immunologic recognition of bacteria bearing these structures.

The outer membrane contains a variety of proteins that are not associated with the cytoplasmic membrane. In addition to previously mentioned porins, proteins that contribute to bacterial attachment are also found associated with the outer membrane. Braun's lipoprotein is covalently attached at its amino terminus to a lipid that inserts into the inner leaflet of the outer membrane. This protein is covalently attached at its carboxy terminus to the peptidoglycan tetrapeptide and thus functionally "tethers" the cell wall to the gram-negative outer membrane (see Figure 1-4).

Between the outer membrane and the cytoplasmic membrane lies the periplasmic space. The periplasmic space can represent up to 40% of the cellular volume and, as such, is a significant cellular compartment. Rather than having a discrete chemical structure, the periplasm can be thought of as the inside of a bag, with the cytoplasmic and outer membranes restricting the free diffusion of periplasmic contents. The composition of the periplasm is a gel-like solution of proteins and oligosaccharides. The periplasm contains nutrient-binding proteins that function in the transport of specific growth-essential compounds (e.g., amino acids, sugars, vitamins, ions). It also contains hydrolytic enzymes (e.g., alkaline phosphatase) that break down nontransportable substrates, converting them into transportable nutrients.

One might wonder why gram-negative bacteria have evolved such a complicated organization. The presence of an outer membrane confers several advantages to these bacteria. First, the outer membrane creates a periplasm housing digestive and protective enzymes, as well as transport proteins, in the immediate juxtaposition of the cytoplasmic membrane. Second, the outer membrane provides a primary permeability barrier against dangerous molecules, such as host lysozyme, bile salts, and many antibiotics (see Chapters 4 and 5). Third, the outer membrane presents an outer surface with a strong negative charge, which is important for evading host phagocytosis and the action of complement.

Medically Important Pathogens Unreactive to Gram Stain

Not all bacteria can be classified as gram-negative or gram-positive. These exceptions either have a unique biology or are too small to be observed by conventional high-power light microscopy. They are, however, causative agents of significant medical diseases.

Mycobacteria. These represent an important group of pathogenic bacteria that do not reliably stain with the Gram-stain procedure. Instead, these bacteria are identified using an acid-fast stain. The nature of this staining procedure relies upon the bacteria to retain the dye carbolfuchsin even when decolorized using extreme conditions (e.g., heat, hydrochloric acid in the presence of alcohol). Because of their special staining characteristics, these bacteria are sometimes referred to as the acid-fast bacilli. Acid-fast pathogens notably include the Mycobacteria: *Mycobacterium tuberculosis*, the causative agent of tuberculosis, is a disease on the rise in the United States (see Chapter 22); and *Mycobacterium leprae* is the causative agent of leprosy. Although leprosy is not a disease of First World importance, it is a disease of the Third World and of historical significance (see Chapter 25). In terms of their cell envelope, both *M. tuberculosis* and *M. leprae* contain a single membrane and a peptidoglycan cell wall. However, unlike gram-positive or gram-negative organisms, the mycobacterial cell wall also contains covalently linked β-hydroxy fatty acids, which give rise to a waxy cell envelope (Figure 1-9) and renders these organisms highly resistant to germicides and drying. The waxy composition of the mycobacterial cell wall is responsible for the acid-fast staining properties of these bacteria.

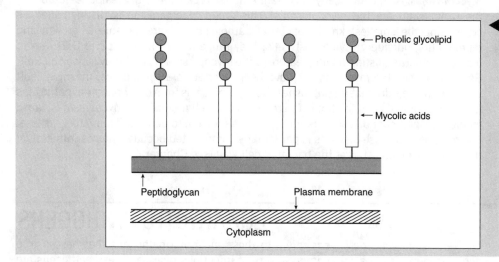

◀ **FIGURE 1-9**
Simplified Structure of Acid-fast Mycobacteria

Rickettsiae and Chlamydiae. These represent two medically significant families of atypical bacteria (for specific descriptions of these pathogens, see Chapters 8 and 9, respectively). Both of these organisms are considered obligate intracellular pathogens and are characterized by their small size (< 1 μm at their extreme dimensions). Like gram-negative bacteria, they contain a cell envelope that is organized with two membranes encompassing a thin peptidoglycan cell wall. Given this property, why are these organisms not classified by the Gram-stain reaction? One explanation is that they are too small to be visualized by high-power light microscopy. As described in Chapter 8, *Rickettsia rickettsii* is the etiologic agent of Rocky Mountain spotted fever (among other diseases), which is a disease of low morbidity and high mortality. By contrast, the sexually transmitted diseases caused by *Chlamydia trachomatis* have a high morbidity and low mortality (see Chapter 9). Regardless of their level of morbidity or mortality, both rickettsiae and chlamydiae are considered important bacterial pathogens.

Spirochetes. Another class of medically significant bacterial pathogens that cannot be visualized with the Gram stain are the spirochetes (also known as treponemes). Like gram-negative bacteria, the spirochetes have an LPS-containing outer membrane as well as a cell wall that is composed of a thin peptidoglycan layer. The spiral, or cork-screw, arrangement of these organisms characterizes this morphologic group, which includes *Treponema pallidum*, the causative agent of syphilis (see Chapter 25), and *Borrelia*

Morbidity refers to the number of occurrences of a specific disease within a given population. *Mortality* refers to the number of deaths that occur within a given population as a result of a specific disease.

burgdorferi, the causative agent of Lyme disease (see Chapter 8). This characteristic morphology results from the placement of their flagella within the periplasmic space; most flagella-expressing bacterial pathogens organize these structures external to their cell envelope. Spirochetes are not detectable by Gram stain because the width of these organisms lies beyond the limits of high-power light microscopy (Figure 1-10). Instead, these organisms have to be identified by special techniques such as dark-field microscopy or fluorescent microscopy.

FIGURE 1-10 ▶
Morphologic Structure and Biologic Organization of Spirochetes

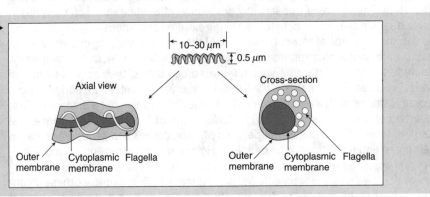

Mycoplasmas. A final medically important group of organisms that are not detectable by the Gram stain are the mycoplasmas. This group of organisms is distinguished as comprising the smallest known bacterial pathogens that are capable of growth and reproduction outside of living host cells; they range in size from 0.12 to 0.25 μm in diameter. Another distinguishing feature of the mycoplasmas is that they lack a cell wall. Because of this, the mycoplasmas have been referred to as mollicutes, meaning "soft skin." A final feature that distinguishes the mycoplasmas from other bacterial pathogens is the presence of complex lipids (sterols) in their cell membrane. Mycoplasmas cause medically significant diseases, ranging from pneumonia to pelvic inflammatory disease. The treatment of these diseases is particularly complicated because many antimicrobial therapies specifically target the bacterial cell wall (see Chapter 4).

EUKARYOTIC PATHOGENS

The term *eukaryotic pathogens* refers to those microbial pathogens that have a true nucleus and that are also common agents of infectious disease. These pathogens are biologically quite diverse and therefore difficult to characterize systematically. However, the convention of medical microbiology has been to categorize the eukaryotic pathogens as either fungi or parasites.

Fungi

There are more than 200,000 species of fungi, most of which function in the environmental decomposition of organic material. Fewer than 100 fungal species have been implicated in human disease (referred to as mycoses), and of these, only 10–15 are considered to be major pathogenic fungi (see Chapter 28).

Common to both fungal pathogens and classic eukaryotes is the existence of a cytoplasmic membrane, a nuclear membrane, and other internal organelles. In addition, the fungal cytoplasmic membrane contains complex sterols as part of their membrane composition. However, in contrast to human cells, the predominant fungal cytoplasmic membrane sterol is ergosterol, a complex membrane lipid unique to many fungi. In addition, fungi contain a rigid cell wall that is markedly different in biochemical composition from that found in the bacterial cell envelope. This cell wall consists of the chemical constituents unique to fungi. These constituents include the polysaccharides mannan, glucan, and chitin, which interact with each other and with membrane proteins to form the fungal cell wall.

A single fungal cell can be as small as a bacterium (1 μm) or as large as a red blood cell (RBC) [100 μm]. Fungi can exist as single cells or in complex colonies; the common mushroom is an example of the complex morphology that can be assumed by some fungi. Fortunately, the fungi of medical significance are not as complex as mushrooms; rather, pathogenic fungi can be described in general terms as being either yeasts or molds.

Yeasts are individual cells that result from parental cell budding to form a progeny cell. Alternatively, fungi may also grow through the formation of hyphae, which are essentially filamentous extensions of the fungal cell wall oriented in a single dimension. This type of fungal growth generally results in septa that divide the hypha into discrete cellular units, aligned one after another in a chain. Less frequently, hyphae may be nonseptate, which is essentially a single continuous filamentous fungal cell (Figure 1-11). A mass of fungal hyphae form a mycelium, which in turn forms larger masses that are referred to as molds. Some pathogenic fungi can grow either as yeasts or as molds and are correspondingly referred to as dimorphic fungi. Usually, whether dimorphic fungi exist as yeasts or molds is influenced by temperature, such that dimorphic human fungal pathogens exist as yeasts within infected human tissues, whereas at ambient temperatures outside of the human host they exist as molds.

Common Molecular Constituents of Fungal Cell Walls
- **Mannan** is a mannose-based polymer found on the surface and in the structural matrix of the fungal cell coat, where it can be covalently attached to proteins.
- **Glucans** are glucosyl polymers, some of which form fibrils that increase the strength of the fungal cell coat.
- **Chitin** is composed of long polymers of N-acetylglucosamine that is associated with the cell coat of many fungi.

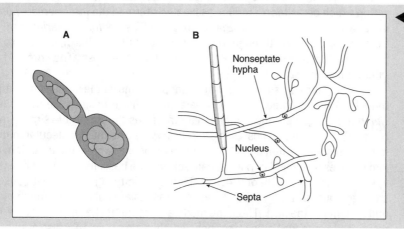

FIGURE 1-11
General Diagram of a Septate and Nonseptate Fungal Hyphae. (A) *Budding yeast.* (B) *Fungal mycelium with septate and nonseptate hyphae.*

Pathogenic fungi are taxonomically classified based upon complex criteria, including the nature of their reproductive elements and septation of hyphae. A detailed description of this classification requires an in-depth understanding of mycology, which is beyond the scope of this text. What should be appreciated by the student is that fungal infections are of increasing medical significance, not only globally but also in the United States. They are major causes of dermatologic infection in all human populations and also represent important causative agents of life-threatening illnesses in immunocompromised populations (see Chapter 28). A list of fungal pathogens causing mycoses within the United States is given in Table 1-3. In addition to causing mycoses,

TABLE 1-3
Medically Important Fungal Pathogens

Compartment	Fungal Agent	Morphology during Infection	Morphology at Room Temperature
Systemic	*Coccidioides immitis*	Yeast-like	Mycelia
	Histoplasma capsulatum	Yeast	Mycelia
	Blastomyces dermatitidis	Yeast	Mycelia
	Cryptococcus neoformans	Yeast	Yeast
	Candida albicans	Yeast and hyphae	Yeast
	Aspergillus spp.	Mycelia	Mycelia
Subcutaneous	*Sporothrix schenckii*	Yeast	Mycelia
Cutaneous	*Microsporum* spp.	Mycelia	Mycelia
	Trichophyton spp.	Mycelia	Mycelia
	Epidermophyton spp.	Mycelia	Mycelia

fungi also are major causes of allergies and can cause intoxications (e.g., mushroom poisoning). The unique biology of fungi requires unique antifungal therapies as opposed to antibacterial strategies (see Chapter 4). Antifungal strategies are often quite toxic to the human host because of the similarities between the eukaryotic biology of fungal pathogens and host cells.

Parasites

The term parasite refers to a complex group of pathogens that share few common properties aside from being nonfungal, eukaryotic, human pathogens. Parasites differ from fungi by their lack of a cell wall. Parasites also may be motile, whereas fungi are nonmotile. Parasites hold particular medical significance in underdeveloped countries; however, they also are of medical significance in the United States. For example, *Giardia lamblia* is the causative agent of giardiasis, a common disease of the gastrointestinal tract caused by the ingestion of contaminated fresh water (see Chapter 6).

One feature that is relatively unique to the parasites is that many of these pathogens require two or more host species to complete their life cycle. Convention refers to the host within which the parasite reproduces sexually as the *definitive host*, whereas the host within which parasites reproduce asexually is termed the *intermediate host*. For example, malaria is caused by a protozoal pathogen (*Plasmodium malariae*) and is transmitted from person to person through the bite of a mosquito. In this disease, sexual reproduction occurs within the insect, making it the definitive host. The infected human is the intermediate host.

Pathogenic parasites pose significant problems for the human host, largely because of the similarities between host and parasitic cells. Parasites use molecular mimicry, in which a pathogen produces molecular structures that resemble similar molecular structures within the human host (see Chapter 16). As a result of molecular mimicry, a vigorous immune response often does not ensue in response to parasitic infection. A second problem involves treatment of parasitic infection. The basis for antimicrobial or antiviral therapy, as described in Chapter 4, is selective toxicity, a process that causes damage to a pathogen but not to the host. Because parasites are eukaryotes, much of their biology is quite similar to the host. Thus, the medical community has a limited arsenal of treatment regimens to manage these infections, which is a problem that also applies to treating the mycoses. One final problem that parasites often pose for the human host is the existence of multiple life forms. For example *Plasmodium falciparum*, the causative agent of malaria, takes on a variety of forms depending on the tissue it infects. Plasmodiae exist as sporozoites when infecting the liver, trophozoites when infecting RBCs, and merozoites when infecting mosquitoes. These multiple forms represent the challenging equivalent of a "moving target" for the immune system of the human host.

The complexity of parasites makes them difficult to discuss in general terms, and it is the focus of a subspecialty of medical microbiology referred to as parasitology. Tables 1-4 and 1-5 list many of the medically important parasites, the diseases that they cause, and any notable characteristics associated with these pathogens. At a minimum, the student should be familiar with the important parasitic pathogens described in these tables. As described below, the parasites can generally be categorized into two groups— protozoa or helminths.

Parasites *are generally classified either as* **protozoa** *or as* **helminths***.*

Protozoa. Protozoa are microscopic and unicellular organisms that morphologically resemble fungal yeasts, especially with regard to size. Protozoa range in size from 2 μm to larger than 100 μm and are organized with the typical complexity of eukaryotic cells. Like fungi, many protozoal species (more than 40,000) exist within the general environment but only a relative few are of medical significance (see Table 1-4). In general, the overall structure of most protozoa consists of a cytoplasmic membrane and an endoplasm (referring to the inner part of the cytoplasm), within which nuclei, mitochondria, and other structures typical of eukaryotes reside. In addition, an outer ectoplasm layer containing organelles of motility (e.g., flagellar structures) may be present. Protozoal flagella are of a much different organization and composition than the prokaryotic flagella that were described earlier in this chapter; however, both eukaryotic and prokaryotic flagella function similarly in motility.

◀ TABLE 1-4
Medically Important Protozoal Pathogens

Class	Locomotive Organelle	Representative Pathogenic Protozoa	Disease	Disease Distribution
Rhizopods	Pseudopods	Entamoeba histolytica	Intestinal amebiasis (intestinal ulcers and liver abscesses)	Worldwide
Flagellates	Flagella	Trypanosoma cruzi	Chaga's disease	Epidemic in South America
		Trypanosoma brucei	African sleeping sickness	Epidemic in Africa
		Leishmania spp.	Cutaneous and subcutaneous lesions	Generally associated with underdeveloped countries
		Trichomonas vaginalis	Protozoal vaginosis	Significant worldwide sexually transmitted disease
		Giardia lamblia	Giardiasis	Significant worldwide gastrointestinal disease
Sporozoa	None	Plasmodium spp.	Malaria	Worldwide
		Toxoplasma gondii	Toxoplasmosis	Important disease worldwide

Protozoal pathogens are classified largely based upon their organelles of locomotion (see Table 1-4). Rhizopods (amebas), such as *Entamoeba histolytica*, cause disease by invading tissue using finger-like projections referred to as pseudopodia (false feet) as their locomotive organelle. The ciliates use cilia as their mode of locomotion and are of limited medical significance. Flagellates include the genera of *Trypanosoma, Leishmania, Trichimonas*, and *Giardia*, and they are responsible for many significant human diseases. As their name implies, these organisms use flagella as their means of locomotion. The sporozoans such as *Plasmodium* and *Toxoplasma*, the agents of malaria and toxoplasmosis, lack an organelle that facilitates motility.

◀ TABLE 1-5
Medically Important Helminth Pathogens

Class	Morphology	Alimentary Tract	Pathogens	Disease
Roundworm (nematode)	Spindle-shaped	Tubular	Trichinella spiralis	Trichinosis
			Ascaris lumbricoides	Ascariasis
			Wuchereria bancrofti	Elephantiasis
Tapeworm (cestode)	Head with segmented body	None	Taenia spp.	Tapeworm
Fluke (trematode)	Leaf-shaped with oral suckers	Blind	Schistosoma spp.	Schistosomiasis

Helminths. In contrast to the protozoa, the helminths are macroscopic, multicellular, and highly differentiated organisms. The helminths challenge the definition of the science of microbiology because of their large size, which can range between 0.1 mm and 1 M. This diverse group of eukaryotic pathogens are of extreme importance in the context of global medicine, especially in the area of tropical medicine. The biology of the helminths, also referred to as animal parasites or worms, is far too diverse to be addressed by this text. However, the student should be aware that the helminths are generally categorized according to morphology and the type of alimentary tract that they use (see Table 1-5). Using this classification, the helminths can be grouped as round-worms (nematodes), tapeworms, or flukes. Roundworms generally demonstrate a fusiform body and a tubular alimentary tract that runs from the mouth to the anus. The roundworms can be further grouped by the disease that they cause; for example, trichinosis and ascariasis cause gastrointestinal infections, whereas elephantiasis is a cutaneous infection. The tapeworms have flattened, ribbon-shaped bodies, which on one end present defined structures (suckers and hooklets) that function in attachment. This worm lacks an alimentary tract; instead, it absorbs nutrients across its outer layer (cuticle). Flukes are leaf-shaped organisms with a complex alimentary tract that is branched and may not have a defined anal exit for waste. The most medically significant of the flukes are *Schistosoma* spp., which infect between 5% and 10% of the world's population, with as many as 400,000 cases of schistosomiasis occurring annually within the United States (largely associated with the immigrant population). Snails are the definitive host for schistosomes and, as a result, this disease can be controlled by appropriate sanitary measures aimed at controlling snail populations.

Difficult-to-Categorize Eukaryotic Pathogens

Like prokaryotic pathogens, some eukaryotic pathogens do not fit neatly into categories such as yeasts and parasites. A specific example of this is *Pneumocystis carinii*. This organism is responsible for a pneumonia of high mortality in immunocompromised patients, such as premature infants, patients undergoing cancer chemotherapy (see Chapter 28), organ transplant recipients receiving immunosuppressive therapy (see Chapter 10), and patients with AIDS (see Chapter 27). This eukaryotic pathogen was historically classified as a parasitic protozoan based upon its biologic characteristics, such as DNA content and susceptibility to antiprotozoal but not antifungal chemotherapy. However, analysis of *P. carinii* ribosomal RNA sequences suggests that it may be more closely related to fungi. In fact, it is possible that *Pneumocystis* represents an evolutionary bridge between the parasites and the fungi.

RESOLUTION OF CLINICAL CASE

The clinical case described at the beginning of this chapter involved a child with an inner ear infection. The clinical symptoms of this patient were the result of inflammation in response to an infectious agent. The infection itself was probably contracted from the day care contacts experienced by the child. These symptoms represented a classic case of otitis media, which the science of epidemiology suggests is closely associated with bacterial infection (see Chapters 7 and 18). Understanding the epidemiology of otitis media implicates an etiologic agent of bacterial origin, which in turn suggests an antibacterial treatment (see Chapter 4). On the other hand, antibiotic resistance is a major problem in bacterial otitis media (see Chapter 5), and the symptoms often spontaneously resolve within days. Thus, the mother's demand that the child be placed on an antibiotic may do very little to alleviate her son's symptoms, but it may do much harm by selecting for an antibiotic-resistant strain. In this case, the pediatrician patiently explained this to the mother, and the child's symptoms resolved within a few days without antibiotic therapy.

REVIEW QUESTIONS

Directions: For each of the following questions, choose the **one best** answer.

1. Which one of the following bacterial structures by itself can cause septic shock in humans?

    (A) Bacterial capsules

    (B) Bacterial flagella

    (C) Bacterial cell wall

    (D) Bacterial lipopolysaccharide

    (E) Bacterial teichoic acid

2. A child visits the emergency room complaining of symptoms of diarrhea and fever. A stool sample is submitted to the clinical laboratory to identify the pathogen causing the infection. A preliminary Gram-stain result describes the predominant organism associated with the stool sample as a bacillus, staining a faint pink color. Based upon this information, which one of the following etiologic agents is suspected as responsible for this disease?

    (A) The causative agent is a gram-positive rod containing teichoic acid

    (B) The causative agent is a gram-negative rod containing lipopolysaccharide with a highly repeated O antigen associated with its outer membrane

    (C) The causative agent is a gram-negative rod that has lipooligosaccharide associated with its outer membrane

    (D) The causative agent is a gram-negative rod that has a highly repeated teichoic acid species on its cell surface

    (E) Because the organism stains pink by the Gram stain, the causative agent is more likely to be an acid-fast bacilli

3. Which one of the following organisms placed in the conditions described would be most sensitive to the antibacterial action of lysozyme?

    (A) Gram-positive rods in a hypotonic solution

    (B) Gram-negative cocci in a hypotonic solution

    (C) Gram-positive cocci in an isotonic solution

    (D) Gram-negative rods in an isotonic solution

    (E) Acid-fast bacilli in a hypotonic solution

4. Which one of the following statements best describes the unique chemical composition of the fungal cell wall?

    (A) It contains mannans, peptidoglycan, and a capsule

    (B) It contains glucans, mannans, and chitin

    (C) It contains glucans, mannans, and teichoic acids

    (D) It contains glucans, ketodeoxyoctulonate, and chitin

    (E) It contains peptidoglycan, lipopolysaccharide, and teichoic acids

5. An important microbial pathogen has been found to have the following characteristics: it is approximately 15 μm in size; it lacks peptidoglycan, chitin, mannan, and glucans in its cell wall; it has an 80S ribosome; and it has mitochondria associated with the cytosol. Which one of the following terms would be most correct when describing this pathogen to colleagues?

    (A) Virus

    (B) Bacteria

    (C) Fungi

    (D) Parasite

    (E) Mycobacteria

ANSWERS AND EXPLANATIONS

1. **The answer is D.** Bacterial lipopolysaccharide is the clear answer because humans are extremely susceptible to this molecule. Because of its toxicity, this molecule is also known as endotoxin. Option A is incorrect because the bacterial capsule is typically associated with antiphagocytic activity. Option B is incorrect because bacterial flagella are involved in motility. Option C is incorrect because the bacterial cell wall is associated with bacterial resistance to osmotic lysis. Option E is incorrect because lipoteichoic acids are associated with gram-positive bacteria and may be involved in attachment.

2. **The answer is B.** Gram-negative rods (bacilli) would stain pink and would have lipopolysaccharide associated with them. Options A, C, D, and E are incorrect because a gram-positive organism would stain purple; gram-negative organisms expressing lipo-oligosaccharide are generally not found in the gut; gram-negative organisms do not express teichoic acids; and acid-fast bacteria do not stain well using the Gram stain, respectively.

3. **The answer is A.** Hydrolysis of the cell wall under hypotonic conditions results in cellular disruption because of osmotic lysis of the protoplast created by lysozyme treatment. This experiment is described in Figure 1-6. The existence of an outer membrane in gram-negative bacteria generally protects the cell wall from lysozyme hydrolysis, thereby excluding options B (gram-negative cocci in a hypotonic solution) and D (gram-negative rods in an isotonic solution). Acid-fast bacilli have a waxy cell coat that protects them from lysozyme interaction, thereby excluding option E (acid-fast bacilli in a hypotonic solution). Option C is incorrect because hydrolysis of the bacterial cell wall under isotonic conditions results in the formation of protoplasts but does not functionally kill the cells.

4. **The answer is B.** The fungal cell wall has three unique components—glucans, mannan, and chitin. The other options included chemical structures that are found in bacteria or are not considered part of the cell wall (e.g., a capsule).

5. **The answer is D.** The relatively large size of this pathogen (approximately 15 μm) implicated it as being a parasite. One can exclude viruses and bacteria (options A, B, and E) based upon the size of the pathogen and the presence of an 80S ribosome. The fact that the cell wall contained no chitin, mannan, or glucans eliminates fungi (option D).

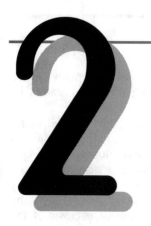

BACTERIAL GROWTH AND PHYSIOLOGY

CHAPTER OUTLINE

Introduction of Clinical Case
Growth of Prokaryotes
• Measurement of Growth
• Bacterial Physiology and Growth In Vivo
Anaerobic Bacteria
• Sensitivity to Oxygen
• Locations in the Body
Nonclostridial versus Clostridial Anaerobic Infections
• Nonclostridial Anaerobic Infections
• Clostridial Diseases
Illustrative Pathogen: *Bacteroides*-like Group
• Biologic Characteristics
• Reservoir and Transmission
• Virulence Factors
• Pathogenesis
• Diagnosis
• Prevention and Treatment
Illustrative Pathogen: Histotoxic clostridia
• Biologic Characteristics
• Reservoir and Transmission
• Virulence Factors
• Pathogenesis
• Diagnosis
• Prevention and Treatment

Bacterial Endospores
• Importance of Spores for Medicine
Illustrative Pathogen: *Bacillus anthracis*
• Biologic Characteristics
• Reservoir and Transmission
• Virulence Factors
• Pathogenesis
• Diagnosis
• Prevention and Treatment
Illustrative Pathogen: *Clostridium tetani*
• Biologic Characteristics
• Reservoir and Transmission
• Virulence Factors
• Pathogenesis
• Diagnosis
• Prevention and Treatment
Resolution of Clinical Case
Review Questions

INTRODUCTION OF CLINICAL CASE

A 70-year-old man who had suffered a stroke that left him with weakness on his right side that limited his mobility, but who still was able to live independently, was found lying in his bed covered with feces. He was admitted to the hospital because of the presence of multiple decubitus ulcers. Examination at the hospital revealed a somnolent but arousable man who had

> **Decubitus ulcers** are caused by prolonged pressure to a relatively small area and are usually produced by lying in one position for a long time.

two large decubitus ulcers, one on the left sacral area that was approximately 8 × 6 cm, and one on the right side that was approximately 12 × 15 cm and very deep. The right

Ticarcillin/clavulanate *is a combination of an extended-spectrum penicillin plus a β-lactamase inhibitor (see Chapter 4) that has activity against a broad range of anaerobes (as well as gram-negative aerobes and facultative anaerobes).*

Metronidazole *is an antimicrobial agent that is active (see Chapter 4) against anaerobes (including* Clostridia *species) and some protozoa.*

Crepitus *is gas in tissue.*

ulcer extended inferiorly over the gluteal area and seemed to involve the superior portion of the right leg. Two blood cultures were obtained, and the patient was started on ticarcillin/clavulanate.

Eighteen hours later, one of the two blood cultures grew a large, brick-shaped, gram-positive bacillus under anaerobic culture conditions. Consequently, metronidazole was added to the patient's therapy. Re-examination of the patient's decubitus ulcers revealed crepitus at the top of the right leg posteriorly and a gray, watery ("dishwater") fluid draining from the right decubitus ulcer. A Gram stain of the fluid showed no inflammatory cells but many large, brick-shaped, gram-positive rods. The patient was taken to the operating room, where the left sacral area was debrided. Extensive necrosis of the muscles (myonecrosis) was noted over the hip and down the posterior aspect of the man's right leg; infection extended to the superior femur, which was also necrotic.

GROWTH OF PROKARYOTES

Generally, prokaryotes grow more quickly than eukaryotic cells. For example, under optimal growth conditions in the laboratory, *Escherichia coli* replicates in as few as 20 minutes, whereas a mammalian cell requires 1 day or longer to double. The ability of many (but not all) prokaryotes to reproduce relatively quickly probably contributes to the pathogenesis of many infectious diseases, particularly acute bacterial infections (e.g., septic shock caused by gram-negative bacteria). Once inside the body, fast-growing pathogens can often rapidly multiply and cause symptomatic damage before specific host defenses are induced. However, there are some pathogenic bacteria that grow much more slowly (e.g., *Mycobacterium tuberculosis*, which doubles approximately once per day). These slow-growing prokaryotes tend to cause chronic infections, in part because they require time after colonizing the body to replicate to the levels necessary to induce pathophysiologic effects.

Bacterial growth is an exponential process involving binary fission, in which a single bacterial cell divides into two progeny cells. The precise amount of time required for any bacterium to double depends on both its genetic background and environmental conditions. Environmental factors known to influence bacterial growth include:

- Temperature (note that many human pathogens grow optimally at 37°C)
- pH
- Nutrient availability (e.g., ions, energy sources, carbon and nitrogen sources)
- Oxygen availability
- Osmolarity

Turbidity *is a property related to the amount of* cell mass *present in a liquid (broth) bacterial culture. When placed in a spectrophotometer, intact bacterial cells (both living and dead) scatter a focused light beam more than their surrounding medium. Therefore, as the biomass of a bacterial culture increases (i.e., as the culture becomes more "turbid"), the culture exhibits more and more light-scattering properties, which can be detected by the spectrophotometer. When a culture increases in cell mass (becomes more turbid), this usually correlates with an increase in the number of total (viable and nonviable) cells present in that culture.*

Measurement of Growth

Growth of prokaryotes can be easily studied in vitro by measuring either the total number of bacterial cells or the number of viable bacterial cells present in a culture. Total bacterial number (i.e., the number of both viable and nonviable bacteria present in a culture) can be determined using spectrophotometric techniques that measure the turbidity of a culture. Alternatively, the number of viable bacteria in a culture can be estimated by performing colony counts, a method in which known dilutions of a culture are aseptically transferred and spread onto the sterile surface of solid media poured into Petri plates (see Appendix 1). Because only the viable cells present in an inoculum can give rise to colonies on the Petri plates, the number of viable bacteria that was present per milliliter of the original culture can be deduced simply by counting the number of colonies that develop after suitable incubation on the plates and multiplying this number by the dilution factor used, if any, to dilute the inoculum added to the plates.

Bacterial Growth Curve. As shown in Figure 2-1, results from in vitro growth experiments can be plotted on a semi-log graph to yield a bacterial growth curve. Bacterial growth curves exhibit several characteristic phases:

- Lag phase: a period when the bacterial cells are preparing (e.g., increasing enzyme synthesis) for growth.
- Exponential or log phase: a period when bacterial cells are actively growing at their maximal rate.
- Stationary phase: a period when growth slows because of the depletion of nutrients from the medium or an accumulation of toxic by-products of growth in the medium.
- Death phase: a period when bacteria start to die as the culture increasingly suffers from nutrient depletion or accumulation of toxic by-products. The numbers of total versus viable bacteria most significantly diverge during the death phase.

Aseptic transfer refers to the process of inoculating microbes found in a specimen into a new medium, without any contamination from the microbes always present in the background environment (e.g., in the air or on a microbiologist's hands). Aseptic transfer depends upon using good sterile technique (see Appendix 1).

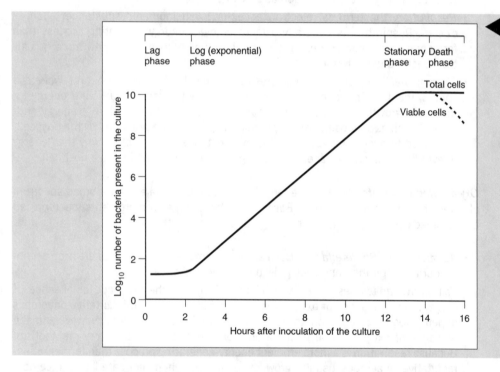

◀ FIGURE 2-1
Typical Bacterial Growth Curve

One important piece of information that can be gleaned from a growth curve is the doubling time (also called the generation time) of a bacterium under a particular set of environmental growth conditions. Any college-level microbiology text can be consulted for an explanation of the mathematical basis for calculating doubling times using data such as those shown in Figure 2-1.

Bacterial Physiology and Growth In Vivo

Although insights can be gained from studying bacterial growth in vitro, one must appreciate that bacteria typically face a considerably more hostile growth environment inside the human body than in a laboratory flask. For example, when present inside the human body, a pathogen faces nutrient competition from both normal flora microbes and mammalian cells. Furthermore, considerable fluctuations in the amounts of nutrients available for bacterial growth often occur inside the body (e.g., bacteria in the colon are transiently flooded with nutrients when the ileocecal valve opens). Finally, the presence of specific and nonspecific host defense mechanisms in the human body offer significant obstacles that can inhibit the growth of many bacteria.

Iron. Because iron is an important cofactor for bacterial metabolism, it is an essential nutrient for bacterial growth. Considering this, it is not surprising that one of the important host defense mechanisms of the human body is the restriction of iron availability to pathogens. Most extracellular iron in the body is sequestered by host iron-binding proteins, including transferrin and lactoferrin. Unfortunately, some pathogens have been able to develop successful strategies for acquiring iron in vivo despite these host attempts to restrict iron availability. For example, pathogenic *Neisseria* spp. have developed specific receptors on their surfaces that enable them to bind transferrin and lactoferrin. Once the human iron-binding proteins become bound to the surface of these pathogens, iron is removed and used for growth of the neisserial cell. Alternatively, some bacteria (particularly enteric bacteria) excrete small organic molecules called siderophores that bind iron with high affinity. After siderophores bind the iron, the iron:siderophore complexes bind to siderophore receptors on the bacterial cell surface, where these bacteria can access the bound iron for their growth.

Energy. There are several mechanisms by which prokaryotes obtain energy for growth:

- *Fermentation:* involves a biochemical pathway in which the terminal electron acceptor is an organic substance, such as pyruvate.
- *Respiration:* the terminal electron acceptor is an inorganic substance, such as oxygen. Respiration is generally a more efficient energy-generating process than fermentation, so bacteria using a respiratory metabolism often grow more quickly than bacteria using fermentation.
- *"Energy theft":* a group of prokaryotes (including all *Chlamydia* spp. and *Rickettsia* spp.) without the metabolic machinery necessary to produce sufficient energy for their own growth grow inside mammalian cells and utilize ("steal") energy substrates, such as adenosine triphosphate (ATP), as they are produced by the host cell. This need to access intracellular energy substrates helps explain why the "energy thieves" are obligate intracellular pathogens that must exist inside a host cell.

Oxygen Requirements. Related to energy production, bacteria exhibit a broad spectrum of oxygen requirements for growth. Based upon these oxygen requirements, bacteria can be classified according to the following groups:

- *Aerobes:* (e.g., *Bordetella pertussis*) always use oxygen as a terminal electron acceptor during respiration and thus grow only in the presence of oxygen.
- *Facultative anaerobes:* (e.g., *E. coli*) grow in either the presence or absence of oxygen. In the absence of oxygen (i.e., anaerobic conditions), facultative anaerobes depend upon fermentation to generate energy for their growth. However, in the presence of oxygen, these bacteria are able to shift to a respiratory metabolism. Because respiration is a more efficient energy-generating process than fermentation, facultative anaerobes usually grow more quickly when incubated under aerobic rather than under anaerobic conditions.
- *Aerotolerants:* (e.g., *Streptococcus pyogenes*) are also able to grow under either aerobic or anaerobic conditions. However, these prokaryotes differ from facultative anaerobes in that aerotolerant bacteria always use the same fermentation pathway to produce energy, whether they are growing in the presence or absence of oxygen. In other words, these bacteria cannot shift their metabolism to perform respiration when their environment contains oxygen.
- *Strict anaerobes:* (e.g., *Clostridium tetani*) also must use fermentation to obtain energy for their growth but are distinguished from the aerotolerants because they are sensitive to the presence of oxygen (for reasons explained below) and thus are unable to grow under aerobic conditions.
- *Microaerophiles:* includes the medically important genera *Campylobacter* and *Helicobacter*, requires the presence of some oxygen for growth, but this oxygen must be present at less-than-normal atmospheric concentrations. These organisms typically obtain their energy through a respiratory-type metabolism.

ANAEROBIC BACTERIA

Sensitivity to Oxygen

Why are strict anaerobes sensitive to the presence of oxygen? Probably no single explanation applies to all anaerobes. However, exposing any cell (prokaryotic or eukaryotic) to oxygen is known to create highly reactive toxic by-products, such as peroxides and superoxides, that can damage DNA and other cellular constituents. Aerobes, facultative anaerobes, and aerotolerants (as well as mammalian cells) are able to produce enzymes, such as catalase, peroxidase, and superoxide dismutase, that can detoxify these oxygen by-products. The absence of these enzymes from many (but not all) strict anaerobes apparently makes them much more sensitive than other bacteria to oxygen-induced damage. Alternatively, some anaerobes apparently are able to produce catalase (or peroxidase) and superoxide dismutase but are still sensitive to oxygen because some of their other essential enzymes function properly only in a highly reduced environment, such as exists in the absence of oxygen.

Redox Potential. Whatever the particular explanation for their sensitivity to oxygen, all strict anaerobes require a low redox potential environment (i.e., a reduced environment) for growth. Although the minimum redox potential necessary for growth varies among anaerobes, the redox potential of healthy human tissue is too high to support the growth of strict anaerobes. However, numerous in vivo conditions can lower tissue redox conditions and thus predispose an individual to anaerobic infection. For example, medical conditions that lead to poor circulation can limit oxygen delivery to tissue, thereby lowering the redox potential and creating a more favorable environment for anaerobic infection. If facultative anaerobes are introduced into tissue simultaneously with strict anaerobes, the facultative anaerobes may consume sufficient amounts of oxygen to lower tissue redox potential to levels permitting anaerobic growth.

Locations in the Body

Although anaerobes might seem fairly exotic, these bacteria represent the majority of the normal flora present at several body locations (Table 2-1); in fact, anaerobes colonize virtually all mucosal surfaces. Although some of these body sites (e.g., the skin) might not appear at first glance to be particularly favorable for anaerobic growth, the sites are able to support the growth of anaerobes because of the presence of sizable populations of normal flora facultative anaerobes that consume oxygen and create a low redox potential microenvironment, or the production of body secretions that contribute to creating the reduced microenvironment needed, or both.

Superoxide dismutase is an enzyme that detoxifies highly reactive free radical forms of oxygen, using the following reaction:

$$2\ O_2^- + 2\ H^+ \xrightarrow[\text{dismutase}]{\text{superoxide}} O_2 + H_2O_2$$

Hydrogen peroxide (H_2O_2) is also highly toxic, but *catalase* (if available) can detoxify it by the following reaction:

$$H_2O_2 + H_2O_2 \xrightarrow[\text{catalase}]{} 2\ H_2O + O_2$$

Peroxidases also detoxify hydrogen peroxide but use a reductant (R) other than hydrogen peroxide to accomplish this:

$$H_2O_2 + H_2R \xrightarrow[\text{peroxidase}]{} 2\ H_2O + R$$

If unfamiliar with the concept of *redox potential*, consult a good biochemistry or chemistry text. For the purpose of understanding redox potential in the context of anaerobic microbiology, one need only appreciate that: (1) a low redox potential environment corresponds to a highly reduced environment, whereas a high redox potential environment is a highly oxidized environment; and (2) the introduction of oxygen into an environment usually raises that environment's redox potential (i.e., a strict anaerobe seeking a highly reduced, low redox potential environment will not flourish in the presence of oxygen).

◀ **TABLE 2-1**
Body Sites Normally Colonized by Anaerobes

Bacteria	Body Site			
	Mouth and Pharynx	**Intestines[a] (particularly the colon)**	**Urogenital Tract (particularly the vagina)**	**Skin**
Bacteroides spp.	−	+	+	−
Prevotella spp.	+	+	+	−
Clostridium spp.	−	+	+/−	−
Fusobacterium spp.	+	+	+	−
Peptostreptococcus spp. (and related gram-positive anaerobic cocci)	+	+	+	+/−
Propionibacterium spp.	−	−	−	+

Note: + = presence; − = absence.
[a] Contrary to common belief, *Escherichia coli* (a facultative anaerobe) is not the predominant microorganism in the normal intestinal flora. The majority of the intestinal flora is anaerobic. Anaerobes outnumber facultative anaerobes by 1000 to 1 in the gut. Anaerobes are also the predominant flora in the mouth, skin, upper respiratory tract, and lower female genital tract.

NONCLOSTRIDIAL VERSUS CLOSTRIDIAL ANAEROBIC INFECTIONS

Numerous anaerobic species are occasionally involved in human infections, but the most important causes of anaerobic infections are listed in Table 2-2.

TABLE 2-2 ▶

Anaerobic Bacteria of Greatest Medical Significance

	Morphology	Genus
Gram positive		
	Spore-forming rods	Clostridium
	Non–spore-forming rods	Actinomyces
	Non–spore-forming cocci	Peptostreptococcus (and related gram-positive cocci such as Peptococcus)
Gram negative		
	Spore-forming rods	None
	Non–spore-forming rods	Bacteroides-like group (Bacteroides spp., Prevotella, Porphyromonas)
		Fusobacterium
	Non–spore-forming cocci	Veillonella

Although both normal flora clostridial and nonclostridial anaerobes may sometimes be present together in an infection, consideration of nonclostridial anaerobic infections separately from clostridial infections is usually helpful. Nonclostridial anaerobic infections are almost always endogenous infections caused by normal flora. The nonclostridial anaerobes are characterized by their inability to form endospores and by the fact that protein toxins are not usually important in their pathogenesis. Infections involving nonclostridial anaerobes are more common than those involving clostridia and are almost always opportunistic in nature, as explained below.

In contrast, clostridial diseases have more heterogeneous origins. Clostridial diseases may result from endogenous infections (which may also involve nonclostridial anaerobes) involving normal flora clostridia, from exogenous infections, or from intoxication. Clostridial infections involve endospore-forming anaerobes whose pathogenesis is heavily dependent on the production of potent protein toxins. Although some clostridial diseases (e.g., *Clostridium difficile* infections of the gastrointestinal tract) have an opportunistic component because they almost always affect compromised individuals, other clostridial diseases (e.g., food-borne botulism) affect individuals previously in good health.

Nonclostridial Anaerobic Infections

When normal flora nonclostridial anaerobes are restricted to their normal body sites, they usually do not cause illness. (In fact, these normal flora bacteria may actually help protect against infection by exogenous pathogens [see Chapter 11]). However, if some event, for example, a bite, wound, or perforation of the intestine, allows normal flora nonclostridial (or clostridial) anaerobes access to normally inaccessible body sites, and tissue redox conditions are sufficiently low for anaerobic growth (either because of co-introduction of facultative anaerobes into the contaminated tissue or as a result of some medical condition favoring development of a lowered redox environment), these anaerobes can establish infection. Although nonclostridial anaerobes often have low virulence (i.e., many of these bacteria are required to start an infection), infections involving these bacteria can be quite serious, even fatal, once they are initiated.

Polymicrobic Contamination. An important characteristic of many anaerobic infections, particularly those involving nonclostridial anaerobes, is their polymicrobic nature. The normal microbial flora present at many body sites represents a complex mixture including many species of both anaerobic and facultative anaerobic bacteria, as well as other microorganisms such as yeasts (see Chapter 11). Therefore, if a bite, perforation, or other trauma occurs, a number of different microbial species often simultaneously enter previously inaccessible body sites. As mentioned, this polymicrobic contamination often contributes to the establishment of infections involving anaerobes by allowing normal flora facultative anaerobes to consume oxygen, thereby lowering the tissue redox potential to levels acceptable for anaerobic growth. Further, the polymicrobic nature of most infections involving the nonclostridial anaerobes has important therapeutic consequences. Because these infections often involve several different bacterial species, they often require the use of multiple types of antibiotics for effective treatment. Therapy of nonclostridial anaerobic infections is further complicated by the fact that many of these anaerobes (particularly gram-negative anaerobes such as *Bacteroides fragilis*) are often highly resistant to antibiotics.

Two important concepts regarding nonclostridial anaerobic infections (Table 2-3) merit emphasis. First, some nonclostridial anaerobes (e.g., *B. fragilis*, the anaerobic species most commonly involved in human infections) are isolated from human infections in disproportionate number relative to their representation in normal flora. This implies that some nonclostridial anaerobes are more pathogenic than others, although the virulence factors used by these anaerobes are, with few exceptions, still not well understood. Second, the nonclostridial anaerobes are very important causes of abscess formation. These anaerobic abscesses, which can form in virtually any organ in the body, usually do not respond to antibiotic therapy alone and often require surgical drainage and prolonged antibiotic therapy.

> An **abscess** is a localized collection of pus.

Bites	Oral and sinus infections
Aspiration pneumonia	Postabortion and puerperal infections
Postsurgical infections (particularly after bowel or gynecologic surgery)	Appendicitis
Septicemias (particularly in patients suffering from cancer and diabetes)	Septic thrombophlebitis
Localized abscesses (common sites include cranium, lungs, liver, and female genital tract)	

a These infections also simultaneously may involve normal flora clostridia, facultative anaerobes, or both.

◄ **TABLE 2-3**
Human Infections Commonly Involving Nonclostridial Anaerobes[a]

Gas Production. Both in vivo and in vitro, nonclostridial anaerobes are often slow growing and have fastidious nutritional requirements. Consequently, clinical specimens from infections suspected of involving nonclostridial (or clostridial) anaerobes often must be cultivated on rich media for several days or longer to demonstrate the presence of anaerobic bacteria (see Appendix 1 for information regarding cultivation of anaerobes). Further, because anaerobes use gas-producing fermentations for their energy production, anaerobic infections often produce foul-smelling gases in the involved tissue. Therefore, whenever an infection involving gas and unpleasant odor is encountered, the possibility of anaerobic infection should be considered.

> **Fastidious bacteria** are bacteria with complex nutritional requirements, and they will not grow on simple media.

Clostridial Diseases

The clostridia are gram-positive, spore-forming, anaerobic rods responsible for a number of significant human diseases (Table 2-4). Although some clostridial diseases may have an endogenous origin (e.g., some cases of clostridial myonecrosis), many clostridial diseases (e.g., tetanus) have an exogenous origin. Some clostridial illnesses involve an infection, whereas others involve an intoxication. The most important single principle uniting the clostridial diseases is that symptoms of these diseases result from the ability of pathogenic clostridia to produce very potent protein exotoxins (see Table 2-4).

TABLE 2-4 ▶

Major Clostridial Diseases of Humans

Species and Disease Caused	Symptoms	Virulence Factor	Reference
Clostridium difficile			
Antibiotic-associated pseudomembranous colitis[a,b]	Diarrhea (often with blood); fever	Toxin A (enterotoxin) Toxin B (cytotoxin)	Chapter 11
C. botulinum			
Botulism[c]	Flaccid paralysis	Botulinum neurotoxin	Chapter 20
Histotoxic clostridia (most notably *C. perfringens*) Wound infections[b]			
Myonecrosis	Fever; pain; foul smell; gas in tissue; necrosis	α-Toxin[d]	Chapter 2
Anaerobic cellulitis	Foul smell; gas in tissue; less pain and necrosis than in myonecrosis	α-Toxin[d]	Chapter 2
Superficial wound contamination	Little pain; little gas	α-Toxin[d]	Chapter 2
C. perfringens type A Food poisoning[b]	Diarrhea; abdominal cramps	*C. perfringens* enterotoxin	Chapters 2 and 6
C. tetani Tetanus[b]	Spastic paralysis; muscle contractions of jaw, back, extremeties	Tetanus toxin	Chapter 2

[a] Both *C. difficile* and *C. perfringens* can also cause antibiotic-associated diarrhea, which is a less severe diarrheal illness than antibiotic-associated pseudomembranous colitis.
[b] Infections.
[c] There are multiple forms of botulism (see Chapter 20); the most common form—food-borne botulism—can be an intoxication.
[d] α-Toxin is the most important toxin for wound and soft tissue infections by *C. perfringens*; however, other *C. perfringens'* toxins also contribute to the pathogenesis of these infections.

ILLUSTRATIVE PATHOGEN: *Bacteroides*-like Group

Biologic Characteristics

The *Bacteroides*-like group of bacteria include a number of species that recently underwent a taxonomic reorganization. Although all bacteria in this group are anaerobic, gram-negative rods that share certain biochemical characteristics, this group, once all considered *Bacteroides* spp., has now been subdivided into the nonpigmented genus *Bacteroides* and the pigmented genera *Porphyromonas* and *Prevotella* (which can be differentiated using additional biochemical tests).

Reservoir and Transmission

Usually no transmission of the *Bacteroides*-like group to the host is necessary because these bacteria are already present as normal flora in the body; that is, infections with these opportunistic bacteria usually have an endogenous origin. Individual species within the *Bacteroides*-like group of nonclostridial anaerobes often have a predilection for specific body locations (e.g., colon, vagina, or mouth). This contributes to the tendency for certain members of the group to be associated with disease in particular organs (note, however, that these associations are not absolute and that nonclostridial infections also can cause generalized septicemias). For example, because *B. fragilis* is an important member of the normal colonic flora, this bacterium has a greater likelihood than *Prevotella* spp., which primarily reside in the mouth or respiratory tract, of entering the peritoneal cavity following some trauma or colonic malignancy and causing peritonitis. Conversely, *Prevotella* spp. are more often the cause of dental and lung infections (resulting from the aspiration of sputum into the lungs) than is *B. fragilis*.

Virulence Factors

The *Bacteroides*-like group produces enzymes such as collagenase, neuraminidase, and DNase, that contribute to pathogenesis by allowing these bacteria to penetrate into tissues. Several species of the *Bacteroides*-like group, most notably *B. fragilis*, produce a capsule with antiphagocytic properties. This capsule also appears to contribute to abscess formation through an incompletely understood process. Although the lipopolysaccharide (LPS) of *B. fragilis* has only weak endotoxic activity, the LPS made by some of the pigmented members of the *Bacteroides*-like group elicits significant endotoxic effects. Furthermore, the LPS made by members of the *Bacteroides*-like group (including *B. fragilis*) appears to contribute to abscess formation. Protein toxins are not considered to be important in the virulence of the *Bacteroides*-like bacteria, with the exception of an enterotoxin produced by some strains of *B. fragilis* that may be involved in childhood diarrheas.

> An **enterotoxin** is a toxin active in the gastrointestinal tract.

Pathogenesis

Typical of nonclostridial anaerobes, the pathogenesis of the *Bacteroides*-like group of anaerobes often involves the introduction of these bacteria into new habitats in the body (e.g., an abdominal stab or gunshot wound perforating the colon may allow normal intestinal flora to enter the peritoneal cavity), followed by growth if redox conditions permit. The *Bacteroides*-like anaerobes then produce tissue damage, using the degradative enzymes mentioned above, and induce an inflammatory response that may result in abscess formation.

Diagnosis

Clinical observation of foul-smelling discharges, gas in tissues, or the location of an infection near a mucosal surface provides a physician with helpful clues that *Bacteroides*-like bacteria are involved in an infection. Direct Gram stains of clinical specimens also can provide useful information because these bacteria are often pleomorphic and pale staining. Preliminary suspicion of their involvement can then be confirmed by culturing the organisms anaerobically and by performing additional biochemical tests, such as gas-liquid chromatography, which can identify the distinctive fermentation end-products that are made by different species belonging to the *Bacteroides*-like group (see Appendix 1 for anaerobic culturing techniques). Because the *Bacteroides*-like group consists of normal flora present in many body sites, clinical specimens for anaerobic cultivation must be collected extremely carefully; otherwise, contamination of the specimen with normal flora may produce false-positive results.

> **Pleomorphic** means that the bacteria of a given species are not all the same size and shape.

Prevention and Treatment

Effective treatment of infections (including abscesses) involving the *Bacteroides*-like group of bacteria often involves a combination of antimicrobial therapy and surgery, which includes drainage of abscesses and excision of necrotic tissue. Antimicrobial therapy of these infections is complicated by the polymicrobic nature of many of them, as well as by their high degree of antibiotic resistance, especially in the case of *B. fragilis*. Therefore, combinations of antibiotics are often used to treat these infections.

Physicians can take steps to prevent the development of anaerobic infections, particularly in obviously susceptible individuals. For example, prophylactic antimicrobial therapy may be administered to a patient before bowel or gynecologic surgery, and steps can be taken to minimize aspiration of oral material into the lungs of individuals with swallowing difficulties.

ILLUSTRATIVE PATHOGEN: Histotoxic clostridia

Biologic Characteristics

Like all clostridia, the histotoxic clostridia are gram-positive, anaerobic, spore-forming rods whose pathogenesis involves exotoxin production. They are distinguished from other clostridia by their ability to cause wound and soft tissue infections.

The histotoxic clostridia include several species. Of these, *C. perfringens* is the single most important because it is isolated in approximately 90% of infections involving histotoxic clostridia. Other important species include *C. septicum*, which is a common cause of infection in patients suffering from cancer of the gastrointestinal tract, *C. histolyticum*, and *C. novyi*.

Reservoir and Transmission

The histotoxic clostridia have a widespread distribution in the environment. Histotoxic clostridia (e.g., *C. perfringens*) are present in soil and as part of the normal intestinal flora. Consequently, infections involving them can have either an endogenous origin (e.g., from fecal contamination of a wound) or an exogenous origin (e.g., from soil contamination of a wound). The ability of the histotoxic clostridia to form endospores allows these bacteria to persist in the soil for long periods of time before entering a wound and causing infection. Once implanted in a wound, these endospores may germinate if conditions permit. Infection also can occur if vegetative cells of the histotoxic clostridia enter wounds.

Virulence Factors

Each species of the histotoxic clostridia is capable of producing a number of different toxins. For example, *C. perfringens* can make at least 13 different kinds of toxins. The single most important of these 13 toxins in wound infections appears to be α-*toxin*, which has phospholipase properties and contributes to hemolysis, necrosis, and inhibition of phagocyte function. *C. perfringens* also makes a capsule, although the role of this capsule in infections is unclear.

Pathogenesis

Infection by the histotoxic clostridia is a multistep process. First, cells or spores of the histotoxic clostridia need to enter the target tissue. This entry can be accomplished through a wound or any condition that disrupts mucosal integrity (e.g., by a tumor). Low redox conditions then must develop (e.g., as a result of necrosis at a wound site) for multiplication of the histotoxic clostridial cells in the wound to occur. Once infection is initiated, growing cells begin producing protein toxins, which induce the characteristic pathologic consequences described below.

Gas gangrene (myonecrosis): In this wound infection, histotoxic clostridia grow in muscle, which provides an excellent environment for growth because of its low redox conditions due to acid production from muscle contractions. As toxins are produced by the clostridia, necrosis occurs, providing additional low redox habitats for anaerobic growth. As a result, this infection progressively spreads unless stopped by surgery. Gas, as a by-product of clostridial fermentation, and edema are produced in muscle tissue as a consequence of clostridial growth and toxin-induced necrosis. The toxins produced also have potent inhibitory or lethal effects on phagocytes, which limit effective host defense responses. As these toxins accumulate in the body, some eventually enter the circulation and affect distant organs, such as the heart. As a result of these toxin-induced processes, myonecrosis is rapidly fatal unless effective therapy is promptly initiated.

Anaerobic cellulitis: This illness is usually less serious than myonecrosis because it involves only subcutaneous and cutaneous tissues, which provide less favorable habitats than muscle for growth of histotoxic clostridia.

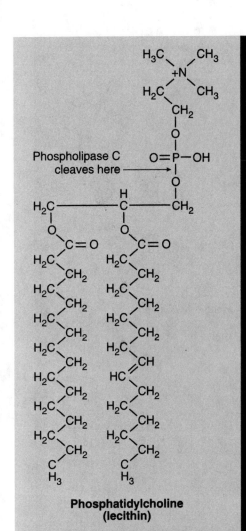

Phospholipase C cleaves here ⟶

Phosphatidylcholine (lecithin)

C. perfringens α-toxin has phospholipase C enzymatic properties. *This enzymatic activity probably weakens the integrity of the mammalian plasma membrane, making this membrane more susceptible to lysis. Some recent studies also suggest that α-toxin may activate eukaryotic phospholipases present in the plasma membranes of mammalian cells.*

Simple wound infection: This is the least serious wound infection involving the histotoxic clostridia. Infection is limited to cutaneous tissue.

Other infections involving the histotoxic clostridia include:

Uterine infection: This is a special type of myonecrosis, usually involving the gravid (pregnant) uterus. Uterine infections by *C. perfringens* were particularly common in the era of illegal abortions but are also associated with childbirth. The uterine infections have a greater tendency than other cases of *C. perfringens*-associated myonecrosis to cause septicemia and thus typically spread quickly and have a high fatality rate.

Septicemia: *C. septicum* or *C. perfringens* can enter the bloodstream of individuals with a malignancy. Death can occur rapidly without proper diagnosis and treatment.

***C. perfringens* food poisonings:** *C. perfringens* causes two different types of food poisoning. The first type, *C. perfringens* type A food poisoning, is a very common illness in the United States and Europe. This disease results from ingestion of *C. perfringens* cells that sporulate in the intestines and produce an enterotoxin which causes abdominal cramps and diarrhea (see Chapters 6 and 20). The second type of *C. perfringens* foodborne disease is called necrotizing enteritis (also known as Pig-Bel). This illness is more serious but is much less common in the United States than *C. perfringens* type A food poisoning. It is most common in New Guinea due to local dietary customs, including the consumption of undercooked pork. Necrotizing enteritis involves extensive damage to the intestinal mucosa that is mediated by β-toxin, whose molecular action is not clear.

Diagnosis

Because an early diagnosis is essential for survival from myonecrosis, as well as from uterine infections and septicemias associated with the histotoxic clostridia, diagnosis of these illnesses must be based primarily on clinical signs (e.g., the presence of gas and edema in tissues). Gram stains of specimens from affected tissues also can provide important clues for the differential diagnosis of these illnesses. Bacteriologic analysis then can be used to provide confirmation of the presumptive diagnosis.

Prevention and Treatment

Treatment for myonecrosis is difficult. Antibiotic therapy alone is not effective. Instead, the primary therapy for myonecrosis involves surgical removal of affected necrotic tissue, often by amputation, if possible. Antibiotic therapy is given as adjunctive therapy. Mortality rates for patients who have myonecrosis vary from 15% to 30%, with the outcome largely depending on the anatomic location of the myonecrosis. Thus, if gas gangrene develops in muscles of the trunk, where amputation is not possible, the prognosis is poor.

Therapy for anaerobic cellulitis also involves surgery to remove necrotic tissue, as well as the administration of antibiotics. Simple wound infections usually can be treated by surgical removal of necrotic tissue and cleansing of the wound. Antibiotics are not usually required.

Hyperbaric oxygen, which is intended to raise tissue redox conditions and thereby inhibit growth of anaerobic clostridia, is sometimes used as adjunctive therapy for serious infections involving the histotoxic clostridia. The best strategy for preventing wound infection by the histotoxic clostridia is proper cleaning and debridement of wounds, when necessary.

BACTERIAL ENDOSPORES

When some bacteria encounter suboptimal environments (e.g., an environment with limited nutrients), they respond by forming endospores. Because only one endospore forms per vegetative mother cell, bacterial sporulation is a survival strategy, not a reproductive response. Only two medically important bacterial genera are able to form endospores: *Bacillus* and *Clostridium*. These two spore formers can be easily distinguished in the laboratory because *Bacillus* spp. are aerobes (or facultative anaerobes), whereas *Clostridium* spp. are anaerobes.

Importance of Spores for Medicine

Endospore formation is medically important for two reasons. First, bacterial endospores are the most resistant life forms known. Mature bacterial spores are exceptionally resistant to heat, radiation, chemicals, and drying because they are packed internally with a highly protective compound called calcium dipicolinate. Consequently, conditions for sterilizing surgical instruments must be designed to ensure killing of endospores (see Appendix 2 for sterilization and disinfection techniques). Second, endospores are medically important due to their role in disease transmission. Because they contain virtually no internal water, they are essentially metabolically inert. Consequently, an endospore can persist for a long period (perhaps 100 years or more) before it germinates into a new growing cell. Therefore, endospores can survive for a long time in the environment before entering the human body and causing disease. Several human diseases commonly result from implantation or inhalation of spores, including anthrax (caused by *B. anthracis*), tetanus (caused by *C. tetani*), and infections involving the histotoxic clostridia (e.g., *C. perfringens*).

> Bacterial **sporulation** refers to the process during which a bacterial cell gives rise to a spore. **Germination** refers to the process by which an endospore develops into a new, growing cell.

ILLUSTRATIVE PATHOGEN: *Bacillus anthracis*

Biologic Characteristics

Anthrax is caused by *B. anthracis*, a gram-positive, nonmotile, aerobic, spore-forming rod that is found in soil and in contaminated farm animals and their products (e.g., wool).

Reservoir and Transmission

B. anthracis can enter the body through several mechanisms, including (1) inhalation of spores or cells present in soil-containing dust, (2) entrance of spores or cells into wounds, or (3) ingestion of spores or cells (rare). The ability of *B. anthracis* to form spores allows it to persist in soil or animal products for long periods before causing infection.

Virulence Factors

B. anthracis pathogenesis involves two essential virulence factors: a polypeptide capsule with antiphagocytic properties and a toxin complex. The toxin complex consists of three separate proteins: protective antigen (PA), which binds to mammalian receptors; lethal factor (LF), which kills mammalian cells through a still unknown mechanism; and edema factor (EF), which is an adenylate cyclase that causes edema by elevating cyclic adenosine monophosphate (cAMP) levels in mammalian cells. The toxin complex works through a three-step process: (1) PA binds to mammalian receptors, (2) bound PA is proteolytically activated so it binds LF and EF to mammalian cells, and (3) LF and EF actions are expressed in mammalian cells.

Pathogenesis

The initial symptoms of each of the three forms of anthrax are directly related to bacterial entry into the body:

Cutaneous anthrax: initially involves formation of an inflammatory sore, called an eschar or malignant pustule, at the site of entry of *B. anthracis* spores or cells into the skin.

Pulmonary anthrax: follows inhalation of *B. anthracis* spores or cells and initially resembles a respiratory illness, with symptoms including fever and cough (known as "wool-sorters disease").

Gastrointestinal anthrax: follows ingestion of food (usually meat) contaminated with *B. anthracis* spores or cells and initially involves gastrointestinal symptoms, including nausea, vomiting, and diarrhea.

B. anthracis cells may disseminate throughout the body in all three forms of anthrax, although this occurrence is less common with cutaneous anthrax, which often spontaneously resolves. Disseminated anthrax often leads to fatal shock. The antiphagocytic capsule helps *B. anthracis* resist host defenses and, therefore, contributes to the establishment and continuance of infection. The toxin complex induces pathophysiologic responses, such as shock, by triggering immune cells (e.g., macrophages) to release tumor necrosis factor (TNF) and other pro-inflammatory molecules.

Diagnosis

Initial presumptive diagnosis of cutaneous anthrax is usually based on clinical grounds (e.g., by identification of the characteristic eschar), although the diagnosis is complicated by the rarity of this illness. (Most physicians in industrialized countries have never seen a case of anthrax.) Gram stains of a specimen from the eschar also can provide helpful clues to the diagnosis. The presumptive diagnosis of cutaneous anthrax then can be confirmed in the laboratory by culturing, further staining, and serologic testing. Pulmonary and gastrointestinal anthrax are often misdiagnosed, which results in a high fatality rate, because of their rarity and lack of specific symptoms.

Prevention and Treatment

Antibiotic therapy (e.g., penicillin) is effective, if initiated promptly. Because anthrax has a zoonotic reservoir (see Chapter 8), control of human anthrax also requires control of anthrax in animals and animal products. Infected domestic animals are usually sacrificed, and their burned, disinfected carcasses are buried deep in the ground to prevent the spread of spores into the top soil. Wool and other animal products coming from contaminated areas need to be gas sterilized for safety. A live-spore vaccine (derived from a nonencapsulated *B. anthracis* strain) is available for animal vaccination against anthrax, whereas a nonliving anthrax vaccine may be used to protect humans at high risk, such as farmers or animal-product workers in countries where anthrax is endemic. Public health control measures have made anthrax rare in the United States, but the disease is more significant in Third World countries. Currently, there is considerable concern about the potential use of anthrax spores as a biologic warfare agent.

> A **zoonotic reservoir** means that a pathogen is carried by some animals besides, or in addition to, humans.

ILLUSTRATIVE PATHOGEN: *Clostridium tetani*

Biologic Characteristics

Tetanus is caused by *C. tetani*, a gram-positive, spore-forming, anaerobic rod.

Reservoir and Transmission

Spores of *C. tetani* are found in soils throughout the world, providing an excellent reservoir for tetanus. Entry of *C. tetani* into the body usually involves implantation of spores into a wound. If the redox potential of the surrounding tissue is sufficiently low, the implanted spore germinates into a new vegetative cell that multiplies and produces tetanus toxin in the wound. After implantation into a wound, *C. tetani* spores can persist in the body for quite a while, perhaps months, waiting for the proper low redox growth conditions to develop before germinating into actively growing cells. Consequently, the incubation period for the development of tetanus symptoms is variable, but averages approximately 1 week.

Virulence Factors

The virulence factor responsible for the symptoms of tetanus is tetanus toxin, also called tetanospasmin, which is an extremely lethal neurotoxin. Tetanus toxin induces spastic paralysis by inhibiting the release of inhibitory neurotransmitters (e.g., glycine) in the central nervous system (CNS), using a molecular mechanism described in Chapter 20. The physiologic consequence of tetanus toxin is uncontrolled muscle contractions.

Pathogenesis

As growing cells of *C. tetani* produce tetanus toxin at the wound site, the toxin starts to migrate along nerves into the CNS (using a process called retrograde axonal transport), where it blocks the release of inhibitory neurotransmitters. As a consequence, muscles are overstimulated to contract, causing spastic paralysis. An individual suffering from tetanus undergoes convulsive muscle contractions of the jaw (called trismus, or lockjaw), back, and extremities (Figure 2-2). These contractions may become so violent that bone fractures occur. Unfortunately, the affected individual is conscious throughout this illness but cannot stop these contractions. Death often results from cardiac and respiratory effects or secondary complications.

FIGURE 2-2 ▶

Sir Charles Bell's Painting of a Soldier with Generalized Tetanus. Note the spastic paralysis, which includes a clenched jaw (referred to as trismus), giving tetanus its common name, "lockjaw." (Source: Reproduced with permission of the President and Fellows of the Royal College of Surgeons of Edinburgh, Scotland.)

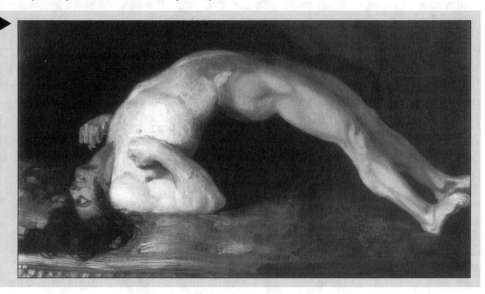

Diagnosis

Tetanus is suspected upon exposure to a bite or a puncture wound. The disease is not common in the United States because of vaccination, but a few cases still occur each year, primarily in individuals who have not received proper booster vaccines. Tetanus is still very common in Third World countries, where it causes several hundred thousand deaths per year. Many of these deaths involve neonatal tetanus that develops when the umbilical cord is unsterilely cut.

Prevention and Treatment

Treatment of tetanus is difficult once symptoms have developed. Tetanus antitoxin is administered, along with muscle relaxants and symptomatic therapy (e.g., assisted ventilation). If recovery does occur, there are usually no long-term side effects. However, recovered individuals do not develop natural immunity against the infection because too little tetanus toxin is produced during the disease to induce a protective immune response.

Because of the seriousness of tetanus and the availability of a very effective tetanus vaccine, control of tetanus emphasizes prevention rather than treatment. Tetanus immunity is achieved using formalinized tetanus toxoid. This toxoid is administered as part of the childhood diphtheria-pertussis-tetanus (DPT) vaccine (see Chapter 29). After the initial series of childhood DPT immunizations, adults need to be re-immunized every 10 years with a booster dose of tetanus (or tetanus-diphtheria) toxoid vaccine.

RESOLUTION OF CLINICAL CASE

When the 70-year-old man was taken to the operating room and his left sacral area was debrided, extensive necrosis of the muscles (myonecrosis) was noted over his hip and down the posterior aspect of his right leg, as well as infection extending to the superior femur, which was also necrotic. The upper fifth of the femur was resected, and virtually all of the superficial and deep muscles around the hip were removed. Hip disarticulation was recommended for the patient, but his family would not consent to this procedure.

This case is quite typical of gas gangrene (clostridial myonecrosis), which occurs when histotoxic *Clostridium* spp. gain access to tissue in which anaerobic conditions prevail. Gas gangrene usually occurs following the inoculation of a traumatic wound with dirt containing clostridial spores. However, it may occur even after "clean" surgery because the spores are ubiquitous. The present case occurred when some histotoxic clostridial species that were normal flora of the gastrointestinal tract entered (through fecal contamination) a deep ulcer where anaerobic conditions prevailed. A diagnosis of myonecrosis is usually entertained when a patient has pain in a wound and systemic toxicity out of proportion to the extent of an injury or surgical wound. The finding of crepitus should heighten suspicion because clostridia produce large amounts of gas in human tissue. The "dishwater" drainage (edema) contained no polymorphonuclear leukocytes because histotoxic clostridia produce toxins that lyse these cells. In gas gangrene, only gram-positive rods are visible by microscopic examination, whereas mixed flora, including both anaerobes and facultative anaerobes are commonly involved in other forms of cellulitis and fasciitis. Antibiotic therapy plays only an adjunct role in gas gangrene because antibiotics cannot reach the ischemic, necrotic tissue where the bacteria are, and many antibiotics are ineffective in an anaerobic environment anyway. Definitive therapy requires complete removal of all infected tissue, including all necrotic muscle. If the process is caught early enough, amputation of a limb may be curative. However, if gas gangrene reaches or starts on the trunk, cure is usually impossible and the patient soon dies (death was the most likely prognosis for the patient in our case). Recovery also is quite unlikely once blood cultures become positive for histotoxic clostridia, that is, once generalized septicemia occurs.

REVIEW QUESTIONS

Directions: For each of the following questions, choose the **one best** answer.

Questions 1 and 2

Rebound tenderness is pain that occurs on the sudden release of pressure from an examiner's hand; it is usually an indication of peritonitis, an inflammation of the peritoneum which lines the abdominal cavity.

A 14-year-old boy is brought to the emergency department with a single gunshot wound in the left lower quadrant of the abdomen. There is no exit wound. He is started on ticarcillin, clindamycin, and gentamicin and is taken directly to the operating room. The surgeon finds that the bullet has penetrated the large bowel twice and the small bowel once. The bowel perforations are closed, and the peritoneal cavity is irrigated with saline. The patient does well for 5 days following surgery. On the sixth day, however, his temperature rises to 102°F, and he complains of abdominal pain, particularly in the left lower quadrant. On examination, there is tenderness in the left lower quadrant and generalized rebound tenderness. A computerized tomography scan of the abdomen reveals the probable presence of an abscess. The patient is returned to the operating room, where a large abscess is drained.

1. Considering this information, which one of the following statements is most likely to be correct?
    - **(A)** The abscess is unlikely to involve anaerobic bacteria
    - **(B)** The abscess probably involves a single bacterial species
    - **(C)** Endotoxin is probably not involved in eliciting the patient's fever
    - **(D)** *Bacteroides* spp. are probably involved in this infection
    - **(E)** The bacteria involved in this abscess are unlikely to be antibiotic resistant

2. Microscopic examination of a Gram-stained sample of pus drained from this patient's abscess shows the presence of polymorphonuclear leukocytes and bacteria, including large pink rods and pale-staining pink rods, some of which have pointy ends, and some of which have irregular shapes. When a sample of this drained abscess material is aseptically cultured, several different types of colonies are observed. Some of the colonies grow only under anaerobic conditions; at least one colony grows under both aerobic and anaerobic conditions. The patient's abscess is most likely to involve
    - **(A)** *Bacteroides*-like spp. only
    - **(B)** *Fusobacterium* spp. only
    - **(C)** *Escherichia coli* only
    - **(D)** *Bacteroides*-like spp. and *E. coli*
    - **(E)** *Bacteroides*-like spp., *Fusobacterium* spp., and *E. coli*

3. In the laboratory, pure cultures of *Bacteroides fragilis, Bacillus cereus, Clostridium botulinum, Escherichia coli*, and *Staphylococcus aureus* are mixed together, boiled for 10 minutes, and inoculated onto a sterile agar plate. The plate is then incubated overnight on the desktop. The next morning, colonies are growing on the plate. Assuming the sterile technique was beyond reproach (i.e., no contamination occurred), the growth on this plate is most probably
    - **(A)** *B. fragilis*
    - **(B)** *B. cereus*
    - **(C)** *C. botulinum*
    - **(D)** *E. coli*
    - **(E)** *S. aureus*

4. Which of the following statements regarding anaerobes and anaerobic infections is correct?

    (A) Anaerobes often produce catalase (or peroxidases), superoxide dismutase, or both

    (B) Anaerobes are often fast growing

    (C) Anaerobes are more abundant in normal colonic flora than coliforms (e.g., *Escherichia coli*-like, facultative anaerobes)

    (D) Anaerobes grow well under the tissue redox conditions present in healthy tissue

    (E) Anaerobes are rarely involved in polymicrobic infections that culminate in abscess formation

5. In the laboratory, a microbiologist decides to compare, under identical environmental conditions, the growth of two strains, 1 and 2, of *Escherichia coli*. Using plate count techniques, she obtains the results shown in the figure below. Which of the following statements about these results is correct?

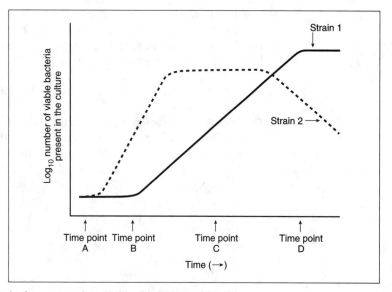

    (A) Strain 1 was growing optimally at time point B

    (B) Strain 2 was increasing in number at time point C, which corresponds to the log phase of growth

    (C) Strain 2 has a more rapid optimal doubling time than strain 1

    (D) At maximum growth, there were more viable cells of strain 2 than of strain 1

    (E) At time point D, strain 1 is in the death phase

6. Tetanus is best described by which one of the following statements?

    (A) It is usually an intoxication rather than an infection

    (B) It involves a flaccid paralysis

    (C) It results from stimulation of inhibitory neurotransmitter release

    (D) It primarily affects the neuromuscular junctions

    (E) It often results from germination of spores inside a wound

ANSWERS AND EXPLANATIONS

1 and 2. The answers are: 1-D, 2-E. *Bacteroides* species (particularly *B. fragilis*) are often involved in abdominal abscesses. The likely presence of anaerobes in this abscess could be confirmed by anaerobically culturing a specimen from the abscess. Infections resulting from perforation of the intestines often are polymicrobic. Although the lipopolysaccharide (LPS) of *B. fragilis* has only weak endotoxic activity, the likely polymicrobic nature of the patient's infection makes it probable that other gram-negative bacteria, with more strongly endotoxic LPS molecules, are also present. Many anaerobes are extremely antibiotic resistant.

The information presented in question 2 is consistent with the abscess involving both gram-negative facultative anaerobes (e.g., *E. coli*) and multiple types of gram-negative strict anaerobes (e.g., *Bacteroides*-like species and *Fusobacterium* species). The presence of at least two anaerobes would not be surprising because abdominal abscesses often are polymicrobic.

3. The answer is B. The bacterium most likely to be growing on this plate is *B. cereus*. Options A, D, and E are incorrect because only the spore-forming bacteria such as *Bacillus* and *Clostridium* spp. are likely to survive boiling because of their ability to form highly heat-resistant endospores. Of the two spore formers present in the mixture, only *B. cereus* is able to grow aerobically. Option C, *C. botulinum*, is anaerobic and thus would not grow on a plate left on a desktop.

4. The answer is C. Anaerobes are the predominant normal flora present in the colon, as well as in most other mucosal surfaces. Options A and B are incorrect because anaerobes often do not produce catalase (peroxidases) or superoxide dismutase and are often slow growing and astidious. Options D and E are incorrect because anaerobes grow best under low redox conditions that are absent in healthy tissue, and they are often involved in polymicrobic infections that result in abscess formation.

5. The answer is C. Because during log growth the slope of strain 2 is steeper than the slope of strain 1, strain 2 is the faster growing under the environmental conditions used in the experiment. Option A is incorrect because strain 1 was in the log phase of growth at time point B. Option B is incorrect because strain 2 was in the stationary phase (no growth) at time point C. Option D is incorrect because comparison of *y*-axis values indicates that there were more viable bacteria of strain 1 than of strain 2 at the maximal growth of both strains. Option E is incorrect because strain 1 is in the stationary phase at time point D. Strain 2 is in the death phase, however, at point D.

6. The answer is E. Tetanus is an infection that develops from the presence of viable tetanus-toxin–producing *Clostridium tetani* cells in the body. Option B is incorrect because tetanus evokes a spastic paralysis that may be so severe that bone fractures occur. Tetanus involves an inhibition (not stimulation, option C) of the release of inhibitory neurotransmitters in the central nervous system, and it does not affect neuromuscular junctions (option D).

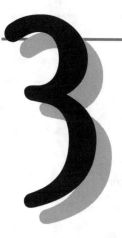

GROWTH OF VIRUSES

CHAPTER OUTLINE

Introduction of Clinical Case
Characteristics of Viruses
• Composition and Architecture of Viruses
• Classification of Viruses
• Virus Growth Cycle: An Overview
• Kinds of Virus Infections
Replication Strategies
• DNA Viruses
• RNA Viruses
• Viruses Using a Reverse Transcriptase
Virus Adaptation
• Point Mutations
• Recombination
• Viral Resistance, Antigenic Drift, and Antigenic Shift
Resolution of Clinical Case
Review Questions

INTRODUCTION OF CLINICAL CASE

In February, a 32-year-old Boston businessman visited his family physician with complaints of malaise, a scratchy sore throat, and chronic nasal congestion and discharge (rhinorrhea) severe enough to cause restless sleep. The patient had no other complaints, and a physical examination revealed no evidence of lower respiratory disease. The man was otherwise in good health. The physician prescribed a decongestant and suggested the use of an over-the-counter nasal spray before bedtime, if needed. The patient demanded an antibiotic to ensure he would be fit for a lengthy air trip the following week. The physician prescribed a broad-spectrum antibiotic. Six days later, the patient reported that his respiratory symptoms had subsided and that he was ready to travel abroad, but he noted that he had experienced diarrhea for the past several days.

CHARACTERISTICS OF VIRUSES

Composition and Architecture of Viruses

Viruses are truly remarkable pathogens, exhibiting features quite unique when compared to prokaryotes or eukaryotes (Table 3-1). Their most striking attribute is their modus operandi of replication. Instead of reproducing by binary fission, viruses deliver their nucleic acid genome into cells and commandeer the transcriptional and translational

TABLE 3-1 ▶
Viruses as Distinguished from Cells

Feature	Viruses	Cells
Nucleic acids	DNA or RNA	DNA and RNA
Mode of replication	Directed synthesis and assembly of component parts	Binary fission
Possession of enzymes	None or limited to nucleic acid polymerases, kinases, etc.; no enzymes for generating energy as ATP	Extensive enzymatic machinery, usually including that generating energy in the form of ATP
Protein synthesis	Requires host cell machinery	Yes

Note. ATP = adenosine triphosphate.

machinery of the cell to direct the synthesis and assembly of virus components—a remarkable example of parasitism at the level of macromolecules.

Virus Genomes. The genome of a virus is either a DNA molecule or one or more molecules of RNA. The viral genome is always enclosed within a protein shell called a capsid. Capsids may or may not be composed of capsomeres, which are defined as morphologic subunits of the capsid discernible by electron microscopy. They are created by the specific clustering of capsid proteins.

Virus Particles. Virus particles come in two forms (Figure 3-1). Nonenveloped viruses are composed of a viral genome molecule or molecules enclosed within a capsid. These particles are sometimes called naked nucleocapsids. Enveloped viruses are composed of nucleocapsids surrounded by a lipid-containing membrane. This viral membrane, or envelope, is a crucial part of an enveloped virus particle; its denaturation or destruction renders the virus particle noninfectious. Viral envelopes always have virus-specific proteins embedded in them. Neutralizing antibodies interfere with the ability of a virus to enter a cell if they react with one or more specific capsid proteins of a nucleocapsid virus or any of the envelope proteins of an enveloped virus.

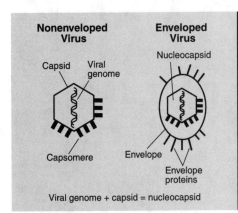

FIGURE 3-1 ▶
Computer-Enhanced Electron Micrographs of Representative Nonenveloped (A–C) and Enveloped (D–F) Viruses. (A) Poliovirus (30-nm diameter), a picornavirus. (B) Bovine papillomavirus (55-nm diameter), a papovavirus. (C) An adenovirus (75-nm diameter). (D) A coronavirus (pleomorphic, approximately 120-nm diameter). (E) Influenzavirus (pleomorphic, 100-nm diameter), an orthomyxovirus. (F) Herpes simplex virus (approximately 180-nm diameter). Note that the relative sizes of the viruses to each other are approximately correct. (Sources: Figure A—courtesy of B. A. Phillips and John Cardamone, Jr., University of Pittsburgh School of Medicine, Pittsburgh, Pennsylvania; Figure B—original photo provided by Dr. Robert Garcia, University of Colorado School of Medicine, Denver, Colorado; Figures C, D, F—digitized computer files reproduced with permission of Dr. M. Stewart McNulty, Department of Agriculture, Veterinary Sciences Division, Belfast, Northern Ireland; Figure E—original photo provided by J. S. Younger and John Cardamone, Jr., University of Pittsburgh School of Medicine, Pittsburgh, Pennsylvania.)

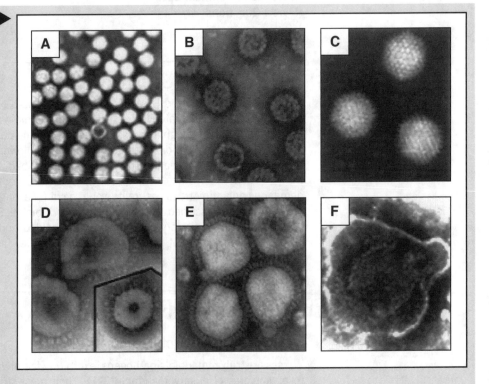

Classification of Viruses

There are seven families of DNA animal viruses, six of which are important to human medicine; the thirteen RNA animal virus families all contain important human pathogens (Table 3-2).

The current virus classification scheme is based on the nature of the virus genome,

◀ **TABLE 3-2**
Animal DNA and RNA Viruses

DNA Viruses[a]

Family	Size (nm)	Nucleic Acid	Capsomeres	Nucleocapsid Symmetry	Envelope
Parvoviruses	25	Linear, ssDNA [+ or −]	12	Icosahedron	No
Papovaviruses	50	Circular, dsDNA	72	Icosahedron	No
Adenoviruses	75	Linear, dsDNA	252	Icosahedron	No
Herpesviruses	180–200	Linear, dsDNA	162	Icosahedron	Yes
Poxviruses	200 x 400 (175–275)[b]	Linear, dsDNA	None	Complex	Yes
Hepadnaviruses	42	Partially overlapping, circular, dsDNA with ssDNA regions	~ 32	Icosahedron	Yes
Iridoviruses[c]	125–300	Linear, dsDNA	~ 2000	Icosahedron	Yes and no

RNA Viruses[d]

Family	Size (nm)	Nucleic Acid	Capsomeres	Nucleocapsid Symmetry	Envelope	Some Human Viruses
Picornaviruses	30	Linear, ss [+] RNA	None	Icosahedron	No	Polioviruses; rhinoviruses; hepatitis A
Togaviruses[e]	50–70	Linear, ss [+] RNA	42	Icosahedron	Yes	Rubella; encephalitis viruses
Flaviviruses[e]	40–50	Linear, ss [+] RNA	32	Icosahedron	Yes	Dengue; hepatitis C
Coronaviruses	100	Linear, ss [+] RNA	None	Icosahedron	Yes	Respiratory viruses
Caliciviruses	40	Linear, ss [+] RNA	32	Icosahedron	No	Norwalk; hepatitis E
Paramyxoviruses	200 ± 50	Linear, ss [−] RNA	None	Helical	Yes	Measles; mumps; RSV
Rhabdoviruses	70 x 180	Linear, ss [−] RNA	None	Helical	Yes	Rabies
Filoviruses	50 x ~850	Linear, ss [−] RNA	None	Helical	Yes	Ebola
Bunyaviruses[e]	100	Linear, ss [−] RNA; 3–5 segments	None	Helical	Yes	Hantaviruses; encephalitis viruses
Orthomyxoviruses	100	Linear, ss [−] RNA; 8 segments	None	Helical	Yes	Influenza viruses
Arenaviruses	130	ss RNAs; 2 segments, one [−] and one ambisense [+ and −]	None	Helical	Yes	Lassa fever; hemorrhagic fever viruses
Reoviruses	70	Linear, dsRNA; 10–12 segments	32 (inner shell)	Icosahedron	No	Rotaviruses
Retroviruses	150	2 linear, ss [+] RNA molecules (diploid)	32	Icosahedron	Yes	HTLV-1; HIV

Note. ss = single stranded; ds = double stranded; [+] = positive sense (or polarity); [−] = negative sense; RSV = respiratory synctial virus; HTLV-1 = humanT-lymphotropic virus-1; HIV = human immunodeficiency virus.
[a] The initial letters of the DNA virus families spell HHAPPPI.
[b] Dimensions of the parapoxvirus genus.
[c] There are no currently no known human pathogens among the iridoviruses.
[d] The initial letters of the thirteen virus families create the mnemonic "2 Pcs FOR BARTeR" (i.e., PPCCFORBARTR). The "e" represents ebola virus, the most egregarious of the filoviruses.
[e] Members may be arboviruses (arthopod-borne viruses).

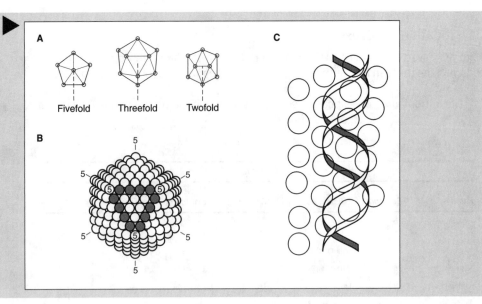

FIGURE 3-2

Most Virus Capsids Exhibit One of Two Kinds of Symmetry. (A) Views along the fivefold, threefold, and twofold rotational axes of an icosahedral particle with a capsomere at each of its 12 vertices. (B) The view along the threefold axis exhibited by the capsomeres of the icosahedral adenovirus particle. (Note capsomeres at apices have five neighboring capsomeres, whereas all others have six neighbors.) (C) Schematic diagram of the protein subunits (each circle) arranged in a helical structure. The superimposition of a DNA molecule is to illustrate further the helicity of the resulting protein capsid.

properties of the virus capsid, the presence or absence of an envelope, and unique aspects of the replication cycle.

Nature of the Virus Genome. The genome of a virus can be DNA or RNA, and the nucleic acid may be double stranded (ds) or single stranded (ss). The viral genome may be linear, circular, or superhelical, and the number of genome segments may vary. The polarity (sense) of the genome may be positive [+] or negative [−].

Properties of the Virus Capsid. Protein subunits may be organized to form a rod-shaped capsid with helical symmetry or a spherical capsid with icosahedral symmetry. The number of capsomeres comprising the capsid varies according to rules governing the symmetry of the capsid (Figure 3-2).

Unique Aspects of the Replication Strategy. Replication may require reverse transcriptases (e.g., for retroviruses and hepadnaviruses) or synthesis of subgenomic mRNA molecules (e.g., for togaviruses and caliciviruses).

Virus Growth Cycle: An Overview

The virus growth cycle proceeds through a series of well-defined steps.

Attachment or Adsorption. During attachment, the earliest interaction, a virus particle encounters and binds to a specific receptor on the plasma membrane of a cell. For some viruses (but not all), tropism is determined solely by the presence or absence of specific cell receptors (Table 3-4). The term "tropism," as applied to a virus, is often used to refer to the target organ, the dysfunction of which accounts for the predominant features of the disease the virus produces. For example, a poliomyelitis virus is clearly a neurotropic virus, but its ability to spread to the spinal column, brain, or both requires initial infection of lymphoid or epithelial cells that must possess common receptors.

Penetration. Penetration is the translocation of the entire viral particle or its nucleocapsid into the cell's cytoplasm. Viruses use two mechanisms to gain entry into a cell: *receptor-mediated endocytosis*, whereby the virus is engulfed into endocytic vesicles and delivered into the cytoplasm, and *direct fusion* between the envelope of a virus particle and the cell's plasma membrane. For example, viral-specific envelope proteins mediate the fusion of the envelopes of paramyxoviruses and certain retroviruses (e.g., human immunodeficiency virus [HIV]) with the host cell's plasma membrane. Concurrent with penetration, or shortly thereafter, the modified virus particle is further dissociated; that is, the genome is uncoated, which allows the expression of viral genes.

Synthesis and Assembly of Viral Constituents. Once the viral genome is uncoated, the expression of viral-specific genes ensues. For most DNA viruses, the viral genome (probably still associated with capsid proteins) is transported to the nucleus, where a

*A **positive-polarity** [+] DNA or RNA strand encodes the information for making protein; a **negative-polarity** [−] strand does not.*

***Tropism** describes the cell types a given virus can infect.*

***Viral tropism** helps explain why viruses cause specific diseases.*

◀ **TABLE 3-4**
Examples of Virus Receptors[a]

Virus	Receptor[a]	Cells Expressing the Receptor
Polioviruses	IgG superfamily protein; function unknown	Gut, Peyer's patches, neurons of CNS
Rhinoviruses	Intercellular adhesion molecules (e.g., I-CAM1)	Nasopharyngeal epithelium
Human coronaviruses	Aminopeptidase (CD[b]13)	Nasopharyngeal epithelium
Adenoviruses	α_v-Integrin	Nasopharyngeal epithelium
Influenza and parainfluenza viruses	Sialic acid moieties of plasma membrane proteins	Pharyngeal and bronchial epithelium
Measles virus	CD[b]46 (Moesin)	Epithelial
Herpes simplex type 1 virus	Heparin sulfate; complement receptor CR1 (CD[b]35)	Wide variety of cell types
Epstein-Barr virus	Complement receptor CR2 (CD[b]21)	B lymphocytes
Rabies virus	Acetylcholine receptor? Others?	Epithelial, muscle, neurons of parasympathetic nervous system and CNS
Parvovirus B19	Erythrocyte P antigen	Erythroid cell precursors
HIV	CD[b]4	Helper T lymphocytes

Note. CNS = central nervous system; HIV = human immunodeficiency virus.
[a] The presence or absence of receptors may explain the tropism of a given virus (e.g., polioviruses). However, the presence of a receptor does not ensure that virus growth will occur within the cell; that is, that the cell is permissive.
[b] CD identifies cluster designations; these are cell surface markers, and they are identified by monoclonal antibodies.

select set of RNA transcripts are synthesized by cellular enzymes. These transcripts are modified by host capping, splicing, and polyadenylation reactions and are shipped to the cytoplasm as messenger RNA (mRNA) molecules for translation into viral proteins. Invariably, at least one of these early proteins is required for viral DNA replication and consequently must be transported to the nucleus. Once copies of the virus genome have been synthesized, transcripts made from them are processed into the mRNA molecules encoding the structural components of the virus. These mRNA molecules are translated in the cytoplasm, and the proteins are ferried back to the nucleus, where they combine with virus genome molecules to form nucleocapsids.

RNA viruses replicate in eukaryotic cells, which lack the enzyme machinery for synthesizing RNA from RNA. Thus, all RNA virus genomes contain one or more genes encoding one or more RNA-dependent RNA-polymerase activities. This enzyme system often accomplishes two separate viral functions: the synthesis of mRNA molecules (transcription) and the synthesis of new viral genome molecules (replication). Upon formation of new genome molecules and the synthesis of the viral structural proteins, assembly of new virions occurs.

Release. Release is the process by which virus particles gain access to the extracellular environment. If virus infection is cytotoxic to the cell, release occurs upon lysis of the cell. For enveloped viruses that obtain their envelope (bud) from the host cell's plasma membrane, the release and the formation of virions is one and the same process. Mechanisms (e.g., exocytosis) exist so that some viruses—enveloped or nonenveloped—are released from cells without any virus-induced cytopathology.

A feature of virus infections that originally baffled early virologists is that no infectious virus particles (virions) can be recovered from disrupted infected cells immediately after penetration until newly synthesized viral genomes and structural components assemble to form progeny virions. This time period originally was dubbed the "eclipse phase." For nonenveloped viruses and enveloped viruses that obtain their envelope from intracellular membranes, the eclipse phase ends when the first progeny virions form

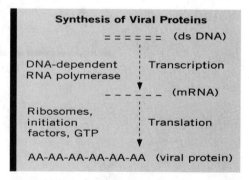

Synthesis of Viral Proteins

====== (ds DNA)

DNA-dependent RNA polymerase ┆ Transcription

------ (mRNA)

Ribosomes, initiation factors, GTP ┆ Translation

AA-AA-AA-AA-AA-AA (viral protein)

All RNA viruses encode the polymerase enzymes for replicating their genomes.

In this book, **virion** *is defined as an* **infectious virus particle.**

inside the cell. In contrast, some enveloped viruses obtain their envelope from the plasma membrane and consequently become virions only upon exiting the cell with a portion of the cell's modified plasma membrane as their envelope. Thus, such viruses, exemplified by retroviruses, orthomyxoviruses, and paramyxoviruses, do not accumulate intracellularly, and the eclipse phase ends upon the formation of the first extracellular virions.

Kinds of Virus Infections

The consequence of many virus infections is cell death. However, both in vivo and in vitro, other outcomes are possible. An abortive virus infection results when a particular virus penetrates a cell but fails to express all of its genes because that cell is lacking a crucial factor (e.g., protein) or contains an inhibitory factor. For that particular virus, such cells are nonpermissive because no progeny virions are produced. Thus, a cell lacking receptors for a particular virus is nonpermissive for that virus. In contrast, a permissive cell is defined as one that produces progeny virions; that is, it gives rise to a productive virus infection. Permissive and nonpermissive cells may or may not survive the virus infection.

Persistent virus infections occur when virus replication does not directly harm the viability of the host cell. For example, hepatitis B virus (HBV) can cause a persistent virus infection in 10% of its victims, resulting in chronic HBV. Herpesviruses are notorious for causing latent infections in which the viral DNA genome becomes quiescent in the infected cell's nucleus, and no viral proteins are made.

Finally, certain viruses are able to infect cells and either induce cell hyperplasia (e.g., warts caused by human papillomavirus) or transform the cells into cancer cells (e.g., tumors caused by certain retroviruses). In nonpermissive cells, transforming infections can occur only if one or a limited number of early viral proteins are synthesized and possess transforming activity (see Chapter 26). In permissive cells, transformation can occur if virus production does not kill the cell.

Hyperplasia is the abnormal enlargement or multiplication of normal cells.

REPLICATION STRATEGIES

DNA Viruses

With the exception of the poxviruses, all DNA viruses replicate in the cell's nucleus, which is reasonable given the presence there of the cell's DNA synthesizing machinery on which viruses rely. Most DNA viruses temporally regulate the expression of their genes. For example, depending on whether a single papovavirus's early gene's transcript is spliced, one or two different mRNA molecules are made. One of these mRNA molecules encodes the large T antigen (T-Ag). Although not a DNA polymerase, T-Ag is a multifunctional protein required for viral DNA replication. Furthermore, in nonpermissive cells, it can act as a viral oncogene. In permissive cells, after replication of the viral genome, synthesis of the early transcripts ceases, and late RNA transcripts are made. These transcripts are spliced into mRNA molecules that direct the synthesis of the capsid proteins, which are subsequently transported into the nucleus where they combine with newly made viral genomes to form progeny nucleocapsid virions (Figure 3-3). Although they do not transform cells, parvoviruses resemble papovaviruses in their replication strategy.

A viral oncogene is a viral gene, the product of which can transform a normal cell into a cancer cell.

In the case of adenoviruses, early gene expression involves at least 26 mRNA molecules and proteins, all of which are synthesized prior to genome duplication. One of these proteins is a viral-specific DNA polymerase, without which viral DNA cannot be replicated. Apparently using progeny DNA genomes as templates, the 18 late genes are transcribed; these encode all the structural components of the adenovirus particle. Assembly of progeny virions takes place in the nucleus and may or may not kill the infected cell.

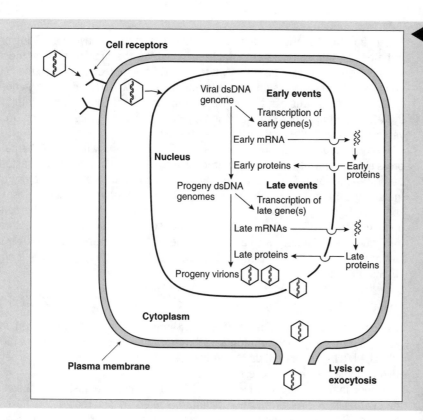

FIGURE 3-3
Replication of Nonenveloped DNA Viruses. The replication strategy of even simple nucleocapsid DNA viruses, such as papovaviruses and adenoviruses, involves the temporal regulation of viral genes.

Herpesviruses, with a DNA genome approximately four times larger than that of adenoviruses, exhibit a more complex pattern of gene expression that is temporally divided into three classes: immediate early, early, and late. In a productive growth cycle, five immediate early genes function primarily to modulate cellular functions and induce the expression of the early and late genes. The early genes (approximately 20) encode for a viral DNA polymerase and other proteins needed for genome replication. Newly copied DNA genome molecules in turn express most of the 55 late genes, which encode the capsid and envelope proteins required for the assembly of new herpes virions (Figure 3-4).

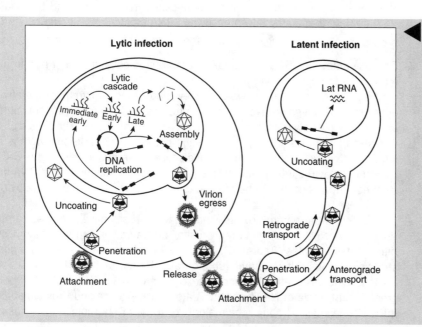

FIGURE 3-4
Herpes Simplex Virus Type 1 Lytic Infection of Epithelial Cell and Latent Infection of Sensory Neuron. The function of latent (Lat) RNA molecules, which are not mRNA molecules, remains unknown. Herpesviruses are unique in obtaining their envelopes from the nuclear membrane.

In addition to productive infections, all herpesviruses have the unique propensity to initiate in certain cells a latent infection. In latency, the viral DNA enters the nucleus and becomes dormant, expressing only latent (Lat) RNA molecules, which may play a role in suppressing the expression of the immediate early, early, and late genes. However, latently infected cells can be "activated" by a variety of conditions to enter a productive cycle of infection. For example, when chickenpox virus (varicella-zoster virus) is reactivated in an adult, the result is shingles (herpes zoster).

As noted above, parvoviruses, papovaviruses, adenoviruses, and herpesviruses express at least one early protein required for viral DNA replication. In contrast, the poxvirus particle—the largest of the animal viruses—carries into a cell an array of enzymes, including a preformed RNA transcriptase (DNA-dependent RNA polymerase) and accessory factors for synthesizing mRNA molecules in the cytoplasm of the cell. Encoding approximately 185 genes, poxviruses establish a virus-synthesizing factory, a kind of mini-nucleus (complete with a virus-encoded DNA polymerase and RNA transcriptase) within which viral transcription, translation, genome replication, and assembly of new virions take place.

RNA Viruses

Because of the diverse nature of RNA virus genomes and the different mechanisms required for their replication, four categories can be delineated: (1) ss [+] RNA viruses, (2) ss [−] RNA viruses, (3) dsRNA viruses, and (4) the retroviruses, which have an ss [+] RNA genome but rely on reverse transcription for growth.

Once in the cytoplasm of a cell, [+] RNA genomes use host-cell ribosomes to direct the synthesis of viral proteins. A hallmark shared by picornaviruses, flaviviruses, caliciviruses, togaviruses, and coronaviruses is that their purified [+] RNA genomes are infectious when transfected directly into a cell; therefore, these viruses do not need to carry any preformed enzymes. Despite possessing a [+] genome, retroviruses are an exception because they employ a unique replication scheme (see below).

Although the order of their genes (i.e., their genetic maps) is different, picornaviruses and flaviviruses replicate by a common mechanism, the primary features of which are:

> *A [+] RNA genome is a functional mRNA molecule.*

- Synthesis of viral precursor proteins from the infecting virus genome, because it acts like a mRNA molecule
- Proteolytic processing of the precursor proteins to form nonstructural (viral polymerase proteins) and capsid proteins (Figure 3-5A)
- Synthesis by the viral polymerase of a full-length complementary RNA (cRNA), which in this instance is a negative-sense RNA strand, and the use of this as a template for making new progeny [+] RNA molecules (see Figure 3-5B)
- Assembly of the progeny genome molecules and capsid proteins into nucleocapsids

Because a flavivirus is an enveloped virus, its nucleocapsid must bud from the plasma membrane to become a virion.

Togaviruses and caliciviruses have evolved a mechanism to temporally regulate the expression of their genes. Nonstructural proteins, including the viral polymerase proteins, are synthesized only from the parental virus genome molecule. The capsid proteins and, in the case of the togaviruses, the envelope proteins are made only from a subgenomic-length mRNA synthesized from negative-sense cRNA molecules (Figure 3-6).

> *A subgenomic mRNA is a mRNA molecule of less than genomic length, synthesized from a negative-sense RNA molecule acting as a template.*

In coronavirus infections, at least eight different subgenomic mRNA molecules are synthesized, and each may be replicated using its own cRNA template by the viral RNA polymerase.

Although the paramyxoviruses and rhabdoviruses have genomes composed of one ssRNA molecule, and orthomyxoviruses, bunyaviruses, and arenaviruses have segmented genomes (see Table 3-2), all ss [−] RNA viruses share a common replication strategy. Because they cannot function as mRNAs, ss [−] RNA viruses must carry a nucleocapsid-associated transcriptase (i.e., an RNA-dependent RNA polymerase) in order to synthesize cRNA strands that are positive-sense and thus capable of acting as mRNA molecules. Although the majority of these cRNA molecules act as mRNA mole-

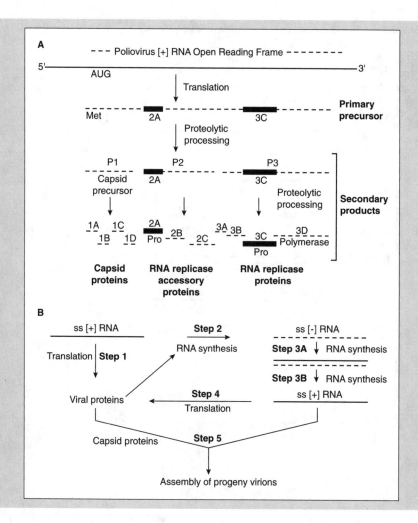

A

- - - Poliovirus [+] RNA Open Reading Frame - - - - - - -

5'————————————————————————————3'

AUG

↓ Translation

Primary precursor

Met   2A   3C

↓ Proteolytic processing

P1   P2   P3

Capsid   2A   3C
precursor

↓ Proteolytic processing   **Secondary products**

1A 1C   2A   3A 3B   3D
  1B 1D   Pro --2B--   --2C--   3A 3B 3C 3D Polymerase
                                       Pro

**Capsid   RNA replicase   RNA replicase
proteins   accessory   proteins
            proteins**

B

ss [+] RNA   **Step 2**   ss [-] RNA
                           RNA synthesis
Translation | **Step 1**   **Step 3A** ↓ RNA synthesis

Viral proteins   **Step 3B** ↓ RNA synthesis
              ←—— **Step 4** ——   ss [+] RNA
                  Translation

Capsid proteins   **Step 5**

                 Assembly of progeny virions

FIGURE 3-5
Replication of the Picornaviruses. *(A) The process involves the synthesis of a primary polypeptide precursor that is processed by viral-encoded proteases (i.e., proteins 2A/Pro and 3C/Pro) to form all the capsid and nonstructural proteins, including (B) a viral RNA-dependent RNA polymerase system that synthesizes a limited number of ss [−] RNA strands as templates for making copies of the viral ss [+] RNA genome.*

cules, full-length [+] cRNA strands are also required as templates for the synthesis of full-length, negative-sense genome molecules. Thus, the viral polymerase performs three important tasks: (1) the synthesis of viral mRNA molecules (transcription), (2) the synthesis of full-length [+] cRNA molecules as replication templates, and (3) the synthesis of new negative-sense genome molecules. These last two steps are part of the genome replication process (Figure 3-7). How the various viral polymerase activities are regulated is still unclear.

The reoviruses, characterized by a genome composed of 10–12 dsRNA molecules (each one a gene), is the only viral family whose particles contain a dsRNA genome. Yet their replication scheme is akin to that of the ss [−] RNA viruses in that each particle must bring into the cell a preformed virion transcriptase (a dsRNA-dependent RNA polymerase) in order to synthesize viral mRNA molecules. Although the mechanism is poorly understood, this enzyme also is responsible for replicating the dsRNA genome molecules.

Viruses Using a Reverse Transcriptase

Two animal virus families—the retroviruses and the hepadnaviruses—employ reverse transcription, the synthesis of a DNA molecule from a RNA template, in their growth cycles. Reverse transcriptases (RT) are enzymes that perform several different activities as part of a single protein complex. The most prominent of these enzymatic activities are: (1) a RNA-dependent DNA polymerase that synthesizes a complementary DNA (cDNA) strand from the ssRNA genome molecules; (2) a RNase H activity digests the RNA strand of a RNA–DNA hybrid duplex; and (3) a DNA-dependent DNA polymerase responsible for synthesizing a second DNA strand using the cDNA strand as a template. Thus, the original ssRNA retroviral genome is converted into a dsDNA molecule called a *proviral DNA*. In this process, a short terminal repeat (STR) sequence in the genomic ss [+] RNA

*A [−] **RNA genome** is an antisense molecule; cRNAs act as mRNA molecules or as templates for making new viral genomes.*

FIGURE 3-6 ▶
Replication Cycle of a Togavirus or Calicivirus. This process involves the synthesis of a subgenomic mRNA responsible for the synthesis of all the viral structural proteins. The open rectangle denotes a strong stop codon that restricts ribosomes from translating the sequences encoding the viral structural proteins from the viral genome molecule.

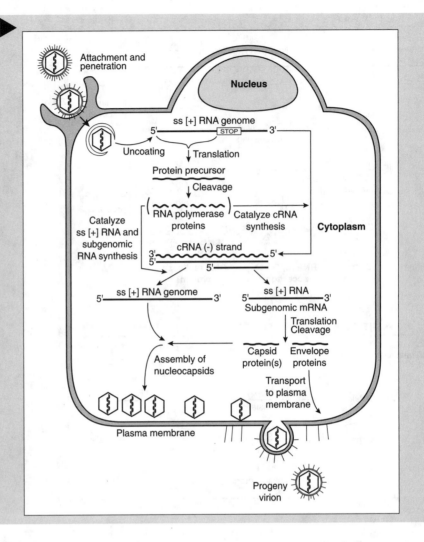

FIGURE 3-7 ▶
Critical Events in the Replication Cycle of a Single-Stranded, Negative-Sense (ss [−]) RNA Virus. (1) Primary transcription of the genome by the viral transcriptase. (2) Replication of the virus genome. (3) Secondary transcription using newly replicated viral genome molecules as templates. (4) Assembly of virus genome (segments) to form progeny virions.

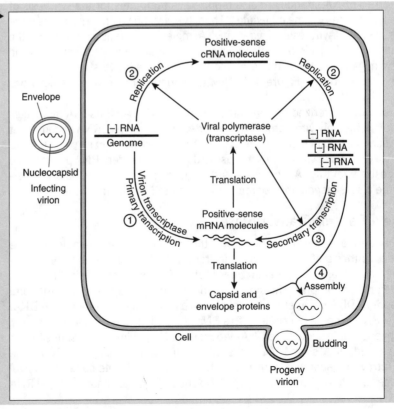

is reiterated and juxtaposed to form a crucial regulatory sequence, the long terminal repeat (LTR), at both ends of the proviral DNA. Once integrated into the cell's chromosomal DNA, the proviral DNA is referred to as a *provirus*.

Upon penetration into a cell, the retroviral RT, packaged in the viral nucleocapsid, must convert the viral RNA genome into proviral DNA for viral genes to be expressed. Thus, unlike all other ss [+] RNA viruses, the retroviral genome introduced *by itself* into a cell by transfection is not infectious; that is, it cannot produce virus particles because retroviral genes can be expressed only from the provirus. The splicing of RNA transcripts and the cleavage of viral precursor proteins, as discussed earlier, play important roles in the formation of retrovirus particles (Figure 3-8).

Retrovirions form when nucleocapsids, containing two full-length genomic ss [+] RNA molecules and newly synthesized RT molecules, bud from the plasma membrane. In the case of HIV, particle infectivity requires not only budding but subsequent proteolytic alteration of the nucleocapsid in situ by the virus-encoded protease.

Hepadnaviruses are the only DNA animal viruses that rely on reverse transcription. However, the role played by the hepadnaviral RT is very different from that of the retroviral RT. Once inside the nucleus, the infecting viral DNA genome (and, later in the growth cycle, a copy of it) is used to synthesize viral mRNA molecules responsible for making the RT and capsid proteins. One particular viral RNA transcript is the *pregenomic RNA* (Figure 3-9). Maturation of virus particles inside the cell begins with the packaging of this pregenomic RNA molecule into a capsid along with one or more RT molecules. Inside this nucleocapsid, the RT synthesizes a cDNA strand using the pregenomic RNA as a template. The RNase H activity hydrolyzes the RNA strand. Finally, a

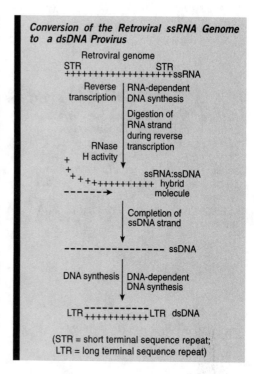

Conversion of the Retroviral ssRNA Genome to a dsDNA Provirus

(STR = short terminal sequence repeat; LTR = long terminal sequence repeat)

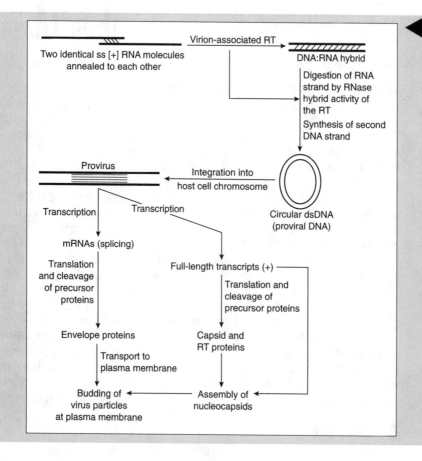

FIGURE 3-8

Expression of Retroviral Genes. *The expression of retroviral genes requires reverse transcription of a viral ss [+] RNA genome into a proviral dsDNA and integration of the proviral DNA into a host cell chromosome. RT = reverse transcriptase; ss = single stranded; ds = double stranded.*

portion of a second cDNA strand is synthesized to form the circular dsDNA hepadnavirus genome. Budding from intracellular membranes completes the formation of virions.

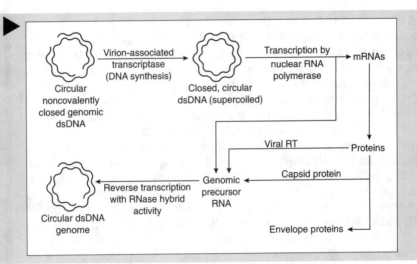

FIGURE 3-9 ▶

Replication of Hepadnaviruses. The replication cycle of the hepadnaviruses involves the transcription and assembly of a pregenomic, single-stranded, positive-sense RNA molecule into an immature particle and the use of a viral-encoded reverse transcriptase to convert it into a circular, partially double-stranded (ds) DNA molecule.

VIRUS ADAPTATION

Point Mutations

Virus genomes mutate by the same mechanisms described for other microorganisms. Given the rate and extent of virus nucleic acid duplications, the fact that mutants are formed constantly is not surprising; their survivability is determined by natural selection. The mutation rates of most DNA viruses approximate those for cells because viral DNA synthesis (except for poxviruses) occurs in the nucleus, where cellular enzymes can repair mismatched base pairs. In contrast, all RNA viruses employ RNA template-dependent polymerases that are highly prone to errors (approximately one mistake in 10^4–10^5 nucleotide incorporations). In addition, no proofreading repair processes are associated with the synthesis of DNA or RNA from RNA templates. Thus, the retroviral RT makes a base-pairing mistake approximately once every time it reverse transcribes its genome into proviral DNA. As a consequence of these considerations, an RNA virus population, even if derived from the growth of a single virion infecting a cell population, is often described as a quasi-species to indicate the expected heterogeneity of viral genomes in the particle population.

Having noted that RNA-dependent RNA polymerases and reverse transcriptases generate great diversity among viral genomes, how these mutational changes actually affect virus viability must be considered. Thus, for example, HIV tolerates an extraordinary number of amino acid substitutions in its outermost surface-envelope glycoprotein, allowing the mutants to escape neutralization by antibodies. In contrast, measles virus exists as a single serotype, suggesting that its viral envelope protein loses some essential function if altered so that it no longer reacts with neutralizing antibodies.

Recombination

In addition to point mutations, both DNA and RNA viruses can undergo recombination in which portions of viral genomes are exchanged with one another. The frequency of recombination among single-molecule RNA genomes (e.g., picornaviruses) is relatively low, occurring perhaps once in every 10^5–10^6 genomes copied. On the other hand, herpesviruses and poxviruses undergo recombination rates of 10% or higher, depending on the distance between genetic markers.

Reassortment. Viruses with segmented genomes, like orthomyxoviruses or reoviruses (see Table 3-3), can undergo a special kind of recombination called *reassortment*. For example, a cell co-infected with two different influenza virus strains can give rise to a novel virion containing gene segments from each of the parental viruses. The frequency of reassortment between two different influenza A viruses or between two strains of reoviruses can be as high as 50%.

Viral Resistance, Antigenic Drift, and Antigenic Shift

Spontaneous mutation, recombination, and reassortment permit virus populations to evolve in response to the selective pressures exerted by chemotherapeutic agents or host immune responses. For example, the random generation of mutant RTs during HIV growth creates strains resistant to azidothymidine (AZT) and other anti-RT drugs. Likewise, spontaneous mutations in genes coding for the envelope proteins of influenza A viruses propel the gradual evolution of virus strains capable of escaping previous host antibody responses. This process is known as antigenic drift. Drift is the primary reason why new influenza virus strain proteins are introduced into the "flu vaccine" on an almost yearly basis. However, because of their segmented genomes, influenza A viruses are also capable of sudden, dramatic alterations in their antigenicity (antigenic shift) by the process of genetic reassortment. Assume that two different influenza virus strains co-infect the same cell in the same animal (probably swine or fowl). During assembly, some nucleocapsids form with one (or more) genomic segment obtained from one parental virus and one (or more) from the other. These bud to become reassortant virions. Among these reassortants, some virus particles with unique envelope proteins may emerge (Figure 3-10).

Unique influenza virus serotypes that arise by antigenic shift are capable of causing pandemics such as those that occurred in 1918–19, 1957, and 1968; in these cases, encounters with previous influenza strains did not evoke protective immune responses against infections with the novel, reassortant virus (see Chapter 17).

> ***Reassorted viruses*** are viruses produced upon infection of a single cell by two different viruses with segmented genomes that encode viral proteins on their multiple genomic segments. Reassortment of the various genomic segments during infection of a cell by two different rotavirus serotypes can give rise to viruses of new generic composition that may encode new combinations of viral surface antigens. The introduction of new antigens results in antigenic shift and enbles the virus to temporarily avoid host immuneserveillence (see Chapter 17).

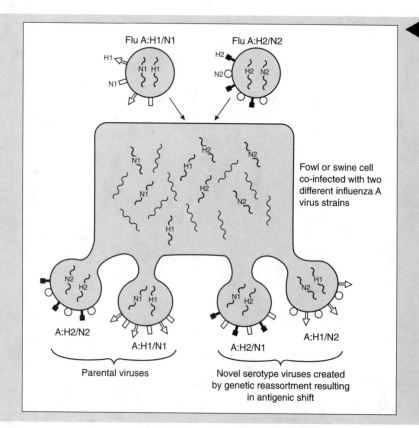

◀ **FIGURE 3-10**
Reassortment of Virus Genes. *If a cell is infected with two different influenza A virus serotypes, novel virus serotypes can arise by the reassortment of virus genes coding for viral envelope proteins. H = envelope hemagglutinin protein; N = envelope neuraminidase protein.*

RESOLUTION OF CLINICAL CASE

The businessman from Boston almost certainly was suffering from a common cold, for which antibacterial drugs provide no effective treatment. In healthy individuals, common colds can be assumed to be self-limiting. Physicians should understand that the targets of antibiotics (e.g., prokaryotic ribosomes and bacterial cell walls and membranes, see Chapter 4) are immaterial in virus infections. Furthermore, the antibiotic prescribed at the patient's request probably altered the patient's intestinal flora and caused his diarrhea (see Chapter 11). Given a rapidly increasing understanding of the molecular events in the virus growth cycle, the future holds promise for drugs that will more specifically inhibit chemical reactions unique to viruses (e.g., RNA-dependent RNA polymerases, reverse transcriptases, viral proteases).

REVIEW QUESTIONS

Directions: For each of the following questions, choose the **one best** answer.

1. Cells are distinguishable from viruses because cells
    - **(A)** encode enzymes for replicating their genomes
    - **(B)** contain transcriptases
    - **(C)** encode and direct the synthesis of membrane proteins with unique antigenic specificities
    - **(D)** divide by binary fission
    - **(E)** depend on adenosine triphosphate (ATP) for energy

2. The most important and unique characteristic of positive-polarity [+] RNA viruses is that
    - **(A)** they always possess an envelope
    - **(B)** they do not carry a transcriptase
    - **(C)** they have a genome that can act as messenger RNA (mRNA)
    - **(D)** they are virtually always cytotoxic to cells
    - **(E)** they enter into cells by receptor-mediated endocytosis

3. The primary reason viruses develop resistance to chemotherapeutic agents is because of
    - **(A)** mutations in the viral genome
    - **(B)** indiscriminate use of chemotherapeutic agents
    - **(C)** the synthesis of novel viral enzymes that destroy the agents
    - **(D)** the rapid growth of viruses
    - **(E)** the preferential use of chemotherapeutic agents by the host cell

4. The reason a single-stranded negative-polarity (ss [−]) RNA virus possesses a transcriptase in its virus particle is that
    - **(A)** the viral genome cannot otherwise express its genes
    - **(B)** ribosomes cannot translate the viral genomic RNA molecule unless the transcriptase is attached
    - **(C)** the viral transcriptase functions to ensure expression of cellular genes needed for virus replication
    - **(D)** the transcriptase is required to synthesize the proviral DNA

5. In 2 succeeding years (1993–1994 and 1994–1995), the prevalent influenza virus type A strains used in the influenza virus vaccine were hemagglutinin protein 1, neuraminidase protein 1 (H1/N1) Beijing/32/92-like and H1/N1 Shangdong/9/93-like, respectively. The most likely explanation for needing to change the subtypes in the vaccine is
    - **(A)** antigenic shift
    - **(B)** antigenic drift
    - **(C)** deletions in the 1993–1994 H1/N1 genome
    - **(D)** loss of one or more RNA genome segments in one of the viruses
    - **(E)** alterations in viral RNA transcriptases

ANSWERS AND EXPLANATIONS

1. **The answer is D.** What distinguishes cells from viruses is that viruses do not grow by binary fission. Both cells and viruses encode protein enzymes needed for duplication (option A) and expression of their genes (option B). Additionally, they both encode structural proteins, using cellular translational machinery to make them (option C), and use ATP to catalyze many of these reactions (option E).

2. **The answer is C.** Only [+] RNA viruses have genomes that can function directly as mRNA molecules. Not all [+] RNA viruses have envelopes (option A), and retroviruses have a reverse transcriptase (option B). No strict correlation exists between either viral cytotoxicity (option D) or the mechanism of penetration and the polarity of the viral genome (option E).

3. **The answer is A.** Resistance to chemotherapeutic agents arises primarily by chance mutations. The indiscriminate use of antiviral drugs (option B), their preferential use by host cells (option E), and the rapid growth of viruses (option D), even if factual statements, would fail to explain how virus resistance arises. Viruses cannot be induced to synthesize novel hydrolytic enzymes (option C).

4. **The answer is A.** Single-stranded [−] RNA genomes cannot act as messenger RNA (mRNA) molecules and therefore require a viral-encoded transcriptase to make complementary (cRNA) strands that serve as mRNA molecules. Viral transcriptases are not part of the translational machinery; therefore, option B is invalid. Virus growth does not require cellular genes transcribed by *viral* transcriptases, making option C invalid. Option D is wrong because ss [−] RNA viruses do not use reverse transcriptases.

5. **The answer is B.** Because both viruses are H1/N1, the need to change the subtypes in the vaccine is a result of small changes in envelope proteins due to point mutations. This is the definition of antigenic drift. If an antigenic shift had occurred, the H numbers, N numbers, or both of the 1993–1994 and 1994–1995 viruses would be different from each other (option A). Genome deletions, if not lethal, would not necessarily explain strain differences (option C). Loss of RNA genome segments would render an influenza virus noninfectious (option D). Antigenic differences depend on altered envelope proteins not altered viral transcriptases (option E).

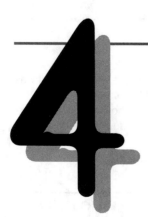

ANTIMICROBIAL THERAPY

CHAPTER OUTLINE

Introduction of Clinical Case
Therapy of Infections Involving Nonviral Pathogens: General Concepts and Principles
• Selective Toxicity
• Bactericidal versus Bacteriostatic Agents
• Other Principles
Antibacterial Therapy
• Bacterial Structure
• Mechanism of Action of Antibacterial Antibiotics
Antifungal Therapy
• Membrane-Active Antifungal Agents
• Other Antifungal Agents
Antiviral Therapy
• Background
• Agents and Actions
Illustrative Pathogen: *Mycoplasma pneumoniae*
• Biologic Characteristics
• Reservoir and Transmission
• Virulence Factors
• Pathogenesis
• Diagnosis
• Prevention and Treatment
Resolution of Clinical Case
Review Questions

INTRODUCTION OF CLINICAL CASE

A 25-year-old man presented with a persistent cough. He was well until approximately 1 week ago, when a headache and a mild sore throat developed. During the past few days he had developed a dry, hacking cough, which had increased in frequency and awakened him at night. He stated that during the past month or so, several of his children were ill with headaches, sore throats, and earaches, and 2 weeks ago his wife also developed a nonproductive cough, which had persisted.

Examination revealed a temperature of 100°F, minimal injection of the phar-

> *Injection of the pharynx* refers to the erythema (redness) that can be seen when the pharynx is involved in an inflammatory reaction, usually of an infectious origin. *Rales* are unique sounds heard with a stethoscope that are made by air passing through fluid in the alveoli or terminal bronchioles. The fluid may or may not be caused by an infection such as pneumonia.

ynx, normal-sized tonsils, and fine rales heard over the left lower lung field posteriorly. A "bedside test" for cold agglutinins was positive (a cold agglutinin titer of > 1:512). Chest roentgenogram revealed a patchy infiltrate in the left lower lobe. The leukocyte count was 9400/mm³, and the differential was normal. The patient could not produce sputum for stain or culture. He was started on oral erythromycin and sent home. His wife was examined the next day, and although both her physical examination and chest roentgenogram were unremarkable, she was also started on erythromycin.

THERAPY OF INFECTIONS INVOLVING NONVIRAL PATHOGENS: GENERAL CONCEPTS AND PRINCIPLES

Historically the term antibiotic *refers only to those antimicrobial agents that have a natural biologic origin. (Interestingly, most antibiotics used medically are produced by relatively nonpathogenic fungi and bacteria.) Antimicrobial agents are a broader group of agents, including the true antibiotics as well as chemically synthesized agents.*

The concept of using chemotherapy to treat infectious diseases was first proposed in the early 20th century by the German physician and scientist Paul Ehrlich. Antimicrobial chemotherapy progressed from dreams to reality in 1935, when the sulfonamides were introduced to fight bacterial infections successfully. Pharmaceutical companies now have developed an array of antimicrobials for use against bacterial, fungal, parasitic, and viral infections. Although the success of antimicrobial therapy is now threatened by the development of antibiotic resistance (see Chapter 5), the development of antimicrobial chemotherapy certainly ranks among the foremost miracles of modern medicine.

Before discussing specific antimicrobials and their actions, a few basic concepts and principles regarding antibiotic therapy of nonviral pathogens must be introduced. More details on these and related subjects (e.g., the routes of administration of different antimicrobials) can be obtained in good pharmacology or infectious diseases textbooks.

Selective Toxicity

The most fundamental concept or principle of all antimicrobial chemotherapy (whether for viral or nonviral pathogens) is selective toxicity, which means that a useful antimicrobial must kill or inhibit the pathogen against which it is used without (seriously) harming the host.

Bactericidal versus Bacteriostatic Agents

Another important concept or principle is that antimicrobial agents used for treating infections involving nonviral pathogens do not always kill these pathogens. Antibiotics that are capable of killing bacteria (or fungi) at achievable concentrations are said to possess a bactericidal or fungicidal action; antibiotics that cannot kill bacteria or fungi but instead inhibit their growth are said to have a bacteriostatic or fungistatic action.

Knowing whether an antibiotic has bactericidal or bacteriostatic properties is important for a physician. For example, when a patient is treated with a bacteriostatic agent, that antibiotic stops the pathogen's multiplication, but it does not, by itself, remove the viable pathogen from the body. The therapy is buying the patient time by inhibiting further growth of the pathogen, but the patient's own defense system must ultimately clear the infection. Problems can arise, therefore, if a patient treated with a bacteriostatic drug is immunocompromised. If the patient's impaired host defense system is unable to clear the pathogen from the body, and the antimicrobial is then withdrawn, the pathogen may begin growing once more, and the original infection can redevelop. This example illustrates the need for a physician to consider the host defense status of a patient when choosing appropriate antibiotic therapy.

Other Principles

Some other important concepts and principles of antimicrobials include the following:

1. Some antibiotic agents (e.g., the aminoglycosides) do not efficiently penetrate mammalian cells. Antimicrobials that do not efficiently enter mammalian cells have diminished effectiveness for treating infections involving intracellular pathogens.

2. The site of infection and pharmacologic properties of antibiotics must be considered when designing a therapeutic regimen because inhibitory concentrations of all antibiotics cannot be achieved at every body site.

3. Two or more antibiotics often must be used in combination during therapy. There are several reasons why such combination therapy may be necessary:

   • Some pathogens can exist at several different locations in the body (e.g., *Mycobacterium tuberculosis* can exist extracellularly in lesions but also exist intracellularly inside phagocytes). To treat infections involving such pathogens effectively, simultaneous administration of several different types of antibiotics, each of which is geared toward fighting the pathogen at a specific location, may be necessary.

   • Some pathogens (e.g., *M. tuberculosis*) are notorious for their ability to develop antibiotic resistance. Therapy against infections involving these highly resistant pathogens usually relies upon the simultaneous administration of multiple types of antibiotics so that an agent that works against the particular strain of pathogen causing a patient's infection is included in the regimen. This approach also limits the development of further antibiotic resistance because it is considerably more difficult for a pathogen to develop resistance simultaneously to several different antimicrobial agents than to a single agent (although multiple drug resistance does occur [see Chapter 5]).

   • Combined use of different antimicrobials may provide synergistic inhibitory effects that provide enhanced therapeutic benefits. As discussed later in this chapter, combining certain antibiotics in therapy can have antagonistic effects on their antimicrobial activity.

   • Multiple types of antibiotics may need to be given to patients suffering from life-threatening infections when it is not possible to wait for laboratory results identifying the infecting agent and its antimicrobial sensitivity.

   • Multiple types of antibiotics may be necessary to combat a polymicrobic infection.

4. Not all antibacterial agents have broad-spectrum activity (i.e., work equally effectively against many different types of bacteria). For example, there are some narrow-spectrum antibiotics that work better against gram-positive bacteria than against gram-negative bacteria, often because of difficulty crossing the outer membrane of the gram-negative bacterial cell. Chemists can sometimes alter the structure of these agents to give them a broader spectrum of activity or other properties.

5. The environment also can affect the activity of an antimicrobial agent. For example, some antimicrobial agents, such as aminoglycosides, do not work well in an anaerobic environment, as mentioned in Chapter 3.

ANTIBACTERIAL THERAPY

Bacterial Structure

Selective toxicity, the foremost principle of antimicrobial therapy, is best achieved by identifying agents that recognize and exploit differences in structure or metabolism between microbial pathogens and human cells. Considering this, a review of the structure of a bacterial cell is useful before discussing antibiotic actions. A "typical" bacterial cell is shown in Figure 4-1. Regions of this cell include the following structures.

CYTOPLASM

The cytoplasm contains genetic material (both chromosomal and plasmid-borne DNA) and ribosomes, which are involved in protein synthesis. The cytoplasm is also the site of some energy production (e.g., glycolysis) and intermediary metabolism, which produces components needed for growth.

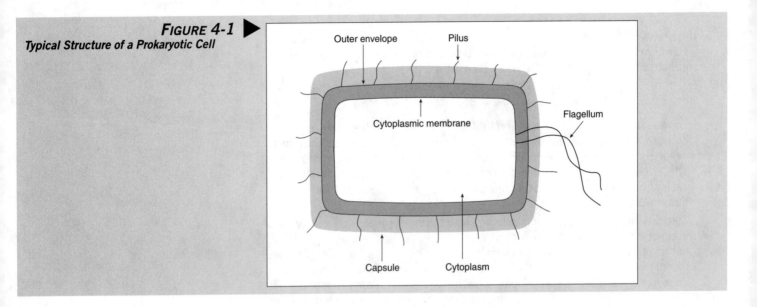

FIGURE 4-1 ▶
Typical Structure of a Prokaryotic Cell

CELL ENVELOPE

This consists of two parts: the cytoplasmic membrane and the outer envelope.

Cytoplasmic Membrane. The cytoplasmic membrane is involved in transport and secretion, some energy production (if present, the electron transport chain used during respiration is located here), and some synthetic pathways (e.g., cell wall synthesis).

Outer Envelope. The outer envelope was described in detail in Chapter 1. Key points about the outer envelope include the following:

- In gram-positive bacteria, the outer envelope is comprised of a single, thick layer of cell wall. This cell wall mostly contains peptidoglycan, along with some lipoteichoic or teichoic acids.

- In gram-negative bacteria, the outer envelope contains a thin cell wall layer of peptidoglycan (without teichoic or lipoteichoic acids) and an outer membrane containing lipopolysaccharide, which has endotoxic activity. The space between the cytoplasmic membrane and the outer membrane is called the periplasmic space.

- The outer envelope provides strength to protect the gram-positive and gram-negative bacterial cell against osmotic lysis and also provides a protective permeability barrier for gram-negative bacteria.

PILI

Also called fimbriae, pili are shorter and finer appendages than flagella. There are often many pili per bacterial cell. Pili are composed mostly of repeating subunits of a protein called pilin. There can be two types of pili:

Common Pili. These pili help to mediate attachment of bacteria to mammalian tissue. In some cases (e.g., *Neisseria gonorrhoeae*), pili can also have antiphagocytic properties.

Sex Pili. These pili are present in some gram-negative bacterial cells and function to bring donor and recipient cells together during conjugation (see Chapter 5).

FLAGELLA

These structures, composed of flagellin protein, are important for bacterial motility. The number and location of flagella per motile bacterium varies. Nonmotile bacteria lack these appendages.

CAPSULE

The capsule is usually composed of polysaccharides. The exception is the capsule of *Bacillus anthracis*, which is composed of polymerized D-glutamic acid. Capsules often have antiphagoctyic properties (see Chapter 18). Some capsules can also help mediate attachment.

Mechanism of Action of Antibacterial Antibiotics

The action of the major antibacterial antibiotics is discussed within the context of the bacterial target sites or bacterial actions that are affected by these agents (Table 4-1).

Site or Action	Mechanism of Action	Agents	Effect of Agents
Inhibition of cell wall synthesis	Inhibits transpeptidation	Penicillins	BC
		Cephalosporins	BC
	Inhibits incorporation of disaccharide into growing peptidoglycan	Vancomycin	BC
	Inhibits recycling of lipid carrier for cell-wall synthesis	Bacitracin	BC
Inhibition of membrane function	Affects bacterial membrane permeability	Polymyxin	BC
	Affects fungal membrane permeability:		
	• Binds ergosterol	Polyenes[a]	FC
	• Blocks ergosterol synthesis	Azoles[b]	FC or FS
Inhibition of nucleic acid synthesis	Inhibits bacterial DNA synthesis	Quinolones[c]	BC
		Metronidazole	BC
	Inhibits bacterial RNA synthesis	Rifampin	BC
	Inhibits fungal RNA (and DNA) synthesis	Flucytosine	FS or FC
Inhibition of protein synthesis	Acts on 30S ribosomal subunit	Aminoglycosides[d]	BC
		Tetracyclines	BS
	Acts on 50S ribosomal subunit	Chloramphenicol	BS
		Erythromycin	BS or BC
		Clindamycin	BS
Inhibition of metabolism	Inhibition of tetrahydrofolate synthesis:		
	• Inhibitors of dihydropteroate synthesis	Sulfonamides	BS
	• Inhibitors of dihydrofolate conversion to tetra-hydrofolate	Trimethoprim	BS
	Inhibition of mycolic acid synthesis	Isoniazid	BS or BC

Note. BC = bactericidal; BS = bacteriostatic; FC = fungicidal; FS = fungistatic.
[a] Major polyenes include amphotericin B and nystatin.
[b] Examples of azoles include ketoconazole, miconazole, and fluconazole.
[c] Examples of quinolones include ciprofloxacin and norfloxacin.
[d] Examples of aminoglycosides include streptomycin and gentamicin.

◀ **TABLE 4-1**
Brief Summary of the Action of Some Major Antibacterial and Antifungal Antimicrobial Agents

The five major sites in or actions of the bacterial cell that serve as points of attack for currently used antibacterial antibiotics include:

- Cell walls
- Membranes
- Nucleic acid synthesis
- Ribosomes (protein synthesis)
- Intermediary metabolism

CELL WALL SYNTHESIS INHIBITORS

Before discussing the action of antibiotics that inhibit cell wall synthesis, one must review how bacteria make their cell wall. As mentioned earlier, the bacterial cell wall is composed primarily of peptidoglycan (also called murein), which is made up of layers of a repeating disaccharide (consisting of *N*-acetylglucosamine linked to *N*-acetylmuramic acid). To provide structural strength to the cell wall (the primary function of the cell wall), the different layers of peptidoglycan containing this repeating disaccharide are then cross-linked via amino acid side chains that are present on *N*-acetylmuramic acid, as shown diagramatically below (see Chapter 1, Figure 1-3).

(M = *N*-acetylmuramic acid; . . . = crosslinks; and G = *N*-acetylglucosamine):

M-G-M-G-M-G-M-G-M-G
          .   .
          .   .
M-G-M-G-M-G-M-G-M-G

Bacteria construct their cell wall in three stages (Figure 4-2):

1. Cytoplasmic Stage: In the cytoplasm, *N*-acetylmuramic acid and *N*-acetylglucosamine are attached to uridine diphosphate (UDP) carrier molecules. The five amino acids that comprise the side chain are then sequentially added to *N*-acetylmuramic acid.

2. Plasma Membrane Stage: At the cytoplasmic membrane, *N*-acetylmuramic acid (now containing the added pentapeptide) is transferred from UDP to a lipid carrier

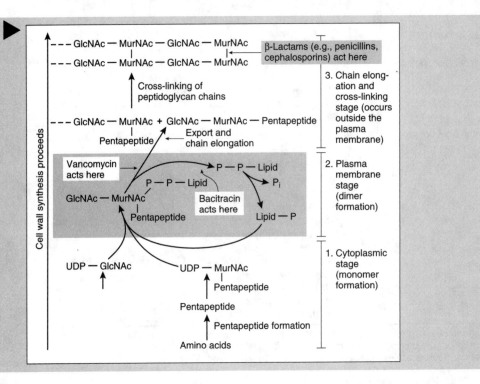

FIGURE 4-2 ▶

Bacterial Cell Wall Synthesis. *MurNAc = N-acetylmuramic acid; GlcNAc = N-acetylglucosamine; UDP = uridine diphosphate; P-P-lipid = disaccharide-lipid carrier complex; P_i = inorganic phosphate.*

*Some bacteria use a **bridge for cross-linking**; an example of this is shown in Figure 4-4. In other bacteria, there is direct linkage, without a bridge, between peptide side chains of N-acetylmuramic acid residues in different peptidoglycan layers.*

(named undecaprenol or bactoprenol). *N*-Acetylglucosamine is then added to form a disaccharide; if the bacteria use a peptide bridge for cross-linking the peptidoglycan, it also is added at this point. The resultant disaccharide–lipid carrier complex then moves to the outer surface of the membrane, where the disaccharide transfers from the lipid carrier to the growing end of a layer of peptidoglycan outside the membrane. During this transfer, the lipid carrier (now in a pyrophosphate form) loses a phosphate and then recycles back to the cytoplasmic side of the membrane, where it can accept another *N*-acetylmuramic acid.

3. Chain Growth and Cross-linking Stage: After transfer from the membrane, the disaccharide is incorporated into the growing chain of peptidoglycan. Different layers of this peptidoglycan are then cross-linked by bacterial enzymes called transpeptidases. These enzymes catalyze the formation of a peptide bond between A D-alanine residue attached to a *N*-acetylmuramic acid in one layer of peptidoglycan and another amino acid attached to a *N*-acetylmuramic acid located in another layer of polysaccharide. Because this reaction occurs outside the bacterial mem-

brane, where no adenosine triphosphate (ATP) is available to drive this cross-linking, energy for transpeptidation comes from cleavage of the terminal D-alanine residue, which is subsequently lost from the cross-linked structure. This process is repeated many times, producing a highly cross-linked—and very strong—cell wall.

β-Lactam Antibiotics. The penicillin and cephalosporin families of antibiotics are among the most commonly used agents for antibacterial therapy. These agents (along with the more recently introduced carbapenems and monobactams) contain a β-lactam ring in their structure (Figure 4-3). Because this β-lactam ring has a three-dimensional structure resembling the D-alanine-D-alanine present on the peptide bridge of *N*-acetylmuramic acid, the β-lactam antibiotics inhibit the ability of transpeptidases to catalyze

> A rarely used antimicrobial agent, **cycloserine**, resembles D-alanine and therefore competitively inhibits the completion of synthesis of the amino acid side chain that should be added to N-acetylmuramic acid. The exact sequence or composition of this five-amino acid side chain varies among different bacteria, except for the invariable presence of the two terminal D-alanine residues.

◄ **FIGURE 4-3**
Basic Structure of β-Lactam Antibiotics. The circled number 1 shows the location of the β-lactam ring; 2 shows the site of β-lactamase cleavage, if any; and 3 shows the location of side chains that distinguish individual types of penicillins.

the final cross-linking step of cell wall synthesis (Figure 4-4) and thus render the growing bacterial cell susceptible to lysis. Thus, these antimicrobials have bactericidal effects. Note that the β-lactam antibiotics will not affect existing cross-linked peptidoglycan; they work only on growing cells that are actively synthesizing new cell wall. Because of this, bacteriostatic antibiotics antagonize the action of the β-lactams and should not be used in combination with these agents.

Bacteria are not necessarily defenseless against the β-lactam antibiotics. A number of pathogens are able to produce β-lactamases, which are enzymes that can cleave the essential β-lactam ring of many β-lactam antibiotics, thus destroying the antimicrobial activity of these agents (see Figure 4-3 and Chapter 5). In response, pharmaceutical chemists have modified the β-lactam structure of many penicillins and cephalosporins to make them more resistant to β-lactamases.

One approach to deal with the problem of β-lactamases has been the development of agents, such as clavulanic acid and sulbactam, that bind to and specifically inhibit β-lactamases. Clavulanic acid and sulbactam do not themselves kill or inhibit bacteria but are used in combination with β-lactam agents to protect these antibiotics from β-lactamases. (For an example of the clinical use of these agents, see the clinical case in

FIGURE 4-4 ▶
Cross-Linking of Individual Peptidoglycan Layers. *During the cross-linking reaction shown in this figure, the bond between the terminal D-Ala-D-Ala residues is cleaved to provide energy. As a result, the terminal D-Ala is lost from the final cross-linked product. Note that β-lactam antibiotics structurally resemble D-Ala-D-Ala. Not all bacteria have the pentaglycine bridge shown in this figure (i.e., small variations in the precise chemical nature of the cross links occur among different bacterial species), but the terminal D-Ala-D-Ala residues are always involved in the cross-linking reaction. GlcNAc = N-acetylglucosamine; MurNAc = N-acetylmuramic acid.*

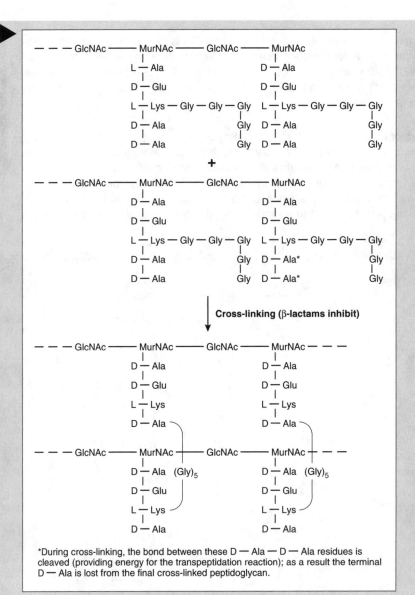

Chapter 2.) Pharmaceutical chemists have produced a number of penicillin and cephalosporin derivatives that have a broader spectrum of activity and allow for different routes of administration.

Vancomycin. This agent binds to the lipid-disaccharide complex formed during the plasma membrane stage of cell wall synthesis, thus preventing the disaccharide from transferring outside the membrane to the growing layer of peptidoglycan. It is a bactericidal antibiotic that works only against gram-positive bacteria. In fact, because nearly all gram-positive bacteria were sensitive to vancomycin, one of the traditional uses of this agent was as a "last resort" therapy for gram-positive infections that were unresponsive to any other antibiotics. Unfortunately, vancomycin-resistance is now developing, particularly in gram-positive cocci such as the enterococci (see Chapter 5).

Bacitracin. Recycling of the lipid carrier at the completion of the plasma membrane stage of cell wall synthesis is essential for continuation of the process. Otherwise, the bacterial cell quickly runs out of lipid carrier. Bacitracin binds to the lipid carrier after it has released the disaccharide and prevents recycling of this carrier. Bacitracin is bactericidal and is used only topically because of its toxicity.

AGENTS THAT AFFECT BACTERIAL MEMBRANES

The polymyxins have a detergent-like effect on cell membranes, causing a breakdown in their permeability properties. These bactericidal agents are useful topically against gram-negative bacteria, which have an outer membrane, but cannot be given systemically because of their toxicity. If given internally, they cause damage to the membranes of mammalian cells, resulting in neurotoxicity and nephrotoxicity.

NUCLEIC ACID SYNTHESIS INHIBITORS

Inhibitors of Bacterial DNA Synthesis. The class of antimicrobials called the quinolones are bactericidal agents that inhibit bacterial DNA synthesis by interfering with bacterial DNA gyrase A, an enzyme humans do not have. Nalidixic acid was the first quinolone to be used therapeutically, but it was useful only against urinary tract infections because therapeutic levels could be reached only in the urine. However, recent chemical modifications that created the fluoroquinolone derivatives (e.g., norfloxacin and ciprofloxacin) have significantly enhanced the efficacy and spectrum of the quinolones.

Metronidazole is taken up and modified inside anaerobic bacteria (and some protozoa). The activated drug is thought to produce a bactericidal effect by inducing strand breaks in DNA, thereby inhibiting DNA replication.

Inhibitors of Bacterial RNA Synthesis. Rifampin (a rifamycin) is a bactericidal antibiotic that forms a complex with bacterial RNA polymerase. (Human RNA polymerases do not bind with this agent). The effect of rifampin binding to RNA polymerase is inhibition of bacterial transcription. Rifampin is a front-line drug for the treatment of tuberculosis; it is particularly useful because it is effective against both intracellular and extracellular *M. tuberculosis* (see Chapters 22 and 25).

AGENTS THAT INHIBIT BACTERIAL PROTEIN SYNTHESIS

As mentioned in Chapter 1, there are fundamental structural differences between the 70S prokaryotic ribosome, which is composed of 30S and 50S subunits, and the 80S eukaryotic ribosome, which is composed of 40S and 60S subunits. These structural differences provide the basis for the selective toxicity of a number of antibiotics that affect bacterial protein synthesis. Some of these bacterial protein synthesis–inhibiting antibiotics interact primarily with the 30S ribosomal subunit, whereas others affect primarily the 50S subunit.

Antibiotics That Interact with the 30S Ribosomal Subunit. Aminoglycosides and tetracyclines are the two major classes of agents that interact with the 30S subunit of prokaryotic ribosomes.

The aminoglycosides (e.g., streptomycin, gentamicin) are bactericidal agents that bind to the 30S ribosomal subunit and cause deleterious effects such as misreading of mRNA and premature termination of translation. The aminoglycosides are often used for treatment of *Pseudomonas* infections. Because oxidative phosphorylation is required for the uptake of aminoglycosides into a bacterial cell, these agents are ineffective against strict anaerobes, aerotolerants (e.g., streptococci), and facultative anaerobes growing in an anaerobic environment (see Chapter 2). All aminoglycosides have some inherent neurotoxicity and nephrotoxicity, and levels of these agents thus must be closely monitored during clinical use.

The tetracyclines are broad-spectrum bacteriostatic agents that also interact with the 30S ribosomal subunit, causing an inhibition of bacterial protein synthesis. Because tetracyclines effectively enter the mammalian cell, they are useful for treating infections involving obligate intracellular pathogens such as *Rickettsia* and *Chlamydia*. They also are useful against mycoplasmal organisms, which cannot be treated with β-lactam agents because they lack a cell wall.

Antibiotics That Interact with the 50S Ribosomal Subunit. Several clinically useful antibiotics inhibit bacterial protein synthesis by interacting with the 50S ribosomal subunit, including chloramphenicol, erythromycin, and clindamycin.

Chloramphenicol is a broad-spectrum antibiotic with a bacteriostatic action. It has been used for infections involving intracellular pathogens, typhoid fever, meningitis caused by ampicillin-resistant *Haemophilus influenzae* or β-lactam–resistant pyogenic gram-positive cocci, and infections involving gram-negative anaerobes. The usage of chloramphenicol has been declining because the drug inhibits blood-cell formation in the bone marrow.

Erythromycin, which belongs chemically to the macrolide family, is another broad-spectrum agent with primarily a bacteriostatic effect (although it may have a bactericidal effect in certain circumstances against some bacteria). This usually nontoxic agent is considered the drug of choice for treating Legionnaire's disease, and it has numerous other clinical applications. The macrolide family also includes some recently introduced agents such as clarithromycin and azithromycin, which may be used to treat chlamydial infections, Lyme disease, and acquired immunodeficiency syndrome (AIDS)-related infections involving *Mycobacterium avium*.

Clindamycin is another bacteriostatic inhibitor of protein synthesis that interacts with the 50S ribosomal subunit. It is effective against many anaerobes but, because it disturbs the normal anaerobic flora of the gut, can induce antibiotic-associated pseudomembranous colitis caused by *Clostridium difficile* (see Chapter 11).

AGENTS THAT AFFECT INTERMEDIARY METABOLISM

Several clinically useful antimicrobials, including folate-synthesis inhibitors and isoniazid, interfere with bacterial metabolism.

Folate-Synthesis Inhibitors. Tetrahydrofolate is an essential molecule for conducting one-carbon transfer reactions in both eukaryotes and prokaryotes. The pathway for tetrahydrofolate synthesis is shown in Figure 4-5. The sulfonamide class of antimicrobials structurally resembles para-aminobenzoic acid (PABA), one of the initial precursors in the microbial tetrahydrofolate synthesis pathway. Because of this structural resemblance, the sulfonamides competitively inhibit enzymes involved in the synthesis of dihydropteroate. Trimethoprim, another antimicrobial, inhibits dihydrofolate reductase, the enzyme catalyzing the conversion of dihydropteroate to tetrahydrofolate; mammalian dihydrofolate reductase does not bind trimethoprim.

To obtain a synergistic effect (and limit the development of resistance), trimethoprim and sulfamethoxazole often are given in combination for therapy (e.g., as the trade preparation Bactrim). This combined bacteriostatic therapy is often used for *Escherichia coli* urinary tract infections and also is useful against the eukaryotic pathogen *Pneumocystis carinii*.

Isoniazid. Isoniazid is a front-line antituberculosis agent that structurally resembles pyridoxine. It is believed to inhibit the synthesis of mycolic acids necessary for synthesis of the mycobacterial cell envelope. Isoniazid is generally considered to be bactericidal, but some investigators believe that it only has weak bactericidal or bacteriostatic activity against nonreplicating *M. tuberculosis*.

> *One-carbon transfer reactions* are critical for many biosynthetic processes, including purine synthesis and the synthesis of some amino acids.

FIGURE 4-5 ▶

Action of the Sulfonamide and Trimethoprim Antimetabolites. Note that bacteria and some other microorganisms (e.g., some parasites) carry out the entire pathway shown in this figure, whereas humans acquire dihydropteroate—the immediate precursor for tetrahydrofolate synthesis—from their diet. PABA = para-aminobenzoic acid.

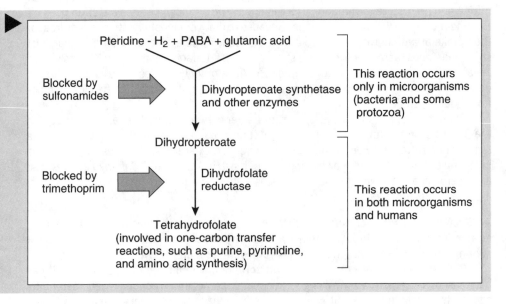

Pteridine - H₂ + PABA + glutamic acid

Blocked by sulfonamides

Dihydropteroate synthetase and other enzymes

This reaction occurs only in microorganisms (bacteria and some protozoa)

Dihydropteroate

Blocked by trimethoprim

Dihydrofolate reductase

Tetrahydrofolate
(involved in one-carbon transfer reactions, such as purine, pyrimidine, and amino acid synthesis)

This reaction occurs in both microorganisms and humans

ANTIFUNGAL THERAPY

Because fungi are eukaryotic, they share many more structural and metabolic similarities with human cells than do the bacteria. Consequently, there are significantly fewer antifungal agents available for therapy, and toxicity is often a significant problem (see Table 4-1).

Membrane-Active Antifungal Agents

Antifungal therapy for most serious fungal infections exploits structural differences between the fungal and mammalian plasma membranes. Typical of eukaryotes, fungi contain sterols in their membranes. However, whereas cholesterol is the predominant plasma membrane sterol in mammalian cells, ergosterol is the major sterol of the fungal membrane and is essential for the proper functioning of this membrane.

Two major groups of membrane-active antifungal antibiotics currently exist, the polyenes and the azoles. The polyenes (e.g., amphotericin B and nystatin) are fungicidal agents that bind to ergosterol in the fungal membrane, disrupting the membrane's permeability properties. Despite having toxic side effects, amphotericin B has been a traditional mainstay for the treatment of life-threatening mycoses. Nystatin is so toxic that it can be used only topically.

The azoles are a group of structurally related agents (including ketoconazole, miconazole, fluconazole) that produce either fungistatic or fungicidal effects by inhibiting ergosterol synthesis. With lowered levels of ergosterol, the functioning of the fungal membrane breaks down.

Other Antifungal Agents

Several other antifungal agents also exist, the most important of which include flucytosine and griseofulvin.

Flucytosine. Flucytosine is an agent with fungistatic or fungicidal properties that inhibits nucleic acid synthesis in some fungi. It is often used against fungi that can grow only as yeasts (e.g., *Cryptococcus neoformans*).

Griseofulvin. Griseofulvin is a fungistatic agent that inhibits fungal mitosis and has traditionally been used for infections involving the dermatophytes (see Chapter 2).

ANTIVIRAL THERAPY

Background

As with other antimicrobial therapies, the ultimate goal of antiviral therapy is to achieve the elimination of infectious virus particles from the body. Current antiviral drugs (Table 4-2) do not inactivate free virus particles or destroy infected cells. Instead, they interrupt (with varying degrees of efficacy) the growth of viruses within cells by interfering with the entry of the viral genome into the cell's cytoplasm (uncoating), the replication of the viral genome, or the proteolytic processing of viral precursor proteins. Remember that the immune system's antibodies must ultimately neutralize free virus particles, and its activated T lymphocytes must destroy virus-infected cells. Destructive action against infected cells, although it can elicit or exacerbate disease symptoms, is crucial because these infected cells are the factories producing virions. Any kind of immunosuppression makes successful antiviral therapy much more difficult.

Unlike the many antibiotic therapies that can cure bacterial or fungal infections, most antiviral therapies cannot cure a virus infection. For example, acyclovir ameliorates the severity of primary herpes simplex virus type 1 (HSV-1) lesions but does not prevent latent infection or recurrent disease. AZT can reduce the amount of HIV (i.e., the virus burden) in AIDS patients, but it cannot eliminate the virus. In addition, virtually all

TABLE 4-2 ▶

Antiviral Therapeutic Agents

Drug	Active Form	Clinical Indications	Inhibits	Primary Toxicity
Amantadine	Itself	Influenza A viruses	Intracellular uncoating	Nontoxic
Rimantadine	Itself			
Zidovudine (AZT)	AZT-TP	HIV	Reverse transcriptase	Anemia
Didanosine (DDI)	DDI-TP			
Acyclovir (Acv)	Acv-TP	HSV-1, HSV-2, and VZV	Viral genome synthesis	Nontoxic
Ganciclovir (Gcv)*a*	Gcv-TP	CMV		Neutropenia
Famciclovir	Pcv-TP*b*	VZV		Unknown
Cidofovir (Cdv)*a*	Cdv-diP	CMV		Nephrotoxic
Ribavirin (Rbv)	Rbv-TP	Respiratory syncytial virus and hantaviruses	Viral genome synthesis	Nontoxic as aerosol
Vidarabine (Vdb)	Vdb-TP	HSV- and CMV-encephalitis	Viral genome synthesis	Nephrotoxic
Foscarnet*a*	Itself	HSV and CMV	Viral genome synthesis	Nephrotoxic
Ritonavir*c*	Itself	HIV	Protein cleavage	Nausea and hepatotoxic
Nevirapine	Itself	HIV	Reverse transcriptase	Rash

Note. AZT = azidothymidine, now known as zidovudine; TP = triphosphate; HIV = human immunodeficiency virus; diP = diphosphate; HSV-1 = herpes simplex virus type 1; CMV = cytomegalovirus; VZV = varicella zoster virus.
a Signifies drugs currently licensed for treatment of AIDS-associated retinitis caused by cytomegalovirus.
b Penciclovir TP is the antiviral metabolite formed from famciclovir in vivo.
c One of four drugs that block the activity of the HIV protease.

antiviral drugs invariably select for drug-resistant virus strains, which leads to a loss in antiviral effect.

Agents and Actions

AGENTS THAT BLOCK THE REPLICATION OF VIRAL GENOMES

Most antiviral drugs are nucleoside analogues that act by interfering with viral-specific nucleic acid synthesis, either by being incorporated into a viral nucleic acid strand and terminating further synthesis or by directly inhibiting the activity of the viral nucleic acid polymerase (Figure 4-6). With the exception of a newly introduced antiherpesvirus drug—cidofovir—nucleoside analogues cannot block virus replication until they are phosphorylated by viral-specific and/or host-cell kinases, thereby becoming direct substrates (i.e., nucleoside triphosphates) for the viral DNA or RNA polymerases.

For example, azidothymidine (AZT, also known as zidovudine) must be converted to azidothymidine triphosphate before it can be incorporated by the retroviral reverse transcriptase into proviral DNA. Because AZT (and other similar compounds) lacks an oxygen molecule on the 3′ carbon of its deoxyribose moiety, further polymerization of nucleotides is blocked. Agents acting in this fashion are called strand terminators.

Acyclovir and ganciclovir, which are guanosine analogues effective against primary acute infections caused by HSV and cytomegalovirus (CMV), respectively, also can act as strand terminators. In contrast, other nucleoside analogues, such as ribavirin, seem to act by binding to the viral polymerase and blocking its enzymatic (i.e., polymerization) activity or, like idoxuridine, are incorporated into viral genomes where they can cause mutations and thus defective viral genomes. These antiviral actions are not mutually exclusive; acyclovir may act as a strand terminator and a direct inhibitor of the herpesvirus DNA polymerase, depending, in part, on dosage.

Most drugs cause toxic side effects, and patient monitoring, particularly when drugs are delivered intravenously, is very important.

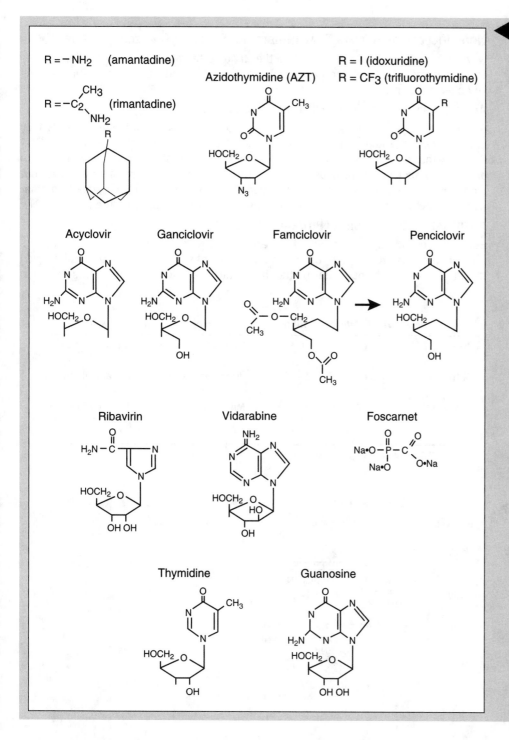

FIGURE 4-6
Some Antiviral Drugs Currently Used to Treat Human Viral Infections. Most drugs are analogues of natural ribonucleosides (e.g., guanosine) or deoxyribonucleosides (e.g., thymidine). Note that famciclovir (although not an active antiviral drug itself) after introduction into the body is converted to the active antiherpesvirus compound penciclovir. Two natural nucleosides are shown at the bottom.

AGENTS THAT ACT ON EARLY STAGES OF VIRUS INFECTION

Amantadine and rimantadine are unusual antiviral drugs because they themselves, unmodified, are antiviral; they inhibit only influenza A virus infections, not the replication of influenza B or C viruses; and they block a critical uncoating step required for the transport of the viral nucleocapsid to the nucleus where the viral genome is replicated. Although not commonly used in the United States, amantadine and rimantidine are relatively nontoxic and 50%–75% effective in preventing or ameliorating disease when administered at least 48 hours prior to influenza symptoms. Some studies suggest that they reduce the severity of disease even when administered at the onset of influenza symptoms. They are particularly useful drugs in institutions where the elderly or other highly susceptible populations exist in close quarters.

Non-Nucleoside Agents That Inhibit the Reverse Transcriptase of HIV

Nevivapine interferes with the activity of the HIV reverse transcriptase by binding directly to this enzyme. This inhibitor may be included with AZT and a protease inhibitor during HIV chemotherapy.

Agents That Block Viral Protein Processing

A new class of therapeutic agents, called protease inhibitors, block the growth of HIV by interfering with the proteolytic cleavage of HIV structural precursor proteins—GAG and GAG POL—by the HIV-encoded protease (see Figure 4-7). Combining a protease inhibitor with one or more nucleoside analogues not only exerts a greater inhibition of virus growth but reduces the likelihood that virus mutants resistant to both types of drugs will arise. Combination drug therapy for HIV infection is called highly active antiretroviral therapy (HAART).

Antiviral Therapy Using Natural Products

Currently, several human viral infections are treated with interferon (IFN) preparations. IFNs are proteins produced in response to a number of stimuli, including virus infection itself (Table 4-3). IFN molecules neither inactivate free virions nor block virus growth in

TABLE 4-3 ▶
Properties of Human Interferons (IFNs)

IFN	Type	Acid Stability	Subtypes[a]	Induced by	Produced by
IFN-α	1	Stable	20+	Viruses and other stimulants	Virtually all cells
IFN-β	1	Stable	1	Viruses and other stimulants	Virtually all cells
IFN-γ	2	Unstable	1	Mitogens	Activated T-lymphocytes and natural killer cells

[a] Each subtype is encoded by a different gene and is antigenically distinct.

FIGURE 4-7 ▶
Role of the Retroviral Reverse Transcriptase (RT) and Protease (Pro), as Well as Cellular Enzymes, in the Growth and Maturation of Retroviruses. *Current drug regimens are most effective against the RT and Pro, but the development of agents that can inhibit other viral-specific targets (e.g., the viral integrase [Int]) is under way. GAG = capsid precursor protein; POL = precursor protein of RT, Pro, and Int; ENV = envelope proteins; ▲ = translational stop signal in unspliced mRNA molecule; MA, CA, NC = nucleocapsid-associated proteins; TM = transmembrane protein; SU = surface unit protein.*

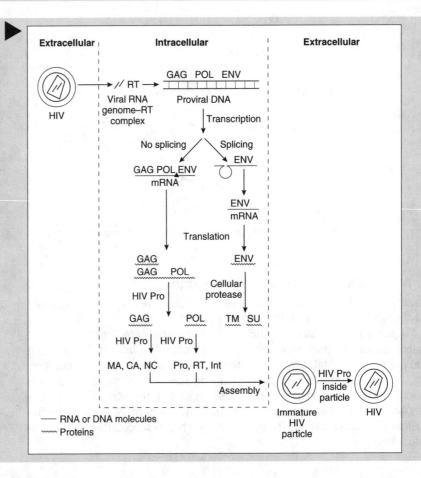

cells not previously exposed to interferon. Conceptually, IFN action is divided into two steps: a stimulus that results in the synthesis and release of IFN molecules by cells and the induction of an antiviral state in uninfected cells by newly made IFN molecules.

IFN synthesis can be induced in animals within hours of the introduction of a variety of substances, including bacterial products such as lipopolysaccharide, double-stranded RNA and anionic polymers. When a susceptible cell binds one or more IFN molecules, a virus-resistant state is induced usually within hours. This resistance can last for several days. Although virions may infect, and even kill, interferon-treated cells, few or no progeny viruses are produced. Thus, the virus burden in the patient is reduced. IFNs provide a major natural defense against virus infections and, with the capacity to produce IFN from cloned human genes, highly concentrated IFN is available to treat virus diseases such as hepatitis B. However, interferon treatment is often accompanied by serious, influenza-like reactions, and patient monitoring during treatment is important. Like other antiviral drugs, IFNs may ameliorate disease but they rarely cure them.

ILLUSTRATIVE PATHOGEN: *Mycoplasma pneumoniae*

Biologic Characteristics

The mycoplasmas are very small, prokaryotic pathogens that are distinguished by their lack of a cell wall and the presence of sterols in their plasma membrane. They are extracellular pathogens that can grow (although slowly) on an artificial medium. In addition to *M. pneumoniae*, other mycoplasmas (e.g., *M. hominis*) and related species (e.g., *Ureaplasma urealyticum*, which is similar to *Mycoplasma* species except it produces urease) are opportunists that can cause genitourinary tract infections (see Appendix 3).

Reservoir and Transmission

Several *Mycoplasma* species (and related prokaryotes) have been isolated from both animals and humans. However, *M. pneumoniae* appears to have a primarily human reservoir, although it is not considered part of the normal flora of the respiratory tract. Transmission of *M. pneumoniae* results from close contact (e.g., from inhalation of aerosol droplets), so it often spreads through families.

Virulence Factors

An adhesin (named P1 protein) helps mediate attachment of *M. pneumoniae* to bronchial epithelial cells. Metabolic by-products (e.g., hydrogen peroxide) also contribute to illness. For example, hydrogen peroxide can inhibit the ciliary escalator, facilitating the persistence of *M. pneumoniae* in the respiratory tract.

Pathogenesis

M. pneumoniae attaches to the ciliary bronchial epithelium and inhibits ciliary function through its metabolic by-products. It is not highly destructive to the respiratory epithelium but instead induces an inflammatory response (via its metabolic products) that causes the typical symptoms of *M. pneumoniae* infection (i.e., fever, cough, headache, and malaise). Colonization by *M. pneumoniae* can be asymptomatic or result in illness ranging from a pharyngitis to bronchitis and pneumonia. Pneumonia caused by *M. pneumoniae* is known as primary atypical pneumonia (or, commonly, as walking pneumonia because most affected patients do not require hospitalization) and may account for 20% of all pneumonias. This illness is unusual for its prevalence among older children and teenagers. Primary atypical pneumonia is usually less severe than pneumococcal pneumonia (Table 4-4).

TABLE 4-4 ▶
Some Differential Diagnostic Features of Pneumococcal Versus Mycoplasmal Pneumonias

Feature	Pneumococcal pneumonia	Mycoplasmal pneumonia
Onset	Sudden	Gradual
Rigors	Single chill	"Chilliness"
White blood cells	> 15,000/mm^3	< 15,000/mm^3
Temperature	> 103°F	< 103°F
Gram stain	Cocci and many neutrophils	Mixed normal flora and some mononuclear cells
Chest radiographs	Lobar infiltrate	Patchy infiltrate

Diagnosis

The initial diagnosis of mycoplasmal pneumonia is usually based on clinical grounds, with later confirmation by laboratory tests. Gram stains of sputum show mononuclear cells but not *M. pneumoniae*, which does not Gram stain because it lacks a cell wall. Because *M. pneumoniae* grows slowly (i.e., culture results are not available for 1 week or longer), serologic tests (e.g., complement fixation) are often used to confirm an initial clinical diagnosis of primary atypical pneumonia. Demonstrating high titers of cold agglutinins in a patient's serum is often used as a simple, but relatively nonspecific, indicator of possible infection by *M. pneumoniae*.

Prevention and Treatment

No vaccine is currently available. Treatment with antibiotics such as erythromycin or tetracycline is usually effective. Because *Mycoplasma* species lack a cell wall, they are not sensitive to β-lactam antibiotics (e.g., penicillins, cephalosporin). However, they do have 70S ribosomes, so they are sensitive to prokaryotic protein-synthesis inhibitors (e.g., erythromycin, tetracycline).

A *lobar infiltrate* is a more or less uniform density that occupies one or more lobes of the lung. A *patchy infiltrate* is not uniform, follows the bronchioles, and does not occupy an entire lobe.

RESOLUTION OF CLINICAL CASE

Both the husband and wife in this case were suffering from infection with *M. pneumoniae*. They both improved slowly during a 2-week period, and the husband's chest radiograph showed clearing.

The incidence of *M. pneumoniae* infections is highest among children between 5 and 14 years of age. Young children tend to manifest nonspecific upper respiratory tract syndromes, whereas older children and young adults more frequently have tracheobronchitis and pneumonia. Because the transmission of *M. pneumoniae* from person to person by infected respiratory secretions requires close and prolonged contact, secondary cases are most commonly seen in groups such as families, college dormitory roommates, and military recruits.

Cold-agglutinin–induced hemolysis is one of the most frequent nonrespiratory manifestations of mycoplasmal pneumonia. Apparently, *M. pneumoniae* alters the erythrocyte I antigen, changing it into an immunogen. As a result, complement-fixing, temperature-sensitive immunoglobulin M antibodies that react against the erythrocyte I antigen are produced. Approximately 50%–60% of patients show a fourfold or greater rise in the cold agglutinin titer for type O erythrocytes or have a single titer of 1:128 or higher. The more severe the illness, the more likely an increase in cold agglutinins. Although cold agglutinins may be found in 50% of patients with mycoplasmal pneumonia, clinically significant hemolysis is rare. The presence of cold agglutinins obviously lacks sensitivity for the diagnosis of *Mycoplasma* pneumonia, and specificity is also low, as cold agglutinins may also be seen in pneumonias caused by adenovirus or influenza virus and in infectious mononucleosis and lymphoma. However, titers of 1:128 or more are highly suggestive of mycoplasmal pneumonia. The diagnosis can be confirmed by a fourfold or greater increase in anti-*M. pneumoniae* antibodies in convalescent serum compared to acute serum, and the causative organism can be isolated from the pharynx or sputum. However, because the results of either antibody titers or isolation attempts are not available for weeks, a tentative diagnosis often must be made based on the clinical and epidemiologic characteristics, and erythromycin or tetracycline must be started empirically. Although *M. pneumoniae* is insensitive to cell wall synthesis–inhibiting antibiotics such as penicillin, it is a prokaryotic organism containing 70S ribosomes and is sensitive to antibacterial protein-synthesis inhibitors.

REVIEW QUESTIONS

Directions: For each of the following questions, choose the **one best** answer.

1. A new prokaryotic pathogen is isolated at the Centers for Disease Control and Prevention. Biochemical analysis of this pathogen gives the following results:

Compound/Constituent	Presence in New Organism
Peptidoglycan	+
Teichoic acid	+
DNA	+
70S ribosomes	+
Sterols	−
Phenolic glycolipid	−

   Based upon these analytic results, the new organism most closely resembles which of the previously characterized organisms?

   (A) *Mycoplasma pneumoniae*

   (B) *Mycobacterium leprae*

   (C) *Escherichia coli*

   (D) *Pseudomonas aeruginosa*

   (E) *Staphylococcus aureus*

2. Which of the following is an antimicrobial agent that inhibits bacterial cell wall synthesis by blocking the recycling of the lipid carrier?

   (A) Cephalosporin

   (B) Streptomycin

   (C) Bacitracin

   (D) Vancomycin

   (E) Polymyxin

3. Considering only cellular structure, which of the following organisms should be most resistant to therapy with cephalosporin?

   (A) *Escherichia coli*

   (B) *Bacteroides fragilis*

   (C) *Staphylococcus aureus*

   (D) *Corynebacterium diphtheriae*

   (E) *Mycoplasma pneumoniae*

4. Which of the following statements best describes sulfonamides?

   (A) They are bactericidal

   (B) They often are used in combination with trimethoprim

   (C) They act by inhibiting dihydrofolate reductase

   (D) They are cell wall synthesis inhibitors

   (E) They block folic acid synthesis in humans

5. Zidovudine, originally known as azidothymidine (AZT), blocks HIV-1 replication by specifically inhibiting which of the following steps in the life cycle of the virus?

(A) Binding to the CD4 cell receptor

(B) Viral penetration and uncoating

(C) Reverse transcription

(D) Integration

(E) Virus assembly

6. The reason for using triple drug combination therapy in the treatment of a patient with AIDS is that

(A) the deoxynucleoside inhibitor will block the virus replicating inside the cell, whereas the protease inhibitor will inactivate extracellular virus

(B) the likelihood of a mutant arising that is resistant to all three drugs is much lower than that of a mutant arising that is resistant to only one or two of the drugs

(C) resistance to deoxynucleoside analogues is common, whereas resistance to protease inhibitors is unknown

(D) deoxynucleoside analogues are effective early in AIDS, whereas protease inhibitors act later in the disease

(E) all drugs directly affect different domains of the viral reverse transcriptase

7. An infectious disease physician is treating two patients suffering from nonviral pneumonias. One of the patients is an elderly man with pneumococcal pneumonia, and the other patient is a teenager with primary atypical pneumonia caused by *Mycoplasma pneumoniae*. Which of the following statements about the illnesses affecting these two patients is correct?

(A) The elderly patient's illness is more likely to have had a gradual onset than the teenager's illness

(B) A Gram stain of sputum from the teenager would show the infecting mycoplasmas as small blue cocci

(C) A penicillin or cephalosporin would be appropriate therapy for either of these patients

(D) The elderly patient probably experienced a lower fever than did the teenager

(E) The laboratory may be able to culture the pathogens responsible for both patients' pneumonia

8. A new antibiotic sharing the same action as amphotericin B is isolated by a pharmaceutical company. The new drug is most likely to be effective against which of the following pathogens?

(A) *Clostridium tetani*

(B) *Cryptococcus neoformans*

(C) *Rickettsia prowazekii*

(D) *Escherichia coli*

(E) *Staphylococcus aureus*

ANSWERS AND EXPLANATIONS

1. **The answer is E.** The new organism has all the characteristics of a gram-positive bacterium such as *Staphylococcus aureus* (see Chapter 1). The new microbe does not resemble a *Mycoplasma* species (option A) for two reasons: it contains peptidoglycan, which is found in the cell wall that mycoplasmas lack; and, it does not contain sterols (as a *Mycoplasma* would). The new pathogen is dissimilar from *Mycobacterium* spp. (option B) because it lacks phenolic glycolipids, and it does not resemble a gram-negative species (e.g., options C and D) because it contains teichoic acid, which is not found in gram-negative bacteria.

2. **The answer is C.** Only bacitracin inhibits bacterial cell wall synthesis by blocking the recycling of the lipid carrier. Table 4-1 lists the actions of cephalosporin, streptomycin, vancomycin, and polymyxin.

3. **The answer is E.** *Mycoplasma* spp. lack a cell wall; therefore, they are not sensitive to any antibiotic that acts by inhibiting cell wall synthesis, (e.g., the cephalosporins). All of the other bacteria listed have a peptidoglycan-containing cell wall.

4. **The answer is B.** Sulfa drugs are often combined with trimethoprim to generate a double block in the bacterial tetrahydrofolate synthesis pathway in order to reduce the likelihood of the development of antimicrobial resistance and increase antimicrobial activity. Option A is incorrect because sulfonamides are bacteriostatic when administered alone. Option C is incorrect because the listed action is the way in which trimethoprim, not the sulfa drugs, works to inhibit the folic acid synthesis pathway. Humans do not carry out the step in folic acid synthesis blocked by the sulfa drugs, so option E is incorrect. Sulfonamides do not inhibit cell wall synthesis, so option D is incorrect.

5. **The answer is C.** Zidovudine is a nucleoside analogue that inhibits synthesis of proviral DNA during reverse transcription of HIV RNA (see Chapters 3 and 27 for a further explanation of this process).

6. **The answer is B.** Zidovudine (azidothymidine) and protease inhibitors are combined for HIV therapy to reduce the likelihood that virus mutants resistant to both types of drugs will arise. There are no chemotherapeutic agents that inactivate retrovirions (option A). Viral mutants arise that are resistant to protease inhibitors (option C). There are no drugs that act only early or late in AIDS (option D). Protease inhibitors do not directly affect the reverse transcriptase (option E).

7. **The answer is E.** Both *Streptococcus pneumoniae* and *Mycoplasma pneumoniae* can be cultured. Pneumococcal pneumonia typically has a very sudden onset (faster than that of primary atypical pneumonia caused by *M. pneumoniae*). *M. pneumoniae* does not Gram stain because it lacks a cell wall (and is very small). β-lactams (e.g., penicillins, cephalosporin), which act by inhibiting cell wall synthesis, are not effective against *M. pneumoniae* because it lacks a cell wall. Patients typically experience a higher fever with pneumococcal pneumonia than with pneumonia caused by *M. pneumoniae*.

8. **The answer is B.** Amphotericin B is active against fungal pathogens, such as *Cryptococcus neoformans*. It is inactive against prokaryotic pathogens such as *Clostridium tetani, Rickettsia prowazekii, Escherichia coli*, and *Staphylococcus aureus* (options A, C, D, and E, respectively) because these microorganisms do not have ergosterol in their plasma membranes. Amphotericin B is a polyene that acts by binding to ergosterol, causing changes in the permeability of a fungal cell's plasma membrane.

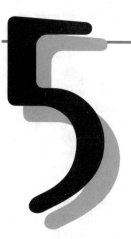

RESISTANCE TO ANTIMICROBIAL AGENTS

Saleem A. Khan, Ph.D.

CHAPTER OUTLINE

Introduction of Clinical Cases
Importance of Antimicrobial Resistance
Mechanisms of Antimicrobial Resistance
- Alteration of the Antimicrobial Site of Action
- Overproduction of the Target
- Production of a New Enzyme to Bypass the Targeted Site of Action
- Limiting Access of the Antimicrobial Agent to Its Site of Action
- Modification of the Antimicrobial Agent

Genetic Basis for Antimicrobial Resistance
Illustrative Pathogen: *Pseudomonas aeruginosa*
- Biologic Characteristics
- Reservoir and Transmission
- Virulence Factors
- Pathogenesis
- Diagnosis
- Prevention and Treatment

Illustrative Pathogen: *Enterococcus faecalis*
- Biologic Characteristics
- Reservoir and Transmission
- Virulence Factors
- Pathogenesis
- Diagnosis
- Prevention and Treatment

Prevention of the Spread of Antimicrobial Resistance
Resolution of Clinical Cases
Review Questions

INTRODUCTION OF CLINICAL CASES

Case 1

A 46-year-old obese woman had two distinct attacks of acute cholecystitis in the past 3 years, one of which occurred last month and required hospitalization. On both occasions, right upper quadrant abdominal sonograms showed stones in the gallbladder (i.e., cholelithiasis). The patient was advised to have a cholecystectomy, but she refused. Three days ago, approximately 8 hours after eating a large dinner of corned beef and cabbage, she was awakened from sleep by what she thought to be a gallbladder attack. Her symptoms included nausea,

> **Acute cholecystitis** is an acute infection of the gallbladder that results in an inflammatory response that occurs at this organ site.

vomiting, and abdominal pain. The next day she was admitted to the hospital, placed on nasogastric suction, given intravenous fluids, and administered meperidine for pain relief. Upon admission, she had a low-grade fever (100.4°F) and was started on piperacillin, an extended-spectrum penicillin-type antibiotic. After 2 days in the hospital, the patient's temperature rose to 102.2°F, and she began to experience chills with shaking. One blood culture drawn prior to antibiotic therapy was positive for bacterial growth. A second blood culture drawn after admission and antibiotic therapy was also positive for growth. A Gram stain evaluation of both cultures demonstrated gram-positive cocci in pairs and short chains. Organisms isolated from these blood cultures grew on agar containing 6.5% sodium chloride (NaCl) at 45°C, grew on agar containing bile salts, and were typed as group D streptococci. Based on these microbiologic characteristics, the organism was identified as *Enterococcus faecalis*.

- Why is it notable that bacteria were cultured from the patient's blood?
- Why is the patient experiencing pain and fever despite antimicrobial therapy?

Case 2

An 87-year-old man was brought to the hospital from a nursing home because of fever and disorientation. Two months before, the patient had undergone a transurethral resection of the prostate gland because of longstanding difficulty in voiding caused by benign prostatic hypertrophy. At the time of that admission, he had been catheterized to relieve the obstruction and scheduled for prostate surgery to correct his difficulty in voiding. At the time of catheterization, urine culture grew gram-negative rods on MacConkey agar that were lactose and oxidase negative. Based on this information, the clinical laboratory identified this isolate as *Escherichia coli*. To control this urinary tract infection, the patient was started on a 2-week course of ampicillin. An attempt to remove the catheter 1 week after surgery was unsuccessful because of urinary retention, and another Foley catheter had to be installed in its place.

Two weeks after surgery, the patient still required a catheter. At this time, the patient developed fever, chills, and hypotension and was treated with fluid administration. Suspecting antimicrobial resistance to the ampicillin, the physician prescribed a combination therapy of ticarcillin (an extended-spectrum penicillin) and gentamicin (a well-tolerated aminoglycoside). Blood cultures grew out *Enterobacter cloacae*, which was susceptible to third-generation cephalosporins (e.g., cefotaxime) and aminoglycosides (e.g., gentamicin) but not ticarcillin. Cefotaxime was substituted for ticarcillin, and the patient was stabilized after 7 days, at which time the gentamicin component of this dual antibiotic regimen was stopped.

One month after surgery, the patient remained on cefotaxime but was discharged to a nursing home. At this time, it was still not possible to remove the Foley catheter. The patient showed no symptoms for 10 days. He then developed a low-grade fever, and his temperature escalated during the course of 4 days until it was 103°F. Because of these symptoms, the patient was immediately readmitted to the hospital with notable signs of confusion and disorientation in addition to his fever. Microscopic examination of his urine revealed white blood cells too numerous to count and 4–5 red blood cells per high-power field. A Gram stain of the urine demonstrated numerous thin, faintly staining gram-negative bacilli. Both urine and blood culture on MacConkey agar grew lactose-negative, oxidase-positive, gram-negative bacilli. These organisms demonstrated a green pigment upon extended culture and were able to grow at 42°C. Based on these microbiologic characteristics, the patient's isolate was identified as *Pseudomonas aeruginosa*. Antibiotic-resistant profiles of this isolate indicated that it was resistant to both gentamicin and cefotaxime (as well as many other antibiotics) but was sensitive to piperacillin and tobramycin; the patient was immediately placed on this combination therapy.

IMPORTANCE OF ANTIMICROBIAL RESISTANCE

Antimicrobial resistance is an important consideration in contemporary medicine. When the "antibiotic era" (see Chapter 4) began in this century, most bacteria were sensitive to each antibiotic as it was introduced to the medical community. However, with the continued use of each antibiotic (and sometimes as a result of misuse), antimicrobial resistance has developed, sometimes quite rapidly and with serious consequences. For example, when benzylpenicillin (penicillin G) was first utilized in the 1940s, nearly all infections caused by pathogenic staphylococci responded to this relatively inexpensive antibiotic. By 1950, approximately 70% of staphylococcal strains isolated within hospitals were resistant. In today's hospital environment, nearly 85% of staphylococcal strains are resistant, and many of these are resistant to antibiotics other than benzylpenicillin. In response to the emergence of resistance to benzylpenicillin, the medical community has developed second- and third-generation penicillins that are effective against staphylococcal and other bacterial infections.

Note that the data above concerning antibiotic resistance were obtained from hospital isolates. It is important to emphasize that many microbial pathogens isolated for these studies were actually acquired in the hospital, which is a concept known as *nosocomial infection. Community-acquired infection* refers to infection outside of the hospital environment. Because of the intensive use of antibiotics within medical facilities, antibiotic resistance patterns of nosocomially acquired infections tend to be much different from those of community-acquired infections. An appreciation for where a bacterial isolate may have been contracted (or transmitted) is one aspect of the science of epidemiology and is often overlooked in the management of infectious disease. Relating this epidemiologic concept back to Case 1, should the prior medical history of the patient be considered when prescribing the antimicrobial regimen? After all, the patient had been hospitalized within the past month. Did she acquire this antibiotic-resistant organism during that time? A single, albeit extended-spectrum, antibiotic was prescribed for her latest episode. However, should the possibility of nosocomially derived, multiple antibiotic-resistant bacteria have been considered in the design of her treatment regimen, in light of her recent hospitalization?

MECHANISMS OF ANTIMICROBIAL RESISTANCE

As described in Chapter 4, antimicrobial therapy can be categorized by the site of action that the antimicrobial agent targets (e.g., cell wall synthesis, membrane synthesis and integrity, nucleic acid synthesis, ribosomal translation, or intermediary metabolism). In turn, general mechanisms responsible for antibiotic resistance can be categorized by the general strategies used to facilitate resistance to a given antimicrobial. These strategies include:

- Altering the targeted site of action
- Overproduction of the target
- Production of a new enzyme to bypass the targeted site of action
- Limiting access of the antibiotic to the targeted site of action
- Modifying the antibiotic to render it ineffective against the site of action.

Specific examples of how different antimicrobial strategies are utilized against different antibiotics are given in Table 5-1.

Alteration of the Antimicrobial Site of Action

This is typically accomplished by subtly changing the "targeted site of action" in such a way that the target can still perform its function (although perhaps not quite as well) but is not as sensitive to antimicrobial therapy. A specific example is resistance to bacterial cell wall inhibitors (see Chapter 4). Some enzymes (e.g., transpeptidases) that participate in the process of cell wall synthesis bind to and are inhibited by the penicillins. These proteins are referred to as the penicillin-binding proteins (PBPs). Single amino acid changes on the part of a PBP can significantly decrease the PBPs' affinity for a particular penicillin. The net result of this is that, although the bacteria become somewhat less efficient at producing a cell wall, they can now survive in the presence of

TABLE 5-1 ▶

Examples of Bacterial Resistance to Specific Classes of Antimicrobials

Antimicrobial Class	Antimicrobial Resistance Strategy		
	Alter Site of Action	Alter Antimicrobial Access[a]	Modify Antimicrobial Target
Cell wall inhibitors	Change in PBPs Overproduction of PBPs	Porin alteration Alter membrane composition	β-lactam hydrolysis
Physiologic inhibitors	Overproduction of dihydropteroate synthase (sulfonamides) or dihydrofolate reductase (trimethoprim)	Porin alteration	None reported
Membrane inhibitors	Alter membrane composition	Porin alteration	Proteolysis or hydrolytic cleavage
Nucleic acid inhibitors	Change in enzyme (e.g., DNA gyrase mutations)	Porin alteration Alter membrane composition	Aminoglycoside acetylation, phosporylation, or adenylation
Protein synthesis inhibitors	Ribosomal modification by genetic mutation or post-translational modification	Porin alteration Efflux pumps	Chloramphenicol transacetylase Erythromycin rRNA methylase

Note. PBP = penicillin-binding protein.

[a] One important difference that should be noted for the alteration of access to antimicrobial targets is the presence or absence of the outer membrane, which is a principal permeability barrier of gram-negative bacteria but does not exist for gram-positive bacteria. Thus, alterations in gram-negative porin or outer membrane lipid composition can significantly affect access to the antimicrobial target.

penicillin. Another illustration of antimicrobial target alteration is a mutation that causes single amino acid or nucleic acid changes in ribosome structure. For example, resistance to spectinomycin commonly results from a change in the amino acid composition of the ribosomal 5S protein.

Altering an antimicrobial target is a strategy not only confined to bacterial pathogens; viral and eukaryotic pathogens also employ this strategy. For example, prolonged treatment of chronically infected human immunodeficiency virus type 1 (HIV-1) patients with the antiviral drug azidothymidine (AZT) commonly selects for viral variants that are resistant to this form of therapy as a result of specific alterations in their reverse transcriptase enzyme (see Chapter 27).

Overproduction of the Target

Instead of altering the sequence (nucleic acid or protein) of the antimicrobial target, it is possible to alter (increase) the copy number of the target so that the effective drug concentration required to inhibit a specific process is increased. A clear example of this is the case of para-aminobenzoic acid (PABA) conversion to dihydropteric acid. Bacteria and parasites can overexpress enzymes such as dihydropteroate synthase and therefore minimize their susceptibility to sulfonamides.

Production of a New Enzyme to Bypass the Targeted Site of Action

Some bacteria, such as members of Enterobacteriaceae and *Staphylococcus aureus*, can synthesize entirely new enzymes, which can carry out the PABA-to-dihydropteroate conversion. These enzymes have a significantly decreased affinity for trimethoprim or the sulfonamides. As a result, these organisms are no longer sensitive to these antimicrobials.

Limiting Access of the Antimicrobial Agent to Its Site of Action

This mechanism of action is recognized as playing a significant role in bacterial resistance, particularly for gram-negative bacteria, which have an outer membrane as their principal permeability barrier. Alterations in porin structure confer low-level multiple drug resistance to *Neisseria gonorrhoeae, Pseudomonas aeruginosa,* and other gram-negative bacteria. In contrast to hydrophilic antibiotics that diffuse through pores, lipophilic antibiotics (e.g., erythromycin) generally gain access to gram-negative bacteria by diffusing through the outer membrane. In these cases, changes in the lipid composition of the outer membrane may significantly contribute to resistance.

The expression of specific transporters is another way that bacteria limit access of an antimicrobial agent to its site of action. For example, an energy-dependent efflux transporter that is specific for tetracycline effectively "pumps" this antibiotic out of some bacteria, thereby preventing it from reaching its intracellular ribosomal target. Other less specific efflux systems are being increasingly recognized (e.g., the multiple resistance locus [mtr] of *N. gonorrhoeae*). Drug resistance problems caused by these efflux strategies are not limited to bacteria. Treatment failure in cancer chemotherapy commonly results from multidrug resistance that occurs because of P-glycoprotein amplification (P-glycoprotein is an ATP-dependent efflux transporter that pumps a variety of nonpolar, planer molecules out of cells).

Modification of the Antimicrobial Agent

A general strategy for rendering a bacterium resistant to an antimicrobial agent is to covalently modify the chemical structure of the antimicrobial in such a way that this agent ineffectively interacts with its target. This can be accomplished in at least two different ways: by chemical breakdown (hydrolysis) of the antibiotic or by chemical substitution of the antibiotic.

One example of this strategy includes the bacterial β-lactamases, which can hydrolyze the β-lactam ring that is essential for penicillin and cephalosporin antimicrobial activity (see Chapter 4). Whether a given β-lactamase is active against a particular β-lactam antibiotic depends on the structure of the antibiotic (e.g., β-lactamases are unable to access the target β-lactam ring of some penicillins and cephalosporins because these antibiotics contain side groups that physically block β-lactamase [see Chapter 4]).

Another important mechanism of antibiotic resistance is the pathogen's ability to modify an antibiotic by chemical substitution so that the antibiotic can no longer interact with its targeted site of action. Examples of this include the acetylation of chloramphenicol by the enzyme chloramphenicol acetyltransferase and the acetylation, adenylation, and phosphorylation of aminoglycoside antibiotics by other bacterial enzymes.

Understanding the basic strategies of antimicrobial resistance is an important first step in learning the many specific mechanisms of resistance. It is equally important for clinicians to appreciate the genetic basis that encode these antibiotic resistance strategies. This knowledge allows for the design of more effective antimicrobial regimens and limits the further spread of resistance.

GENETIC BASIS FOR ANTIMICROBIAL RESISTANCE

To understand the genetic basis for antibiotic resistance, it is first necessary to have a basic understanding of the mechanisms of gene transfer in bacteria. Antibiotic resistance genes (as well as other genes) can be transferred between different bacteria by three distinct processes: genetic transformation, transduction, or conjugation (Figure 5-1).

1. **Genetic transformation:** the process by which a recipient cell takes up naked DNA released by a donor cell. Natural transformation occurs in a number of bacterial pathogens, including *Streptococcus* spp., *Haemophilus* spp., and *Neisseria* spp. In this process, a single strand of DNA (generally derived upon lysis of a homologous donor cell) enters a recipient cell and is integrated into the homologous region of

FIGURE 5-1

Basic Mechanisms of Genetic Exchange: Transformation, Transduction, and Conjugation. During the process of transformation, naked DNA is liberated from the donor bacteria upon lysis and is taken up by the recipient bacteria. Transduction utilizes bacteriophage to transfer DNA from a donor to a recipient. Neither of these mechanisms require cell-to-cell contact, which is a necessary property for conjugation. Conjugative transfer occurs between bacteria through highly differentiated structures known as sex pili.

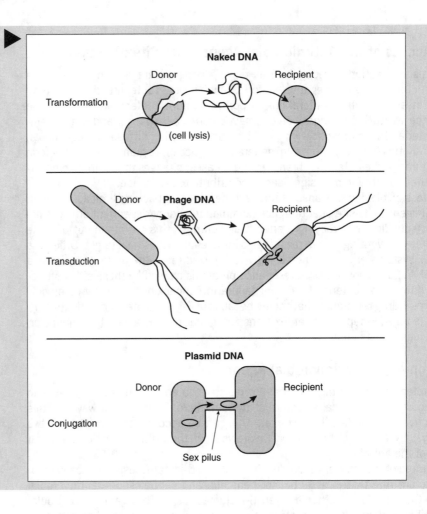

Classification of Plasmids Based on Three Encoded Functions
*Fertility/sex factors (F factors) carry genes that encode the ability of bacteria to undergo **conjugal** transfer of genetic information.*
Resistance factors (R factors) carry genes that make bacteria resistant to one or more antibiotics and can also undergo conjugative transfer.
Virulence plasmids carry genes that encode toxins and other virulence factors.

recipient DNA, replacing the recipient allele. Natural transformation is a highly efficient process in contrast to artificially induced transformation, which can be achieved only by using special procedures in the laboratory; even under laboratory conditions this type of transformation occurs with low efficiency relative to natural transformation. Because of its inherent inefficiency, artificially induced transformation is thought to occur infrequently in nature.

2. **Transduction:** the process involving a bacteriophage (a bacterial virus) that mediates gene transfer from a donor cell to a recipient cell. This type of genetic exchange is quite common among members of gram-negative Enterobacteriaceae; it is also of importance for some gram-positive pathogens, such as *Staphylococcus aureus* and *Corynebacterium diphtheriae*, which utilize a bacteriophage to mobilize the diphtheria toxin gene to strains of *C. diphtheriae* that do not carry the gene. Transduction can be either generalized (i.e., random fragments of the donor bacterial chromosome can be transferred to the recipient) or specialized (i.e., specific chromosomal DNA segments are transferred from donor to recipient).

3. **Conjugation:** the process of genetic exchange mediated by plasmids, which are extrachromosomal elements in bacterial cells that replicate independently of the host chromosome. Unlike transformation and transduction, conjugation generally requires cell-to-cell contact to accomplish the process of gene transfer. All plasmids contain genes that allow them to replicate independently in bacterial cells. The replication region of plasmids usually includes a gene encoding a replication initiator protein, an origin of replication that contains the start site for DNA replication, and a copy control gene that controls the replication and copy number (the ratio of plasmid molecules per bacterial chromosome). Some plasmids are referred to as *conjugative* plasmids because they carry genes encoding a sex pilus, which is required for DNA transfer between donor and recipient cells. Conjugative plasmids present in the donor ("male") bacteria encode the sex pilus, which forms a bridge

with the recipient ("female") bacteria. This allows the conjugative plasmids, which sometimes include regions of chromosomal DNA, to transfer genes from the donor to the recipient cells without exposure to the extracellular environment.

Conjugative plasmids that encode resistance to one or more antibiotics are of particular significance for understanding the genetic basis of antibiotic resistance; these plasmids are referred to as R plasmids or R factors. R factors can be found in almost all major human bacterial pathogens and express proteins that can confer resistance to several different types of antibiotics. Often, a single R factor encodes simultaneous resistance to multiple types of antibiotics. In addition, many R factors have a broad host range, allowing them to be transferred to and replicated within diverse bacterial pathogens. This attribute significantly facilitates the spread of antibiotic resistance among different bacterial species.

The misuse of antibiotics has contributed to the selection of antibiotic-resistant strains. As evidence, R factors specifying resistance to new drugs are often detected shortly after their routine inclusion in animal feeds. Similarly, a large number of the bacterial pathogens encountered in the hospital environment are resistant to multiple antibiotics. This results from the continuous heavy use of standard antimicrobial regimens without rotation. It is because of this that nosocomial infections are resistant to multiple antimicrobials and are very difficult to manage.

It should be appreciated that R factors, as well as bacterial chromosomes, frequently contain transposons. Transposons (also known as jumping genes) are specific DNA sequences (usually larger than 5000 bp) containing one or more antibiotic-resistance genes. Transposons can repeatedly insert at many different sites within a chromosomal genome or plasmid, a process referred to as transposition. Insertion sequences are DNA elements (usually 750–1500 bp) that are similar to transposons, except that they do not carry antibiotic-resistance genes. Transposons either can move between two autonomously replicating genetic elements (e.g., from a chromosome to a plasmid) or they can jump to different locations within a particular chromosome or plasmid. Transposition can either be replicative or nonreplicative. Replicative transposition involves replication of the transposon and results in the duplication of the transposable element; as a consequence, it is present in multiple copies within the cell. Nonreplicative transposition involves simple excision of the transposon from the donor site and insertion at the new target site. The two ends of transposons contain identical DNA sequences present in an inverted orientation; these sequences are termed inverted repeats (IRs). The IRs are recognized by transposon-encoded transposase enzymes that function in the movement of these genetic elements. Many diverse transposons are associated with bacterial genomes, and a large number of different transposons associated with R factors contain multiple antibiotic-resistance genes. The mechanism of transposition allows a single R factor to acquire multiple antibiotic-resistance genes and therefore significantly contribute to bacterial antimicrobial resistance.

Antimicrobial resistance is becoming increasingly problematic for nearly all medically significant bacterial infections. Two pathogens that illustrate the problems posed by antimicrobial resistance include *Pseudomonas aeruginosa* and *Enterococcus faecalis*. Both of these opportunistic pathogens are important causes of nosocomial infection, and the management of these infections is complicated by the widespread antimicrobial resistance encountered within the hospital setting.

ILLUSTRATIVE PATHOGEN: *Pseudomonas aeruginosa*

Biologic Characteristics

As a group, the Pseudomonadaceae are motile, gram-negative bacilli that require an aerobic environment for growth. It is notable that these organisms grow on media containing bile salts (i.e., MacConkey agar; see Chapter 12), which is a characteristic generally associated with members of Enterobacteriaceae (see Chapters 12, 13, and

Morphology of the Pseudomonadaceae

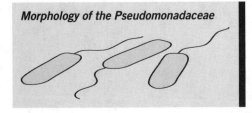

24). However, pseudomonads can be distinguished from Enterobacteriaceae on the basis of their production of large quantities of cytochrome oxidase in the oxidase test. In this test, all *Pseudomonas* spp. are oxidase positive, whereas all members of Enterobacteriaceae are oxidase negative. *P. aeruginosa* is the major human pathogen of the pseudomonad group.

Reservoir and Transmission

Pseudomonads (including *P. aeruginosa*) occur widely in soil, in water, and on vegetation. *P. aeruginosa* is also frequently found in small numbers on the skin, within the oral cavity, and within the intestines of healthy humans, where it causes no disease. It is an opportunistic pathogen found more frequently among unhealthy, hospitalized patients. Another related pseudomonad that causes opportunistic infection is *Pseudomonas cepacia* (recently renamed *Burkholderia cepacia*). Although it causes disease less frequently than *P. aeruginosa*, it is clinically significant because more than 90% of *P. cepacia* isolates are resistant to aminoglycoside antibiotics. In contrast, only 20% of *P. aeruginosa* isolates are resistant to the aminoglycoside antibiotics.

Virulence Factors

Virulence Factors Associated with *P. aeruginosa* Disease Isolates
Versatile growth requirements that allow this organism to exist within both the environment and the host
Broad-host range conjugative plasmids
Motility
Pili
Endotoxin (lipopolysaccharide)
Exotoxin A
Exotoxin S
Elastase
Collagenase
Phospholipase C
Alginate

Arguably, the most important virulence factor of *P. aeruginosa* is its ability to survive and grow in diverse environments ranging from the human host to drinking water. Because this pathogen can exist in diverse environments, it is always poised to take advantage of any shortcoming in host defenses. In addition, the polar flagellum of *P. aeruginosa* allows it to chemotactically migrate to the most favorable growth environment. The pili expressed by *P. aeruginosa* allow these bacteria to adhere to certain host tissues; therefore, when this organism breaches the natural defenses of the host, it can then begin the process of colonization. In addition to expression of common pili that participate in attachment, disease isolates of *P. aeruginosa* often express sex pili encoded by broad-host range conjugative plasmids that facilitate the development of strains with multiple antimicrobial resistance.

P. aeruginosa produces a number of conventional virulence factors that play a significant role in disease. All disease and nondisease isolates produce endotoxin (lipopolysaccharide), although on a per-molecule basis, the endotoxic activity of *Pseudomonas* lipopolysaccharide is weaker than the endotoxin activity of the lipopolysaccharide expressed by most other gram-negative pathogens. Significantly, more than 90% of disease-associated isolates of *P. aeruginosa* secrete a protein toxin termed exotoxin A. This toxin gains access to the cytoplasmic compartment of eukaryotic cells and catalyzes the adenosine diphosphate (ADP)-ribosylation of elongation factor 2, leading to a shutdown of protein synthesis and the death of the cell. The mechanism of exotoxin A action is identical to diphtheria toxin (see Chapter 23), although these two toxins share no amino acid sequence similarities. Another exotoxin produced by some strains of *P. aeruginosa* is termed exotoxin S. This exotoxin also has ADP-ribosylation activity, although its physiologic target is not clear.

Several hydrolytic enzymes are also produced by clinical isolates of *P. aeruginosa*. Two secreted proteases, elastase and collagenase, contribute to disease by degrading host connective tissue as well as other host proteins associated with an immune response (e.g., IgA and complement proteins). Phospolipase C hydrolyzes host membrane lipids and is known to induce a marked inflammatory response. Collectively, these hydrolytic enzymes contribute to the tissue destruction associated with disease caused by *P. aeruginosa*.

Some strains of *P. aeruginosa* express alginate, a carbohydrate glycocalyx, which is a copolymer of mannuronic acid and glucuronic acid. This extracellular polysaccharide promotes adherence to respiratory epithelium and confers resistance to phagocytosis upon *P. aeruginosa* strains.

Pathogenesis

Examples of Types of Infections Produced by *P. aeruginosa*
Burns and environmentally contaminated wounds
Ulcerative keratitis from contaminated contact lenses or eye drops
Foliculitis of skin from soaking in contaminated hot tubs
Otitis externa (swimmer's ear)
Urinary tract infections
Septic arthritis
Endocarditis
Pneumonia associated with patients on respirators
Lung infections in cystic fibrosis (CF) patients

Because *P. aeruginosa* is an opportunistic pathogen, there is a relationship between how this bacterium gains access to the host and the type of disease that ensues. *P. aeruginosa* is known to cause disease in skin, wounds, the urinary tract, burns, eyes, and ears. While respiratory tract infections are rare, they do occur in healthy individuals. Within healthy individuals, these infections can progress to systemic infection, although this is very rare. Rather, infection caused by *P. aeruginosa* is much more common in immunocompromised individuals and, thus, is often associated with hospitalized patients. (A classic case of disseminated *P. aeruginosa* infection is illustrated in Case 2.)

Cystic Fibrosis (CF) and Infection Caused by P. aeruginosa. CF patients are particularly susceptible to infection caused by *P. aeruginosa*. CF is a disease that manifests with excessive mucus in the smaller respiratory passages as well as increased chloride levels within the lung. *P. aeruginosa* is routinely introduced into the respiratory tract of these individuals by aerosols. The respiratory epithelium of these patients favors attachment of *P. aeruginosa* compared to normal individuals. Furthermore, a high proportion of *P. aeruginosa* isolates from CF patients produce alginate (often abundantly), which also assists colonization. Besides facilitating colonization, alginate renders the organisms resistant to phagocytosis and to drying and also helps to form a biofilm, which complicates antibiotic access, within the bronchi. The high chloride environment of the cystic lung reduces the effectiveness of innate immune mechanisms of the lung epithelium. Meanwhile, the potent exotoxins and hydrolytic enzymes produced by *P. aeruginosa* damage the lung. The cumulative effect of repeated *P. aeruginosa* infection can eventually cause lung failure and death of the patient with CF.

Biofilm refers to the growth of bacteria as a thick, interconnected film that coats a discrete surface. Because of their numbers and their proximity, bacteria existing in this growth pattern from a closed ecologic community can limit access of certain molecules (e.g., antibiotics). In the case of a P. aeruginosa-infected CF patient, biofilms are often established within the bronchi.

Diagnosis

Culture of *P. aeruginosa* from the site of infection is important in establishing it as the responsible etiologic agent. *P. aeruginosa* grows readily on many types of media, sometimes (but not always) producing a fruity, grape-like odor. Many (but not all) *P. aeruginosa* isolates produce water-soluble pigments that include pyocyanin, pyoverdin, pyorubin, or pyomelanin, which diffuse into the agar and often give rise to characteristic blue-green pigmented colonies. Alginate-expressing strains give rise to mucoid colonies when cultivated on agar medium. Culture of *P. aeruginosa* from the infected site and identification by Gram stain, oxidase test, pigment formation, mucoid colony morphology, growth at 42°C, and other biochemical tests, are used to diagnose disease caused by this organism.

Prevention and Treatment

P. aeruginosa is routinely resistant to antimicrobial therapy. To a large extent, this resistance is accomplished by limiting the diffusion of many antibiotics through the outer membrane, although *P. aeruginosa* also employs other antimicrobial resistance mechanisms, as described previously. Tests to identify antimicrobial patterns of resistance of *P. aeruginosa* isolates are typically performed to determine an appropriate treatment regimen, which usually involves a combination of antibiotics. This practice also limits the spread of further antibiotic resistance.

Experimental vaccination using an inactivated form of exotoxin A has been shown to be effective in certain high-risk populations. However, this vaccine is still experimental, and its use is further complicated by defining the population that would receive it. Perhaps the most effective means of disease prevention is to limit the number of times a susceptible individual encounters potential pathogens such as *P. aeruginosa*. These encounters can be minimized by appropriate sanitary measures and by behavior-modification strategies, but they can never be entirely eliminated.

ILLUSTRATIVE PATHOGEN: *Enterococcus faecalis*

Biologic Characteristics

Enterococcus is a genus of bacteria that includes the important human opportunistic pathogen *Enterococcus faecalis*. These organisms are gram-positive cocci occurring in pairs or as short chains. They are closely related to the streptococci and, in fact, were once known as *Streptococcus faecalis* because they classically typed as group D by the Lancefield typing system used to classify the streptococci (see Chapter 18). However, enterococci differ from other streptococci in that they can grow in the presence of 6.5%

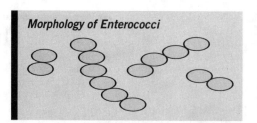

Morphology of Enterococci

NaCl and in the presence of bile salts. Furthermore, they actively grow at 45°C and are not killed by temperatures as high as 60°C.

Reservoir and Transmission

Enterococci commonly inhabit the gastrointestinal and the genitourinary tracts of humans and, as such, are considered normal flora. Like *P. aeruginosa*, they cause opportunistic infections in unhealthy individuals.

Virulence Factors

Enterococci are considered normal flora of the human intestine and therefore are constantly in a position to cause any infection from an enteric portal of entry in a compromised human. Enterococci produce few recognized virulence factors outside of those that allow them to outcompete other members of the natural flora for opportunistic infection.

Pathogenesis

Enterococci typically invade deeper tissues by breaching normal host immune barriers. As a member of the normal intestinal flora, enterococci are strategically positioned to cause opportunistic urinary tract infections, wound and soft tissue infections, infections resulting from surgical contamination, bacteremia associated with malignancies, biliary tract disease, and gastrointestinal disease. Significantly, bacteremia resulting from enterococcal infection can result in the development of bacterial endocarditis.

Diagnosis

Infections caused by enterococci are generally identified by culture of specimens derived from the infected site. Gram stain and growth on high-salt agar and at high temperatures are suggestive of an infection caused by enterococci. Other biochemical tests can be performed to more definitively define the organism as *E. faecalis*. This, in conjunction with a patient history consistent with an immunocompromised status and an enteric portal of entry, is generally enough evidence to implicate enterococci as the agent responsible for disease.

Prevention and Treatment

Enterococci are generally resistant to aminoglycosides because they do not take up this antibiotic class. They are also inherently more resistant to the penicillins than the closely related streptococci, probably because of the nature of their PBPs. However, at penicillin concentrations that do not inhibit enterococci, aminoglycoside antibiotic uptake is no longer inhibited by enterococci. This renders enterococci susceptible to the aminoglycoside. The mechanistic basis for this antimicrobial synergism has yet to be defined, but, based on this observation, enterococcal infections are typically managed using this combination antibiotic therapy (i.e., employing both a penicillin or vancomycin and an aminoglycoside). Complicating this combination antimicrobial therapy is the emergence of β-lactamase–producing enterococcal strains and individuals that are allergic to penicillin. For either of these complications, the nonpenicillin, cell-wall inhibitor vancomycin has been used instead of penicillin. However, recent reports of vancomycin-resistant enterococci are creating considerable concern in the medical community and have sparked renewed interest in the development of new antimicrobial agents. Prevention is discussed in the following section.

> **Infections Produced by Enterococci**
> *Urinary tract infections*
> *Wound and soft-tissue infections*
> *Bacteremia associated with malignancies, biliary tract disease, and gastrointestinal disease*
> *Endocarditis*

PREVENTION OF THE SPREAD OF ANTIMICROBIAL RESISTANCE

There is clearly a medical basis for the increase of antimicrobial resistance to antibiotics. Studies have shown that the extent of nosocomially derived antimicrobial resistance is proportional to the extent of antimicrobial usage. In turn, the extent of resistant isolates to a given antibiotic quickly decreases upon removing a given antimicrobial regimen from a defined hospital setting. The extent to which this decrease in antibiotic resistance extends to community-acquired infections is variable. Some resistant phenotypes are so stabilized among bacterial pathogens that these pathogens no longer revert to sensitive phenotypes in the environmental absence of a given antibiotic (e.g., penicillin as a treatment for gonorrhea; see Chapter 17).

An appreciation of the basic mechanisms and historical importance of antimicrobial resistance can lead to measures that prevent its spread. Many of these measures are denoted in the margin note. Generally, the physician responsible for dispensing antimicrobials must have a basic knowledge of the mechanisms of antimicrobial resistance as well as an awareness of the medical and behavioral consequences of ill-considered antimicrobial therapy. The informed and conservative prescription of antibiotics for the management of infectious disease can extend the currently available antimicrobial therapies for years to come and will limit the challenges to disease management such as those presented by the *P. aeruginosa* and *E. faecalis* infections.

> *Physician Control of Antimicrobial Resistance*
> *1. Avoid the spread of nosocomial, antimicrobial resistant bacteria through the use of proper sanitary measures.*
> *2. Be epidemiologically informed of hospital or practice trends with regard to antimicrobial pathogen resistance patterns.*
> *3. Consider antimicrobial therapy as a conservative approach to managing infectious disease. Use this option with the following considerations:*
> *• Design antimicrobial therapy regimens with consideration to the characteristics of the organism causing infection (as determined through the clinical microbiology laboratory), in conjunction with an informed history of the organism's antimicrobial resistance patterns*
> *• Consider using a narrow-spectrum antibiotic in contrast to a broad-spectrum antibiotic*
> *• Ensure that the dosage prescribed is adequate and that there are adequate assurances that the patient will comply with the course of the prescription*

RESOLUTION OF CLINICAL CASES

Case 1

Recall that the case presented at the opening of this chapter involved bloodborne *E. faecalis* in an individual with a history of gallbladder disease. The gallbladder is often colonized by bacteria derived from the intestine. The intestinal flora comprises a broad array of bacteria (see Chapter 11) including the enteric gram-negative bacilli, especially *E. coli* (see Chapter 12); gram-positive cocci (e.g., enterococci); and anaerobes (see Chapter 2). Bacteria can spread from the large bile ducts to the gallbladder, and from the gallbladder they can progress up the intrahepatic bile ducts and into the bloodstream. This process is termed ascending cholangitis, and it frequently occurs when the common bile duct is blocked by a stone or by stricture. Blood is normally sterile, so that the presence of any bacteria in this compartment is abnormal and is referred to as sepsis. The patient's symptomology is a response to the presence of bloodborne bacteria that were derived from the biliary tract.

Because organisms causing ascending cholangitis demonstrate considerable variation in their susceptibility to different antibiotics, these cases are particularly difficult to manage by antimicrobial therapy. This is why the extended-spectrum antibiotic piperacillin was prescribed for the patient. Despite this, the patient became increasingly ill because of ineffective antimicrobial therapy. This case illustrates how antimicrobial therapy is routinely used in the management of infectious diseases; it also illustrates how it can fail to manage infectious disease.

In the end, it is difficult for the infectious disease physician to devise a combination antibiotic regimen that effectively manages an infectious disease as complex as ascending cholangitis. One antibiotic regimen that can be utilized is an extended-spectrum penicillin, such as ticarcillin or piperacillin, in combination with an aminoglycoside, usually gentamicin. The extended-spectrum penicillin and gentamicin generally provide excellent coverage for the enteric gram-negative bacilli; the combination of a penicillin and an aminoglycoside enable synergistic killing of most enterococci. This is clearly aided by the effective use of a microbiology laboratory, both with regard to identifying the bacterial agent in the blood as an enterococcus and by determining the antimicrobial susceptibility pattern of this organism. The importance of the clinical laboratory for the management of antimicrobial-resistant infections and in the control of the spread of antimicrobial resistance cannot be overstated.

Case 2

In this case, *P. aeruginosa* has gained access to an immunocompromised patient's bloodstream by way of a urinary tract infection. The patient's age alone (87 years), regardless of his health status, is enough to suspect a certain lowering of his immune status. This situation is further exacerbated when the urinary tract is compromised by obstruction, foreign bodies (e.g., urinary catheters or stones), or surgery, which often results in bacteriuria that cannot be eliminated by antimicrobial agents alone. In this case, an antibiotic was administered at the time of surgery to prevent the *E. coli* within the patient's urinary tract from invading the bloodstream. The *E. coli* may have been suppressed by this treatment. The suppression of *E. coli* in conjunction with the presence of the urinary catheter created a scenario in which a more resistant organism, *E. cloacae*, established itself within the urinary tract. At this point, a switch to broad-spectrum antibiotics was necessary. However, as long as the urinary catheter was in place, this therapy was, in many ways, counterproductive because it allowed for the emergence of a new bacterium, *P. aeruginosa*, that progressed to sepsis. This frustrating problem of escalation to ever more resistant bacteria, and then to fungi, is a common one in modern medicine.

Bacteriuria is the presence of bacteria in the urine.

Sepsis refers to a systemic inflammatory response syndrome (SIRS) that can be initiated by the presence of bacteria in the bloodstream (see Chapter 21).

REVIEW QUESTIONS

Directions: For each of the following questions, choose the **one best** answer.

1. Which one of the following statements is most true about multiple antimicrobial resistant bacteria?

   (A) Resistance arises in the absence of antimicrobial selection

   (B) Alteration of the antibiotic (e.g., by chloramphenicol transacetylase) can lead to multiple antibiotic resistance

   (C) Limiting access of the antimicrobial agent (e.g., by porin alteration) can allow a pathogen to become resistant to multiple antibiotics

   (D) Somatic mutation rather than exchange of genetic information is the most common mechanism in the emergence of multiple antimicrobial resistance

   (E) As new generation antimicrobial agents are developed, the emergence of multiple antimicrobial resistant bacteria strains is decreasing

2. R factors in *Escherichia coli* are best described by which one of the following statements?

   (A) They can control their transfer from cell to cell and carry multiple transposable elements

   (B) They are absolutely required for bacterial growth in the absence of an antimicrobial agent

   (C) They are moved between bacteria by transposons only

   (D) They are disappearing from nature because of the use of new antibiotics

   (E) They can be easily controlled in a nosocomial environment

3. Transposons in bacteria have which one of the following functions?

   (A) They transpose to a number of different sites in a genome and contain inverted repeats at their ends

   (B) They replicate autonomously (independently) in host cells

   (C) They do not carry genetic information; rather, they inactivate essential genes by genetic insertion

   (D) They are essential for the replication of the plasmids on which they reside

   (E) They can be spread between bacterial cells in the absence of conjugation, transformation, or transduction

4. Antibiotic resistance is best described by which one of the following statements?

   (A) It is always caused by the degradation of the drug by the bacteria

   (B) It is found only in gram-positive bacteria

   (C) It can be genetically transferred between bacterial cells by the process of conjugation

   (D) It is never encoded for by chromosomal elements

   (E) It is never transferred between different bacterial species

5. A 20-year-old cystic fibrosis (CF) patient dies as a result of pulmonary collapse. The most likely reason for the death of this individual is best described by which one of the following statements?

   (A) The consequences of chloride deposition within the cystic fibrotic lung could not be overcome by the patient

   (B) A single pulmonary infection caused by a *Pseudomonas aeruginosa* isolate expressing pili, alginate, exotoxin A, exotoxin S, proteases, and other hydrolases overwhelmed this immunocompromised individual, resulting in death

   (C) A single pulmonary infection caused by a virulent organism that was resistant to multiple antibiotics overwhelmed this immunocompromised individual because the organism did not respond to antimicrobial therapy

   (D) Repeated infection of the patient's lung by *P. aeruginosa* predisposed the patient to lung collapse that resulted in death

   (E) *P. aeruginosa* conjugative phage encoding a transposon integrated in a lung cell of this patient causing spread to adjacent cells and the pulmonary collapse

ANSWERS AND EXPLANATIONS

1. **The answer is C.** Option A is incorrect since resistance to antibiotics is selected for by antimicrobial therapy. Option B is true in that enzymatic actions such as chloramphenicol transacetylase can result in resistance to chloramphenicol. However, the answer is incorrect as it relates to multiple antibiotic resistance because this mechanism is specific for chloramphenicol. Porin alteration restricts the transport of many antibiotics to their site of action (see Table 5-1). Genetic exchange between bacteria is a major mechanism of spreading multiple antibiotic resistance, thus option D is incorrect. Likewise, option E is incorrect because the emergence of multiple antibiotic-resistant organisms is well documented.

2. **The answer is A.** R factors typically express genes for the transfer of DNA between cells. Option B is incorrect because plasmids and R factors are considered "dispensable genetic information;" thus, the organism can survive quite well without these R factors. Transposons facilitate the spread of R factors onto chromosomal or plasmid elements within a cell, but eventually the genetic information has to get to another cell. This is accomplished by transformation, transduction, or conjugation. R factors are increasing in their occurrence because of antimicrobial use. And, within the hospital environment, R factors are particularly important because of the intensive use of antimicrobials within this setting.

3. **The answer is A.** Transposons lack an active replication system and, therefore, must integrate into a plasmid or chromosome for replication. Transposons can transpose to a number of different sites in a genome, and they contain inverted repeats at their ends. However, they cannot self-replicate. Transposons do carry genetic information, often encoding antimicrobial resistance genes. Transposons generally are not essential for the plasmids on which they reside. Finally, transposons cannot replicate, and therefore be spread, in the absence of a chromosome or a plasmid.

4. **The answer is C.** Option A is incorrect because there are multiple mechanisms for antibiotic resistance; degradation of the antibiotic is just one mechanism. Option B is incorrect because antibiotic resistance is found throughout the bacterial kingdom. Genetic exchange between bacteria of the same species, of different species within the same genera, and even between different genera is common. Antibiotic resistance can be encoded for by chromosomal as well as episomal (plasmid) elements. Finally, transfer between bacterial species, although rare, does occur and is a major contributor to the spread of antimicrobial resistance.

5. **The answer is D.** Multiple infections by *P. aeruginosa* are typical in a CF patient and are generally thought to result in pulmonary failure. This occurs because of the ubiquitous nature of *P. aeruginosa* within the environment encountered by the CF patient and the elaboration of virulence components by this organism. Option A is not correct because although chloride levels cause dysfunction, these levels are typically tolerated by the patient. Options B and C are not correct because CF patients typically experience multiple episodes of *P. aeruginosa* infection. Option E is incorrect because it does not describe the typical interaction between a bacterium and a host cell.

PART II: ESTABLISHMENT OF INFECTIOUS DISEASES: TRANSMISSION AND COLONIZATION

OVERVIEW

INTRODUCTION

Human infectious diseases almost always result from the presence of a microbial pathogen in the human host (i.e., from infection). The outcome of microbial infection depends on complex interactions between the infectious agent and the human host. Conse-

quently, one cannot appreciate human infectious disease without understanding both the biology of microbial pathogens and the biology of the host. The overview for Part I describes a general algorithm for infectious disease involving four steps:

> ***Steps of the Pathogenic Cycle***
> *1. Gain access*
> *2. Colonize*
> *3. Cause pathology*
> *4. Disseminate*

gaining access to the host, colonization of the host, causing pathology to the host, and dissemination to a new host. To be sure, not all infectious diseases can be described within the context of this algorithm. For example, there are diseases such as microbial foodborne intoxication (Chapters 6 and 20) or asymptomatic sexually transmitted diseases (STDs) [Chapter 9] that do not fit neatly into this algorithm. However, these diseases represent the exception and not the rule.

Within the context of this general algorithm, dissemination and access constitute transmission; this forms the basis by which much of this section is organized. Chapters within this section include transmission by ingestion (Chapter 6), by inhalation (Chapter 7), from animal to man (zoonosis) [Chapter 8], by sexual contact (Chapter 9), and by bloodborne or transplantation vectors (Chapter 10). Once transmitted, the microbial pathogen typically establishes a site of infection within the human host through a process referred to as colonization (as described in Chapter 11). In some cases, colonization requires that microbial pathogens confine themselves to a specific host, sometimes directly invading host cells (Chapter 13).

The term *infection* is somewhat ambiguous in that it is often used to describe the proliferation of a microbial pathogen (viral, bacterial, or parasitic) within humans, irrespective of whether disease pathology ensues. For example, commensal organisms (also referred to as local flora) "infect" a human host but do not cause disease (Chapter 11). Other microbial pathogens that infect and cause no disease in a particular host (asymptomatic or subacute infection) may be transmitted to other hosts in which they can cause disease. Latent infection refers to a microbial pathogen that infects a host but causes no apparent disease until later. Other infectious disease patterns are described as chronic or persistent (mild but persists within the host for a long time), or acute (overt and debilitating symptoms occur soon after infection). Thus, an infection can have any of several different pathologic outcomes. Within this text, the term infection is typically used to describe overt disease caused by a microbial entity, unless this term is qualified by the type of infection (e.g., asymptomatic, latent, subacute, chronic, or persistent).

Transmission

One useful way to organize infectious diseases is by the site of infection. The general sites of infection and the types of infection that ensue are described in Table II-1. What should be appreciated from this table is that where a microbial pathogen gains access to the human host is often predictive of symptomatology. For example, microbial pathogens that gain access to the host by inhalation often result in respiratory symptoms; microbial pathogens that gain access to the host by sexual transmission typically result in genitourinary complications, and so forth. Thus, an awareness of how an organism is transmitted to a host can make the difficult task of remembering what microbial pathogens cause what symptomatology much more manageable.

TABLE II-1 ▶

Types of Diseases Associated with Transmission Patterns

Site of Infection (Mode of Transmission)	Example
Lung (person-to-person)	Respiratory tract infection caused by *Haemophilus influenzae*, *Bordetella pertussis*, influenza virus, and so on
Eye (self-inoculation)	Conjunctivitis caused by *Moraxella* spp., *H. influenzae*, *Serratia marcescens*, *Streptococcus pneumoniae*, and so on
Intestine (self-inoculation)	Diarrhea or other gastrointestinal symptoms caused by *Clostridium* spp., *Staphylococcus aureus*, *Bacillus cereus*, enteroviruses, and so on
Skin penetration (animal-to-person)	Cellulitis caused by *Pasteurella haemolytica*, *Francisella tularensis*, and so on
Genitourinary tract (self-inoculation, nosocomial)	Sexually transmitted diseases and urinary tract infection caused by a variety of microbial pathogens
Blood (self-inoculation, nosocomial, animal-to-person)	Systemic infection (e.g., Lyme disease caused by *Borrelia burgdorferi*, rabies, and so on)

Transmission of infectious disease typically occurs by one of four characteristic modes: (1) self-inoculation, as in the case for foodborne infection; (2) person-to-person transmission, as in the case for diseases caused by inhalation or sexual contact; (3) animal-to-person, as in the case of zoonotic disease; or (4) as a consequence of nosocomial (hospital-related) disease. Understanding the transmission patterns of infectious diseases is important because interrupting transmission is arguably one of the most powerful means we have for controlling disease. For example, Chapter 6 describes several gastrointestinal illnesses that can be controlled by proper food handling and sanitary measures. Chapter 8 describes zoonotic infections that can be effectively brought under control by eliminating or managing the insect vector or the animal reservoir. Acceptance of the sexual transmission of diseases like acquired immunodeficiency syndrome (AIDS) or gonorrhea (Chapter 9) has encouraged the use of condoms as a barrier to disease transmission. These are but a few examples discussed in this section of how a working knowledge of disease transmission can be used for disease management.

Colonization

Colonization is the establishment of a critical mass of microbial pathogens at a site of the human host. However, colonization does not necessarily result in disease. For example, *Haemophilus influenzae* often transiently colonize the respiratory tract of humans without causing disease (Chapter 9). Because of this colonization pattern, *H. influenzae* is able to be spread from person to person and survives only within humans. The process of colonization implies that a given microbial pathogen has gained access to a particular

Colonization
1. Adherence
2. Multiplication
3. Invasion (in some cases)

body compartment and that this pathogen has been able to attach to and multiply within this compartment. In some cases, these organisms are able to invade host cells as part of the process of colonization.

The body has natural processes designed to prevent colonization. For example, we often think of the voiding of urine as a means to eliminate breakdown products from our body. However, this process plays an additional role by washing away most non-pathogenic microorganisms that have gained access to the urinary tract, keeping this body compartment sterile. Bacterial pathogens that cause urinary tract infections often express adhesins that allow them to stick to host cell surfaces, thereby preventing their elimination by natural host defenses such as urination (Chapter 12). This process is referred to as *adherence*, and this is a common theme in the pathogenesis of many infectious diseases.

In addition to attaching to a surface, microbial pathogens must also be able to *multiply* at the site of colonization. This is not a trivial matter, as the human host is armed with an arsenal of specific and nonspecific defense mechanisms. The most obvious is the host immune system. Less obvious are nonspecific host factors that prevent the growth of nonpathogenic bacteria. For example, we often consider that the host serum iron-binding protein transferrin plays a primary role in the transport of iron throughout the body. However, transferrin also plays a secondary role in host defense by binding iron so tightly as to render this element unavailable to nonpathogenic bacteria. Iron is absolutely required for the growth of all prokaryotic and eukaryotic pathogens. In order for pathogenic bacteria to cause disease within the bloodstream, they must solve the problem of obtaining iron from host transferrin. They do this by expressing specific high-affinity iron-transport processes that allow them to multiply aggressively within the bloodstream. As stated above, the ability of a limited number of bacteria to gain access to a site within the body typically does not give rise to disease symptoms. Rather, multiplication at the colonized site allows a critical mass of products, such as toxins, to be produced, giving rise to disease pathology. Microbial pathogens need not produce toxins to cause disease; rather, the presence of microbial pathogens in sufficient quantities can stimulate a host immune response that damages host tissues. This is described in greater detail in Part III.

A final process that may or may not occur during colonization is *invasion*. As described in Part I, Overview, microbial pathogens can be classified as intracellular or extracellular. Intracellular pathogens are referred to as such because they have invaded host cells. The process of invasion is typically an active process on the part of the microbial pathogen. For example, *Shigella dysenteriae* is a facultative intracellular pathogen because it can live both within a host cell or outside the host cell. This pathogen expresses specific proteins that facilitate the invasion of host intestinal cells (Chapter 13). Other microbes are obligate intracellular pathogens and cannot grow outside the host cell. The rickettsiae (Chapter 8) and the chlamydiae (Chapter 9) are two obligate intracellular pathogens that are described in Part II. These organisms gain at least two benefits from invasion: (1) they escape immune surveillance, and (2) they derive preformed nutrients (e.g., ATP) from the intracellular environment of the host cell. Of course, viruses by definition are all obligate intracellular pathogens and must invade cells in order to establish an infection.

Like transmission, an understanding of colonization is useful in the management of infectious disease. For example, knowing that chlamydiae are obligate intracellular pathogens should influence the treatment options for infection caused by this organism, that is, by confining treatment to an antibiotic that can effectively get inside a eukaryotic cell. In another example, cranberry juice is often used to treat urinary tract infections, both because it decreases the pH of the urine, making it difficult for bacteria to multiply, and because specific sugars are voided in soluble form that act as competitive antagonists of cell-bound receptors (Chapter 12). Thus, a working knowledge of colonization can provide a rationale for the management of infectious diseases.

Transmission and colonization are critical to the process of the establishment of infectious diseases. These concepts form the basis for a principles-oriented understanding of infectious disease. Considering infectious disease in this context will provide a strong foundation for understanding the diversity of infectious diseases in the years to come.

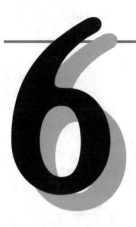

INFECTIOUS DISEASES ACQUIRED BY INGESTION

CHAPTER OUTLINE

Introduction of Clinical Case
Ingestion-Acquired Diseases
- Infections
- Intoxications

Transmission
- Fecal-Oral Route
- Foodborne Route
- Waterborne Route

Defenses in the GI Tract
- Physical and Chemical Defenses
- Immune Defenses
- Normal Microbial Flora

Illustrative Pathogen: Human rotavirus
- Biologic Characteristics
- Reservoir and Transmission
- Virulence Factors
- Pathogenesis
- Diagnosis
- Prevention and Treatment

Illustrative Pathogen: Hepatitis A virus
- Biologic Characteristics
- Reservoir and Transmission
- Virulence Factors
- Pathogenesis
- Diagnosis
- Prevention and Treatment

Illustrative Pathogen: *Campylobacter jejuni*
- Biologic Characteristics
- Reservoir and Transmission
- Virulence Factors
- Pathogenesis
- Diagnosis
- Prevention and Treatment

Illustrative Pathogen: *Giardia lamblia*
- Biologic Characteristics
- Reservoir and Transmission
- Virulence Factors
- Pathogenesis
- Diagnosis
- Prevention and Treatment

Illustrative Pathogen: *Cryptospirodium parvum*
- Biologic Characteristics
- Reservoir and Transmission
- Virulence Factors
- Pathogenesis
- Diagnosis
- Prevention and Treatment

Resolution of Clinical Case
Review Questions

INTRODUCTION OF CLINICAL CASE

A 24-year-old male first-year medical student went to the emergency department because of diarrhea. He had been well until the day before, when he developed cramping abdominal pain in the "center" of his stomach. As the pain increased in intensity during the day, the patient began experiencing symptoms of diarrhea. After the first bowel movement, the diarrhea consisted of nearly clear fluid with little, if any, solid material. By that night, he was febrile to 101.2°F, had constant periumbilical pain,

> *The absence of organomegaly means that no organs were enlarged on physical examination.*

and was having a diarrheal bowel movement about once every hour. Physical examination revealed signs of modest dehydration. His temperature was 101°F, his blood pressure was 105/65 mm Hg, and his pulse was 103 beats/min. His abdomen was tender in the periumbilical region; there was no rebound tenderness or organomegaly. The stool was not grossly bloody, but contained hemoglobin by dipstick examination. Unstained stool revealed both leukocytes and erythrocytes. A Gram stain showed numerous neutrophils and gull-wing–shaped gram-negative rods (Figure 6-1), in addition to normal bowel flora. On fecal culture these organisms were determined to be fastidious and microaerophilic.

FIGURE 6-1 ▶

Gull-Wing–Shaped Bacteria

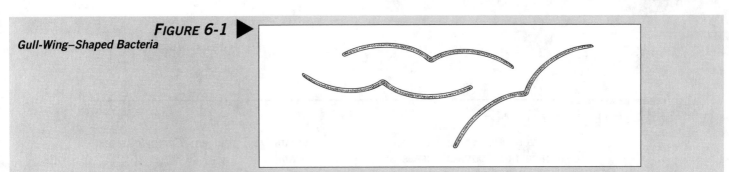

Later that day, several other first-year medical students experiencing similar symptoms were seen in the same emergency room. When questioned, all mentioned attending the medical school orientation picnic the previous day and remembered eating barbecued chicken at the picnic.

- What illness are these students suffering from?
- What microorganism causes this illness?
- How is this illness usually acquired?
- How is this illness treated?
- What is the likely outcome for these students?

INGESTION-ACQUIRED DISEASES

Ingestion is a major transmission route for infectious disease. Ingestion-acquired infectious diseases can be either true *infections* (where illness results from the ingestion of viable microorganisms into the body) or *intoxications* (where illness results directly from the ingestion of a microbial toxin). Ingestion-acquired infections or intoxications are responsible for most diarrheal illnesses, which is reasonable because the gastrointestinal (GI) tract encounters these ingestion-acquired pathogens or toxins first. However, a few ingestion-acquired pathogens or toxins cause primarily extraintestinal disease. For example, foodborne botulism causes a flaccid paralysis of the neuromuscular system, while hepatitis A virus (HAV) affects the liver.

Infections

Most ingestion-associated diseases (e.g., cholera and typhoid fever) are true infections, that is, no pathology develops unless viable pathogens colonize and multiply within the GI tract. Ingestion-acquired pathogens typically use one of two strategies to cause these infections: invasion or in vivo toxin production.

Invasion. Many ingestion-acquired bacteria (e.g., *Salmonella* spp. [see Chapter 24], *Shigella* spp. [see Chapter 13]) and all ingestion-acquired viruses (e.g., rotavirus) must invade the intestinal epithelium in order to cause disease. This intestinal invasion often results in damage to intestinal enterocytes or in a significant inflammatory response from the gastrointestinal-associated lymphoid tissue (GALT, discussed further below), producing the GI symptoms (e.g., diarrhea, cramping) associated with many ingestion-associated diseases. Inflammation induced by bacterial invasion of the intestinal epithelium often results in the presence of elevated levels of fecal leukocytes, an effect which can be diagnostically useful (see Resolution of Clinical Case, below, and Chapter 13).

Besides commonly causing GI symptoms (e.g., diarrhea, abdominal cramps), many invasive, ingestion-acquired pathogens induce more generalized symptoms (e.g., fever and effects on other organ systems), particularly if the pathogen evokes a strong cytokine response or is able to disseminate to body locations outside the GI tract after invasion. Two examples of ingestion-acquired bacteria that invade the intestinal epithelium and then disseminate to other body sites are *Salmonella typhi*, the cause of typhoid fever (see Chapter 24), and *Listeria monocytogenes*, the cause of listeriosis (see Chapter 15). Two examples of ingestion-acquired viruses that disseminate beyond the GI tract are hepatitis A virus (HAV) [see below], which disseminates to the liver after ingestion, and polioviruses (see Chapter 29), which can disseminate to the brain after invading the intestinal mucosa.

In Vivo Toxin Production. The pathogenesis of several ingestion-acquired bacterial infections requires the introduction of viable pathogens into the GI tract, where they subsequently produce exotoxins. For example, the disease cholera develops following the ingestion of *Vibrio cholerae* in contaminated water or food; having gained access to the small intestine, this bacterium attaches to the epithelium, multiplies, and secretes cholera enterotoxin (see Chapter 20). Two other examples of ingestion-acquired bacteria whose pathogenesis clearly involves in vivo toxin production are *Escherichia coli* O157:H7 and enterotoxigenic *E. coli* (see Chapter 12).

Most ingestion-acquired bacteria that produce exotoxins in vivo are noninvasive, extracellular pathogens. However, invasion and in vivo toxin production are not always exclusive events. For example, many strains of the invasive bacterium *Shigella dysenteriae* produce the potent shiga toxin (see Chapters 13 and 20).

While GI symptoms are the most common consequence of in vivo toxin production by ingestion-acquired pathogens, toxins produced in vivo can sometimes affect other body systems as well. For example, although *E. coli* O157:H7 remains in the GI tract after ingestion (i.e., does not invade the intestinal epithelium), it causes hemolytic uremic syndrome (a disease involving the kidneys; see Chapter 12) as well as hemorrhagic colitis. Hemolytic uremic syndrome develops when shiga toxin, which is produced by *E. coli* O157:H7 cells in the GI tract, is absorbed into the circulation and then transported to the kidney.

Other Mechanisms. As might be expected, a few ingestion-acquired infections do not appear to involve either toxin production or extensive invasion of the intestinal epithelium. For example, enteropathogenic *E. coli* appears to cause GI illness by binding to the intestinal epithelium and somehow inducing cytoskeletal rearrangements in enterocytes (see Chapter 12 for more details).

Intoxications

Several ingestion-associated illnesses (e.g., foodborne botulism, staphylococcal food poisoning, and the emetic form of *Bacillus cereus* food poisoning) can be true intoxications. That is, these illnesses can result simply from a microbial toxin preformed in foods or water before ingestion. Consequently, no viable microorganisms need be ingested for these intoxications to be contracted. The ability of toxins preformed in foods to cause staphylococcal and *B. cereus* emetic food poisonings helps explain why the vomiting (and to a lesser extent diarrheal) symptoms of both these intoxications typically develop rapidly (i.e., within 6 hours). Because the toxins responsible for these two illnesses are already present in contaminated foods, they are immediately available to act on their intestinal targets when contaminated food is ingested (see Chapters 19 and 20). In contrast, the pathogens responsible for ingestion-acquired infections usually must attach, multiply, invade, and/or produce toxin in vivo before inducing pathology, so symptoms of ingestion-acquired infections usually take more than 10 hours to develop.

Foodborne botulism is one ingestion-acquired intoxication whose symptoms do not develop quickly. Symptoms of foodborne botulism usually develop 12–18 hours after ingesting toxin-contaminated foods. The relatively long time required for the onset of

> There are two forms of Bacillus cereus food poisoning. These forms are differentiated on the basis of their symptoms: the "emetic" form involves mostly vomiting, while the "diarrheal" form needs no explanation.

foodborne botulism symptoms (relative to other foodborne intoxications) stems from the fact that botulinum toxin's target lies outside the GI tract (in contrast to the GI tract targets of *B. cereus* emetic toxin and staphylococcal enterotoxins). Therefore, botulinum toxin must be absorbed into the blood and transported to its target (the neuromuscular junction; see Chapter 20) before any pathologic effects develop.

TRANSMISSION

Fecal-Oral Route

A large percentage of ingestion-acquired infectious disease is transmitted by foodborne (Table 6-1) or waterborne routes. In some cases, a particular ingestion-acquired infectious disease has become specifically associated with either the foodborne or waterborne transmission route; for example, foodborne botulism, as implied by its name, is rarely if ever acquired by ingestion of contaminated water. However, such distinctions frequently become blurred in the real world; for example, HAV is often acquired by eating food that had been washed with fecally contaminated water; under these circumstances, should this virus be considered a foodborne or waterborne pathogen? Further, identifying the route of entry for an individual case of ingestion-acquired infectious disease often becomes difficult when the responsible pathogen can be transmitted via multiple routes; for example, *Shigella* spp. can be acquired by ingesting contaminated food or water, or by placing fecally contaminated objects (e.g., fingers) in the mouth.

Many ingestion-acquired infectious diseases (e.g., shigellosis; see Chapter 13) result from fecal-oral transmission mechanisms; that is, these illnesses develop after ingestion of fecally contaminated food or water or from placing fecally contaminated objects (e.g., fingers) into the mouth. Depending on the particular pathogen involved, this fecal contamination may be of human (e.g., *S. typhi*) or zoonotic origin (e.g., *Campylobacter jejuni*).

However, a number of ingestion-acquired illnesses do not typically result from fecal-oral transmission. For example, foodborne botulism usually results from ingestion of foods contaminated with *Clostridium botulinum*, a soil bacterium. Similarly, enterotoxin-producing *Staphylococcus aureus* is often introduced into foods from the skin of food handlers.

Foodborne Route

It is estimated that foodborne disease kills approximately 9000 people each year in the United States.

Young children are particularly susceptible to the dehydration and electrolyte loss induced by severe diarrheal disease.

It is estimated that tens of millions of cases of food poisoning occur every year in the United States. Even this enormous estimate may understate the true incidence of foodborne illness, as many cases involve only relatively mild symptoms and thus go unrecognized. While morbidity is the most common outcome of foodborne disease in industrialized countries, foodborne illnesses still cause a significant number of deaths in these societies, with the elderly and compromised individuals being particularly susceptible. In developing countries, food poisoning and waterborne disease represent a much more serious public health problem, causing millions of deaths each year, primarily of young children.

Foodborne diseases can be caused by either chemicals or microorganisms (or their toxins); however, approximately 75% of foodborne disease cases in the United States have a microbial origin. The major pathogens responsible for foodborne disease in the United States are listed in Table 6-1. When considering the relative frequency of involvement of individual microorganisms in food poisoning, it should be appreciated that the numbers shown in Table 6-1 represent estimates since the causative pathogen or toxin is successfully identified in only approximately 50% of all food poisoning cases.

Finally, Table 6-1 shows that most (but not all) foodborne illnesses involve GI symptoms such as diarrhea and vomiting, with fever also being fairly common (particularly for invasive gram-negative bacteria, which commonly induce a significant inflammatory response).

TABLE 6-1
Common Foodborne Microbial Pathogens

Organism	Mechanism	Frequency[a]	Incubation Period	Common Food Vehicles	Typical Clinical Symptoms[b]
I. Bacteria intoxications					
Staphylococcus aureus	Heat-stable enterotoxin	~15%	1–6 hr	Ham and baked goods (pastry)	Vomiting
Bacillus cereus (emetic form)	Heat-stable enterotoxin	~1%	1–6 hr	Fried rice	Vomiting
Clostridium botulinum	Heat-labile enterotoxin	<1%	12–72 hr	Home-preserved foods	Flaccid paralysis
In vivo toxin production					
Clostridium perfringens	Heat-labile enterotoxin	15%–20%	~12 hr	Beef, poultry, and gravy	Diarrhea
Bacillus cereus (diarrheal form)	Heat-labile enterotoxin	~1%	~12 hr	Cream sauce	Diarrhea
Escherichia coli O157:H7	Shiga-like toxin	~1%–2%	16–48 hr	Beef and apple cider	Fever and diarrhea
Enterotoxigenic *E. coli*	Heat-labile and heat-stable enterotoxins	~1%	16–72 hr	Salads	Diarrhea
Invasion					
Nontyphoid *Salmonella* spp.	Invasion and inflammation	45%–50%	12–48 hr	Chicken, beef, eggs, and milk	Fever and diarrhea
Shigella spp.	Invasion and inflammation	~15%	16–72 hr	Variable	Dysentery and fever
Campylobacter jejuni	Invasion and inflammation	5%–10%	3–5 days	Chicken, beef	Fever and diarrhea
Yersinia enterocolitica	Invasion and inflammation	~1%	~72 hr	Milk and tofu	Diarrhea
Listeria monocytogenes	Invasion and inflammation	~1%	Several days	Milk and cheese	Influenza-like
Unclear mechanism					
Vibrio parahemolyticus[c]	Unknown	~1%	10–24 hr	Shellfish	Fever and diarrhea
II. Viruses					
Hepatitis A virus	Necrosis	2%	10–45 days	Shellfish	Fever and malaise, then hepatitis
Norwalk-like viruses	Necrosis	2%	24–48 hr	Shellfish	Vomiting and diarrhea
III. Parasites[d]					
Trichinella spiralis	Invasion	1%	3–30 days	Meat (especially pork)	Fever and myalgia

[a] "Frequency" refers to the percentage of all identified microbial foodborne diseases in the United States that have been attributed to that pathogen. Numbers shown are based on data from the Centers for Disease Control from the 1970s–1980s; these percentages are likely to underestimate significantly the frequency of more recently recognized pathogens such as *E. coli* O157:H7 and *C. jejuni*.
[b] Note that nearly all foodborne illnesses involving diarrhea and vomiting also involve abdominal cramps and pain (not shown).
[c] Note that other *Vibrio* spp. (e.g., *V. vulnificus*) are increasingly important in foodborne disease.
[d] Other parasites (e.g., *Giardia lamblia*) collectively account for ~1% of microbial foodborne diseases.

Waterborne Route

Waterborne diseases are an increasing problem in the United States. For example, in 1993 over 350,000 people became ill from a single outbreak of cryptosporidiosis in Milwaukee, Wisconsin. Increasing problems with waterborne diseases result, at least

Some experts believe that even when used properly, existing chlorination and filtration technology may not completely rid drinking water of highly resistant pathogens (e.g., Cryptosporidium parvum).

in part, from the advancing age of many municipal water treatment facilities. Given the resistance of many waterborne pathogens to chlorination, a water treatment facility must perform at optimal levels, using a combination of chlorination and filtration approaches, in order to prevent the occurrence of waterborne disease outbreaks.

The immense size of the recent Milwaukee cryptosporidiosis outbreak illustrates another important point regarding waterborne disease outbreaks. Outbreaks of waterborne disease often represent an even greater threat to public health than food poisoning outbreaks since virtually everyone in a community ingests municipal water, whereas only a limited number of people typically consume a contaminated food item.

In industrialized countries possessing relatively good water treatment programs, waterborne microbial diseases are usually relatively self-limiting GI illnesses for immunocompetent individuals. However, as mentioned earlier, waterborne illnesses often have fatal outcomes (particularly for children) in Third World countries lacking adequate water treatment facilities. Even in industrialized countries, waterborne illness are typically serious or life-threatening for immunocompromised individuals. For example, a number of patients with acquired immunodeficiency syndrome (AIDS) died following the Milwaukee cryptosporidiosis outbreak (see discussion later in this chapter).

A variety of microorganisms commonly cause waterborne illness (Table 6-2), but the two waterborne pathogens becoming most important in the United States are both parasites, namely *Cryptosporidium parvum* and *Giardia lamblia*. The increasing waterborne disease problems associated with these two parasites stem, in large part, from their relatively high resistance to chlorination. Furthermore, as discussed later in this chapter, treatment of infections involving these parasites is often difficult or ineffective.

TABLE 6-2 ▶
Common Waterborne Microbial Pathogens

Pathogen	Incubation Period	Disease
Bacteria		
Vibrio cholerae[a]	Usually 2–3 days	Cholera: life-threatening diarrhea
Other gram-negative pathogens, including *Escherichia coli*[a], *Salmonella*[a] spp., *Shigella*[b] spp., and *Campylobacter jejuni*[a]	As shown in Table 6-1	Fever and diarrhea
Parasites		
Giardia lamblia[a,b]	1–4 weeks	Chronic diarrhea, fatigue, cramps, and weight loss
Entamoeba histolytica[b]	2–4 weeks	Variable, from mild diarrhea and cramps to severe dysentery; more serious in the immunocompromised patient
Cryptosporidium spp.[a,b]	5–10 days	Variable, from mild diarrhea and cramps to severe diarrhea in the immunocompromised patient
Viruses		
Hepatitis A virus[a,b]	10–45 days	Fever and vomiting, then hepatitis
Norwalk and Norwalk-like virus[a,b]	24–48 hours	Diarrhea, vomiting, and cramps
Rotavirus[b]	24–72 hours	Diarrhea, dysentery, cramps, and dehydration in young children
Enterovirus[b]	5–10 days	Gastrointestinal and other illnesses, e.g., poliomyelitis

[a] Also spread by ingestion of contaminated foods.
[b] Also spread by direct fecal-oral contamination.

DEFENSES IN THE GI TRACT

Once present in the host's GI tract, a pathogen or toxin responsible for ingestion-acquired illness encounters numerous defenses, including constitutive physical and chemical defense mechanisms, immune defense mechanisms, and the normal microbial flora of the GI tract. These GI defenses must be overcome for ingestion-acquired infectious disease to occur.

Physical and Chemical Defenses

A number of constitutive physical and chemical defense mechanisms offer the GI tract nonspecific protection against ingestion-acquired microorganisms. Immediately after ingestion, a microorganism encounters the acidity of the stomach, which kills many of these microbes before they can cause problems further down the GI tract. The ability of the stomach to help control many ingested pathogens is obvious from laboratory studies with human volunteers. These laboratory studies demonstrated that 10,000-fold fewer *V. cholerae* cells need be ingested to develop cholera when these bacteria are ingested in a sodium bicarbonate solution (which raises the pH of the stomach).

Even if a pathogen successfully passes through the stomach, several other constitutive physical and chemical defense mechanisms await further down the GI tract, including:

Bile. Many nonenteric bacteria are strongly inhibited by bile, which can act as a detergent against the plasma membrane of susceptible bacteria.

Proteolytic enzymes. The upper GI tract is bathed in large concentrations of proteases such as trypsin and chymotrypsin that can inhibit or kill microbes.

Mucus. The intestines are rich in mucus, which helps protect the intestinal epithelium by acting as a shield against microorganisms.

Intestinal motility. The constant movement of material through and eventually out of the GI tract helps to clear microorganisms.

Pathogens use several strategies to overcome the physical and chemical defenses of the GI tract. To overcome the acidity barrier of the stomach, enteric pathogens may:

1. Rely upon their being ingested in large numbers (e.g., cholera usually develops after ingestion of heavily contaminated water), which increases the probability that at least some ingested pathogens will survive their transit through the stomach.
2. Develop innate resistance to acid (e.g., ingestion-acquired viruses such as hepatitis A and poliovirus are highly acid resistant, as are *Shigella* spp.).
3. Rely upon their being ingested in food particles, which physically protects the microbe from direct exposure to the acidity of the stomach.
4. Rely upon their being ingested in foods (e.g., milk) that buffer the natural acidity of the stomach.
5. Produce enzymes such as urease that raise the pH of the pathogen's microenvironment (e.g., *Helicobacter pylori*; see Chapter 14).
6. Seek shelter on the epithelial side of the stomach's mucous layer; gastric mucus shields the gastric epithelium from the acidity of the stomach and has a buffering capacity (e.g., *H. pylori*; see Chapter 14).

Similarly, pathogens acquired by ingestion are often innately bile resistant. For example, enteric gram-negative bacteria are usually protected against the detergent effects of bile by their lipopolysaccharides, which serve as a shield to keep bile away from their otherwise detergent-sensitive outer and cytoplasmic membranes. To overcome the protective effects of mucus, many ingestion-acquired pathogens use motility to move themselves through the mucus of the GI tract to the intestinal epithelium or to produce enzymes (e.g., neuraminidase) that degrade intestinal mucus. Finally, many ingestion-acquired pathogens resist the clearing action of peristalsis by adhering to the GI tract.

The physical and chemical defenses of the GI tract also present a potential barrier to the preformed toxins responsible for foodborne intoxications. Consequently, in order to cause illness these preformed toxins must be fairly resistant molecules. For example, although the staphylococcal enterotoxins and *B. cereus* emetic toxin are proteins, both are highly resistant to intestinal proteases. In fact, these two proteins are not only resistant to the many stresses of the GI tract, they are also relatively *heat stable*, which helps them retain activity after incomplete cooking of foods. In contrast, botulinum toxin (a relatively labile molecule) uses a different strategy to resist the stresses of the GI tract. This toxin is ingested as part of a large complex, composed of several non-neurotoxic *C. botulinum* proteins that surround, and thereby protect, the botulinum toxin molecule from intestinal proteases, acidity, and other defenses. Once absorbed into the blood, this complex dissociates, releasing the neurotoxin to induce its pathologic effects.

> *Botulinum toxin can be inactivated by 5 minutes of boiling.*

Immune Defenses

The GI tract is primarily protected by two immune defense mechanisms. First, the body secretes large amounts of immunoglobulin A (IgA) into the intestinal lumen. IgA can neutralize toxins, prevent adhesion, and promote clearance; IgA often traps pathogens in mucus, which can then be cleared from the GI tract by peristalsis. However, a lag usually occurs before sufficient levels of IgA are present in the GI tract to protect against a newly ingested pathogen. This lag need not occur if the individual's GALT has recently been exposed to the same pathogen.

Besides producing intestinal IgA, the follicles of the GALT (called Peyer's patches) are also involved in providing cell-mediated immunity for the GI tract. Peyer's patches contain M cells (present in the intestinal epithelium), macrophages (which immediately underlie the M cells), B cells, and T cells. The role of M cells is to ingest pathogens and toxins and pass these along to the underlying macrophages. The macrophages then process these antigens and present the processed antigen to B and T cells, inducing IgA production and activation of cell-mediated immune responses.

Intestinal cell-mediated immune responses are particularly important for protection against invasive pathogens; unfortunately, several ingestion-acquired pathogens have developed strategies to take advantage of being ingested by M cells. Consequently, M cells actually facilitate passage of several pathogens through the intestinal epithelium (see Chapter 13). In addition, while GALT cell-mediated immune responses are clearly important for controlling many GI infections, cell-mediated immune responses also frequently result in the inflammation that leads to the symptoms associated with many ingestion-acquired invasive pathogens (see Chapter 13).

Normal Microbial Flora

The lower small intestine and large intestine of healthy people are heavily colonized with microorganisms. These normal GI flora organisms protect against many ingestion-acquired pathogens by inhibiting pathogen colonization and producing inhibitory substances that can affect pathogen growth. The effectiveness of the normal GI flora as a defense mechanism is evident from clinical observations indicating that patients receiving antibiotic therapy often develop diarrhea, which can sometimes be life-threatening (see Chapter 11).

Many successful ingestion-acquired pathogens have developed strategies to overcome the protection of the normal GI flora and thus are able to cause disease in healthy people. For example, to avoid intense competition for intestinal adherence sites with the resident flora, many ingestion-acquired pathogens produce novel adhesins, allowing these pathogens to attach to previously unoccupied sites in the GI tract. This point is illustrated by the enterotoxigenic *E. coli*, which produce not only the type 1 common pili found in normal flora strains of *E. coli*, but also unique adhesins named colonization factor antigens (CFAs). CFAs are pili that recognize different intestinal binding sites than the type 1 pili. Therefore, these CFA-producing enterotoxigenic *E. coli* strains can bind to sites in the human intestine that were not previously occupied by normal flora *E. coli*.

ILLUSTRATIVE PATHOGEN: Human rotavirus

Biologic Characteristics

Rotaviruses comprise a genus within the *Reovirus* family (see Chapter 3). This family is characterized by a genome composed of 10–12 segments of double-stranded RNA (dsRNA) molecule; rotaviruses typically possess 11 segments. Rotaviruses contain, along with their genome, a dsRNA-dependent RNA polymerase (i.e., a transcriptase) enclosed in an icosahedral capsid comprised of two layers. These viruses have no envelope. There are five serotypes of human rotaviruses as defined by antigenic determinants present in the outer capsid.

Reservoir and Transmission

Humans are the reservoir for human rotaviruses. With respect to transmission, the rotaviruses resemble other enteric viruses in that they can withstand the acidity of the stomach and pass into the intestinal tract. There they replicate in the intestinal mucosa, with or without accompanying disease. Rotaviruses are secreted into the stool, leading to transmission by the fecal-oral route. Respiratory spread of rotaviruses is suspected, but not proven.

Rotaviruses are the most common cause of infectious diarrhea in the very young, that is, children up to 2 years of age. Outbreaks involving this virus are particularly common in crowded surroundings such as hospitals and nurseries.

Virulence Factors

One of the purified rotaviral-specific, nonstructural proteins (NSP4) elicits diarrhea in newborn mice. This suggests that at least some rotaviruses encode an enterotoxin-like molecule that can dramatically affect the transport of water and ions across the intestinal mucosa.

> A viral nonstructural protein is a viral-encoded protein that is synthesized in virally infected host cells but is not present in the mature virus particle.

Pathogenesis

After ingestion, rotaviruses can induce symptoms within 48 hours in babies or very young children, while the incubation period may be 24–48 hours longer in adults. Rotaviral pathogenesis has been enigmatic because viral-induced histopathologic changes in the intestinal mucosa do not correlate well with diarrhea or other clinical features of rotaviral disease.

Compared to diarrheal illnesses of nonrotaviral etiology, rotaviruses generally cause a more prolonged and severe diarrhea, often preceded by vomiting. Severe dehydration can result from rotaviral-induced diarrhea; if not treated efficaciously, this dehydration can be fatal (particularly in infants and very young children). Rotavirus infections are nosocomially acquired infections accompanied by severe, dehydrating diarrhea that result in greater than 750,000 child deaths per year worldwide, primarily in countries lacking an adequate medical infrastructure. In the United States alone, rotavirus infection of children results in more than 500,000 physician visits, over 50,000 hospitalizations, and 20–40 deaths per year. Natural infection reduces both the incidence and severity of the disease. A rotavirus vaccine would make a major contribution to child health both in the United States and worldwide.

While the mechanisms of immune protection against rotavirus infection remain obscure, the presence of neutralizing antibodies in the intestinal lumen, either plasma derived or produced locally, seems to provide some protection against reinfection. It remains a mystery why some neonates can shed virus in their stools yet remain symptom free.

Diagnosis

Rotavirus disease cannot be diagnosed solely by its clinical symptomology. Electron microscopy of centrifuged stool samples is up to 90% effective in diagnosing rotaviruses on the basis of their distinct, multilayered capsid morphology. An enzyme-linked immunosorbent assay (ELISA) specific for a rotavirus antigen is available for testing fecal samples. Complement fixation tests and other techniques are available for demonstrating rotavirus-specific antibodies but are of limited value except for epidemiological studies.

Prevention and Treatment

The Centers for Disease Control and Prevention have recommended the inclusion of a recently developed rotavirus vaccine as part of the childhood vaccination regimen to be given at 2, 4, and 6 months of age. The live rhesus rotavirus tetravalent (RRV-TV) vaccine is composed of the rhesus G3 serotype and reassortments of the G1, G2, and G4 serotypes of rhesus and humans. The G1–G4 serotypes represent the most common of the seven rotavirus serotypes. In clinical trials, the vaccine has demonstrated 80% efficacy against severe disease and has been 48%–68% effective in patients with a more mild form of the illness; adverse side effects have been minimal. Although the vaccine has not shown 100% efficacy, this discrepancy may be due to the fact that it targets serotypes G1–G4 and may be either less effective or nonprotective in individuals infected with serotypes G5–G7. Replacement of water and electrolytes lost through diarrhea and vomiting constitutes the primary treatment for rotaviral-induced illness.

ILLUSTRATIVE PATHOGEN: Hepatitis A virus

Biologic Characteristics

HAV belongs to the family Picornaviridae and is the only virus in the genus Heptoviruses. At this time, there is only one serotype of HAV. All picornaviruses are non-enveloped, icosahedral nucleocapsids, with each particle containing a single-stranded RNA (ssRNA) molecule of positive polarity.

Reservoir and Transmission

Humans are the sole reservoir for HAV. As a typical enteric virus, this virus is transmitted via the fecal–oral route, as described for rotaviruses. HAV infection commonly develops following ingestion of fecally contaminated food (e.g., raw shellfish) or water.

Virulence Factors

Specific virulence factors have not been described for HAV. Nevertheless, several features of HAV's biology influence its pathogenicity. Its capsid proteins determine a range of susceptible cells that include hepatocytes and, very likely, cells in the intestinal tract. The cellular receptor or receptors for HAV are unknown. Unlike virtually all other picornaviruses, HAV is a noncytocidal virus. Paradoxically, HAV does not cause a persistent infection or chronic disease in humans, although it might have been predicted to do so.

Pathogenesis

Upon ingestion in contaminated water or food, HAV probably replicates in the gut. Developing relatively abruptly 2–4 weeks after infection, the influenza-like symptoms include low grade fever, malaise, anorexia, and nausea and diarrhea. Abdominal cramping and vomiting may also occur. If the immune system achieves a sufficiently high neutralizing antibody concentration in the blood, liver disease is abrogated. However, in the absence of neutralizing antibody, HAV presumably invades the blood, spreads to the liver, and causes the acute inflammatory disease called hepatitis A. Icterus (jaundice) may or may not accompany clinical disease. Liver damage is thought to be inflicted by cytotoxic lymphocytes, which destroy virus-infected cells. Most hepatitis A infections result in unapparent or very mild nonhepatitic disease with lasting immunity to reinfection. In the vast majority of patients who suffer from hepatitis A, there is complete recovery. In less than 1% of cases, the immune attack causes a fulminant hepatitis that may be fatal. Unlike hepatitis B, C, and D, HAV does not cause persistent infection.

Diagnosis

The viral hepatitides cannot be differentiated from each other solely by clinical signs. To confirm any form of hepatitis, a biochemical determination of liver enzyme (alanine aminotransferase [ALT] and aspartate aminotransferase [AST]) levels in the blood is routinely performed. However, a definitive diagnosis of hepatitis A relies on the measurement of anti-HAV IgM antibodies during clinical disease. Given the frequency of unapparent infections, the presence of immunoglobulin G (IgG) antibodies does not distinguish between a current and a previous HAV infection. For example, 75% of adults in the United States or Europe have IgG antibodies to HAV; hence, detection of these antibodies has no diagnostic value. In some instances, patient history (e.g., virus exposure from intimate association with a known hepatitis A patient) is helpful. In pregnant women, it is important to discriminate between hepatitis A and hepatitis E. Although clinically indistinguishable, only hepatitis E (caused by HEV, a member of the *Calicivirus* genus) can be fatal (in 10%–20% of cases) for these women. The reason for this remains a mystery.

The most relevant liver enzymes measured in the blood of suspected hepatitis patients are ALT (formerly serum glutamic-oxaloacetic transaminase [SGOT]) and AST (formerly serum glutamate pyruvate transaminase [SGPT]).

Prevention and Treatment

There is no chemotherapy for hepatitis A. Prevention can be implemented by two means. In patients recently exposed to HAV, passive immunity can be induced by injecting a pooled immune globulin (IG) preparation rich in anti-HAV antibodies. Presumably, this affords an increased level of neutralizing antibodies in the blood and prevents the virus from infecting the liver. Even if administered 7–10 days after virus exposure, IG can prevent or ameliorate liver disease. For those at risk of HAV exposure, a killed virus vaccine, very similar in nature to the inactivated poliovirus vaccine (see Chapter 29), is available and effective.

ILLUSTRATIVE PATHOGEN: *Campylobacter jejuni*

Biologic Characteristics

Members of the bacterial genus *Campylobacter* are motile, gull-wing shaped, oxidase-positive, gram-negative rods. These fastidious bacteria are grown on special enriched media placed into a microaerophilic environment (i.e., growth of *Campylobacter* spp. requires a CO_2-enriched atmosphere and reduced oxygen concentrations; see Chapter 3). Several species of *Campylobacter* have been associated with human disease. The most notable of the pathogenic *Campylobacter* species are *C. jejuni*, which is an extremely common cause of gastrointestinal disease (see discussion below), and *C. fetus*, which is an opportunistic pathogen that causes systemic infections in immunocompromised individuals (see Appendix 3).

Note that since Campylobacter *spp. are oxidase-positive they are not members of the family Enterobacteriacae (see Appendix 1).*

Reservoir and Transmission

The primary reservoir for *C. jejuni* is animals; humans typically become ill after consuming raw or partially cooked food (particularly poultry) contaminated with this bacterium. The most recent epidemiologic data indicate that *C. jejuni* now ranks among the five most common foodborne pathogens in the United States, causing several million cases of GI illness each year. Additionally, *C. jejuni* can sometimes be acquired by ingestion of contaminated water or from handling a sick household pet.

Virulence Factors

Like the *Shigella* (see Chapter 13), *C. jejuni* is a virulent GI pathogen, that is, ingestion of as few as several hundred *C. jejuni* cells can lead to illness. However, there is currently only limited understanding of the factors contributing to this virulence. Adhesins are believed to be important in the initial binding of *C. jejuni* to the intestinal mucosa. An enterotoxin has been identified, but its relevance to gastrointestinal disease remains unclear. *C. jejuni* produces a lipopolysaccharide (LPS) with endotoxic activity that probably contributes to *C. jejuni*-induced intestinal inflammation.

Pathogenesis

After being ingested in contaminated foods and passing through the stomach, *C. jejuni* adheres to, multiplies in, and invades the epithelium of the lower small intestine (and possibly of the upper colon). This invasion induces an inflammatory response that appears responsible for most of the clinical symptoms of *Campylobacter* enteritis. These symptoms, which begin 1–7 days after ingestion of contaminated foods and usually self-resolve about 5 days later, include fever, abdominal pain, and diarrhea characterized by the presence of leukocytes and red blood cells (RBCs) in the stool.

Diagnosis

Laboratory approaches are important for diagnosing cases of *Campylobacter* enteritis. Isolation and identification of *C. jejuni* can be achieved using special media (e.g., Skirrow's media) that are selective for *Campylobacter* species, followed by biochemical tests.

Prevention and Treatment

The best approach to preventing this illness is rigid adherence to good hygienic procedures, including thorough cooking of foods. *Campylobacter* enteritis is usually self-limiting, that is, most cases resolve without antibiotic therapy. However, antibiotics such as erythromycin may reduce the duration of illness or fecal shedding and thus are sometimes used to treat *Campylobacter* enteritis.

ILLUSTRATIVE PATHOGEN: *Giardia lamblia*

Biologic Characteristics

G. lamblia is a protozoan that exists in two forms (Figure 6-2). The vegetative form is a sting ray–shaped trophozoite containing two nuclei and bearing several flagella. Trophozoites actively multiply in the duodenum by binary fission. In the colon, the trophozoites convert into a cyst form containing four nuclei. These cysts are often excreted in the stool in large numbers and thus represent the infectious form of *G. lamblia*. Once present in the small intestine of a new host, these cysts convert back to trophozoites (with each cyst giving rise to two new trophozoites). As mentioned earlier in this chapter, *G. lamblia* cysts are environmentally resistant; for example, they can survive in untreated water for several months and are also resistant to drinking water treatments.

Reservoir and Transmission

G. lamblia has a zoonotic reservoir that probably includes wild animals, farm animals, and household pets. As mentioned above, *G. lamblia* can be acquired by ingesting untreated or inadequately treated municipal water. Since the 1980s, there have been at least 34 major outbreaks of waterborne giardiasis in the United States involving a total of over 4000 cases. *G. lamblia* is also a common illness in campers and backpackers who drink untreated water contaminated with feces from animals (or other campers). Giardiasis can also result from person-to-person spread via direct fecal-oral ingestion; this transmission mechanism is very common in day care centers and among male homosexuals. Less commonly, *G. lamblia* is acquired by ingestion of contaminated foods.

Virulence Factors

Other than the environmental resistance of the cyst, the virulence factors of *G. lamblia* remain poorly understood.

Pathogenesis

After ingestion, *G. lamblia* cysts develop back into trophozoites, which multiply in the duodenum. In many (perhaps most) people, the presence of these trophozoites is asymptomatic. When disease does develop, it usually begins about 1–3 weeks after exposure. Symptoms of giardiasis typically include an explosive, sudden-onset diarrhea that involves a foul-smelling, greasy-appearing stool devoid of blood or mucus. This diarrhea is typically accompanied by upper abdominal cramps. In adults, the acute symptoms usually resolve in 1–4 weeks, but many adults (particularly immunocompromised individuals) continue to suffer intermittent bouts (i.e., relapses) of soft stools, diarrhea, and flatulence for several weeks or months. In children the acute phase may persist for months, leading to considerable weight loss.

Most *G. lamblia*-triggered GI symptoms apparently result from intestinal malabsorption of fats and carbohydrates. The mechanism by which *G. lamblia* induces this effect remains unclear, although preliminary evidence suggests that intestinal inflammation may be involved.

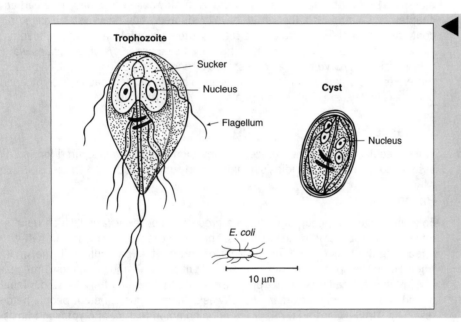

◀ **FIGURE 6-2**
Cysts and Trophozoites of Giardia lamblia.
The sucker helps the trophozoite attach to the gastrointestinal tract, while the flagellum gives the trophozoite motility. Note also the large size of both the cyst and trophozoite relative to bacteria.

Diagnosis

The definitive diagnosis of giardiasis depends on demonstrating the presence of cysts or trophozoites in stool (this becomes more difficult once a patient begins suffering only intermittent bouts of diarrhea).

Prevention and Treatment

Several approaches can be taken to help prevent giardiasis. First, it is essential that municipal water supplies be chlorinated and adequately filtered (filtration is essential since *G. lamblia* is resistant to chlorination). Second, attention to personal hygiene helps control person-to-person spread of *G. lamblia*.

Metronidazole (Flagyl) is commonly used to treat giardiasis, although alternative agents (e.g., quinicrine) can also be used. Because *G. lamblia* can be transmitted directly from person to person by close contact, it is important that family members, playmates, and other close contacts of an individual suffering from giardiasis be examined by a physician.

ILLUSTRATIVE PATHOGEN: *Cryptosporidium parvum*

Biologic Characteristics

Cryptosporidia are small intracellular protozoa. These parasites exhibit alternating sexual and asexual reproduction cycles, both of which occur in the GI tract of the host. Strains of cryptosporidia that affect humans (and dogs) are referred to as *C. parvum*. Inside the host, *C. parvum* follows a complex life cycle involving sporozoites that penetrate intestinal cells and then develop into trophozoites. These trophozoites divide asexually into eight merozoites, which can either be involved in sexual reproduction or oocyst formation. Oocysts are shed from the intestinal epithelium into the intestinal lumen. Once excreted in the stool, these oocytes can infect new hosts.

Reservoir and Transmission

Domestic animals represent an important reservoir for *C. parvum*. This is illustrated by the massive 1993 outbreak of cryptosporidiosis in Milwaukee that was cited earlier in this chapter. This outbreak is thought to have originated when heavy rains washed farm soil containing animal feces into creeks feeding the municipal water supply, leading to the entrance of *C. parvum* oocysts into the Milwaukee water system. Besides waterborne transmission, *C. parvum* can also be spread by person-to-person contact via the fecal-oral route. Person-to-person contact is believed to be the primary cause of cryptosporidiosis outbreaks in day care centers, hospitals, and other institutions.

Virulence Factors

The molecular basis for the intracellular invasion and survival required for and diarrhea associated with cryptosporidiosis remains poorly understood.

Pathogenesis

Following ingestion, oocysts undergo a process called *excystation* which results in the release of sporozoites into the intestines. These sporozoites then invade the cellular region underlying the brush border membranes of enterocytes (particularly in the small intestine). Here, the sporozoites develop into trophozoites. Through unknown mechanisms, this invasion typically results in a profuse diarrhea that begins after a 4–12 day incubation period and lasts for approximately 1–2 weeks in immunocompetent people before self-resolving. Unlike giardiasis, relapse is not a common feature of cryptosporidiosis in the immunocompetent.

Unfortunately, the prognosis for cryptosporidiosis in the immunodeficient is poor. Diarrheal symptoms in these individuals are much more severe, with fluid losses greater than 25 L/day occasionally observed. Unless the patient's immunodeficiency can be reversed, cryptosporidiosis will usually persist for the remainder of the patient's life, causing significant weakness and weight loss. About half of all AIDS patients who contract cryptosporidiosis die within 6 months. While the deaths of these AIDS victims are often directly attributed to some other infection, the malnutrition induced by cryptosporidiosis is usually a major contributing factor.

Diagnosis

Laboratory diagnosis of cryptosporidiosis depends on demonstrating the presence of oocysts in the stool. This is usually accomplished by acid-fast staining stool samples (*C. parvum* oocysts are among the few acid-fast objects found in feces). Other diagnostic assays have also been developed and are under evaluation.

Prevention and Treatment

Control of person-to-person spread of cryptosporidiosis is facilitated by good hygiene (e.g., hand washing, which is effective for preventing illness from any pathogen that is spread in feces). It is very difficult to prevent waterborne cryptosporidiosis because *C. parvum* oocysts are both very small (making them difficult to filter) and very resistant to chlorination (*C. parvum* oocysts are some 20 times more resistant to chlorination than even *G. lamblia* cysts!). New approaches to controlling waterborne cryptosporidiosis are clearly desirable. One short-term approach to prevent the development of serious cryptosporidiosis in immunocompromised individuals is for these individuals to use boiled water for drinking and preparing food (*C. parvum* is sensitive to boiling).

Treatment for cryptosporidiosis is usually unnecessary in the immunocompetent, where this disease has a self-limiting course. Unfortunately, no uniformly effective chemotherapy is available for use in immunocompromised individuals infected with *C. parvum*.

RESOLUTION OF CLINICAL CASE

Infectious diarrhea can be roughly divided into enteritis, which involves the small bowel, and colonic disease. Enteritis tends to cause abdominal pain and clear, watery diarrhea in large volume, whereas colonic pathogens produce urgency and pain on defecation with a stool that often contains mucus, blood, and neutrophils. One pathogen that actually involves the small bowel, but can appear clinically as a colitis, is *C. jejuni*, the causative agent of this clinical case. *C. jejuni* is an extremely common cause of diarrhea. *C. jejuni* is acquired orally, with more than 70% of cases resulting from the ingestion of contaminated poultry (therefore, the barbecued chicken consumed at the orientation picnic is a likely suspect for causing this outbreak of campylobacter enteritis). *C. jejuni* disease usually begins about 3 days after ingestion and typically involves fever, abdominal pain, and watery diarrhea. Bloody stools are reported in about 30% of patients, and the feces of another 30% contain microscopic blood. The stool contains polymorphonuclear leukocytes in about 80% of instances. The illness will resolve without antibiotic therapy, but antibiotics may somewhat reduce both the duration of illness and fecal shedding of *C. jejuni*. Appropriate treatment is with erythromycin or ciprofloxacin, but the latter is not given to children because it produces an arthropathy in young animals. With or without antibiotic therapy, the illness usually resolves within 3–5 days, and there are no long-term sequelae.

REVIEW QUESTIONS

Directions: For each of the following questions, choose the **one best** answer.

1. A 35-year-old female American tourist develops vomiting and an extremely severe (i.e., life-threatening) watery diarrhea while visiting India. During her trip, she has sampled the local foods and drunk the local water. Microscopic examination of her stool does not detect the presence of elevated numbers of leukocytes. Based upon this information, this woman is most likely suffering from an infection caused by which one of the following microorganisms?

   (A) Nontyphoid *Salmonella* spp.

   (B) *Vibrio cholerae*

   (C) *Campylobacter jejuni*

   (D) *Staphylococcus aureus*

   (E) *Shigella dysenteriae*

2. *Cryptosporidium parvum* is best described by which one of the following statements?

   (A) It has only a human reservoir

   (B) It is resistant to boiling

   (C) It is a noninvasive pathogen

   (D) It typically causes only a self-limiting disease in healthy, immunocompetent individuals

   (E) It is easily treated with antimicrobials

3. *Campylobacter jejuni* is one of the most common causes of bacterial food poisoning. Which one of the following statements best describes this microorganism?

   (A) It stains blue on properly prepared Gram stains

   (B) It grows well under normal atmospheric conditions

   (C) It is an invasive pathogen that causes illness primarily by inducing inflammation

   (D) It typically causes symptoms within 6 hours of ingestion

   (E) It rarely induces elevated fecal leukocyte numbers

4. A number of people attending a dinner banquet become sick about 4 hours later. They experience primarily vomiting and stomach pains, but some also have a mild diarrhea. Assuming this illness is of microbial origin, which one of the following statements is true?

   (A) This illness is more likely to have been caused by the food becoming contaminated with a gram-negative versus a gram-positive bacterium

   (B) This illness is most likely the result of in vivo toxin production

   (C) Toxins are probably not involved in this illness

   (D) Appropriate therapy for this illness will involve administration of antibiotics

   (E) None of the above

5. Rotaviral gastroenteritis is best described by which one of the following statements?

   (A) It is caused by a single-stranded, positive-sense RNA (ss[+]RNA) virus

   (B) It primarily affects adults

   (C) It is typically a congenital infection

   (D) It can induce a diarrhea with severe consequences

   (E) It only causes clinical disease once, because of the lifelong immunity induced by infection

ANSWERS AND EXPLANATIONS

1. **The answer is B.** This woman is experiencing the classic severe diarrheal symptoms of cholera. The absence of fecal leukocytes argues against this woman's illness being caused by an invasive bacterium such as nontyphoid *Salmonella* spp., *C. jejuni*, or *S. dysenteriae*. (Note that *V. cholerae* is a noninvasive pathogen.) While staphylococcal food poisoning can involve both vomiting and diarrhea, the diarrhea is not as severe as that experienced by this woman.

2. **The answer is D.** While cryptosporidiosis is a severe diarrheal illness in the immunocompromised, it is usually self-limiting in the immunocompetent. *C. parvum* is vulnerable to boiling, has a zoonotic reservoir, and is an invasive pathogen. Existing antimicrobials are largely (or totally) ineffective against *C. parvum*.

3. **The answer is C.** *C. jejuni* is a gram-negative bacteria, so it stains pink or red on Gram stains. It is microaerophilic so it does not grow well under normal atmospheric conditions. Symptoms of *C. jejuni* enteritis usually take several days to develop (the bacterium must induce an inflammatory response), and this illness usually results in elevated fecal leukocytes, a useful sign for diagnosis.

4. **The answer is E.** The clinical setting indicated in this question strongly suggests a foodborne intoxication involving preformed toxins present in foods (not in vivo toxin production). Assuming this is of microbial origin, it would most likely be either *Bacillus cereus* emetic food poisoning or staphylococcal food poisoning, both of which are caused by gram-positive bacteria. (Note that neither the symptomology nor speed of onset are indicative of botulism, another foodborne intoxication.) Therapy for foodborne intoxications usually is symptomatic. Antibiotics are ineffective because the illness results from preformed toxins in foods, and toxins are not affected by antibiotics.

5. **The answer is D.** The dehydration induced by rotaviral infection can be fatal if untreated. The rotaviruses are members of the *Reovirus* genus, which is characterized by a segmented double-stranded RNA (dsRNA) genome. Clinical rotaviral disease occurs commonly in neonates and babies, only rarely in adults. Neonates do not typically contract this virus during birth. There are five distinct human rotavirus serotypes; infection by any one will not elicit antibodies against the others.

7

PATHOGENS ACQUIRED BY INHALATION

CHAPTER OUTLINE

Introduction of Clinical Case
Pathogens Acquired by Inhalation
- Invasiveness
- Host Defenses of the Respiratory Tract

Strategies to Overcome Respiratory Host Defenses
- Infection of Compromised Hosts
- Infection of Noncompromised Hosts
- Extracellular Pathogens
- Intracellular Pathogens
- Aspiration: Another Mechanism of Entry

Infectious Diseases of the Respiratory Tract
Illustrative Pathogen: Human adenovirus
- Biologic Characteristics
- Reservoir and Transmission
- Virulence Factors
- Pathogenesis
- Diagnosis
- Prevention and Treatment

Illustrative Pathogen: *Haemophilus influenzae* type b
- Biologic Characteristics
- Reservoir and Transmission
- Virulence Factors
- Pathogenesis
- Diagnosis
- Prevention and Treatment

Resolution of Clinical Case
Review Questions

INTRODUCTION OF CLINICAL CASE

A 9-month-old female was brought to the emergency department because of fever, lethargy, irritability, and failure to eat. Although she was the product of a normal delivery and was entirely well until the onset of the present illness, the infant had never been seen by a pediatrician because of the family's financial situation. This infant first exhibited symptoms 3 days ago, when she was noted to be mildly irritable and refused to eat. The mother thought the girl appeared flushed and warm and found her rectal temperature was 100.6°F. The mother assumed the child had the "flu." The infant's condition remained about the same until 12 hours ago, when the child began to cry continuously and could not be comforted. Her rectal temperature at that time was 104.8°F. Six hours ago, the child finally fell into a fitful sleep. A few hours later, the child could not be roused; 911 was called, and a semicomatose infant was brought to the hospital.

At the hospital, the infant's temperature was 104.6°F by ear probe, the pulse was 138 beats/min (normal: 80–160), and the blood pressure was 65/50 mm Hg (average: 85/60). Examination of the skin revealed no lesions. The tympanic membranes were moderately injected but otherwise normal. The mouth and pharynx were unremarkable. The lungs were clear, and no heart murmurs were heard. The abdomen was soft and nontender without organomegaly. The infant was somnolent unless vigorously stimulated. When aroused, the child moved all four extremities. The anterior fontanel was closed. There was moderate resistance to anterior flexion of the neck, which apparently caused pain. The child was immediately started on appropriate doses of ceftriaxone (a third-generation cephalosporin). A spinal tap was performed, which yielded cloudy cerebrospinal fluid (CSF) with the following characteristics: leukocytes, 13,400/mm³, with a differential count of 83% neutrophils, 13% lymphocytes, and 4% mononuclear cells (normal: 0–5 lymphocytes/mm³); protein, 203 mg/dL (normal: 15–40 mg/dL); and glucose, 34 mg/dL (normal: >50 mg/dL). On Gram stains, numerous gram-negative coccobacilli were seen both extracellularly and within neutrophils.

- From what illness is this infant suffering?
- What pathogen is apparently responsible for this illness?
- What is the prognosis for this infant?
- Is there any significance to the age of this infant and the fact that she has never been seen by a pediatrician?

PATHOGENS ACQUIRED BY INHALATION

Inhalation of pathogens into the respiratory tract represents the single most common transmission mechanism for infectious diseases. Person-to-person spread of pathogens transmitted by inhalation is facilitated by sneezing, coughing, or by placing contaminated hands near the face. Crowding also facilitates the spread of diseases involving pathogens acquired through inhalation, helping to explain why many respiratory illnesses (e.g., influenza) are most prevalent during the winter months, when people spend more time together indoors. The prevalence of respiratory diseases during the winter months has also been attributed to (1) the low humidity of heated rooms, which drys the mucous membranes of the respiratory tract and thereby facilitates infection, and (2) the fact that cold weather may hinder the mucociliary escalator.

Invasiveness

It is not surprising that inhalation-acquired pathogens are responsible for nearly all respiratory disease. However, the entrance of pathogens into the body via inhalation sometimes results in disease outside the respiratory tract (e.g., *Neisseria meningitidis* is acquired by inhalation but causes meningitis). The type of disease caused by inhalation-acquired pathogens is (imperfectly) related to each pathogen's "invasiveness" (Table 7-1).

As indicated in Table 7-1, some pathogens acquired by inhalation simply attach to the surface of the respiratory tract and cause illness without penetrating the respiratory epithelium; these pathogens are referred to as noninvasive pathogens. Alternatively, many inhalation-acquired pathogens can invade the respiratory epithelium. Some of these microbes are low-invasive pathogens that stop at the respiratory epithelium, whereas other, highly invasive pathogens move through the respiratory epithelium into subepithelial tissues from which they may further disseminate. Further details about how pathogens invade the epithelium and the mechanisms that invasive pathogens use to disseminate to other body sites are discussed in Chapter 13.

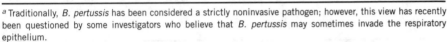

TABLE 7-1
Invasiveness of Some Pathogens That Enter the Body Via Inhalation

Do Not Typically Invade the Respiratory Epithelium	Can Invade the Respiratory Epithelium
Mycoplasma pneumoniae	Influenza virus
Pneumocystis carinii	Rhinoviruses
Bordetella pertussis[a]	*Haemophilus influenzae* type b
Corynebacterium diphtheriae	*Neisseria meningitidis*
	Cryptococcus neoformans

[a] Traditionally, *B. pertussis* has been considered a strictly noninvasive pathogen; however, this view has recently been questioned by some investigators who believe that *B. pertussis* may sometimes invade the respiratory epithelium.

After inhalation, both noninvasive and low-invasive pathogens often cause disease involving primarily respiratory tract symptoms (e.g., rhinoviruses, which invade only the respiratory epithelium and typically cause a sore throat and runny nose). To cause more generalized symptoms, these inhalation-acquired noninvasive or low-invasive pathogens must either (1) induce a strong inflammatory response (e.g., influenza virus) or (2) produce soluble toxins that can affect distant body sites (e.g., *Corynebacterium diphtheriae*). For example, the influenzavirus, which invades only the respiratory epithelium, causes generalized body aches and fever (in addition to respiratory symptoms) because it induces a significant inflammatory response (see Chapter 17). The noninvasive bacterium *C. diphtheriae* produces diphtheria toxin, which can be absorbed from the oropharynx into the circulation, leading to damage in internal organs such as the heart (see Chapter 23).

In contrast, virtually all highly invasive inhalation-acquired pathogens (i.e., pathogens that can invade through the respiratory epithelium into subepithelial tissue and then disseminate beyond the respiratory tract) are able to produce serious disease outside the respiratory tract. For example, *N. meningitidis* (see Chapter 16) and *Haemophilus influenzae* (described in detail later in this chapter) are inhalation-acquired bacteria that can be highly invasive (e.g., they both can cause meningitis). Similarly, the inhalation-acquired measles virus disseminates throughout the body, leading to disease that manifests a plethora of both respiratory and nonrespiratory symptoms, including rash, fever, and conjunctivitis (see Appendix 3).

Host Defenses of the Respiratory Tract

The role of inhalation as the most common portal for infection is somewhat surprising, considering the formidable host defenses present in the respiratory tract. For example, when most microbes are inhaled, they become trapped in the mucus-rich blanket that lines the lower respiratory tract. The mucociliary escalator then moves most of the nonadherent (see Adherence below) mucus-entrapped microbes upward into the throat, where they can be swallowed and killed by the acidity of the stomach. A similar mucociliary defense system is also present in the nares, where it helps clear microbes from the nasopharynx. Although lacking cilia and mucus, the alveoli represent another well-defended site in the respiratory tract, containing large numbers of macrophages and abundant amounts of secretory immunoglobulin A (IgA), which can block pathogen adherence. IgA also facilitates removal of pathogens via the mucociliary escalator because of an affinity between the Fc region of IgA and mucin, a mucus protein. As a result, IgA-coated microorganisms become easily entrapped in mucus, where they can be easily removed by ciliary action. The efficacy of respiratory tract defenses in clearing most microorganisms is evident from estimates that each person inhales an average of 10,000 microorganisms per day, usually without any ill effects.

STRATEGIES TO OVERCOME RESPIRATORY HOST DEFENSES

Infection of Compromised Hosts

To avoid the potent host defenses present in the respiratory tract, a number of inhalation-acquired pathogens (Table 7-2) commonly cause disease by preying, in whole or in part, on compromised people whose respiratory defenses are already weakened by immu-

TABLE 7-2 ▶

Examples of Inhalation-Acquired Pathogens Whose Disease-Causing Ability Can Be Opportunistic

Pneumocystis carinii
Cryptococcus neoformans
Coccidioides immitis
Streptococcus pneumoniae[a]
Myocobacterium tuberculosis[a]

[a] Although *S. pneumoniae* and *M. tuberculosis* are particularly good at causing disease in compromised individuals, they also sometimes cause disease in apparently healthy individuals.

Malnutrition is known to affect the functioning of the immune system.

nodeficiencies or other conditions. For example, although *Streptococcus pneumoniae* (also known as the pneumococcus; see Chapter 18) sometimes causes disease in apparently healthy people, individuals who have recently suffered from a viral infection (e.g., influenza) that damaged their mucociliary escalator are particularly predisposed to secondary infections involving this pathogen. The higher rates of respiratory illness in heavy smokers (whose mucociliary escalator is impaired) is another illustration of the opportunistic nature of many pathogens acquired by inhalation, as are the higher rates of active tuberculosis in malnourished individuals and the common involvement of inhalation-acquired pathogens in opportunistic infections occurring in patients with acquired immunodeficiency syndrome (AIDS). In particular, although fungi and protozoa acquired by inhalation are not a common cause of serious disease in immunocompetent individuals, they represent an increasingly significant cause of infections in immunocompromised people. For example, *Pneumocystis carinii* and *Cryptococcus neoformans* are important causes of infection in individuals with AIDS (see Chapter 28).

However, one of the best examples illustrating the principle that many inhalation-acquired pathogens cause infections with an opportunistic component is the common association of these pathogens with disease in young children and the elderly, two age groups in which the immune system performs suboptimally. An example of the predilection that some inhalation-acquired pathogens have for causing disease in the elderly is the increased incidence of adult pneumococcal pneumonia. Most likely, this association is a reflection of the general waning of the immune system with increasing age. The involvement of inhalation-acquired pathogens in infections of infants and young children is illustrated by the involvement of *H. influenzae* type b (Hib), *N. meningitidis* (see Chapter 16), and *S. pneumoniae* (Chapter 18) as important causes of meningitis in unvaccinated children younger than 5 years. The common involvement of these three inhalation-acquired pathogens in pediatric disease largely stems from the fact that they are all encapsulated bacteria, and it has been established that effective immune responses to all three of these pathogens requires a strong antibody response against their polysaccharide capsules (see Chapters 1 and 18). Unfortunately, producing protective antibodies against polysaccharide capsules presents a real challenge to the immune system of young children during a natural infection because immune responses to polysaccharide antigens generally involve a T-cell independent immune response, which develops slowly in young children (see Part VII).

It is possible to obtain effective capsule antibody responses by coupling a capsule to a protein carrier (see discussion later in this chapter and in Part VII).

Infection of Noncompromised Individuals

Despite the formidable host defenses present in the respiratory tract of noncompromised persons, a number of inhalation-acquired pathogens are still able to cause disease in apparently healthy people (Table 7-3). These pathogens use several effective strategies to resist or overcome the respiratory host defenses present in noncompromised individuals.

Adherence. Once inhaled (or aspirated, see Aspiration) into the respiratory tract, pathogens often attach firmly to respiratory epithelial cells. This attachment provides the pathogen with considerable resistance to the clearing attempts of the mucociliary escalator. For example, *Bordetella pertussis* and *C. diphtheriae* both produce adhesins (see Chapter 12) that firmly attach these two pathogens to respiratory epithelial cells in the bronchii and oropharynx, respectively. Viruses also use this strategy. For example, influenza virus becomes firmly attached to respiratory epithelial cells of the upper and lower respiratory tract via its surface hemagglutinin (see Chapter 17).

Production of Inhibitory Substances. A number of inhalation-acquired pathogens are known to produce substances that directly inhibit the functioning of the mucociliary escalator. For example, *Mycoplasma pneumoniae* produce large amounts of hydrogen peroxide, which is toxic to ciliated cells. Similarly, the tracheal cytotoxin of *B. pertussis* (see Chapter 29) is also thought to paralyze the cilia.

Resistance to Phagocytes. Several respiratory pathogens (particularly those that colonize the macrophage-rich lower respiratory tract) have developed specific strategies for resisting killing or inactivation by phagocytes.

Influenzavirus
Streptococcus pyogenes
Mycoplasma pneumoniae
Rhinovirus
Bordetella pertussis
Corynebacterium diphtheriae
Parainfluenza virus
Respiratory syncytial virus (RSV)

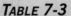

TABLE 7-3
Examples of Inhalation-Acquired Pathogens That Can Cause Disease in Noncompromised Individuals

Extracellular Pathogens

Many inhalation-acquired extracellular pathogens overcome the respiratory host defenses by inhibiting their uptake into phagocytes (where these microbes may be killed). One such commonly used antiphagocytic strategy involves producing an enzyme named IgA protease (see Chapter 19), which cleaves antibodies of the IgA 1 subclass at their hinge region, thus uncoupling the effector region (Fc) from the specificity-determining region (Fab) of these IgA molecules. This can inhibit opsonization because the resultant Fab fragments can still bind to the surface of the IgA protease-producing pathogen (a process sometimes referred to as fabulation), occupying epitopes that could otherwise be recognized by intact antibodies capable of promoting opsonization. The production of IgA protease also contributes to colonization by interfering with clearance of pathogens from the respiratory tract. IgA protease uncouples the Fc region of IgA (which mediates the binding of IgA-coated microorganisms to mucus) from the Fab fragments bound to the microbial surface. As a result, there is diminished entrapment of the IgA protease-producing pathogens in mucus and less subsequent removal of these pathogens via the mucociliary escalator. Another antiphagocytic strategy commonly used by inhalation-acquired extracellular pathogens involves the production of surface factors that inhibit uptake of these microorganisms into phagocytes. The importance of capsules as virulence factors for many pathogenic bacteria (e.g., *S. pneumoniae*, *N. meningitidis*, and *Hib*) entering the body via inhalation has already been mentioned in this chapter. The specific mechanisms by which capsules inhibit the uptake of encapsulated pathogens into phagocytes are described in detail in Chapters 16, 18, and 19. Alternatively, some inhalation-acquired extracellular pathogens produce antiphagocytic surface proteins. For example, *Streptococcus pyogenes*—the cause of streptococcal pharyngitis (strep throat)—resists phagocytosis, in part, by producing a surface protein named M protein (see Chapters 16 and 19).

Many of these encapsulated bacteria also produce IgA protease, which illustrates how successful pathogens may use more than one strategy to defeat the respiratory host defenses.

S. pyogenes not only produces M protein, it also produces an antiphagocytic capsule composed of hyaluronic acid (see Chapter 16).

Intracellular Pathogens

Inhalation-acquired intracellular pathogens generally employ strategies that facilitate their survival inside some phagocytes (see Chapter 15). For example, *Mycobacterium tuberculosis* (the cause of tuberculosis) uses several different mechanisms to survive inside nonactivated macrophages. (The intracellular survival mechanisms used by *M. tuberculosis* are described in Chapter 22.)

Aspiration: Another Mechanism of Entry

Inhalation is not the only mechanism by which microorganisms enter the respiratory tract and cause disease. Microorganisms present in the contents of the oropharyngeal cavity or stomach can also be aspirated into the respiratory tract, which may lead to significant respiratory diseases (e.g., aspiration pneumonia). Aspiration of microorganisms into the lungs represents a significant cause of disease in individuals with medical disorders, leading to unconsciousness, seizures, or swallowing difficulties, as well as in people suffering from alcohol or drug intoxications.

INFECTIOUS DISEASES OF THE RESPIRATORY TRACT

Almost all respiratory disease results from pathogens that directly enter the respiratory tract via inhalation or aspiration. Typically, these pathogens show disease tropisms (i.e., preferences) for specific portions of the respiratory tract (Figure 7-1 and Table 7-4). Although the bases for the tropisms shown in Table 7-4 remain incompletely understood, they likely involve both the particular strategy a pathogen uses to avoid the respiratory

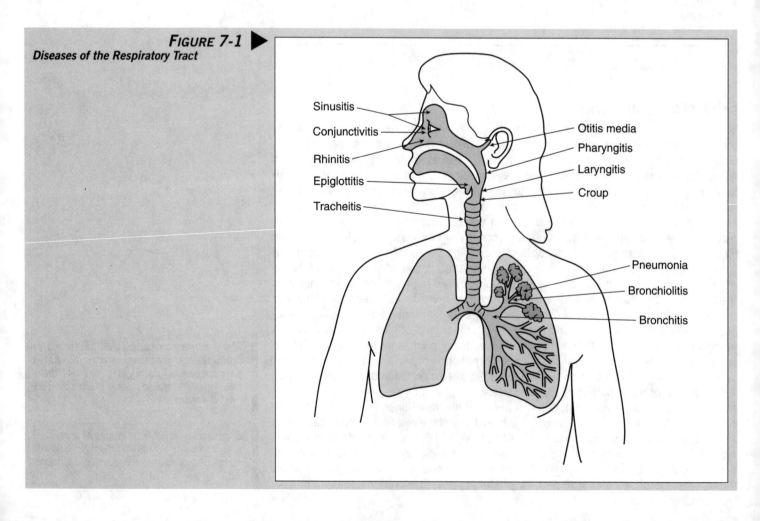

FIGURE 7-1 ▶
Diseases of the Respiratory Tract

Syndrome	Representative Pathogens
Otitis media	*Streptococcus pneumoniae*, nontypeable *Haemophilus influenzae*
Rhinitis	Rhinoviruses, coronaviruses
Acute pharyngitis	*Streptococcus pyogenes*, human adenoviruses
Epiglotittis	*H. influenzae* type b
Acute bronchitis	Influenza virus, *Mycoplasma pneumoniae*, human adenoviruses
Acute pneumonia	*S. pneumoniae*, *M. pneumoniae*, viruses[a] (e.g., influenza, respiratory syncytial virus, adenoviruses), *Legionella pneumophilia*
Chronic pneumonia	*Mycobacterium tuberculosis*[b], fungi (e.g., *Histoplasma capsulatum*, *Coccidioides immitis*, *Cryptococcus neoformans*), *Pneumocystis carinii*

[a] Viruses are a particularly important cause of pneumonia in children younger than 5 years.
[b] Pulmonary tuberculosis.

tract defenses and the pathogen's adherence specificities (i.e., some respiratory pathogens adhere better to particular regions of the respiratory tract).

Respiratory infections exhibit a wide range of severity, from the relatively mild symptoms of the common cold to the high mortality rates associated with pneumococcal pneumonia in the untreated elderly adult. Respiratory diseases (notably the pneumonias) remain among the most common causes of death in the United States as well as in Third World countries (where tuberculosis remains a major cause of mortality).

ILLUSTRATIVE PATHOGEN: Human adenovirus

Biologic Characteristics

Originally isolated from the adenoids of healthy individuals, human adenoviruses are classified into six groups (A–F) based on their DNA sequence homologies, the nature of the disease they cause, their capacity to agglutinate erythrocytes from one or more species, and their potential for causing tumors in nonpermissive hosts. The unenveloped virus particle contains double-stranded DNA (dsDNA) enclosed in an icosahedral capsid. Virus growth occurs in the nucleus, where viral DNA replication and assembly of progeny virions occur. Virus growth in vitro is cytopathic; in vivo, growth of human adenoviruses is usually cytopathic, however the virus may persist in some circumstances.

Although certain adenovirus types are tumorigenic in rodents, there is no evidence to indicate these viruses cause tumors in human beings.

Reservoir and Transmission

As implied by its name the reservoir for human adenoviruses is humans. Adenoviruses are thought to be most commonly transmitted by inhaling contaminated aerosols created by sufferers of respiratory illness. Viral strains that cause gastrointestinal disease are acid stable and survive passage through the stomach. Transference to the eye is typically facilitated by contaminated fingers but may also occur when eyes are exposed to contaminated water (e.g., while swimming in virus-contaminated water).

Virulence Factors

Unlike other DNA viruses, such as the herpesvirus (see Chapter 9), adenovirus is a lytic virus that does not make any overt effort to avoid host immune surveillance. Although the virus can infect almost any cell type of human or animal origin, replication is restricted to certain cell types. The virus can persist in certain cell types in which low levels of virus replication are observed; however, the usual outcome of adenovirus infection is the death of the infected cell with the subsequent release of newly synthesized progeny virus particles. Thus, adenovirus is a very cytopathic virus in nature. The virus encodes many gene products that have multiple functions, some of which increase the virulence of the virus in the host. The immediate early transcriptional regulatory proteins E1A and E1B have been shown to affect cell-cycle progression. While E1A binds the retinoblastoma gene product (Rb) and can induce apoptosis, E1B polypeptides bind the p53 tumor suppressor and may inhibit apoptosis. Since adenovirus is a lytic virus, it does not rely on the host and therefore encodes factors that downregulate host cell macromolecular synthesis. One of the E1B polypeptides as well as one of the E4 early gene proteins inhibit the transport of host cell RNAs and promote the cytoplasmic accumulation of viral RNAs. Adenovirus VA RNAs inhibit the cellular kinase PKR, thereby blocking translation of cellular mRNAs. In addition, the tripartite leader sequence present on all late adenoviral mRNAs enables the efficient translation of viral messages while blocking the translation of host cell mRNAs. Two other late gene products, the L4 and L3 proteins, are involved in blocking host message translation and disrupting the cellular cytokeratin network, respectively. Although the virus is very cytopathic, it does synthesize proteins that affect immune recognition of adeno-infected cells. The E3 early gene product has been shown to affect MHC class I antigen presentation and in conjunction with other E3 polypeptides can protect adeno-infected cells from TNF-mediated lysis.

Pathogenesis

Upon inhalation, groups B, C, and E adenoviruses can infect tonsillar tissue and epithelial cells of the pharynx and lower respiratory tract. If swallowed, viruses of the F group (types 40 and 41) may infect the intestinal epithelium and cause gastroenteritis. Disease resolution relies on both cellular and humoral responses. Although the presence of circulating neutralizing antibodies to adenoviruses prevents the development of clinical disease, it is unclear whether such antibodies actually prevent adenovirus "infection" (i.e., the entrance or replication of adenovirus in any cells of the body). Maternal antibodies almost certainly play an important role in protecting the newborn from both adenovirus infection and disease.

Human adenoviruses cause respiratory diseases, the most prominent of which is acute respiratory disease (ARD) in children and young adults. Certain strains may also cause gastroenteritis, pharyngitis, and conjunctivitis. Hepatitis and meningoencephalitis (as a complication of respiratory disease) are less common consequences of infection by human adenoviruses. For unknown reasons, adenoviral hemorrhagic cystitis occurs more commonly in Japan than in the United States. In immunosuppressed persons, a life-threatening pneumonia may result from adenovirus infection, and pediatric liver transplant recipients are prone to adenoviral hepatitis. However, most people who are infected with adenovirus remain asymptomatic for long periods of time, and virtually all cases of clinical disease are self-limiting unless there is an underlying immunodeficiency.

Diagnosis

Demonstrating the involvement of adenovirus in disease relies on the isolation of the virus from the throat, feces, or other appropriate specimen as well as on its subsequent growth in cultured human cells. Identification can be made using type-specific immunostaining with fluorescent antibodies or by performing antibody neutralization tests. For epidemiologic purposes, it is possible to extract viral DNA, determine a restriction map using specific endonucleases, and identify the group to which the isolated virus belongs. Although not routinely performed in hospital laboratories, anti-adenoviral antibodies can be measured in acute and convalescent sera to verify the cause of disease.

Prevention and Treatment

No effective treatment is currently available for adenoviral infections. Because adenovirus types 4 and 7 can ravage boot camps and troop concentrations by causing ARD, the military currently immunizes recruits, using live, attenuated strains of these two virus serotypes. This vaccination procedure currently is not available for civilian use.

Because adenovirus can infect a wide variety of cell types and its genome has been sequenced and is well characterized, replication-defective adenovirus recombinants have been employed as vectors for gene transfer and gene therapy. Several clinical trials are currently underway using adenovirus vectors to treat a variety of human disorders such as cancer and metabolic diseases such as cystic fibrosis, arthritis, and ornithine transcarbamylase deficiency.

ILLUSTRATIVE PATHOGEN: *Haemophilus influenzae* type b

Biologic Characteristics

The genus *Haemophilus* includes several species of small (1.0–1.5 μm in length), gram-negative coccobacilli that are nonmotile, non-spore-forming, facultative anaerobes (Figure 7-2). These bacteria are considered fastidious because many strains (but not all) require hematin, also referred to as factor X, and nicotinamide adenine dinucleotide (NAD), also referred to as factor V, for growth in culture. Hematin and NAD can be liberated from blood by the gentle lysis of red blood cells. Consequently, *Haemophilus* spp. are often grown on chocolate agar, which is prepared by incorporating gently lysed red blood cells into an agar medium. In fact, the name *Haemophilus* (Gk., *haema* for blood and *philo* for loving) stems from these bacteria usually requiring blood factors, such as X and V, for their growth.

The name **chocolate agar** refers to the rich brown color of this medium.

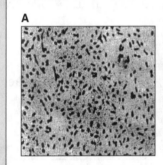 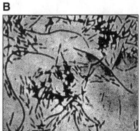 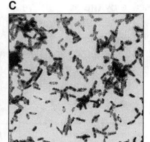

A   B   C

FIGURE 7-2
Microscopic Appearance of **Haemophilus** *spp. Gram stain of encapsulated* H. influenzae *from a primary culture grown on chocolate agar demonstrating their small coccobacilli morphology (A). Gram stain demonstrating the pleomorphic morphology of unencapsulated* H. influenzae *cultured on chocolate agar (B). For comparison, a Gram stain of* Escherichia coli *is demonstrated (C).*

Reservoir and Transmission

The human respiratory tract is considered the primary reservoir of *H. influenzae*, which is the most medically important species of *Haemophilus*. *H. influenzae* carrier rates ranging as high as 80% have been reported for children, and 20%–50% of healthy adults harbor these organisms. Most of these carriers never experience any symptoms of *H. influenzae* disease (i.e., in essence, *H. influenzae* becomes part of the normal upper respiratory tract flora in these carriers). These normal flora *H. influenzae* include both nonencapsulated and encapsulated strains, although asymptomatic carriage of nonencapsulated strains is more common. The presence of *H. influenzae* (even if transient) in so many apparently healthy individuals is undoubtedly important for transmission, which typically occurs through contaminated aerosols or by hand-to-mouth inoculation.

Virulence Factors

The only toxin known to be produced by *H. influenzae* is the endotoxin associated with its lipopolysaccharide. As described earlier in this chapter, *H. influenzae* secretes an IgA protease that may help inhibit opsonization and promote colonization. *H. influenzae* also express pili or fimbria, which are thought to function in host-specific tissue attachment. Outer membrane proteins, named afimbrial adhesins, also contribute to the ability of this pathogen to colonize the respiratory epithelium of the human host.

The most clearly defined virulence factor of *H. influenzae* is a polysaccharide capsule. *H. influenzae* are grouped into six types based on antigenic differences in the composition of this capsule. These six types are designated a, b, c, d, e, and f; a seventh type does not produce a capsule and is thus designated as nontypeable. The antiphagocytic polysaccharide capsule of *H. influenzae* plays an important role in disease by limiting the efficient uptake of this bacterium into phagocytes. The immune system may overcome the presence of this capsule by producing antibodies specific for the capsule, but (as mentioned earlier in the chapter) because polysaccharide capsules are poorly immunogenic, a mature immune response is required to elicit a protective antibody response, explaining, at least in part, why encapsulated *H. influenzae* have traditionally been such an important cause of serious disease in unvaccinated children younger than 5 years.

H. influenzae is also resistant to many antibiotics. In particular, *H. influenzae* is resistant to some β-lactams because it commonly expresses a plasmid-borne β-lactamase. It is also notable that *H. influenzae* uses natural transformation (see Chapter 5), which allows it to share genetic information with other competent members of its species.

Pathogenesis

H. influenzae causes a variety of local respiratory, ear, and eye infections but has also been a major cause of life-threatening cases of epiglottitis, pneumonia, bacteremia, and meningitis (Table 7-5). Prior to the recent introduction of a vaccine (discussed later in this chapter and in Chapter 29), 0.5% of all children developed serious *H. influenzae* disease by the age of 5 years.

As mentioned, the vast majority of both adults and children whose upper respiratory tract becomes colonized with *H. influenzae* remain asymptomatic. However, because of complex interactions between the host environment, host immune status, and the expression of *H. influenzae* virulence factors (Figure 7-3), people (particularly children)

TABLE 7-5 ▶
Important Diseases Caused by Haemophilus influenzae

Invasive Disease[a]	Noninvasive Disease[b]
Meningitis	Otis media
Epiglottitis	Respiratory disease (e.g., bronchitis, pneumonia)
Pneumonia	Conjunctivitis
Bacteremia	

[a] 90% caused by Hib.
[b] Most caused by nontypeable strains.

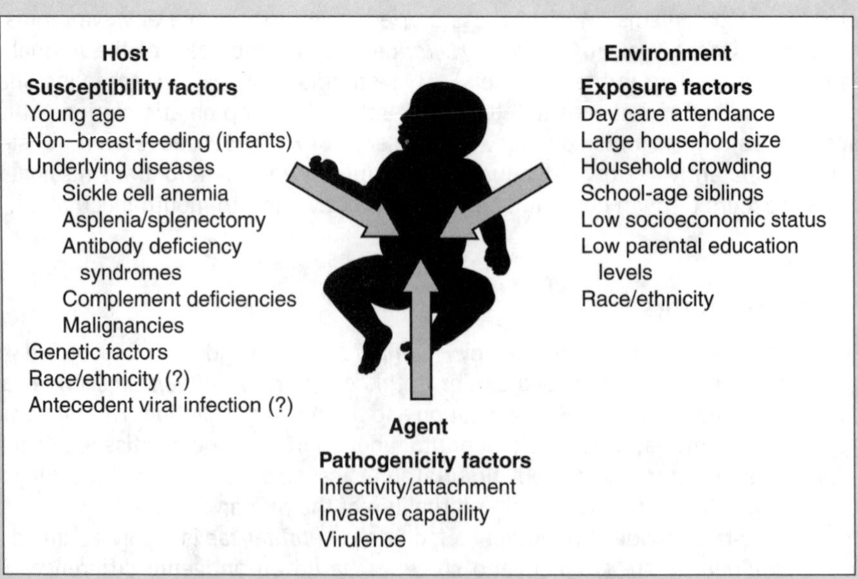

FIGURE 7-3 ▶
Interplay Between Host and Pathogen Factors in Invasive Hib Disease. (*Source: Adapted with permission from Plotkin SA, Mortimer EA, eds. Vaccines, 2nd ed. W. B. Saunders, 1994, p 346.*)

Host
Susceptibility factors
Young age
Non–breast-feeding (infants)
Underlying diseases
    Sickle cell anemia
    Asplenia/splenectomy
    Antibody deficiency
        syndromes
    Complement deficiencies
    Malignancies
Genetic factors
Race/ethnicity (?)
Antecedent viral infection (?)

Environment
Exposure factors
Day care attendance
Large household size
Household crowding
School-age siblings
Low socioeconomic status
Low parental education
    levels
Race/ethnicity

Agent
Pathogenicity factors
Infectivity/attachment
Invasive capability
Virulence

who have been asymptomatically colonized with *H. influenzae* sometimes develop symptomatic disease. As shown in Table 7-5, symptomatic disease caused by *H. influenzae* can be divided into two basic catagories: less serious, noninvasive mucosal disease and life-threatening, disseminated invasive disease.

H. influenzae mucosal disease generally involves the nonencapsulated strains that are commonly present in the oropharynx of many individuals. In mucosal diseases, *H. influenzae* causes pathology primarily by stimulating a local host inflammatory response (triggered, at least in part, by endotoxin). The particular type of disease that ensues depends on the anatomic site where the infection occurs (e.g., if infection and inflammation occur on the inner ear, otitis media results). These infections involving nontypeable (i.e., unencapsulated) *H. influenzae* rarely progress beyond the anatomic site originally infected (see Table 7-5).

In contrast, *H. influenzae* invasive disease almost always involves encapsulated strains, with more than 90% of invasive disease being caused by strains expressing the type b capsular polysaccharide (see Table 7-5). The type b polysaccharide is composed of polyribitolphosphate (PRP) and is poorly immunogenic in young children. Because of its antiphagocytic properties, the PRP capsule allows Hib to invade body compartments, including the bloodstream, epiglottis, and CSF, where its presence induces a strong inflammatory response that triggers disease symptoms.

Before development of the Hib vaccine, diseases involving invasive Hib infections often resulted in fatalities or life-long debilitating sequelae. Hib meningitis was formerly the leading cause of meningitis in young children, causing many fatalities and leading to survivors suffering permanent neural problems. Epiglottitis was another common life-threatening consequence of Hib invasion into the oropharynx. During this disease, the presence of Hib in the epiglottis induced a powerful inflammatory response that often resulted in rapid closure of the airway. Without immediate emergency medical care (e.g., a tracheotomy), the child suffocated. Hib has also been a significant cause of life-threatening respiratory disease (e.g., pneumonia) in children.

Immunity to Hib disease closely correlates with the presence of antibodies to the PRP capsule. Infants are generally protected by maternal antibodies for the first few months of life. Considering the gradual waning of maternal antibody protection in the infant and the problem infants and young children have in responding to polysaccharides (as mentioned previously), it is not surprising that the peak incidence of Hib disease in unvaccinated populations occurs between 6 and 18 months of age. In most unvaccinated individuals, PRP-specific antibody gradually develops on successive exposure of the maturing immune system to Hib strains; consequently, anti-PRP antibodies generally become detectable in sera of unvaccinated people by the age of 10 years. Because protective anti-PRP antibody develops with age, invasive Hib disease is rare in adults.

Before leaving the topic of pathogenesis, it should be noted that *H. influenzae* is not the only pathogenic *Haemophilus* species. *Haemophilus ducreyi* is the causative agent of chancroid, a sporadic sexually transmitted disease (see Chapter 9) that affects older, sexually active individuals. Current opinion is that *H. influenzae* and *H. ducreyi* are probably more distantly related than their common genus name indicates. Although these two bacteria appear similar with regard to their growth requirements and Gram-stain morphology, they cause very different diseases and are biochemically and genetically distinct. Regardless of these taxonomic questions, the important point is that disease resulting from *H. influenzae* is of high morbidity and significant mortality, whereas disease resulting from *H. ducreyi* is of low morbidity and low mortality.

Diagnosis

Because treatment must be immediately initiated for life-threatening Hib disease, presumptive diagnoses are often based on clinical symptoms and Gram stain results of applicable specimens (e.g., CSF in meningitis cases); that is, the treatment of these life-threatening illnesses often cannot wait for culture results to return from the microbiology laboratory. Agglutination tests capable of demonstrating the presence of Hib capsule in CSF also can yield helpful diagnostic information quickly, as can specific CSF tests (e.g., leukocyte counts and protein and glucose levels). However, isolation of gram-negative coccobacilli on chocolate agar is useful for providing confirming evidence of invasive *H.*

influenzae infections, particularly for patients in whom only low numbers of bacteria are present in the CSF.

In contrast, noninvasive *H. influenzae* disease is often difficult to diagnose because of the complexity of the local flora and the fact that most people colonized with *H. influenzae* are asymptomatic.

Prevention and Treatment

At least two factors can contribute to the continuation of inflammation once antibiotics have killed all of the Hib at the site of infection: (1) the dead Hib cells may slowly degrade and, therefore, continue to release soluble endotoxin, which has very proinflammatory effects (see Section 4), and (2) a lag period occurs between removal of any proinflammatory stimulus and a reduction in inflammation.

It is important to appreciate that even if antibiotic therapy is effective at killing Hib during invasive disease, an inflammatory response may continue for some time, possibly leading to permanent neural sequelae. Therefore, prophylaxis for Hib infections is obviously preferable to treatment. Fortunately, a recently developed Hib vaccine has become one of the most significant medical success stories of the past 20 years. The currently used Hib vaccine is a conjugate vaccine prepared using PRP covalently coupled to a protein (see Chapter 29). Conjugation converts the normally T-cell–independent PRP antigen to a T-cell–dependent response, allowing for an adequate immune response to start developing in children as young as 2 months of age (see Section 7 of this book). The Hib conjugate vaccine, which protects infants from both carriage of the organism and Hib disease, has resulted in a dramatic decrease in Hib disease in vaccinated pediatric populations, as shown in Figure 7-4.

H. influenzae is usually susceptible to the newer-generation β-lactam antibiotics (particularly those that are β-lactamase resistant), protein synthesis inhibitors (e.g., chloramphenicol), and sulfonamides. As mentioned earlier, many strains of *H. influenzae* produce a β-lactamase that provides resistance to some β-lactam antibiotics. In addition, chloramphenicol resistance has been reported for some strains.

FIGURE 7-4 ▶
Vaccination Has Reduced the Frequency of Hib Disease. PRP = polyribitolphosphate. (Source: *Adapted with permission from Adams WG, Deaver KA, Cochi SL, et al: Decline of childhood* Haemophilus influenzae *type b (Hib) disease in the Hib vaccine era.* JAMA 269:221–226, 1993.)

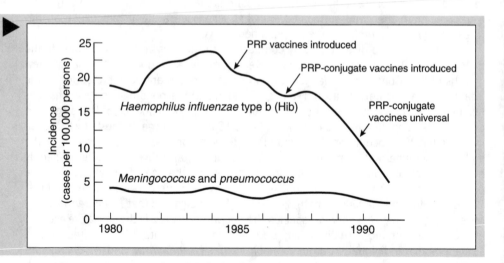

RESOLUTION OF CLINICAL CASE

These CSF findings are indicative of a bacterial meningitis. **Neutrophilic pleocytosis** *means that an elevated number of neutrophils are present.*

Because of the meningismus ("stiff neck") manifested by this child, the clinical diagnosis was some sort of meningitis, most likely bacterial. This diagnosis was confirmed by obtaining CSF, which was pyogenic in character, having a neutrophilic pleocytosis, an elevated protein, and a low level of glucose. In this case, as in most instances of bacterial meningitis, the organism was visualized on Gram stain. The gram-negative coccobacilli seen in this child's CSF are typical of *Haemophilus* spp. and suggests the involvement of *H. influenzae* in this case of infantile meningitis. This etiology would not have been unusual prior to the introduction of vaccination because Hib strains were by far the most common cause of meningitis (and other serious infections, such as epiglottitis and otitis media) in children between the ages of 6 months to 6 years. This pattern of a relatively high frequency of Hib infection and disease in the early years of childhood has been completely disrupted, however, by the widespread use of a vaccine consisting of the type b polysaccharide conjugated to a protein carrier, which can start inducing a protective immune response in infants as young as 2 months of age. Because widespread use of the vaccine has markedly reduced the incidence of Hib disease, why did this child become ill? Remember, that because of financial problems, this infant has not been seen by a pediatrician since birth, implying that she has probably not been vaccinated. The few remaining cases of type b disease in the United States occur in children who have not been vaccinated or have not responded properly to the vaccine.

The choice of ceftriaxone for treating this child was appropriate because Hib is usually sensitive to third-generation cephalosporins, which also penetrate well into the central nervous system, including the brain. However, even with prompt therapy with an appropriate antibiotic, there is concern about the prognosis for this infant. Although the overall mortality rate for patients with Hib is $< 5\%$ with appropriate antibiotic therapy, up to 50% of victims have neurologic sequelae, such as hearing loss, language delay, mental retardation, cerebral palsy, and seizures.

REVIEW QUESTIONS

Directions: For each of the following questions, choose the **one best** answer.

1. Which one of the following statements about *Haemophilus influenzae*-induced epiglottitis is correct?

    (A) No vaccine is currently available to protect against this illness

    (B) *H. influenzae* strains causing epiglottitis are usually nonencapsulated

    (C) This epiglottitis usually results from inflammation caused by invasion of *H. influenzae* in the epiglottis

    (D) This illness is primarily acquired from zoonotic reservoirs

    (E) Antibiotic therapy alone is usually sufficient to treat this illness

2. A patient becomes infected after inhaling an encapsulated bacterium that produces immunoglobulin A (IgA) protease. This bacterium stains blue-purple on a properly performed Gram stain of a fresh culture. This microorganism is most likely

    (A) *Streptococcus pneumoniae*

    (B) *Neisseria meningitidis*

    (C) *Haemophilus influenzae* type b

    (D) *S. pyogenes*

    (E) *N. gonorrhoeae*

3. A defect in B cells that leads to selective immunoglobulin A (IgA) deficiency would primarily predispose a person to which one of the following infections?

    (A) Urinary tract infection

    (B) Gastrointestinal tract infection

    (C) Respiratory tract infection

    (D) Intracellular bacterial infection

    (E) Parasitic infection

4. Immunoglobulin A (IgA) protease is best described by which one of the following statements?

    (A) It is a virulence factor produced only by gram-negative bacteria

    (B) It is often produced by encapsulated bacteria, at least in part, as an additional antiphagocytic virulence factor

    (C) It degrades IgA such that the degraded antibody can no longer bind to the bacterial surface via its effector (Fc) region

    (D) It is made only by pathogens entering the body via the respiratory tract

    (E) It is made predominantly by noninvasive pathogens

5. An 18-month-old boy is brought to the emergency department suffering from emesis (vomiting) and high fever. The boy's parents belong to a religious sect that forbids immunizations. The child becomes increasingly lethargic while in the emergency department, so a lumbar puncture is performed. The boy's cerebrospinal fluid is found to contain many leukocytes and coccobacilli. These bacteria stained pink-red on a properly performed Gram stain. Culturing indicates that this bacteria is fastidious, requiring factor X (hematin) and nicotinamide adenine dinucleotide for growth. Which one of the following statements is correct about the pathogen most likely to be causing this illness?

    (A) It produces a polypeptide capsule

    (B) It correctly Gram stains as a purple coccobacilli

    (C) It produces lipopolysaccharide

    (D) It produces potent exotoxins

    (E) It only causes meningitis

6. In June, a newly recruited Marine, who arrived at boot camp 2 weeks prior, presents to a military doctor with extreme malaise, rhinitis (inflamed nasal mucosa), coryza (profuse nasal discharge), wheezing, and cough. Upon admission to the hospital, he is febrile (103°F). His blood work-up is unremarkable. The most likely etiologic agent for his illness is

    (A) influenzavirus

    (B) respiratory syncytial virus (RSV)

    (C) a rhinovirus

    (D) an adenovirus

    (E) a coronavirus

ANSWERS AND EXPLANATIONS

1. **The answer is C.** The licensed *H. influenzae* type b (Hib) vaccine induces protection against all invasive Hib diseases, including epiglottitis. Epiglottitis is usually caused by encapsulated *H. influenzae* strains belonging to type b. Because Hib is usually transmitted from person to person, option D (zoonotic reservoirs) is incorrect. Although antibiotics may eventually kill the infecting Hib strains, epiglottitis can kill before these antibiotics take effect. Therefore, in addition to antibiotic therapy, other therapies (e.g., a tracheotomy for breathing) are usually necessary immediately after the initial diagnosis.

2. **The answer is A.** *S. pneumoniae*, a gram-positive diplococci, is a major cause of inhalation-acquired infections. Pathogenic strains of *S. pneumoniae* are encapsulated and usually produce IgA protease. Although *S. pyogenes* (option D) is gram-positive, encapsulated (with a hyaluronic acid capsule), and can be acquired by inhalation, it does not produce IgA protease. *N. meningitidis, H. influenzae* type b, and *N. gonorrhoeae* (options B, C, E, respectively) are all gram-negative (also, *N. gonorrhoeae* is not encapsulated, nor is it acquired by inhalation).

3. **The answer is C.** IgA is thought to play its most important protective role against pathogens that enter the body via the respiratory tract. This explains why so many inhalation-acquired pathogens produce IgA protease.

4. **The answer is B.** *Streptococcus pneumoniae*, a gram-positive cocci, produces IgA protease. IgA (or other antibodies) do not productively bind to the bacterial surface via the effector (Fc) region but instead bind via the specificity-determining (Fab) region. Although most bacteria that produce IgA protease enter the body via the respiratory tract, *Neisseria gonorrheae* is a sexually transmitted producer of IgA protease. Most of the IgA protease producers (e.g., *Haemophilus influenzae* type b, *N. meningitidis*) cause invasive disease.

5. **The answer is C.** The case description suggests infection with *Haemophilus influenzae* type b (Hib). In fact, the endotoxic activity of the Hib lipopolysaccharide probably plays a major role in eliciting the inflammation that is associated with invasive Hib disease. Hib produces a polysaccharide capsule and is a gram-negative coccobacillus therefore options A and B are incorrect. Exotoxins (option D) are not known to play any role in Hib disease; symptoms result from inflammation, which can be elicited (at least in part) by endotoxin. Hib causes a number of invasive diseases (most notably epiglottitis and pneumonia) in addition to meningitis (option E).

6. **The answer is D.** The setting of this case (military base), the age of the patient (young adult), and the clinical symptoms described are all typical of an adenovirus infection. Influenzavirus infections (option A) occur predominantly during the winter months (beginning in mid-to-late fall and ending by mid-spring). RSV (option B) preferentially infects infants, not young adults. Rhinoviruses (option C) and coronaviruses (option E) cause common colds, rarely the more severe respiratory disease described in this case.

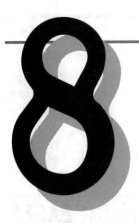

8 ZOONOTIC INFECTIONS

CHAPTER OUTLINE

Introduction of Clinical Case
Zoonotic Diseases
- General Characteristics
- Transmission
- Modes of Entry
- Clinical Manifestations
- Control of Zoonotic Diseases

Illustrative Pathogen: Rabies virus
- Biologic Characteristics
- Reservoir and Transmission
- Virulence Factors
- Pathogenesis
- Diagnosis
- Prevention and Treatment

Illustrative Pathogen: Hantavirus
- Biologic Characteristics
- Reservoir and Transmission
- Virulence Factors
- Pathogenesis
- Diagnosis
- Prevention and Treatment

Illustrative Pathogen: *Yersinia pestis*
- Biologic Characteristics
- Reservoir and Transmission
- Virulence Factors
- Pathogenesis
- Diagnosis
- Prevention and Treatment

Illustrative Pathogen: *Rickettsia rickettsii*
- Biologic Characteristics
- Reservoir and Transmission
- Virulence Factors
- Pathogenesis
- Diagnosis
- Prevention and Treatment

Illustrative Pathogen: *Borrelia burgdorferi*
- Biologic Characteristics
- Reservoir and Transmission
- Virulence Factors
- Pathogenesis
- Diagnosis
- Prevention and Treatment

Resolution of Clinical Case
Review Questions

INTRODUCTION OF CLINICAL CASE

A 39-year-old housewife went to a dermatologist because of a rash on her hip. She stated that the rash began approximately 10 days before, at which time she had a "flu-like" illness consisting of malaise, fatigue, fever, headache, and backache. Initially, the skin rash presented as a round, red, flat lesion no more than one-half inch in diameter. However, the lesion grew markedly in size, prompting the patient's visit. There was a mild burning sensation of the skin but no itching. Examination of the right posterior hip area revealed a 10-cm, annular (ring-shaped), erythematous (red) lesion. The outside edge of the lesion was the most erythematous, and the central area was clear. The entire lesion was macular (flat). On further questioning, the patient stated that she and her husband had been vacationing on Martha's Vineyard during the month of July, returning home approximately 1 week before she noticed the rash. She has no pets and did not recall receiving any bites, except by mosquitoes, during the vacation. A serum specimen was obtained, and the patient was started on an oral course of doxycycline.

- Are the flu-like symptoms and the rash linked?
- If this is an infectious disease, where did she get it, and what agent is responsible?

ZOONOTIC DISEASES

General Characteristics

> **Zoonosis** is derived from the Greek zoon for animal and noses for disease.

Zoonosis refers to an infectious disease that is transferred between vertebrate animals and humans. As will become apparent from this chapter, these diseases are more common than may be publicly perceived, they are difficult to control, and they are of emerging significance. Common sense suggests that individuals having the greatest level of animal exposure are at greatest risk for contracting a zoonotic infection. Farmers, veterinarians, and slaughterhouse workers are particularly vulnerable to these infections. This is especially true now, when the import of animals from one geographic location to another is routine. Another important source of zoonotic infection involves disease transmission from domesticated pets to their owners and other contacts. Consider that there are more than 100 million pet owners in the United States. Although zoonotic disease transmission from pet to owner is rare, more than 30 different zoonotic infections can be acquired in this manner. Simple probability indicates the passage of zoonotic infection between pet and owner is much more common than may be recognized. A final source of zoonotic infection has resulted as a consequence of humans encroaching upon virgin environments. By developing previously pristine habitats, individuals are at risk of contracting zoonotic infections, particularly those carried by insect vectors.

> **Reservoir** refers to the animal or insect in which the etiologic agent resides. **Vector** generally refers to the medium (insect or other) that transfers the etiologic agent between the animal reservoir and its human host.

Transmission

Typically, the animal reservoir component of zoonotic infection experiences either no disease or inapparent (subacute) disease. However, when the infectious agent is transmitted to man, a more severe disease may result. Transmission of zoonotic infection to the human host is accomplished through two characteristic patterns (Figure 8-1). In the first pattern, humans are "dead-end hosts" (i.e., accidental intruders in the animal-to-animal transmission of the microorganism) and cannot transmit the infectious pathogen further (e.g., rabies, Hantavirus, Lyme disease, and rickettsial disease). The second transmission pattern occurs when humans acquire the infectious agent from animals and can then pass it to other humans or animals either directly or by animal or insect vectors (e.g., plague; salmonellosis, Chapter 24; and listeriosis, Chapter 15). Understanding how an organism is transmitted from animals to humans or between humans (once transmitted from an animal) can have profound consequences for the management of disease.

FIGURE 8-1 ▶
Patterns of Zoonotic Infection

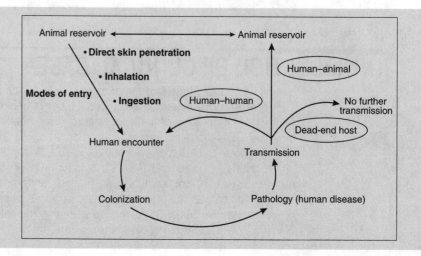

Modes of Entry

The number of medically important zoonotic infections can be overwhelming to the student. Rather than remembering each of these microbial pathogens individually, they can be more easily learned by grouping those that share a common mode of entry into the human host. The student should be familiar with the organisms, diseases, and modes of entry described in Table 8-1, while realizing that not all zoonotic infections are listed. In addition to established infections, zoonoses represent an important source of new or emerging infectious diseases. One example of an emerging zoonosis from the recent literature is mad cow disease.

> **Mad cow disease** (bovine spongiform encephalopathy) is thought to be caused by an infectious protein called a **prion**. Prions are the cause of several human diseases, including Creutzfeldt-Jakob disease. Unlike viruses, bacteria, or eukaryotic cells, prions presumably lack any nucleic acid.

◀ **TABLE 8-1**
Important Zoonotic Diseases Organized by Site of Entry

Disease	Microorganism	Arthropod Vector	Microbial Group	Reservoir
Direct skin penetration				
		Obtained through skin microabrasion		
Anthrax	*Bacillus anthracis*	None	GM+ rod with spores	Domestic mammals
Bubonic plague	*Yersinia pestis*	None	GM+ rod	Flea-to-person spread
Brucellosis	*Brucella* spp.	None	GM− rod	Goats, sheep, cattle, dogs, swine
Leptospirosis	*Leptospira interrogans*	None	Spirochete	Rodents, fox, domestic animals
		Obtained through an arthropod vector		
Lyme disease	*Borrelia burgdorferi*	Tick	Spirochete	Rodents, deer
Bubonic plague	*Yersinia pestis*	Flea	GM− rod	Urban rats
Tularemia	*Francisella tularensis*	Tick, flies	GM− rod	Rodents, rabbits, birds
Rocky Mountain spotted fever	*Rickettsia rickettsii*	Tick	Rickettsia	Wild rodents, dogs
American trypanosomiasis	*Trypanosoma cruzi*	Reduviid bug (kissing bug)	Parasite	Dogs, cats, opossums, armadillos, wild animals
		Obtained through an animal bite		
Pasteurellosis	*Pasteurella multocida*	None	GM− rod	Dogs, cats, birds, wild animals
Rabies	Rabies virus	None	Rhabdovirus	Domestic and wild animals
Inhalation				
Pneumonic plague	*Yersinia pestis*	None	GM+ rod	Person-to-person spread
Anthrax	*Bacillus anthracis*	None	GM+ rod with spores	Spores from wool and animal hides
Psittacosis	*Chlamydia psittaci*	None	Chlamydia	Fecal aerosols of sick birds
Hantavirus pulmonary syndrome	Hantavirus	None	Bunyavirus	Dried rodent feces
Histoplasmosis	*Histoplasma capsulatum*	None	Dimorphic fungus	Microconidia from soil contaminated with droppings from birds and bats
Ingestion				
Listeriosis	*Listeria monocytogenes*	Food	GM+ rod	Vegetables, water, cheese, contaminated with flora from domestic mammals, rodents, and birds
Yersiniosis	*Yersinia pseudotuberculosis*	Food	GM+ rod	Contaminated milk
Yersiniosis	*Yersinia enterocolitica*	Food	GM+ rod	Contaminated milk
Salmonellosis	*Salmonella* spp. (not typhi)	Food	GM− rod	Milk, eggs, meat, poultry and shellfish contaminated with flora of fowl, domestic mammals, turtles, and snakes
Enterohemorrhagic diarrhea	*Escherichia coli*	Food	GM− rod	Contaminated meat products, poor food preparation
Vibriosis	*Vibrio parahemolyticus*	Food	GM−, comma shaped	Contaminated shellfish
Giardiasis	*Giardia lamblia*	Food	Protozoa	Cyst contamination of water by wild animals
Toxoplasmosis	*Toxoplasma gondii*	None	Protozoa	Oocyst contamination from cat feces

Note. GM+ = gram-positive; GM− = gram-negative.

Clinical Manifestations

Most zoonotic diseases are confined to a single mode of entry. Where multiple modes of entry are possible, the different routes of entry may give rise to different clinical symptoms. A classic example illustrating this point is tularemia, which is caused by the gram-negative bacterium *Francisella tularensis*. If humans acquire this organism by handling infected rabbits or muskrats, the bacteria enter through the skin. An ulcerating papule develops at the site of penetration within 1 week. Involvement of the regional lymph node may follow. Introduction of the bacteria into the eye can result in oculoglandular tularemia. In contrast, if the bacteria are inhaled, a severe and acute pneumonia may ensue. Finally, inoculation via an insect (e.g., tick, deer fly) or animal bite can lead to systemic disease characterized by fever, malaise, and pain oriented around the site of the bite. Therefore, knowledge of modes of entry are useful in predicting or recognizing the type of disease caused by a zoonotic pathogen.

Control of Zoonotic Disease

Zoonotic infections present unique challenges for public health control. First, control of mobile animal reservoirs is difficult, if not impossible. Second, a zoonosis typically causes relatively inapparent or benign infections in animal reservoirs that go undetected. Finally, some infectious agents can be transmitted by multiple vectors (e.g., rabies in rodents and bats) making control that much more difficult. In addition to these characteristics, modern medicine has created new scenarios for zoonotic transmission through the transplantation of animal organs to humans, which is a circumstance that could introduce a benign animal pathogen into a naive human host. Because of the complexity of zoonotic diseases, a multidisciplinary approach to their prevention must be used. This approach relies on understanding the characteristics of the pathogen:reservoir:vector:human relationship for each disease. As a result, control measures for the prevention of zoonosis include disease surveillance, veterinary medicine, sanitary engineering, entomologic and wildlife management, and behavioral changes.

Xenozoonosis is a new term alluding to the transmission of an infectious agent via transplantation of an animal organ to a human being.

ILLUSTRATIVE PATHOGEN: Rabies virus

Biologic Characteristics

Rabies virus is the most medically important member of the Rhabdovirus family. It is the causative agent of rabies in humans and infects virtually all mammals. However, only a few of these mammals serve as important animal reservoirs for transmitting disease to humans. All rhabdoviruses possess one single-stranded RNA molecule as their genome. This RNA is enclosed within a helical capsid. The nucleocapsid is enclosed in an envelope containing trimers of a single viral glycoprotein. This glycoprotein is important for binding to cell receptors and for the induction of neutralizing antibodies for disease prevention through vaccination therapy. Because the RNA genome has a negative polarity, it is bound to an RNA-dependent RNA transcriptase that is responsible for transcribing the genome into the five messenger RNAs (mRNAs) that encode the viral proteins.

Vaccinologic therapy describes the administration of a vaccine postexposure with the express purpose of managing the infectious disease. This is particularly useful in slowly progressive diseases in which vaccination can elicit a protective immune response, preventing or limiting disease progression (e.g., rabies, tetanus).

Reservoir and Transmission

In the United States, rabies is rare (generally fewer than 10 cases reported annually). When it is contracted, it is most commonly transmitted through the bite of a rabid rodent or bat. Skunks and raccoons are common reservoirs and are generally ill with rabies encephalitis, resulting in aggressive behavior that often puts humans in harm's way. Bats, on the other hand, are remarkable for transmitting the disease while showing no apparent signs of disease. There is evidence suggesting that rabies, in rare cases, can penetrate mucous membranes (i.e., can be contracted by breathing in aerosols of bat excretions). In developing countries, dogs are a major reservoir for rabies, with hundreds of cases occurring annually. The reason that dogs, cats, and other pets are not a major rabies reservoir in the United States is the public health practice of vaccinating pets against this virus.

Virulence Factors

The major virulence factor of rabies virus is its tropism for and the ability to replicate in neuronal tissue. This allows the virus some measure of protection from immune surveillance and bestows its characteristic pathology within the central nervous system (CNS).

Pathogenesis

Upon gaining access to the host tissues through the animal bite, rabies virus appears to grow in muscle cells. At some point, it infects peripheral (sensory) nerve cells and moves by axonal transport to the CNS, perhaps facilitated by binding of virus to the acetylcholine receptor of neurons. Once it has gained access to the CNS, the virus multiplies in brain cells. During this time, rabies virus migrates down the peripheral nerves to other organs, in particular the salivary glands, where it is poised to be transmitted through a bite. In most vertebrates, an invariably fatal encephalitis develops, with the death of neurons and demyelination of the neuronal sheath. Curiously, the time after initial infection by an animal bite and the time of rabies encephalitis varies from several weeks to many years but typically is 1–2 months. When the bite occurs to the head, a much shorter interval exists between exposure and disease than when the bite occurs to the leg (i.e., the onset of symptomology is proportional to the distance that the virus is required to travel to reach the CNS).

In humans with rabies, initial symptoms include low-grade fever, headache, anorexia, and a change in sensation at the site of the bite. These symptoms often, but not always, are followed by confusion, lethargy, paresis, and increased salivation. In these individuals, behavioral changes, including irrational aggressive actions, often ensue. One characteristic symptom of advanced rabies is hydrophobia, which is an aversion to swallowing water because of painful spasms of the throat and neck. Within several days, seizures, paralysis, and coma may occur. Death as a result of cardiac and respiratory failure is a common consequence of untreated rabies infection.

Diagnosis

The most reliable and rapid diagnostic test for rabies is the detection of viral antigen in cells using specific, antirabies-fluorescent antibodies on tissue specimens. Specimens include biopsied CNS tissue (e.g., hippocampal neurons) as well as skin from the nape of the neck. The detection by tissue staining of Negri bodies in infected cells is still used in developing countries, but it is only 75% reliable. Therefore, the failure to detect Negri bodies does not rule out rabies. Virus recovered from infected individuals can be grown in the brains of suckling mice or in cells cultured in vitro, but this takes time on the order of weeks to months. The clinical history of an animal bite or contact with rabid animals is the single most important reason to suspect rabies exposure. In practice, diagnosis of rabies does not affect treatment, but it does influence the course of postexposure prophylaxis to those not yet experiencing disease.

Negri bodies are viral-induced, perinuclear, eosinophilic, spherical structures formed in rabies-infected cells. These structures can be visualized by cytochemical staining.

Prevention and Treatment

There is no antiviral therapy for rabies. *Pre-exposure immunization* using inactivated virus derived from diploid cells (i.e., human diploid cell vaccine [HDCV]) is recommended for individuals at high risk (e.g., zookeepers and veterinarians). As stated above, mandatory vaccination of pets has significantly limited human rabies in the United States by effectively decreasing its incidence within the animals with which humans have frequent direct contact. *Postexposure rabies immunization* involves the immediate cleansing of the wound and the injection of human rabies immune globulin (HRIG) into the wound site and another site (e.g., the buttocks). At the same time, the patient receives a series of five injections of HDCV vaccine. The decision to proceed with postexposure treatment depends on knowing whether rabies is endemic to the animal community, what animals are infected (e.g., raccoons, squirrels, foxes), and the history of the particular animal inflicting the bite (e.g., if the animal has been previously vaccinated for rabies).

ILLUSTRATIVE PATHOGEN: Hantavirus

Biologic Characteristics

Hantaviruses comprise one of five genera of the family Bunyaviridae. The spherical virus particles possess a nucleocapsid containing three distinct RNA molecules, each having negative polarity. Bound to each of the virion RNAs are a virus-specific transcriptase and multiple copies of a virus-encoded RNA-binding protein. The envelope of the virus particle is derived from intracytoplasmic membranes and presents two different viral glycoproteins on the virion surface. The prototype virus of this group is called Hantaan virus.

Reservoir and Transmission

Hantaviruses persistently infect a variety of rodent species, often causing inapparent infections. Infectious virus particles are found in the urine, saliva, and, in some cases, the feces of infected animals, including mice, rats, and moles. Transmission to human beings occurs by inhaling aerosols containing infectious material. Human-to-human transmission is uncommon. Hantaviral disease is associated with rural settings, but serologic studies have detected anti-Hantavirus antibodies in urban communities throughout the world.

Virulence Factors

The two envelope glycoproteins determine both the host range and hemagglutination properties of Hantavirus particles. Clearly, the capacity to multiply aggressively in the infected host, to be excreted, and to survive dehydration contributes to the pathogenesis of these viruses.

Pathogenesis

It is important to recognize that most Hantavirus-infected humans experience an asymptomatic infection that stimulates lasting immunity to reinfection. However, three distinct diseases may arise from infection by different Hantavirus strains: hemorrhagic fever (HF), hemorrhagic fever with renal syndrome (HFRS), and Hantavirus pulmonary syndrome (HPS). Whereas the mortality rate of HF can be as high as 10%, the mortality rates for HFRS and HPS can be significantly higher. In all these disease syndromes, the virus appears to invade the animal or human host via the respiratory route, where it replicates and spreads—probably via the blood (and possibly within infected blood cells)—to other organs, including the heart, gut, liver, kidney, and CNS. Initial symptoms include fever and any or all of the following: headache, malaise, myalgia, and gastrointestinal distress, including vomiting, diarrhea, or cramping. Once systemically spread, Hantaviruses apparently grow and damage the cells of the vascular endothelium, which results in hemorrhaging. The dysfunction in blood vessel permeability with the accompanying loss of plasma proteins results in hypovolemia, and shock often follows. Hemorrhagic disease complicated by renal shutdown (HFRS) adds to the severity of the disease and further complicates the maintenance of blood volume and electrolyte balance. The role of the immune system in the etiology of hantaviral disease remains obscure.

In 1993, a new Hantavirus serotype, Sin Nombre virus, was isolated from adults living in the southwestern United States who suffered from a severe respiratory infection (later called HPS). Approximately 60% of those that fell ill died. Although HPS is considered a newly emerging disease, it is known that Sin Nombre virus existed prior to 1993 because a similar disease was described in South America prior to this outbreak. One explanation for the emergence of this disease rests on climate changes that affected rodent populations.

Hypovolemia *is an abnormal decrease in the volume of circulating plasma.*

Diagnosis

Diagnosis is made on the basis of clinical history and symptoms. This diagnosis can be confirmed by demonstration of viral RNA in lung tissue using a polymerase chain reaction

(PCR) test, by immunocytochemistry on lung tissue to detect hantaviral antigens, or by a serologic serum test for immunoglobulin M (IgM) antibodies specific for Hantaviruses. Generally, hospitals are not equipped to perform these tests. Instead, these tests are performed by highly specialized laboratories.

Prevention and Treatment

It remains questionable whether the antiviral drug ribavirin can ameliorate Hantavirus diseases. There are reports that the drug decreases the mortality of HF and HFRS, but its effectiveness in treating HPS is unproven. Regardless of antiviral therapy, it is crucial to reverse the dramatic effects of virus infection on vascular permeability by intravenous transfusions of fluid, including electrolytes, and implementing kidney dialysis if renal failure occurs. Prevention involves educating populations at risk (e.g., farmers, campers) to avoid vacant shelters and areas in which rodent infestation is apparent or likely.

> The antiviral agent **ribavirin** (D-ribofuranosyl-1,2,4-triazole-3-carboxamide) is an analog of guanosine. Although its mechanism of action is not fully understood, it can inhibit viral-directed RNA synthesis in cells infected with several different RNA viruses.

ILLUSTRATIVE PATHOGEN: *Yersinia pestis*

Biologic Characteristics

The genus *Yersinia* is a member of the Enterobacteriaceae (see Chapter 12). Three species of *Yersinia* are pathogenic to humans. *Y. enterocolitica* causes a broad range of gastrointestinal syndromes, and *Y. pseudotuberculosis* causes adenitis and septicemia. Both are zoonotic enteric diseases transmitted by ingestion of contaminated food products. *Y. pestis* is the causative agent of plague, also known as the black death.

    Y. pestis is a small, gram-negative rod that is often referred to as the plague bacillus. This organism is nonmotile, non–spore-forming, and it exhibits a unique bipolar staining pattern when stained with Giemsa stain. The organism can grow between the temperatures of 4°C and 40°C, with 28°C being the optimal growth temperature. The temperature at which this organism is cultivated, as well as other environmental considerations (e.g., calcium and iron concentrations), can profoundly affect the expression of its virulence factors. Upon direct inoculation of a patient's specimen on most types of bacteriologic media, *Y. pestis* produces a viscous gray colony indicative of capsular polysaccharide production. This phenotype is lost upon subsequent passage (recall phase variation; Chapter 1).

> The bipolar staining characteristics of Yersinia pestis *can be best visualized using Giemsa stain.*

Bipolar staining

Reservoir and Transmission

The plague bacillus has been endemic in the wild rodents of Europe and Asia for centuries but entered North America in the early 1900s as a result of transcontinental shipping. It is now endemic to rodents in the western United States. Presently, more than 90% of the global incidence of plague occurs in Southeast Asia. As summarized in Figure 8-2, plague is perpetuated in three ways: (1) among commensal rodents using fleas as a vector (referred to as sylvatic plague or wild plague), (2) urban rat plague, which is transmitted by the rat flea (referred to as urban or domestic plague), and (3) human plague, which may be acquired on direct contact with either of the former cycles or through the bite of a tick. Bubonic plague in humans typically manifests itself by the spread to regional lymph nodes, which become swollen and tender, giving rise to buboes, hence, the name bubonic plague. Upon systemic spread throughout the host organs, the plague bacillus can reach the lungs. This gives rise to pneumonic plague, a condition that is approximately 50% fatal. In this form, human-to-human spread occurs by inhalation of septic aerosols.

Virulence Factors

Y. pestis is a facultative intracellular parasite. *Y. pestis* does not grow at 37°C in calcium-deficient media, and the loss of this property correlates with loss of virulence. As described below, sensitivity to calcium concentration is important for these organisms to

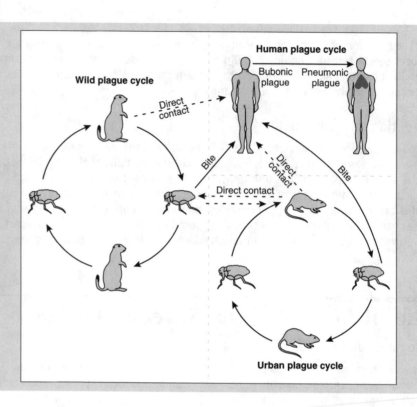

FIGURE 8-2 ▶
Summary of the Wild Plague Cycle, the Human Plague Cycle, and the Urban Plague Cycle

---

Virulence Factors of Y. pestis
- *Calcium, temperature, and iron regulation*
- *Yops*
- *Pigment-binding proteins*
- *Envelope antigens (F-1)*
- *V and W antigens*
- *Pesticin and Pla*

inhibit phagocytosis. These and other properties that appear to facilitate virulence are described in detail below.

Calcium Dependency. In the absence of calcium at 37°C, *Y. pestis* decreases protein synthesis and grows more slowly. Accompanying this low-calcium response (lcr) is an increased expression of several virulence-related proteins, the V and W antigens, and several Yops (see below). This lcr phenotype is mediated by a large plasmid encoding the calcium regulatory protein and several other virulence factors.

Pigment-Binding and Iron-Regulated Surface Proteins. The ability of an organism to acquire iron from the host environment is a recurring theme in the pathogenesis of many microbial pathogens. *Y. pestis* produces siderophores that require other bacterial surface proteins for their uptake. In addition, heme-binding proteins also are found at the organism's surface, enabling it to use heme as a sole source of iron. Virulent *Y. pestis* absorbs heme and other basic dyes at their cell surface during growth at 26°C, forming a pigmented colony. Mutational loss of this phenotype results in organisms that are no longer virulent.

Yersinia Outer Proteins (Yops). *Y. pestis* expresses 11 calcium-derepressible Yops. These proteins collectively function in the translocation of effector molecules across the host plasma cell membrane, causing cellular dysfunction. This process is initiated by the YopB and YopD proteins in conjunction with a contact secretion system, known as a type III secretion system. Upon intimate association between the bacterium and host cell, YopB is inserted into the plasma cell membrane with the help of YopD. YopB facilitates the "injection" of a second group of Yops—known as effectors of host cell response—into the host cell. Examples of these effectors include YopO and YopH, which function in the phosphorylation or dephosphorylation of key components of the host cell signal transduction pathway, and YopE, which is involved in the depolymerization of actin. The net result is Yop-mediated cellular disruption of normal function. In the case of phagocytic cells, this includes the ability to phagocytose *Y. pestis*.

Envelope Antigens. This antigen, also referred to as F-1 antigen, is a soluble glycoprotein mixture associated with the cell surface of *Y. pestis* grown at 37°C. It is antiphagocytic and is thought to play a role during the septicemic phase of the disease. F-1 is highly antigenic, and F-1–specific antibodies protect individuals from disease.

V and W Antigens. These antigens are always produced together. The V antigen is a 38-kD protein, and the W antigen is a 145-kD lipoprotein. The in vivo production of these antigens correlates with the ability of *Y. pestis* to cause an overwhelming septicemia. How this is accomplished is not clear.

Pesticin and Pla. The production of these components is genetically linked and is encoded by a plasmid. They are not regulated by calcium, temperature, or iron. Pesticin is a bacteriocin produced by *Y. pestis* that inhibits the growth of other organisms but not *Y. pestis*, thus giving this organism a competitive edge in colonizing a site. The Pla protease is a plasminogen activator that resides at the bacterial cell surface and also can cleave the complement component C3. Although strains lacking these genes still cause disease, their virulence is attenuated.

> *A* **bacteriocin** is a compound secreted by a bacteria that is toxic to bacteria of other species.

Pathogenesis

The pathogenesis of *Y. pestis* is both complex and fascinating. *Yersinia* infects a flea while the flea takes a blood meal from a bacteremic rodent. The blood clots in the flea's stomach because of the activation of the *Y. pestis* Pla protease. The bacteria are trapped in the fibrin clot and proliferate to large numbers in this nutrient-rich environment. The mass of organisms and the fibrin block the proventriculus of the flea's intestinal tract, and, during its next blood meal, the flea regurgitates the organisms into the next rodent or human host.

Upon gaining access to humans, *Y. pestis* avoids phagocyte ingestion by the production of its envelope antigens, including Yops. In the absence of this phagocytosis, rapid growth ensures spread to regional lymph nodes, causing the characteristic buboe. Dissemination throughout the body may follow. If the bacteria attain high enough levels in the bloodstream, they cause endotoxin-related disease symptoms, such as disseminated intravascular coagulation (DIC) and cutaneous hemorrhages. Pneumonic plague has a similar pathogenesis, except the lungs appear to provide a very efficient portal of entry into the lymphatics in addition to the symptoms of pneumonia. This may explain the high fatality rate of this disease.

Diagnosis

The symptoms and clinical history of the patient, including exposure history, are generally informative. The presence of buboes is the finding in bubonic plague. In pneumonic plague, a general pneumonia ensues and is life threatening. In either disease, septic shock may occur. A Gram stain of a smear or culture of blood or pus from a buboe can confirm the presence of a gram-negative rod but will not narrow a bacterial pneumonia or sepsis case to *Y. pestis*. Fluorescent antibody staining of tissues using antibody specific for *Y. pestis* is an accurate diagnosis. Finally, because of the highly infectious nature of *Y. pestis*, great care must be taken by the physician and laboratory personnel in handling infectious specimens.

Prevention and Treatment

Prevention of plague is most easily achieved by limiting the spread of rats in urban areas and by avoiding both flea bites and contact with dead, wild rodents. Patients with plague must be placed in strict isolation, and antibiotic therapy must be initiated immediately. *Y. pestis* responds well to a combination of streptomycin and tetracycline. No substantial antibiotic resistance has been reported. Because of the rapid progression of the disease, antimicrobial therapy should be initiated prior to bacteriologic culture results. In some cases, close contacts of the patient should also be treated prophylactically with antibiotics and observed for fever. A formalin-killed vaccine for the prevention of bubonic plague is available, but it is not effective against pneumonic plague.

ILLUSTRATIVE PATHOGEN: *Rickettsia rickettsii*

Biologic Characteristics

Rickettsiae are important causes of diseases in the United States and around the world (Table 8-2). They comprise a family of atypical bacteria grouped on the basis of clinical

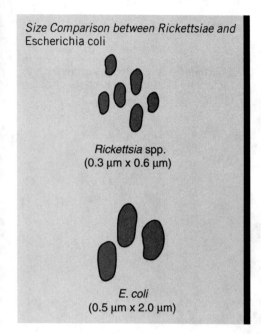

Size Comparison between Rickettsiae and Escherichia coli

Rickettsia spp.
(0.3 μm x 0.6 μm)

E. coli
(0.5 μm x 2.0 μm)

features associated with disease, epidemiologic characteristics, and morphologic properties. Rickettsiae are obligate intracellular pathogens and are characteristically smaller than typical bacteria (600 × 300 nm in size). Like gram-negative bacteria, Rickettsiae possess an outer membrane that contains lipopolysaccharide, a cell wall, and an inner membrane. They are transmitted to humans by way of arthropod vectors—typically, a tick, louse, mite, chigger, or flea. Because of this property, rickettsial disease is typically geographically restricted to the distribution of the arthropod. Rickettsia spp. are generally organized into two antigenically distinct groups that give rise to two different clinical presentations: the spotted fever group, which present initially with a characteristic rash, and the typhus group, which present with more generalized symptoms. Within the United States, Rocky Mountain spotted fever is the most common disease caused by the Rickettsiae, causing 600–1000 annual cases. This section focuses on Rocky Mountain spotted fever; however, it is advisable for students to be aware of other significant rickettsial diseases. Representative examples are listed in Table 8-2.

Reservoir and Transmission

The term "Rocky Mountain spotted fever" is misleading because this disease is distributed throughout North and South America, with the highest frequency in Oklahoma and North Carolina. Ticks of the Dermacentor genus (D. andersoni in the west and D. variabilis in the east) harbor R. rickettsii. This pathogen is maintained within the environment principally by transovarial transmission from infected female ticks to offspring. Less commonly, uninfected ticks become infected after feeding on small mammals experiencing a rickettsitemia. For this mode of transmission to ticks, many different animals can serve as reservoirs in the wild (although rodents and dogs appear to be the most common).

TABLE 8-2 ▶

Diseases Caused by Rickettsia spp.

Disease	Rickettsia Species	Geographic Distribution	Arthropod Vector	Animal Reservoir
Spotted fever group				
Rocky Mountain spotted fever	R. rickettsii	North and South America	Tick	Wild rodents, dogs
Rickettsial pox	R. akari	Global	Mite	Mouse
Typhus group				
Endemic typhus	R. prowazekii	Global	Body louse	Humans, flying squirrel
Murine typhus	R. typhi	Global	Rat flea	Small rodents

Transmission to humans is accomplished by a tick bite. People who have pets or who explore wooded areas are particularly vulnerable to tick exposure.

Virulence Factors

R. rickettsii has the ability to direct actin reorganization within infected cells. This results in the formation of cell projections (filopodia), which can enhance spread between cells that comprise vascular linings (Figure 8-3). Intracellular rickettsial multiplication either directly lyse cells or organize filopodia to facilitate membrane fusion with an adjacent cell. Injury to infected endothelial cells is thought to be due to rickettsial phospholipases, proteases, and membrane peroxidation. As part of their intracellular localization, Rickettsiae have evolved a system that exchanges adenosine diphosphate (ADP) for the higher energy form of adenosine triphosphate (ATP) from the intracellular environment of the host. This confers the advantage of making the host cell support the metabolism of the bacteria, in effect making Rickettsiae energy parasites.

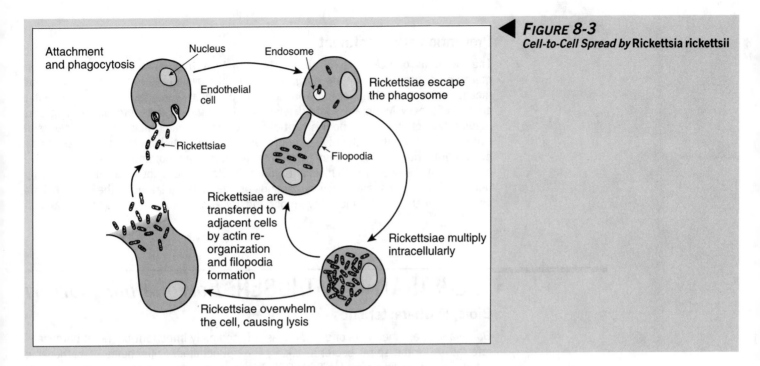

FIGURE 8-3
Cell-to-Cell Spread by **Rickettsia rickettsii**

Pathogenesis

Rocky Mountain spotted fever is among the most severe human infectious diseases, with a mortality rate, when untreated, of 20%–25%. With treatment, the case fatality rate is 4%. Access to the host is obtained by the bite of an infected tick that gives rise to a local vasculitis. Systemic, multiorgan involvement and infection of tissue endothelial beds occurs as Rickettsiae disseminate from the site of infection to the bloodstream. Advanced symptoms of Rocky Mountain spotted fever ultimately reflect damage to the integrity of important vital organs.

After the initial tick bite, the incubation period ranges from 2–12 days. Disease typically begins abruptly with fever, malaise, severe frontal headache, myalgia, and vomiting. Abdominal pain, diarrhea, conjunctivitis, mental confusion, meningitis, respiratory difficulties, renal dysfunction, or myocarditis may follow. A rash develops 2–4 days after the onset of symptoms and is generally localized to the extremities. Rickettsiae readily invade many mammalian cells yet are mainly seen in the vascular endothelium. It is thought that lysis of endothelial cells leads to rupture of capillaries and small vessels. Rash and a state of mental confusion may be a consequence of micro-hemorrhaging in the skin and CNS, respectively.

Diagnosis

Definitive diagnosis of Rocky Mountain spotted fever is a difficult clinical challenge. This diagnosis is typically based on the clinical signs and exposure history. Two problems in isolating and identifying Rickettsiae are that they exhibit fastidious growth requirements, making them difficult to culture, and they do not Gram stain. Furthermore, they are extremely infectious so that isolation by most clinical laboratories places health care professionals at risk. As a result, commonly used tests include immunostaining of patient specimens with antirickettsial antibodies to detect specific rickettsial antigens or measuring specific antirickettsial antibody levels in patient sera. Because of the difficulty in cultivating *R. rickettsii*, cross-reactive antigens from nonrickettsial sources often have been used to perform serologic tests (i.e., the detection of antibody against the infecting organism). This forms the basis for the Weil-Felix test, which uses antigens derived from an unrelated organism (i.e., *Proteus vulgaris*) in lieu of rickettsial antigens. Although this diagnostic test is relatively insensitive and nonspecific, it does have the advantage of being inexpensive. Because of the low incidence of rickettsial disease, there is little incentive to develop a more sensitive and specific diagnostic test.

Prevention and Treatment

The morbidity of rickettsial disease is too low to warrant a vaccine and traditional measures of vector control are not practical. Public awareness is the most important means for its prevention. For individuals exposed to heavily infested tick environments, control of Rocky Mountain spotted fever can be augmented by proper clothing and regular inspection of their bodies for ticks. The time between tick bite and rickettsial transmission is on the order of 1–2 hours, and removal of ticks within this interval can prevent infection. Prompt treatment with tetracyclines or chloramphenicols is effective against early disease. As with most antibiotics, treatment does not kill all of the infecting rickettsial organisms, and recovery depends on the immune status of the patient. This accounts for the greater mortality among elderly and immunosuppressed individuals.

ILLUSTRATIVE PATHOGEN: *Borrelia burgdorferi*

Biologic Characteristics

Borrelia spp. are members of a small class of medically important bacterial pathogens referred to as the spiral bacteria, a.k.a., the spirochetes. Spirochetes of pathogenic significance are summarized in Table 8-3. All spirochetes have an ultrastructure consisting of an outer and inner membrane and an intervening periplasmic space. They differ from gram-negative bacteria by containing several flagellar structures within the periplasm, which typically extend from the surface of bacteria (see Figure 1-2). This gives rise to the characteristic "corkscrew" appearance of the spirochete. Because spirochetes are so thin (0.1–0.2 µm), they cannot be seen by standard light microscopic techniques such as those employed in the Gram-stain procedure. Instead, special stains (e.g., silver impregnation or immunofluorescence) or special lighting conditions (e.g., darkfield microscopy) must be used to visualize these organisms.

TABLE 8-3 ▶
Spirochetes of Pathogenic Significance

Spirochete	Disease Caused by Biologic Agent	Notable Characteristics
Treponema spp.		
	Syphilis caused by *T. pallidum* subspecies *pallidum*	Sexually transmitted disease (see Chapters 9, 25)
	Yaws caused by *T. pallidum* subspecies *pertenue*	Tropical disease, not sexually transmitted but similar in clinical symptomology to syphilis
	Pinta caused by *T. carateum*	Tropical disease acquired by person-to-person contact or through insect bites; causes cutaneous lesions that initially are hyperpigmented but later become depigmented
Borrelia spp.		
	Lyme disease caused by *B. burgdorferi*	Acquired through the bite of a tick; symptoms include a characteristic rash (ECM) followed by arthritis.
	Relapsing fever caused by *B. recurrentis*	Acquired through an insect bite; symptoms are characterized by systemic disease lasting 2–5 days followed by decline, only to recur 4–10 days later
Leptospira spp.		
	Leptospirosis caused by *L. interrogans*	Foodborne illness associated with febrile jaundice and nephritis

B. burgdorferi is the etiologic agent of Lyme disease, or Lyme borreliosis. This is a complex, progressive, and systemic illness that was not recognized in the United States until two housewives in Lyme, Connecticut, brought a peculiar clustering of juvenile rheumatoid arthritis cases to the attention of the health officials. Although the disease has been recognized in the United States for only 20 years, European physicians have described a similar disease under different names since 1883. Within the United States, a total of 16,461 cases of Lyme disease were reported to the Centers for Disease Control and Prevention in 1996, underscoring its significance as a frequent zoonotic infection.

Reservoir and Transmission

Lyme disease is transmitted by a tick bite, typically by a member of the genus *Ixoides*. Although Lyme borreliosis has been described throughout the United States, there are three major endemic foci: the coastal wooded regions of southern New England, New York, and the Middle Atlantic states; areas of Wisconsin, Michigan, and Minnesota; and the coastal and wooded areas of California and Oregon. This distribution is largely a consequence of the distribution and biology of the *Ixoides* tick. These ticks exhibit three seasonal stages in their life cycle: larva, nymph, and adult. All forms can attach to the human host, but only the nymph and adult stages can transmit the disease. Because of the seasonal life cycle of the vector, Lyme disease in the northeastern and north central United States occurs from May through August, peaking in July. In the western region, disease most often occurs from January through May. Human–tick–human and human–human transmission are not known to occur, except for vertical transmission from mother to fetus, which can result in the death of the neonate.

Virulence Factors

Because of the fastidious growth requirements of *B. burgdorferi*, only limited aspects of its biology are known. *B. burgdorferi* expresses important surface proteins, referred to as outer surface proteins (Osps). The Osps are lipoproteins, and several demonstrate antigenic variability that may be important for immune escape (see Chapter 17). Furthermore, these surface proteins are differentially expressed depending on whether the organism is growing in the tick or the human. Osps are thought to be important for tissue attachment and for the activation of *B. burgdorferi* growth in the tick or the human. Plasmids have been associated with *B. burgdorferi*, one of which expresses proteins that correspond to OspA and OspB. How Osps, or other molecules produced by *B. burgdorferi*, contribute to Lyme disease pathology is not understood. However, several Osps form the basis of a promising vaccine for the management of Lyme disease.

Pathogenesis

Nymphal and adult tick forms infected after feeding on a *B. burgdorferi*-infected reservoir pass the organism to humans during a blood meal by regurgitating spirochetes into the bite wound. Transfer of the spirochetes from infected ticks to humans requires a period of 12–24 hours, which is an important factor in disease prevention. *B. burgdorferi* is thought to attach to a proteoglycan receptor on cells at the site of the tick bite where it grows. In 50% of infected individuals, a red macule or papule appears at the site of the bite 3–20 days later. This rash, called erythema chronicum migrans (ECM), can subsequently expand to a large, annular lesion that is 6–16 cm in diameter or even larger. The distinctive ECM lesion may be accompanied by systemic symptoms caused by the dissemination of spirochetes to the bloodstream, where they gain access to the joints, the heart, and the brain (in the case of secondary and tertiary Lyme disease).

During the first 10 days after infection, patients respond with IgM production that is specific for the infecting spirochete. This is quickly followed by an IgG response that persists for years. The humoral immune response to infection is thought to be important. *B. burgdorferi* is predominantly an extracellular pathogen, although it can attach to, and invade, fibroblasts and endothelial cells. This ability may allow it to persist within the host and cause the manifestations of late Lyme disease.

In adults, Lyme disease may display a variety of clinical manifestations, including both physical and mental signs. Generally, the disease follows three stages. The initial stage is characterized by flu-like symptoms, such as mild malaise, nausea, myalgia, fever, and headache. The characteristic rash is associated with 40%–60% of these cases. This rash begins as a red or macular area at the site of the tick bite and expands radially over time, with central clearing (Figure 8-4). These primary symptoms typically resolve without treatment. Secondary stage symptoms occur in approximately 10% of untreated patients. In this stage, the disease reappears weeks to months after the initial infection with symptoms of arthritis, neurologic manifestations, ocular inflammation, CNS involvement, and cardiac involvement. These symptoms also may resolve without treatment. A third (tertiary) stage of disease follows months to years after secondary symptoms and includes migrating episodes of arthritis, multiple ECM lesions, CNS involvement, and cardiac involvement (Table 8-4).

FIGURE 8-4 ▶
Pattern of an Erythema Chronicum Migrans Rash Associated with Lyme Disease

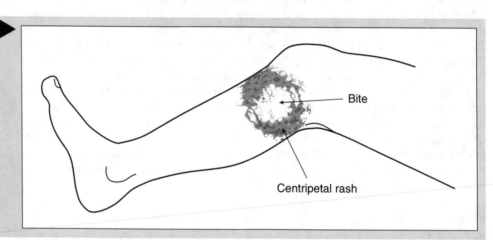

TABLE 8-4 ▶
Clinical Manifestations of Late (Disseminated) Lyme Disease

System	Symptoms
Dermatologic	Secondary (multiple) erythema chronicum migrans lesions
Musculoskeletal	Arthritis (brief attacks of swelling in more than one joint lasting hours to days, recurrent over months to years)
Cardiac	Secondary or tertiary atrioventricular block Myocarditis or pericarditis
Neurologic	Lymphocytic meningitis (headache or stiff neck with ≥ 5 lymphocytes per mm^3 of cerebrospinal fluid) Cranial neuritis Radiculoneuritis (radicular pain with documented motor weakness or sensory loss within a dermatomal distribution; electromyographic evidence of a radiculopathy) Peripheral neuritis (distal paresthesia with electromyographic evidence of an axonal polyneuropathy) Encephalopathy (memory deficit documented by abnormal results of neuropsychologic tests; evidence of intrathecal production of antibodies to *B. burgdorferi* or elevated cerebrospinal fluid protein) Encephalomyelitis (spasticity and magnetic resonance imaging scan or computerized tomographic scan showing abnormalities in the brain or spinal cord; evidence of intrathecal production of antibodies to *B. burgdorferi*)
Ophthalmologic	Keratitis (multiple focal opacities in varying levels of the corneal stroma)

Diagnosis

B. burgdorferi is difficult to grow from clinical specimens such as blood. Therefore, diagnosis is typically made on case history and clinical symptoms and is confirmed serologically. Early serologic tests for Lyme disease had several limitations, including lack of laboratory-to-laboratory standardization, cross-reactivity, and the time required for an individual to seroconvert. More recently, a standardized two-test approach was recommended for the diagnosis of active and previous Lyme disease. The first step uses a sensitive enzyme immunoassay (EIA) or immunofluorescent assay (IFA), each made more specific by the inclusion of flagellar antigens that do not cross-react with other microorganisms. Specimens negative by EIA or IFA need not be tested further. The second step is to confirm a positive test using a standardized Western blot procedure. When this test is used during the first 4 weeks of the disease, procedures to identify both IgM and IgG antibodies should be done. A positive IgM Western blot result alone does not establish active disease in persons with illness of greater than 1 month's duration because of the high likelihood of a false-positive test. If a patient suspected of having early Lyme disease shows a weak Western blot result, serologic evidence of infection is best confirmed by testing the patient's acute- and chronic-phase sera for anti-Borrelia antibodies. Sera from people with disseminated or late-stage Lyme disease almost always shows a strong immunoblot response with IgG to *B. burgdorferi* antigens.

Prevention and Treatment

Environmental modifications to residential properties (e.g., application of insecticides, use of deer fencing, and removal of leaf litter) may help prevent the transmission of Lyme disease to humans. Using personal protection methods recommended for the prevention of all forms of tick-borne diseases is also important. Such measures include wearing light-colored clothing (to detect ticks more readily), tucking long pants into socks, and using insect repellents and acaricides. Performing tick checks daily is perhaps the most important means of prevention because removal of the tick within 1 day of exposure can interrupt disease transmission.

In contrast to rickettsial disease, the high incidence of Lyme disease within the United States makes the development of a vaccine a priority. An experimental vaccine using an Osp formulation is currently under evaluation and may shape the management of Lyme disease in the future. Like rabies, this vaccine may take the form of a preexposure immunization or a postexposure therapy. Until this vaccinologic approach is studied more thoroughly, most people with Lyme disease can be managed with appropriate antibiotic therapy using amoxicillin, doxycycline, or ceftriaxone. Early, localized Lyme disease may be treated with oral doxycycline or amoxicillin. Treatment of the cardiac, neurologic, or rheumatologic manifestations of disseminated Lyme disease should include parenteral administration of either penicillin G or ceftriaxone. For first-degree atrioventricular block, facial palsy without cerebrospinal fluid abnormalities, or mild arthritis, one of the oral regimens should suffice.

RESOLUTION OF CLINICAL CASE

One week after antimicrobial therapy, the patient's rash disappeared. The patient's serology indicated a positive outcome using a Lyme disease-specific EIA. A confirmatory Western blot test indicated that the patient was strongly IgM positive and only weakly IgG positive. Upon completing the course of antibiotic treatment, the rash and systemic symptoms disappeared. A follow-up serologic exam 8 weeks later demonstrated a weak IgM-positive immunoblot result and no IgG response.

This patient most likely experienced a case of primary Lyme disease based on the rash and flu-like symptoms as well as her clinical history of environmental exposure. Supporting this diagnosis was her specific IgM response close to the time she contracted the disease. Administration of antibiotics cleared the disease, which was evident by her follow-up physical examination and serologic findings consistent with a waning immune response to *B. burgdorferi*.

REVIEW QUESTIONS

Directions: For each of the following questions, choose the **one best** answer.

1. A serologic test that is based on cross-reactive antigens of specific strains of *Proteus* spp. is diagnostic for which one of the following zoonotic agents?

    (A) Relapsing fever

    (B) Pinta

    (C) Rocky Mountain spotted fever

    (D) Tularemia

    (E) Rabies

2. Which one of the following statements regarding Lyme disease is accurate?

    (A) It is easily diagnosed by culture of the organism

    (B) It is caused by the spirochete *Treponema pallidum*

    (C) It can commonly result in a migrating arthritis

    (D) The animal reservoir is domesticated animals

    (E) It is typically spread by an animal bite

3. Which one of the following statements about *Rickettsia rickettsii* is true?

    (A) It can survive extracellularly for long periods of time

    (B) Its small size allows it to avoid immune detection

    (C) It efficiently invades and multiplies in mammalian endothelial cells

    (D) It produces "Rickettsia toxin," a potent exotoxin

    (E) It can produce lipoteichoic acid, which facilitates adhesion to the tick gut

4. Psittacosis is a zoonotic lung infection that is associated with which vector-microbial group?

    (A) Dried excrement—*Chlamydia* spp.

    (B) Milk—*Pasteurella* spp.

    (C) Animal wool—*Bacillus* spp.

    (D) Contaminated soil—*Histoplasmosis* spp.

    (E) Tick—*Rickettsia* spp.

5. Twenty-four hours after hiking in the woods in the northeastern United States in late summer, a mother searches her 11-year-old son and notices a tick on his right calf. Removal of the tick is then performed by the mother without incident. Concerned, the mother calls the pediatrician and asks about any potential infectious disease complications that may result from this tick bite. Which one of the following responses would be most accurate on the part of the pediatrician?

  (A) The mother should immediately check the boy's body for the rash that is characteristic of Rocky Mountain spotted fever; if it is not found, the child is at no further risk of infectious complications

  (B) The mother is congratulated for her prompt finding of the tick and told that upon its removal there is no further risk of infectious complications to her child

  (C) The mother is advised to look for a rash in the area of the tick bite in the next couple of days; should such a rash appear, it would result from the complications of Lyme disease

  (D) The mother is advised to watch for abrupt signs of fever, malaise, or rash over the next week; these signs are consistent with Rocky Mountain spotted fever

  (E) The mother is told that the risk of the child having Lyme disease is quite high, and the physician requests that the child be put on prophylactic antibiotics as soon as possible

6. A young boy (age 12 years) who routinely sleeps in an abandoned barn on his parent's farm initially complained of fever, headache, myalgia, vomiting, and diarrhea. Within 2 days of the onset of these symptoms, the child experiences pneumonia-like symptoms and dies of shock caused by hypovolemia. Which one of the following organisms is the most likely causative agent?

  (A) Rabies virus

  (B) Hantavirus

  (C) *Rickettsia rickettsii*

  (D) *Borrelia burgdorferi*

  (E) *Vibrio cholerae*

ANSWERS AND EXPLANATIONS

1. **The answer is C.** *R. rickettsii* exposure elicits antibody that cross-reacts with *P. vulgaris* antigens. In the Weil-Felix test, antibodies from the patient's serum are used to agglutinate antigens from certain strains of *Proteus vulgaris*. This test historically has been an important means of screening individuals infected by *R. rickettsii*. Based on this information, relapsing fever, pinta, tularemia, and rabies (options A, B, D, and E, respectively) can be excluded because these diseases are caused by nonrickettsial sources.

2. **The answer is C.** A common manifestation of secondary and tertiary Lyme disease is migrating arthritis (i.e., can move between joints). Option A is incorrect because *B. burgdorferi* is very difficult to culture from patient specimens and is not the diagnostic test of choice. Option B is incorrect because *Treponema pallidum* is the causative agent of syphilis. Option D is incorrect because deer and mice are the typical reservoirs of *B. burgdorferi*. Option E is incorrect because Lyme disease is spread by the bite of a tick, not an animal.

3. **The answer is C.** *R. rickettsii* efficiently invades and multiplies within endothelial cells. This is thought to result in the characteristic rash associated with Rocky Mountain spotted fever. *R. rickettsii* is an obligate intracellular pathogen, thereby excluding option A. Option B is incorrect because immunologic detection of a foreign body the size of Rickettsiae is routinely accomplished by the human immune system (remember, viruses are smaller than Rickettsiae). Option D is incorrect because no exotoxins are known to be produced by the Rickettsiae. Option E is incorrect because Rickettsiae, although atypical bacteria, are similar in structure to gram-negative bacteria. Lipoteichoic acids are associated with the cell wall of gram-positive bacteria.

4. **The answer is A.** *Chlamydia psittaci* is transmitted to humans upon inhalation of the dried feces of exotic birds. Options B through E are incorrect because they are unrelated to psittacosis.

5. **The answer is D.** It is possible that the tick could have transmitted *R. rickettsii* and that symptoms of Rocky Mountain spotted fever could ensue during the next 7–12 days. Option A is incorrect because the rash associated with Rocky Mountain spotted fever does not arise until 2–12 days after the initial bite. Thus, the lack of clinical findings would not exclude this disease. Option B is incorrect because many tick-borne infections can be transmitted during the period that the tick was attached to the young boy. Option C is incorrect because the time between the tick introduction and removal (approximately 24 hours) is less than the time required to cause Lyme disease (which requires about 2 days). Option E is incorrect because the incidence of the transmission of disease by a tick, in the absence of symptomology, is quite low.

6. **The answer is B.** Hantaviral infections are associated with rapidly progressing and often fatal diseases that have a foci in the lung. Option A is incorrect because rabies is a slow-acting disease that is usually contracted as the result of an animal bite, and it leads to encephalitis. Option C is incorrect because *R. rickettsii* are associated with a tick bite and rash. Likewise, option D is incorrect because disease caused by *B. burgdorferi* typically involves a tick bite and a rash. Furthermore, Lyme disease symptoms are generally not life threatening. Option E is incorrect because *V. cholerae* cause gastrointestinal disease upon ingestion.

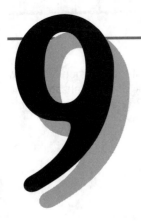

9

SEXUALLY TRANSMITTED DISEASES

William F. Goins, Ph.D.

CHAPTER OUTLINE

Introduction of Clinical Case
Sexually Transmitted Diseases
- General Characteristics
- Limiting Their Spread

Illustrative Pathogen: *Chlamydia trachomatis*
- Biologic Characteristics
- Reservoir and Transmission
- Pathogenesis
- Diagnosis
- Prevention and Treatment

Illustrative Pathogen: Herpes simplex virus
- Biologic Characteristics
- Reservoir and Transmission
- Virulence Factors
- Pathogenesis
- Diagnosis
- Prevention and Treatment

Resolution of Clinical Case
Review Questions

INTRODUCTION OF CLINICAL CASE

A pregnant 19-year-old single woman who had not received any prenatal care was admitted to the hospital following rupture of her membranes in the 35th week of pregnancy. At the time of admission, she was in early labor and progressed to deliver a 6-pound, 7-ounce boy vaginally 17 hours later. The infant appeared normal at birth and was allowed to go home with the mother 2 days later. Ten days after delivery, the mother returned to the hospital because the infant was febrile and irritable. Examination of the child revealed 12 vesicular lesions scattered over his body, as well as bilateral conjunctivitis. Fluid from one of the vesicles was submitted to the clinical laboratory for virus culture. Upon interview, the mother reported three sex partners in the year prior to pregnancy but was unaware of any sexually transmitted disease symptoms. Gynecologic examination of the mother was unremarkable for signs of sexually transmitted diseases; however, because of the infant's symptoms, a cervical swab was taken and submitted to the clinical laboratory for virus culture.

The infant was admitted to the hospital and started on intravenous acyclovir. During the next 48 hours, the number of lesions increased to approximately 30. The infant became lethargic and had a single seizure; he was placed on a drug (phenytoin) to suppress seizure activity. There was evidence of hepatic dysfunction manifested by elevated serum liver enzyme levels. During the second week of hospitalization, the laboratory reported the growth of herpes simplex virus type 2 (HSV-2) from both the infant's vesicular lesion and the mother's cervical culture.

- How did the infant contract this disease?
- Why is the mother not suffering from HSV-related symptoms?
- What is the prognosis for this infant?

SEXUALLY TRANSMITTED DISEASES

General Characteristics

*Historically, STDs have been referred to as **venereal** diseases, a term derived from the Greek* venery, *which, loosely translated, means sexual relations.*

The questions posed at the end of the introduction of the clinical case are largely applicable to any sexually transmitted disease (STD). STDs are unique among the microbial diseases particularly because they link their spread to human procreation. As a consequence of this transmission strategy, humans are generally the sole reservoir for pathogens that cause STDs.

STDs are medically significant and have complex etiologies. An estimated 12 million new cases of STDs occur in the United States annually; 65% of these new infections involve individuals younger than 25 years of age; alarmingly, 20% occur among teenagers. Not including the management of people with human immunodeficiency virus (HIV), the estimated yearly national cost of treating STDs is in excess of $2 billion. More than 25 different microbial pathogens cause STDs, and they are not confined to a single class of microbial pathogens (i.e., viral, prokaryotic, eukaryotic). The most significant STDs are listed in Table 9-1. The student should be familiar with the organisms and diseases associated with these pathogens.

Some STD pathogens, such as HIV-1 (see Chapter 27) and hepatitis B virus (see Chapter 10), cause diseases associated with a high mortality rate and are of obvious medical significance. These STD pathogens represent the exception to the norm, because most STD pathogens cause relatively benign infection and only infrequently result in life-threatening illness. However, because of their morbidity within the population, these STDs are considered a significant public health concern.

__Morbidity__ refers to the incidence of disease within a defined population. __Mortality__ refers to the incidence of death resulting from disease within a defined population.

One other general characteristic of STDs is the bystander effect, in which individuals are inadvertently affected by the behavior of other individuals. This is clearly the case for the child in the HSV case described at the beginning of the chapter, and it may have been the case for the mother as an unsuspecting sexual partner of an infected male. Finally, it should be appreciated that the very nature of the anatomic differences between the male and female reproductive organs often result in two distinct STD pathologies. In males, this is typically manifested as uncomplicated urethritis; in females, urethritis, asymptomatic infection, and ascending disease (e.g., cervicitis, pelvic inflammatory disease [PID], and dissemination) are common symptoms.

Limiting Their Spread

It is remarkable that many STDs are epidemic in the United States because, with exception of the viral STDs, they generally respond well to antimicrobial therapy. Furthermore, their very classification as STDs suggests a practical intervention—abstinence. Ideally, elimination of STDs seems entirely achievable, but realistically, the practical management of STDs can be accomplished only by understanding the basic biology that underlies STD pathogens.

Outside of strict abstinence, the best protection from STDs is to have sex with only one person who is free of infection. This protection can be assured only if sexual partners have previously had, and continue to participate in, a monogamous relationship. At the next level of protection, discussions among partners about their sexual history and whether they have had an STD in the past (considered high-risk behavior) is invaluable. If one or both of the partners has a history of high-risk behavior, or if this information is not available, barrier protection methods (e.g., the use of a condom) can significantly reduce

◀ **TABLE 9-1**
Major Causes of STDs

Microbial Pathogen	Disease	Comments
Viruses		
HSV-1 or HSV-2	Genital herpes	Very common; vesicle formation is caused by cell lysis and inflammatory response.
Human papillomavirus (HPV)	Genital warts (condyloma acuminatum)	Very common; some types are implicated in cervical cancer.
Molluscum contagiosum		This is a poxvirus that causes benign skin lesions.
Human immunodeficiency virus (HIV)	AIDS	This is a retrovirus that ultimately leads to collapse of the immune system.
Hepatitis B virus (HBV)	Liver dysfunction	This hepadenavirus infection can lead to hepatocarcinoma.
Bacteria		
Chlamydia trachomatis	Nongonococcal urethritis (NGU)	This obligate intracellular bacterium is responsible for more than half of all STDs reported in the United States annually. The bacteria cause symptoms similar to gonorrhea (see below). Globally, it is a leading cause of preventable blindness.
Neisseria gonorrhoeae	Gonorrhea	This faculatative intracellular gram-negative bacterium causes acute and more severe urethritis in men and women, chronic pelvic infection in women, and eye infections in newborns.
Treponema palladum	Syphilis	This is a STD of historic significance, which is characterized by a painless chancre upon primary infection; this disease is caused by a spirochete.
Escherichia coli and other enteric (gram-negative or gram-positive) bacteria	Cystitis	*E. coli* can result in dysuria and lower back pain.
Gardnerella vaginalis	Vaginosis	This gram-negative bacterium can cause an infection characterized by a foul-smelling discharge.
Mycoplasma hominis	NGU	*Mycoplasma* spp. lack a cell wall and are resistant to cell wall inhibitors; they cause a purulent discharge similar to gonorrhea.
Ureaplasma urealyticum	NGU	This is also a *Mycoplasma* spp. that lacks a cell wall.
Haemophilus ducreyi	Chancroid	This gram-negative bacterium causes a disease characterized by painful, ulcerative genital lesions and lymph-node suppuration; it is more common in the subtropics but outbreaks in the United States do occur.
Fungi		
Candida albicans	Vulvovaginitis (balanoposthitis in men)	A yellow-green frothy discharge is characteristic in women; asymptomatic vaginal carriage is common.
Protozoa		
Trichomonas vaginalis	Vulvovaginitis (urethritis in men)	This flagellate protozoan causes a characteristic foamy discharge in women.

the risk of contracting STDs. If either partner exhibits symptoms of an STD or suspects that they may have been exposed to an STD, immediate diagnosis and treatment should be sought by both partners. As for any other group of microbial diseases, intervention through education (at the level of STD transmission) has been demonstrated to be an effective means of controlling the spread of these diseases.

ILLUSTRATIVE PATHOGEN: *Chlamydia trachomatis*

C. trachomatis causes sexually transmitted cervicitis and nonspecific urethritis. This organism is representative of the Chlamydiae, a family of bacterial pathogens that have a particular tropism for the columnar epithelium of mucosal surfaces. Human infection caused by *C. trachomatis* primarily involves the genital and ocular mucosa. In the United States, chlamydial infection ranks as the single most prevalent STD, with an estimated 3–4 million cases occurring annually. In men, the disease begins as urethritis and may spread to the epididymis. In women, infection begins in the cervix and urethra and can often spread to the endometrium and fallopian tubes. The inflammatory response to chlamydial infection of the fallopian tubes can result in infertility and life-threatening ectopic pregnancy. Although women acquire the disease by sexual transmission, infants born to mothers with chlamydial infection commonly develop conjunctivitis and pneumonia. Chlamydial trachoma (chronic keratoconjunctivitis), which affects a staggering number of individuals, is the leading cause of preventable blindness. Worldwide, there are 5.5 million people who are blind or at high risk for blindness as a result of trachoma.

> *Ectopic pregnancy* is the implantation of a fertilized egg in a location other than the uterine lining. Scarring of the fallopian tubes can lead to an increased chance of ectopic pregnancy. Undiagnosed and un-treated ectopic pregnancy can result in death.

Chlamydial disease is often referred to as nongonococcal urethritis (NGU). The reason for this is that chlamydial infection typically causes an intense inflammatory response on the genital mucosa that is similar to gonococcal infection (see Chapter 17); however, no organisms can be cultivated on rich agar medium.

Biologic Characteristics

C. trachomatis describes a group of obligate intracellular bacterial pathogens that cause a diverse range of diseases, depending both on the antigenic composition of the insulting pathogenic organism and on the means by which the organism gains access to the host. Rather than being segregated by species, *C. trachomatis* organisms are defined by serovars. The serovar designation of these organisms is correlated with disease pathology. Serovars A–C are associated with trachoma, whereas serovars D–K are most likely to be associated with STDs. Serovars L1–L3 cause lymphogranuloma venereum, a disease localized to the inguinal lymph nodes of infected individuals (Table 9-2).

> *Serovar* refers to the differential reactivity of several isolates within a species to several different antisera preparations. Thus, the term serovar is short for serovariation, meaning that a collection of organisms consistently react with a panel of antisera. Serovars of *C. trachomatis* are grouped by letter.

TABLE 9-2 ▶

Serovars of *Chlamydia trachomatis* and Their Associated Diseases

Serovar	Disease
A–C	Trachoma
D–K	Nongonococcal urethritis, epididymitis, mucopurulent cervicitis, infant pneumonia
L1–L3	Lymphogranuloma venereum

In addition to these diseases, *C. trachomatis* is associated with Reiter's syndrome. Patients with Reiter's syndrome exhibit three characteristic symptoms: (1) conjunctivitis or iridocyclitis (ocular diseases), (2) polyarthritis (arthritis in multiple joints), and (3) genital inflammation. In this syndrome, infection is typically initiated either in the eye or in the genital tract, and the associated arthritis is due to an ensuing autoimmune response to the chlamydial infection. Although other infectious agents also can precipitate Reiter's syndrome, in the United States 50%–65% of these patients have an acute *C. trachomatis* genital infection at the onset of arthritis.

C. trachomatis exists in two distinct morphologic forms as an elementary body (EB)

and as a reticulate body (RB). The EB is a small (approximately 0.3 µm in diameter), dense particle that can exist outside of the host cell. This is the infectious form, but it is physiologically inactive and is not susceptible to antimicrobial agents. The density of the EB is the result of the major outer membrane protein that is highly cross-linked to neighboring proteins by multiple cysteine disulfide bonds. Similar to the *Mycoplasma* spp., *Chlamydia* spp. appear to lack a cell wall. Unlike *Mycoplasma* spp., *Chlamydia* spp. bear a resemblance to gram-negative bacteria by virtue of their two-membrane organization, with lipopolysaccharide (LPS) associated with the outer membrane. The RB is the intracellular form of *C. trachomatis*. In this state, it is metabolically active and is larger (approximately 0.8 µm in diameter) than an EB. Although RBs synthesize their own DNA and membrane structure, they depend on the host for generation of energy in the form of adenosine triphosphate (ATP). As such, these organisms have been referred to as energy parasites. RBs are thought to exist as less-dense particles largely because of the intracellular reducing environment that favors the major outer membrane protein to exist in a non-cross-linked state.

Reservoir and Transmission

The only known reservoir for *C. trachomatis* is humans, and like many STDs, this organism is maintained within the population largely as a consequence of asymptomatic infection of women and men. In roughly 50% of STDs from which gonococci are cultivated, *C. trachomatis* is also present. Because gonorrhea is much easier to diagnose in the laboratory, the true incidence of *Chlamydia* infection may be underreported.

Pathogenesis

Chlamydiae demonstrate a unique life cycle among bacterial pathogens, which is summarized in Figure 9-1. *C. trachomatis* gains access to the host by sexual contact, allowing the passage of metabolically inert EBs from one infected individual to an uninfected individual. Because of their metabolic status and tightly cross-linked outer membrane, EBs are resistant to nonspecific host defense mechanisms. They quickly adsorb to the microvilli of columnar epithelial cells, travel down the microvilli, and localize in the indentations of the host cell's plasma membrane. In this position they are endocytosed

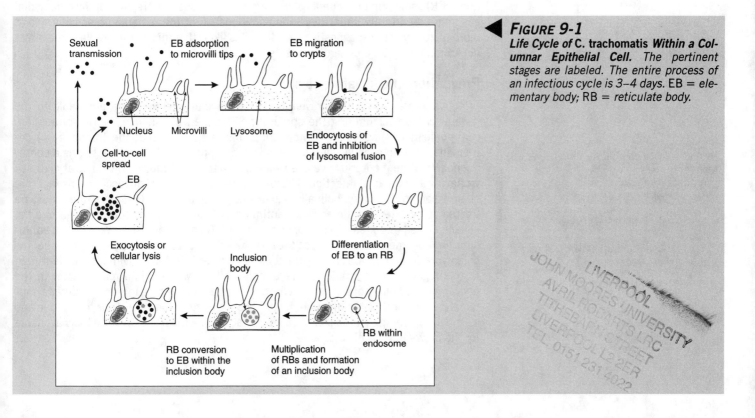

FIGURE 9-1
Life Cycle of C. trachomatis *Within a Columnar Epithelial Cell.* The pertinent stages are labeled. The entire process of an infectious cycle is 3–4 days. EB = elementary body; RB = reticulate body.

within membrane-bound vacuoles. EBs avoid killing the host cell by inhibiting fusion of the infected endosome with lysosomal granules, an event that typically results in bacterial destruction. Rather, inside the endosome *C. trachomatis* convert to metabolically active RBs and multiply into microscopic, intracellular colonies of 100–500 progeny. These intraendosomal inclusions are referred to as inclusion bodies. When the cellular nutrients have been depleted, the RBs convert to EBs and either are exocytosed into the extracellular spaces or are liberated by cell lysis, infecting adjacent cells or another uninfected human host. The process of cellular infection and dissemination takes 72–96 hours per cycle.

Damage from chlamydial infection is largely due to the acute inflammatory response in the area of infection and scarring of the host tissue after infection. The acute inflammatory response may be a consequence of the LPS produced by *C. trachomatis*. Immunity to chlamydial infection seems to be somewhat limited because many individuals suffer repeated episodes of infection by strains from the same serovar. This is referred to as infectious recidivism, and it is a common characteristic of STDs.

Diagnosis

Clinically, chlamydial infections present as a purulent urethral discharge in more than 90% of all men and in roughly 30% of all women; these symptoms by themselves are suggestive of chlamydial infection. Asymptomatic infection or ascending disease requires sensitive laboratory diagnostic tests. This is particularly important for pregnant women because primary infection of the mother represents the major mode of transmission to the neonate.

Chlamydiae cannot be characterized in the laboratory by Gram stain because these organisms lack a cell wall, which is thought to be important in the Gram reaction. Furthermore, because of their small size, detection of individual chlamydiae challenges the limits of light microscopy. Instead, the laboratory diagnosis of *C. trachomatis* infections is accomplished in three ways: (1) direct examination of clinical specimens for chlamydial inclusion bodies by immunofluoresence microscopy, (2) isolation of the infecting organism in cell culture, or (3) detection of specific antibodies against these organisms. These procedures differ significantly in their sensitivity and the level of expertise required by the laboratory personnel to perform them. Polymerase chain reaction (PCR) using primer sequences that target highly conserved regions of the chlamydial genome are currently under development. Because of the remarkable sensitivity and reproducibility of this diagnostic procedure, it is likely that this test will replace the direct detection, cultivation, or serologic tests.

Prevention and Treatment

Effective strategies for the prevention of chlamydial infections are amenable to the general criteria for limiting the spread of STDs (i.e., abstinence, barrier protection, communication, diagnosis). Complicating this is the fact that the frequency of co-transmission with gonococcal disease is very high, as described previously. As a consequence, treatment criteria have been established to reflect those individuals at high risk for having a chlamydial infection. These treatment criteria take into account the fact that chlamydiae are only metabolically active when they exist as RBs; thus, they must be treated using extended therapy with antimicrobial agents that effectively penetrate the eukaryotic cell (e.g., tetracycline or sulfadiazine). Chlamydial resistance to these antibiotics has not emerged, as has been the case for other bacterial pathogens. Consequently, chlamydial infections are entirely treatable, as long as infected individuals are identified. In this regard, asymptomatic carriage, especially in women, is a major factor in the persistence of chlamydial disease. Without an effective vaccine to prevent either symptomatic or asymptomatic infection, this will continue to be the case. Thus, education and sensitive screening methods for at-risk populations are the most powerful tools available for the prevention of this disease.

Who should be treated for chlamydial infection?
- *Patients with gonorrhea*
- *Patients with diseases caused by C. trachomatis*
- *All sexual partners of affected individuals*
- *Neonates born to women with untreated chlamydial infection*

ILLUSTRATIVE PATHOGEN: Herpes simplex virus

Biologic Characteristics

HSV is a complex human viral pathogen that infects a variety of cell types in the body. HSV initially infects epithelial cells of the skin and mucosal membranes; as disease progresses, it can infect the neurons of sensory ganglia and, in limited cases, may infect the brain.

Life Cycle. The HSV life cycle involves transmission by direct contact (usually sexual), with replication at the site of the infected body surface. Penetration into deeper layers typically ensues and involves contact with nerve terminals, where the virus travels by retrograde axonal transport to sensory nerve cell bodies. Infection of the peripheral nervous system (PNS) sensory neurons does not result in cell death but in viral latency (Figure 9-2).

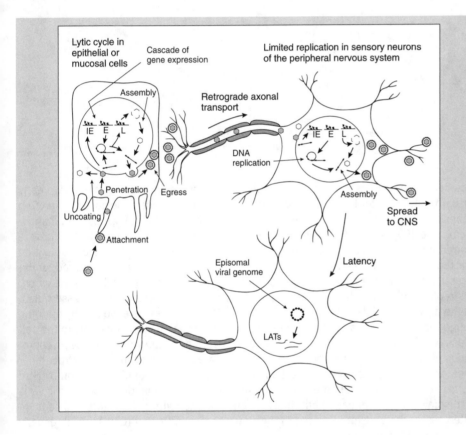

◀ *FIGURE 9-2*
Primary HSV Infection and the Establishment of Latency. The virus encounters and replicates within epithelial or mucosal cells, yielding progeny particles that encounter sensory nerve terminals where the viral capsid is transported to the nerve cell body. Following limited replication, the virus can either invade the CNS or establish a latent infection. IE = immediate early; E = early; L = late; LATs = latency-associated transcripts.

By entering latency, the virus remains dormant, thus escaping immune surveillance. The latent genome can persist for the life of the host as a circular episomal molecule in a histone-associated, chromatin-like structure. Infected individuals may exhibit occasional episodes of spontaneous virus reactivation, which can be caused by a variety of stimuli, including ultraviolet light, emotional stress, surgery, trauma, hormonal regulation, and other factors that generally lead to host immune suppression. Following reactivation the virus displays a limited burst of replication in sensory neurons, where the newly synthesized particles proceed by anterograde transport to susceptible dermal cells. This leads to a productive virus infection and subsequent development of the vesicular lesions that are characteristic of a recrudescent herpes infection (Figure 9-3). It is remarkable that these lesions, in one form or another, affect more than one-third of the global population.

The HSV lytic replication cycle involves a number of intricate processes, accomplished by at least 84 different gene products. Expression of these viral genes is tightly

Latency is a state in which no viral polypeptides are synthesized and the virus genome is transcriptionally silent, except for the expression of latency-associated transcripts. *Reactivation* is a state in which the virus is stimulated to exit latency and enter the lytic portion of the viral reproductive cycle; this includes the production of infectious virus.

FIGURE 9-3 ▶

Reactivation from Latency and Recurrent HSV Infection. *Following stimulation by a variety of factors, the virus reactivates from the latent state, replicates, and spreads to cells at or near the site of primary infection, where subsequent lesions form. LATs = latency-associated transcripts; L = late; E = early; IE = immediate early.*

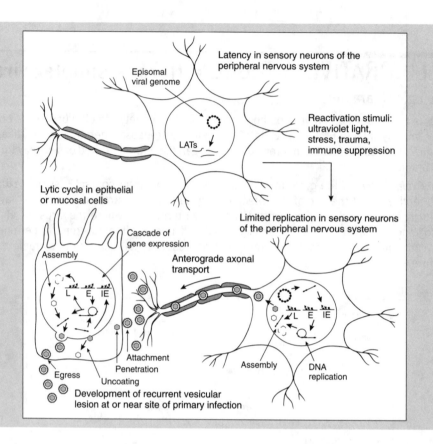

controlled, being expressed in three coordinated waves designated as immediate early (IE), early (E), and late (L). IE genes are expressed in the absence of de novo viral protein synthesis and are responsible for the expression of all remaining HSV genes (i.e., E and L genes). The E genes primarily encode enzymes and DNA-binding proteins that are required for the replication complex or that are involved in the synthesis of nucleotide pools required for viral DNA synthesis. Replication of the viral genome is required for the expression of the L genes, which comprise mostly structural proteins of the mature virion. Virus replication takes place within the nucleus, where the virus capsid is assembled, and the newly synthesized DNA is encapsidated. HSV acquires its envelope by budding through the inner lamellae of the nuclear membrane. The virus then migrates to the cell surface (egress) via the Golgi apparatus, where processing of the viral envelope glycoproteins is accomplished. Infectious, mature virions are exocytosed into the extracellular milieu, where they are poised to infect adjacent cells. Usually, cellular infection by HSV results in cell lysis, except in the case of sensory neuron infection, during which the virus may display limited replication but then may enter latency within these infected cells. In limited cases, the virus may spread to the central nervous system (CNS), which usually results in encephalitis.

Serotypes. Two serotypes of HSV with extensive homology have been identified, yet these serotypes (HSV-1 and HSV-2) possess many intratypic antigenic and biologic differences. HSV-1 is primarily associated with orofacial lesions, whereas HSV-2 is more prevalent in genital herpes infections. Primary HSV-1 infection typically is associated with the production of the characteristic vesicular orofacial herpetic lesions that usually occur on the border of the lip (e.g., cold sores, labialis); it also typically causes gingivostomatitis, conjunctivitis, and encephalitis. Recurrent HSV-1 infection is associated with recurrent labialis and herpetic stromal keratitis. Primary and recurrent HSV-2 infection results in the characteristic lesions associated with genital herpes. HSV-2 infection of the neonate is usually devastating, often leading to multiple organ dissemination, including the CNS.

Primary HSV infection *refers to the initial exposure to HSV in an uninfected host that results in disease.* **Recurrent HSV infection** *refers to repeated infection that recurs as a consequence of reactivation of latent HSV infection.*

Reservoir and Transmission

Humans are the only known reservoir for transmission of HSV. The virus is spread by direct contact between an infected individual and a seronegative person, where the virus particles present in secretions come in contact with mucosal surfaces or epithelial abrasions. The virus infects and replicates within peripheral cells for 1–2 days before being transported to sensory neurons of the PNS. The virus is routinely spread by intimate sexual contact between two individuals, with the rate of transmission of genital herpes directly correlating with the number of sexual partners that an individual has. HSV-1 was previously thought to be primarily associated with orofacial lesions and HSV-2 with genital lesions. However, HSV-1 has now been shown to be the causative agent in 40% of all cases of genital herpes, and HSV-2 is associated with almost 40% of all orofacial cases of herpes. Of interest is the fact that the genital lesions resulting from HSV-1 infection are less severe in nature and their duration is shorter when compared to the corresponding urogenital lesions associated with HSV-2 infection.

Virulence Factors

The severity of HSV infection typically correlates with the neurovirulence of a particular isolate, which in turn correlates with the capacity of the virus to replicate and spread to the nervous system. The severity of acute primary infection generally correlates with the greater frequency and duration of recurrences, which may be the result of the initial viral load. Almost half of the HSV gene products are not essential for virus replication in culture, yet they are important for replication and spread within the host (Table 9-3).

◀ **TABLE 9-3**
Summary of HSV Virulence Factors

Virulence Factor	Effect on Host
Thymidine kinase/ribonucleotide reductase	Maintaining nucleotide pools
γ34.5 gene product	Interferes with neuronal apoptosis
UL41 gene product	Shuts off host protein synthesis
gC gene product	Binds to the C3b
gE:gI gene products	Binding IgG
ICP47 gene product	Interferes with antigen presentation
Latency	Allows the virus to evade the host immune system

Some of these gene products, such as thymidine kinase and ribonucleotide reductase, are responsible for maintaining adequate nucleotide pool levels necessary for the replication of the virus in terminally differentiated nondividing sensory neurons of the PNS or CNS. The HSV-encoded γ34.5 polypeptide interferes with programmed cell death (apoptosis) in neurons. The product of the UL41 gene—designated the virion-derived host shut-off protein—destabilizes cellular messenger RNA (mRNA), thereby enabling the virus to further usurp the machinery of the host cell. Additionally, the virus encodes several gene products during lytic infection that alter the ability of the host to recognize and destroy virus-infected cells effectively in vivo. HSV-1 glycoprotein C (gC) binds to the C3b component of the alternative complement pathway, leading to the inactivation of the complement cascade and a reduction in antibody-dependent cell cytotoxicity (ADCC). Glycoproteins E and I (gE and gI) form a heterodimer capable of binding to the Fc portion of IgG, which also results in a reduction in ADCC. The ICP47 gene product interferes with the transporter associated with antigen presentation, thereby inhibiting major histocompatibility complex (MHC) class I–mediated antigen presentation and HSV-specific cytotoxic lymphocyte (CTL) recognition. Finally, the natural ability of the virus to enter latency allows the virus to evade the host immune system.

Pathogenesis

HSV infection usually results in morphologic changes in an infected cell; these include swelling and rounding, which precede cell lysis. Virus-infected cells also can fuse with neighboring uninfected cells, producing multinucleated giant cells. All of these cytopathic effects, in combination with inflammation from the host immune response, can lead to the formation of vesicular skin lesions or mucosal ulcers. These ulcers can last longer than 3 weeks during primary infection. Fewer and less severe lesions with decreased duration are observed during recurrent infection. During asymptomatic infection, the shedding of the virus is common. The virus replicates in cells of the periphery for several days and can be detected within neurons that innervate the site of primary infection as soon as 1 day postinfection. Within the sensory nerve cell bodies, the virus can display limited replication for 4–6 days prior to the establishment of latency. Virus can be shed from the primary lesions for 7–10 days postinfection, although neutralizing antibodies to the virus can be detected starting at 4–7 days. A strong cell-mediated immune response is more important than the humoral-mediated immune response in clearing the virus; the humoral-mediated immune response does not block recurrence or reinfection but can decrease spread of the virus and limit the severity of the resulting lesions.

Genital HSV infection can be painful yet is normally self-limiting in most healthy individuals. However, it can be a devastating illness in immunocompromised individuals, such as neonates, AIDS patients, and people receiving immunosuppressive therapy. In one-third of all neonatal infections, dissemination to multiple organs such as the liver, lung, and brain is seen, resulting from a viremia via a maternal primary infection. Disseminated disease in neonates produces mortality rates approaching 50% and typically results in multiple sequelae among the survivors. In addition, another third of all affected neonates display CNS involvement in the absence of viremia and disseminated disease. Some of these children display characteristic vesicular lesions; however, in most instances there are no cutaneous signs of HSV infection. Encephalitis in the HSV-infected neonate is approximately 50% fatal, and many children respond poorly to antiviral inhibitory drug treatments. Many neonatal infections result in lesions being present on the skin, eye, or mouth, which can be seen as late as 10 days postpartum. It is believed that these more mild cases of neonatal infection are the result of a recurrent maternal infection. Asymptomatic infection is not a common outcome of neonatal HSV infections.

In some cases, the disease produced by HSV infection is not the direct result of the virus, but it is complicated by the host immune response to infection. For example, primary infection of the eye results in replication of the virus in the corneal epithelial layer, causing conjunctivitis. In these cases, the virus is cleared by the host cell-mediated immune response, and the damage to the epithelial cell layer is rapidly repaired (because this tissue can actively divide [95% recovery in 1 day]). Yet, the virus can establish a latent infection of the ophthalmic branch of the trigeminal ganglion, which innervates the surface of the eye. Upon subsequent reactivation events, virus particles are released from the trigeminal ganglion following anterograde transport. These viruses can enter and replicate within fibroblasts associated with the stromal layer of the eye. The host cell-mediated immune response to these virus-infected cells results in lysis of the infected fibroblasts, which are limited in number and cannot be replaced. Repeated recurrences give rise to corneal opacity, eventually leading to blindness.

Diagnosis

Sensitive methods for the detection of HSV are important for pregnant women because primary infection of the mother represents the major risk factor for infection of the fetus. Most infants with severe disseminated disease are born to women who are asymptomatic virus shedders with no prior history of genital herpes. Sensitive and type-specific serologic tests exist for recognition of HSV. Although the serologic tests are extremely useful for detection of the virus, the definitive diagnosis of HSV has been isolation of virus from vesicular lesions or cerebrospinal fluid, needle biopsy, cell scrapings of the cervix, or cervicovaginal swabs. In the past, microscopic examination of the infected tissue for the presence of intranuclear inclusions and multinucleated giant cells was considered a definitive means for identification of the virus. However, because many human viruses produce similar cytopathic effects, this method is no longer viewed as an effective diagnostic technique. PCR using primer sequences that are specific for highly conserved regions of the HSV genome is now becoming the "gold standard" for detection of HSV from tissue or fluid samples. The extreme sensitivity and reproducibility of this assay can identify one infected cell in 10^6 total cells within a sample. This technique is now routinely used for diagnosis of HSV in larger hospitals and clinics, and further automation should enable the use of HSV PCR kits even in small isolated clinics.

Prevention and Treatment

Increased awareness of HSV as an STD and its route of transmission by intimate sexual contact may limit the spread of this disease. In addition, the use of condoms as barrier protection is effective. This is particularly important because of the prevalence of asymptomatic shedding of HSV.

The use of antiviral drugs that inhibit viral DNA synthesis is an effective treatment regimen for HSV. Treatment with acyclovir has greatly reduced the mortality of disseminated HSV disease by approximately 70% when compared with untreated infections. The outcome with therapy depends heavily on the extent of disease and how early in the course of disease acyclovir therapy is initiated. Cesarean delivery in women with prior history of HSV infection or women who become seropositive during serologic screening can result in decreased spread to the neonate. Considerable effort has been put into the development of vaccines to HSV. However, the effectiveness of a vaccine in treating HSV is questionable because of viral latency and reactivation.

RESOLUTION OF CLINICAL CASE

Approximately 1 in 5000 births within the United States is complicated by HSV infection, typically caused by HSV-2. In this case, HSV was transmitted from an asymptomatic mother to the neonate either secondary to the premature rupture of the membranes or by direct transmission of the virus during passage through an infected genital tract during birth. Primary maternal infections carry a much greater risk of severe disease to the infant than recurrent infections because of the size of the viral load and the immune naivete of both mother and child. Maternal infection is often asymptomatic at the time of delivery, and asymptomatic viral shedding may occur in women with no known history of genital herpes. The mother of this infant was at high risk for contracting an STD because of her age, obvious sexual activity, and history of multiple sexual partners. Her lack of prenatal care was yet another indication that the child's symptoms might be the result of a preexisting maternal STD. For women at high risk for contracting STDs, prenatal care typically involves early screening for the major STD pathogens.

Disseminated infection of the newborn can be apparent upon birth; however, in many cases, both localized and disseminated infection is more typically apparent several days to weeks after delivery. In this case, the infant presented with disease localized to the skin and conjunctiva; these symptoms were followed by signs of neonatal viremia that included neurologic signs such as seizure, cranial nerve palsy, and lethargy (indicative of CNS involvement). Because of the high mortality associated with disseminated HSV infection of neonates, the prognosis for this child is quite poor.

REVIEW QUESTIONS

Directions: For each of the following questions, choose the **one best** answer.

1. Which one of the following general statements about sexually transmitted diseases (STDs) is most accurate?

    (A) STDs are of medical significance only in developing countries

    (B) Nearly all STDs are resistant to current medical therapies

    (C) Prevention and even elimination of many STDs are entirely achievable given the appropriate intervention strategies

    (D) Asymptomatic STD infection of the male urethra is the leading contributor to the worldwide STD epidemic

    (E) STDs are characterized as having high mortality and low morbidity

2. *Chlamydia trachomatis* is an obligate human intracellular pathogen that exists as elementary bodies (EBs) and as reticulate bodies (RBs) during the course of infection. Which one of the following statements is most correct about the biology of EBs and RBs?

    (A) RBs are typically extracellular and metabolically active

    (B) EBs are typically found intracellularly and are not infectious

    (C) RBs are dense particles that are often found associated with microvilli of the mucosal epithelium

    (D) EBs are the infectious form of *C. trachomatis*

    (E) RBs and EBs are both generally found extracellulary and are equally infectious

3. A sexually active man presents at the local STD clinic with a purulent urethral discharge. Laboratory culture of this discharge on rich media that sustains the growth of most fastidious bacteria is ordered. Twenty-four hours later, the laboratory reports the cultivation of gram-negative diplococci that are tentatively identified as *Neisseria gonorrhoeae*. Which one of the following statements is the most likely conclusion that can be drawn from the patient's clinical presentation and laboratory report?

    (A) The patient's urethral infection is most likely the result of herpes simplex virus (HSV) infection, however a diagnosis of syphilis cannot be excluded

    (B) The patient's urethral infection is associated with *N. gonorrhoeae*, however infection with *Chlamydia trachomatis* cannot be excluded

    (C) The patient's urethral infection is associated with *C. trachomatis*, excluding infection caused by *N. gornorrhoeae*

    (D) HSV can be excluded as being responsible for the patient's urethral infection because none of his recent sexual partners are aware of any symptoms of herpes

    (E) There is a greater than 90% chance that the patient's urethral infection is associated only with *N. gonorrhoeae*

4. Which one of following statements is most correct about how a specific herpes simplex virus (HSV) virulence factor increases viral spread or contributes to immune evasion in the host?

   (A) The UL41 gene product interferes with antigen presentation

   (B) The viral capsule acts as an antagonist to macrophage opsonization

   (C) Latency stimulates a hyperimmune humoral antibody response causing autoimmune disease

   (D) Antisense HSV transcripts produced during reactivation shut down host cell synthesis

   (E) HSV-encoded ribonucleotide reductase maintains the nucleotide pools at levels that maximize virus production, enabling the virus to be maintained within the host

5. A recently divorced 42-year-old man presents at his physician's office complaining of a painful penile ulcer that is characteristic of a herpes simplex virus (HSV) lesion. Given this information, the patient demands an explanation for why he appears to have contracted genital herpes. Since his divorce, he has been involved in a monogamous relationship with a 39-year-old woman. Upon obtaining a clinical history from the woman, it is found that she had divorced 5 years earlier and had one brief sexual relationship with an unmarried, sexually active 25-year-old man. The woman assures the physician and partner that a condom was properly used throughout this sexual tryst. Furthermore, the women denies experiencing any STD symptoms and is currently culture negative for all common STD pathogens. Which one of the following statements represents the most likely scenario by which the 42-year-old man acquired this genital HSV infection?

   (A) The 42-year-old man contracted this disease from a contaminated public toilet seat

   (B) The 42-year-old man contracted HSV from the asymptomatically infected woman who contracted HSV from the 25-year-old man

   (C) The woman is an asymptomatic carrier of HSV; her disease was contracted from her first husband

   (D) The woman is an asymptomatic carrier of HSV; her disease was contracted from her mother during birth

   (E) The 42-year-old man is an asymptomatic carrier of HSV that he contracted during birth

ANSWERS AND EXPLANATIONS

1. **The answer is C.** The infectious cycle of STDs can be interrupted at the level of transmission and treatment. The only intervention strategy not currently available for STDs is vaccination. Option A is incorrect because STDs are considered epidemic within the United States and other industrialized countries. Option B is incorrect because, with the exception of some viral STDs, these diseases can be effectively treated using conventional drug therapies. Option D is incorrect because males typically demonstrate overt symptomology, whereas asymptomatic infection is associated with females. Option E is incorrect, with the exception of HIV. STDs generally occur within a given population and cause relatively benign disease. However, because of their high occurrence within a population, the mortality associated with these diseases may be perceived to be relatively high.

2. **The answer is D.** The critical information is that elementary bodies (EBs), which are metabolically inert and extracellular, are the infectious form of *C. trachomatis*. Reticulate bodies (RBs) are the metabolically active form of *C. trachomatis* that are intracellular and noninfectious. Option A is incorrect because RBs are typically intracellular. Option B is incorrect because EBs are typically extracellular and are considered the infectious form. Option C is incorrect because EBs, not RBs, are dense, extracellular, and found associated with microvilli. Finally, option E is incorrect because RBs are generally found intracellularly and are not infectious, and EBs are found extracellularly and are considered the infectious form.

3. **The answer is B.** The important facts about chlamydia that need to be understood to answer this question are that chlamydial infection in males results in a purulent urethral discharge that is often associated with gonococcal coinfection. These symptoms are quite distinct from HSV infection, which results in the formation of herpetic lesions. Finally, chlamydiae are obligate intracellular pathogens that cannot be cultivated on even the richest of bacteriologic media. The clinical presentation is consistent with chlamydial and gonococcal disease, the incidence of coinfection of these diseases, and the observation that only *N. gonorrhoeae* could be propagated on rich bacteriologic medium. Option A is incorrect because the clinical findings are incompatible with either herpes simplex virus (HSV) or syphilis infection. Option C is incorrect because of the finding of *N. gonorrhoeae* by the laboratory, thereby "including infection caused by the gonococcus." Option D is incorrect because the incidence of asymptomatic HSV disease in women is quite prevalent. Finally, one cannot assume that urethral infection of this patient is caused only by *N. gonorrhoeae* because laboratory analysis for the detection of *C. trachomatis* was not performed.

4. **The answer is E.** The demands of viral nucleic acid synthesis require a substantially enhanced nucleotide pool for replication. Option A is incorrect because the UL41 gene product is involved in shutting off host-cell protein synthesis, not inhibiting antigen presentation. Option B is incorrect because HSV does not possess a capsule. Capsules are polysaccharide substances that are typically expressed on the surface of pathogenic bacteria; viruses often express a capsid, which is a protein coat. Option C is incorrect because latency is considered a mechanism of immune evasion that limits the humoral immune response rather than stimulating a hyperimmune humoral antibody response. Option D is not correct because antisense strategies for inhibiting host-cell synthesis during reactivation have not yet been defined.

5. **The answer is C.** It is entirely possible that the woman contracted the disease from her first husband and has remained asymptomatic. The observation that she is culture negative for STDs, including HSV, is quite consistent with this virus existing in a latent state and not manifesting any clinical signs of disease in the asymptomatic carrier. This question explores the student's deductive skills in the context of herpes pathobiology. The clinical scenario involves a man with overt genital herpes simplex virus (HSV) disease who has had two sexual partners (his ex-wife and the 39-year-old woman) and a woman who lacks disease but who has had three previous sexual partners during the past 5 years (her ex-husband, a 25-year-old man with whom she had protected sex, and the 42-year-old infected man). The question posed is how the male patient contracted HSV. Option A is incorrect and is included to reinforce that it is a myth that STDs are transmitted by objects of public hygiene. Option B is probably not correct if, as the woman indicates, a condom was properly used during her sexual affair with the 25-year-old man. Options D and E are incorrect because asymptomatic infection is not a common consequence of HSV acquired by the neonate.

10 BLOODBORNE AND TRANSPLANT-ASSOCIATED INFECTIONS

CHAPTER OUTLINE

Introduction of Clinical Case
Bloodborne Infections
Illustrative Pathogen: Hepatitis B virus
- Biologic Characteristics
- Reservoir and Transmission
- Virulence Factors
- Pathogenesis
- Diagnosis
- Prevention and Treatment

Transplant-Associated Infections
- Viral Immunosuppression

Illustrative Pathogen: Human cytomegalovirus
- Biologic Characteristics
- Reservoir and Transmission
- Virulence Factors
- Pathogenesis
- Diagnosis
- Prevention and Treatment

Resolution of Clinical Case
Review Questions

INTRODUCTION OF CLINICAL CASE

A 26-year-old man, an admitted intravenous drug abuser, presented to a physician in a rural clinic because he experienced weakness and loss of appetite for the past several weeks. His symptoms included periodic bouts of nausea and frequent headaches. He was febrile (101°F). The physician admitted the patient to a hospital for further tests. Blood work revealed a leukocytosis (14,000 white blood cells/mm²) with a normal differential count. Physical examination revealed hepatomegaly as shown by palpation of the liver edge 2 centimeters below the right costal margin and mild jaundice. Liver enzyme levels were approximately five times higher than normal values; that is, his aspartate aminotransferase (AST) level was 200 units/L, and his alanine aminotransferase (ALT) level was 400 units/L. Serologic findings included a positive test for hepatitis B surface antigen (HBsAg) and hepatitis B core antigen (HBcAg) but no detectable anti-HBsAg antibody.

> **HBsAg** is the envelope (i.e., surface) protein antigen of the hepatitis B virus particle; **HBcAg** is the viral capsid antigen.

After an uneventful 2 weeks in the hospital, the patient reported feeling better and was sent home with instructions to maintain bed rest for 2 more weeks and visit his physician after 1 month.

The patient, although feeling well enough to resume work as a butcher, returned to his physician as instructed. His serum was positive for HBsAg; there were no detectable anti-HBsAg antibodies.

- What illness did this patient contract and how?
- What is the interpretation of the serologic findings during acute and convalescent phases of his disease?
- What measures, if any, should be taken to protect the patient's immediate family? What measures, if any, should be taken concerning his work environment?
- What is the prognosis for this patient?

BLOODBORNE INFECTIONS

Discussion in this chapter focuses primarily on infections that follow direct inoculation of infectious agents into the body by blood transfusions (e.g., certain viral hepatitides), as well as those diseases arising as a consequence of immunosuppression of patients. (Human immunodeficiency virus [HIV] infection is discussed in Chapter 27.)

Historically, blood transfusions often caused rejection disease (e.g., erythroblastosis fetalis) as well as infection. Before their etiologies were discovered, bloodborne (or serum) hepatitis and, later, acquired immunodeficiency syndrome (AIDS) were a threat to recipients of blood transfusions. With the advent of tests for screening blood for known adventitious agents, infections from blood transfusions have been greatly reduced. Today, intravenous drug abuse and surgical interventions, including catheterizations, are the most common modes of direct inoculation of infectious agents into the body. Examples of agents involved in these kinds of infections include gram-positive (e.g., *Staphylococcus, Streptococcus, Corynebacterium, Bacillus* spp.) and gram-negative bacteria (e.g., *Pseudomonas, Klebsiella*), fungi (e.g., *Aspergillus*), and viruses (e.g., hepatitis B, hepatitis C, and HIV). A significant percentage of these are nosocomial infections.

> **Nosocomial** refers to a hospital or infirmary. A nosocomial infection is one contracted in a hospital or like environment.

ILLUSTRATIVE PATHOGEN: Hepatitis B virus

Despite the fact that 90% of hepatitis B virus (HBV) infections result in asymptomatic disease and lifelong immunity, this virus can cause acute hepatitis of varying severity and, most importantly, persistent infections with chronic liver disease. Two forms of clinical hepatitis are recognized: (1) persistent chronic hepatitis (PCH), usually with relatively modest liver dysfunction, and (2) chronic active hepatitis (CAH), which is more severe and is likely to progress to cirrhosis and hepatocellular carcinoma (HCC).

Biologic Characteristics

HBV is the prototypic member of the Hepadnavirus family (see Chapter 3, Table 3-2). Also referred to as the Dane particle, the most distinguishing structural features of HBV are a partial dsDNA genome and a lipid envelope possessing a unique viral surface antigen (i.e., HBsAg). The structure and antigenic components shown in Figure 10-1 are important for interpreting the immune response to this infection.

Reservoir and Transmission

Human beings appear to be the only species infected by HBV. Although this virus is clearly hepatotropic, viral particles have been found in other tissues and body fluids. It is spread most commonly by parenteral inoculation. Thus, intravenous drug abusers who share injection paraphernalia comprise a high-risk group. However, because transmission is possible through intimate contact, institutionalized patients in crowded quarters and health care professionals (e.g., those working with kidney dialysis patients) also are at higher-than-normal risk. Transmission by sexual intercourse can occur.

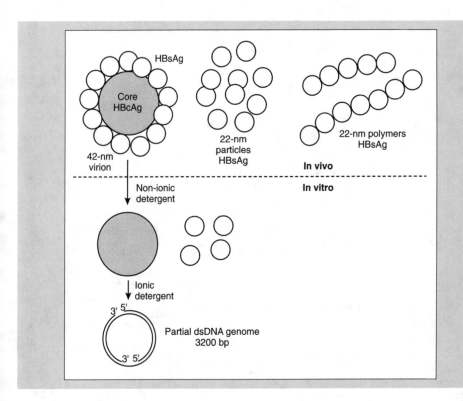

FIGURE 10-1
Forms of Hepatitis B Virus and Its Subviral Particles. The structural features of the hepatitis B virus particle (Dane particle) and various subviral particles formed in vivo and by controlled degradation of the virus in vitro. HBcAg is a form of the hepatitis B core antigen that is masked in the virus particle.

Virulence Factors

The small size of the HBV genome limits the number of factors that this virus is able to encode. One virulence factor is the overproduction of soluble forms of the surface antigen referred to as HbsAg. This antigen aggregates into structures that are noninfectious because they do not associate with viral RNA. These structures may contribute to virulence by acting as decoys, binding HBV-specific antibody and limiting the amount of antibody that could neutralize the truly infectious HBV virion. Other virulence factors certainly include the tropism of HBV for liver cells. This tropism is the consequence of virus attachment to hepatocyte-specific receptors and the ability of this virus to "hijack" hepatocyte-specific transcription factors within the cell.

Pathogenesis

Once in the body, the virus probably is carried to the liver via the blood, where it recognizes hepatocyte receptors and infects cells. Infected cells produce not only infectious HBV (Dane particles) but also secrete enormous quantities ($>10^{13}$ particles/mL) of HBsAg in the form of 22-nm particles and, in lesser concentration, tubular polymers of these particles (see Figure 10-1).

Available evidence suggests that HBV is a noncytopathic virus. If hepatitis results from HBV infection, liver damage apparently results from a cytotoxic T-cell attack directed against infected cells displaying viral antigens on their surfaces. In most cases, the elimination of infected cells resolves the disease process with little or modest liver cell destruction (Figure 10-2). However, in 5%–10% of HBV infections, the immune response fails to eliminate the virus or viral-infected cells, resulting in a persistent HBV infection, the consequences of which can be PCH or CAH (Figure 10-3). In some cases, the clinical symptoms associated with a persistent infection are so mild that the infected individual requires neither hospitalization nor restriction to his or her residence. A carrier may transmit hepatitis B by intimate or sexual contact. As noted above, screening blood donors for evidence of active HBV infection has largely eliminated the threat of transmission via blood transfusion. Because anti-HBsAg antibodies can neutralize HBV infectivity, the synthesis of these antibodies signals the resolution of disease (see Figure 10-2) and immunity to reinfection.

FIGURE 10-2 ▶

Serology of Acute Hepatitis B. *The temporal appearance of HBV-specific antigens and antibodies during a typical case of acute, resolving hepatitis B. The "window" in the upper panel designates a time interval during which viral antigens and antiviral antibodies may be undetectable.*

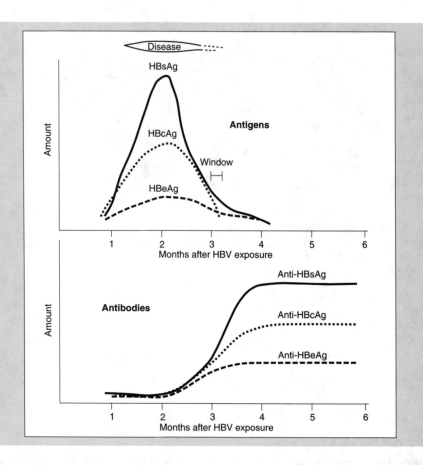

FIGURE 10-3 ▶

Serology of Persistent Chronic (PCH) or Chronic Active (CAH) Hepatitis B. *The temporal appearance of HBV-specific antigens and antibodies during a persistent HBV infection. Persistent infections may result in mild symptoms (carrier state), chronic active hepatitis (CAH), or persistent chronic hepatitis (PCH). Most noteworthy is the prolonged hepatitis B surface (HBs) antigenemia and the absence of protective anti-HBs antibodies.*

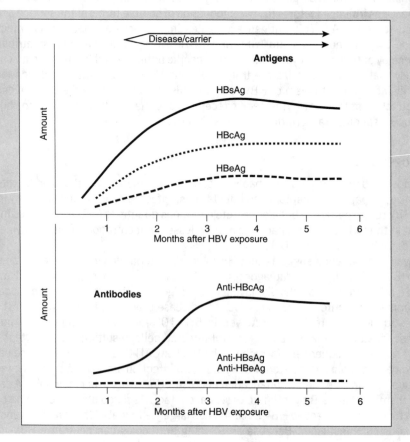

Diagnosis

The clinical symptoms of HBV infection are generally indistinguishable from hepatitis caused by other infectious (e.g., herpesvirus) or noninfectious agents (e.g., alcohol, other hepatotoxic drugs). To diagnose hepatitis B, physicians rely on serologic markers, particularly the detection of HBsAg and various specific anti-HBV antibodies (Table 10-1).

◀ **TABLE 10-1**
Serology of Hepatitis B

HBsAg	Anti-HBsAg (IgG)	Anti-HBcAg (IgG)	Anti-HBeAg (IgG)[a]	Remarks
Positive	Negative	Positive or negative	Positive	Acute or chronic hepatitis B
Negative	Positive	Positive	Positive or negative	Previous infection (immunity exists)
Negative	Negative	Positive	Negative	"Window" or false positive
Negative	Positive	Negative	Negative	Vaccinated with HBsAg
Negative	Negative	Negative	Negative	Not hepatitis B

[a] The appearance of anti-HBeAg antibody during acute infection signals a favorable prognosis.

In addition to HBsAg and HBcAg, another form of the HBcAg, called HBeAg, is produced, which stimulates an anti-HBeAg antibody response. Antibodies to HBeAg generally signal a favorable outcome to HBV infection. In acute hepatitis B, HBsAg is cleared from the blood and replaced by anti-HBsAg antibody (see Figure 10-2). The continued production of HBsAg and the absence of detectable anti-HBsAg antibodies indicates a persistent infection (see Figure 10-3). In all cases, clinical evaluation (and possibly liver biopsy) is necessary to determine the nature and severity of liver involvement.

Certain cases of hepatitis B are complicated by co-infection with a defective RNA virus called hepatitis D virus (HDV). Clinically, HDV infection is diagnosed by detection of anti-HDVAg antibody. Generally, hepatitis D is a more severe disease than hepatitis B.

Prevention and Treatment

Prevention of hepatitis B depends on: (1) screening blood and blood products for HBsAg to prevent inoculations of contaminated materials, (2) educating drug abusers about the risks of sharing contaminated syringes and needles, and (3) vaccinating people who comprise high-risk groups (e.g., men practicing promiscuous homosexual relations, health care professionals routinely exposed to potentially contagious materials, intravenous drug abusers). A safe and effective vaccine, composed of purified HBsAg produced in yeast by recombinant DNA techniques, is available for high-risk individuals and persons accidently exposed to HBV. For patients suffering from chronic, active HBV infection, interferon-α is licensed for treatment. However, a cure is difficult to achieve because the symptomatic improvement accompanying interferon injections usually reverses when treatment ends. Furthermore, interferon-α elicits influenza-like symptoms that may preclude its use. There is no evidence supporting the use of steroids and, in fact, such drugs may be deterimental partly because of their immunosuppressive effects. Only 1% or less of persistent, asymptomatic infections undergo spontaneous cure (i.e., HBsAg is cleared from the blood and replaced with protective anti-HbsAg antibodies).

TRANSPLANT-ASSOCIATED INFECTIONS

Tissue, organ, and bone marrow transplantation are now routine treatments for many diseases. For example, utilizing tissue compatibility matching procedures, meticulous surgical techniques, and the judicious use of immunosuppressive therapy, approximately 75%

Iatrogenic means induced or caused by the actions of a physician. Many iatrogenic infections are nosocomial.

Primary CMV disease is usually more severe when a seronegative recipient is infected with the virus produced from a donor's tissue.

of transplanted kidneys survive for at least 1 year. Thereafter, patient mortality is approximately 5% per year or less. However, the effects of immunosuppression tend to be global because it is not yet possible to prevent tissue rejection while leaving other functions of the immune system untouched. Most immunosuppression is *iatrogenic*, a necessary adjunct to prevent rejection of transplanted organs or the undesirable but inevitable consequence of the chemotherapy used to treat cancers. In bone marrow transplantation, it is an obligatory step in the procedure. The significance of this problem is highlighted by the fact that approximately 80% of transplant recipients experience one or more infections.

Immunosuppression often results when drugs are employed to promote acceptance of donor tissue by a recipient's immune system. The most common diseases occurring within 1 month of transplant surgery are bacterial infections at the surgical site or in the pulmonary or urinary tracts. Infections caused by IV catheters are particularly common. From 1–6 months after surgery, when the maximum desirable immunosuppression is usually attained, the most common infections arise from cytomegalovirus (CMV), usually activated from a latent state in the patient's own cells or from cells of the transplanted organ, and hepatitis C or other non-A, non-B hepatitis viruses. During this period, diseases threatening the patient include those caused by opportunistic microbes such as *Mycobacterium tuberculosis, Cryptococcus neoformans*, and *Pneumocystis carinii*. Some of these diseases represent nosocomial infections.

After 1 year, the major concern centers on chronic diseases such as those caused by CMV (e.g., chorioretinitis, hepatitis, pneumonitis, thrombocytopenia, gastrointestinal ulcers). Other viral diseases of concern include the activation of other herpesviruses such as HSV, varicella zoster virus, and Epstein-Barr virus (EBV), as well as non-A, non-B viral hepatitis. Certain latent human papovaviruses that do not normally cause disease (i.e., BK or JC viruses) may become activated and cause clinical disease. Not only can any of these viral infections compromise the functioning of a transplanted organ, they may exert an immunosuppressive action, exacerbating the patient's susceptibility to other opportunistic organisms.

Viral Immunosuppression

Many infectious diseases, especially in their terminal phases, can suppress the immune system. However, the prototypic infectious immunosuppressive disease is AIDS, wherein HIV infection eventually reduces the concentration of helper CD4+ T lymphocytes below a critical threshold compatible with normal immune system function. Not surprisingly, one of the hallmarks of AIDS is susceptibility to a large number of opportunistic infections, including virtually all those listed above.

ILLUSTRATIVE AGENT: Human cytomegalovirus

Although many bacterial, fungal, and viral agents may cause opportunistic infections, herpesviruses, because of their propensity for latent infection, provide a classic paradigm. In North America, more than 50% (90% in some urban populations) of healthy adults harbor CMV as a latent infection. Human CMV, also called herpesvirus 5, exhibits a narrow species specificity and a predilection for the epithelia of various organs. Although most primary infections of healthy adults result in inapparent disease, CMV can cause an EBV-like infectious mononucleosis in this group. Upon immunosuppression, the growth of CMV is frequently activated from latently infected mononuclear cells, resulting in asymptomatic infection, cytomegalic inclusion disease (CID), or clinical disease in various specific organs such as the liver, lungs, kidneys, or the central nervous system. In newborns, CID may result from a primary (i.e., newly acquired) infection.

Biologic Characteristics

CMV is a member of the human herpesvirus family (see Chapter 9), which includes herpes simplex virus types 1 (HSV-1) and 2 (HSV-2) that cause genital and orofacial lesions; varicella zoster virus (VZV), the causative agent of chicken pox and shingles;

Epstein-Barr virus (EBV), which causes a mononucleosis common in young adults as well as Burkitt's lymphoma and nasopharyngeal carcinoma; and human herpesviruses 6 (HHV-6), 7 (HHV-7), and 8 (HHV-8). HHV-8 is the infectious agent responsible for the induction of Kaposis sarcoma, which is prevalent among AIDS patients.

The CMV virion particle, like the other herpesviruses, is composed of an icosahedral-shaped nucleocapsid surrounded by the electron-dense tegument layer, which is enclosed within a bilayer membrane envelope that is acquired from the host cell. The viral nucleocapsid contains the large (240 Kb) linear double-stranded DNA genome that encodes over 190 viral proteins that are grouped into three kinetic classes designated immediate early, early, and late. The immediate early genes are mainly regulatory in nature and control the expression of the early genes that primarily encode functions involved in viral DNA synthesis. The late genes are expressed following viral genome replication and code for virion structural components. This cascade of viral gene expression is similar to that observed with HSV, except that HSV replication is rapid, resulting in mature particle production within 8-12 hours, while CMV replicates slowly, that is, infectious particles are produced after 3 days and plaques will not develop until 7-14 days postinfection. The reasons for the slow replication rate of CMV may involve the fact that many CMV gene transcripts are spliced by the host cell machinery, while very few HSV genes encode spliced RNAs. Additionally, the CMV immediate early gene functions stimulate host cell macromolecular synthesis, which would be required for proper processing of the many CMV transcripts.

Reservoir and Transmission

Human CMV can replicate only within cells of human origin; thus humans represent the sole reservoir for CMV. In addition, productive infection is restricted to specific cell types within the host. Transmission of the virus occurs via direct or indirect contact between individuals. Virus can be detected in urine, seminal fluid, breast milk, blood, cervical and vaginal secretions, and in oropharyngeal secretions. The virus can be transmitted to a child in utero via the placenta from either a primary or recurrent infection of the mother. Approximately 1% of the population contracts CMV in utero. Though this number seems relatively low, it accounts for more than 35,000 infected infants per year in the United States alone. Up to 60% of the population becomes infected either during birth or during the first few years of life, with the incidence of infection remaining low until adulthood. During adulthood, transmission can occur via the oral-respiratory route, through sexual contact, or by blood transfusion. Finally, transmission occurs in immunosuppressed individuals receiving organ or bone marrow transplants, where latent virus resident either in the transplant tissue or within host immune cells within the tissue can reactivate in the immunocompromised host, resulting in acute infection.

Virulence Factors

CMV can establish a latent state in macrophages, monocytes, and lymphocytes, enabling the virus to avoid host immune surveillance in a manner similar to that of HSV. In culture, CMV infection results in readily visible cytopathic effects (CPE) demonstrated by the margination of cell chromatin, the appearance of membrane vesicles within the cytoplasm, changes in membrane permeability, pyknotic nuclei, and the overall alteration of the cell size. These represent changes to the cell characteristic of CMV infection, as suggested by the name of the virus—"cytomegalo." Several CMV gene products can be classified as virulence factors that contribute to the virus-associated CPE as well as assisting the virus in altering the host response to CMV infection enabling long-term persistence of the virus. The immediate early transcriptional regulatory gene products (IE1 and IE2), in addition to being essential for the expression of viral early and late gene functions, have been shown to regulate cellular cyclins as well as the p53 tumor suppressor gene. Several CMV gene products are involved in the downregulation of antigen presentation associated with CMV infection. The US3 gene product blocks intracellular transport of MHC class I molecules while the US2/US11 complex is involved in the dislocation of MHC class I molecules from the lumen of the endothelial reticulum to the cytosol, where they are rapidly degraded. CMV infection also results in the inhibition of IFNg stimulated MHC class II cell surface expression by disruption of the Jak/Stat pathway. In addition, the UL18 gene product is a homologue of the cellular class I H-chain that binds beta 2-microglobulin acting as a NK cell decoy, thereby mediating NK-mediated clearance of CMV-infected cells. The virus also encodes proteins (US27, US28, US33) with homology to cellular CC chemokine receptors that help the virus sequester chemokines like MCP-1 and RANTES, further compromising host immune surveillance.

Pathogenesis

Virus growth occurs in epithelial cells of many organs such as the salivary glands, liver, kidneys, and in the respiratory tract. Although the mechanisms governing spread of the virus within the body remain obscure, permissive or semipermissive monocytes apparently capable of latent infection, may play a role in viral dissemination. Although CMV is the etiologic agent of a wide variety of human disorders, most CMV infections are asymptomatic except in the immunocompromised host. In this regard, CMV differs from HSV in the relative pathogenecity of viral infection. As noted above, systemic CMV infection in healthy adults can manifest as an infectious mononucleosis. Hepatitis is a common clinical component of mononucleosis.

Because of its frequent role in congenital infections, CMV is the most common infectious cause of developmental birth defects. CID is an extremely serious, sometimes fatal, systemic disease in infants. In utero transmission, usually from a mother with a primary infection, can result in CID in which the infant can display hepatosplenomegaly, petechiae, jaundice, chorioretinitis, low birth size, and prematurity of birth. Only 5% of infected infants develop the clinically detectable symptoms associated with CID. Asymptotic infection of the remaining 95% infected infants may result in hearing loss, depressed IQ, damage to the CNS resulting in severe mental retardation or other sequelae later in life. Although maternal immunity may alter the virulence of the infection, this immunity can be insufficient for protection of the fetus from reactivated virus. The mortality rate is 10%-30% for CID; the remaining infants display CNS complications throughout life. Even subclinical infection in infants may result in various sequelae that manifest during puberty or later in adulthood. Infectious mononucleosis syndrome is the usual outcome of primary infection of normal adolescents or adults, which is not severe in most cases. In immunocompromised individuals such as AIDS patients and individuals receiving transplants, CMV infection manifests either as a mononucleosis syndrome or as pneumonitis. CMV chorioretinitis is the leading cause of blindness in AIDS patients. CMV infection of the immunosuppressed transplant patient results in an increase in both mortality and tissue rejection if left untreated. In immunocompromised individuals, including patients treated with immunosuppressive agents or those suffering from AIDS, disease may follow reactivation of the patient's own latent virus, the introduction of contaminated blood or blood-related products, or the transplantation of organs from a CMV-infected donor. In AIDS patients, CMV produces esophagitis, gastritis, and colitis, and it is a common cause of chorioretinitis.

Neutralizing antibodies do not prevent infection but they may protect against or ameliorate clinical disease. Immune control of CMV seems to rely on the destruction of productively infected cells by cytotoxic T lymphocytes as well as the production of neutralizing antibodies. However, these immune mechanisms do not recognize latently infected cells because these cells do not produce viral antigens.

Diagnosis

A variety of serologic assays can be used to detect CMV-specific antigens in tissues. Isolation of CMV in tissue culture is also performed, but typically requires as long as 1 month to cultivate and identify the virus. Newer generation tests utilizing polymerase chain reaction (PCR) show promise of excellent sensitivity and specificity. However, given the ubiquitous nature of CMV infection, determining the presence of CMV, either directly by virus isolation or indirectly by serologic or biochemical markers, does not alone prove the role of CMV in causing disease. The patient's history and clinical symptoms are at least of equal importance.

Prevention and Treatment

The microbiologic and serologic screening of organ donors for active CMV production can reduce but not eliminate infections caused by its transfer. In allograft patients, prophylaxis with ganciclovir for several months following organ transplantation has proven useful in preventing or ameliorating clinical CMV disease. Foscarnet may be used in conjunction with ganciclovir, except for kidney transplant recipients in whom renal toxicity precludes its use. CMV disease in AIDS patients is particularly difficult to control because extensive virus replication seems to favor the relatively rapid appearance of drug-resistant mutants.

RESOLUTION OF CLINICAL CASE

The patient presented at the start of this chapter almost certainly contracted HBV from intravenous inoculation using shared needles or other drug paraphernalia. His symptoms, biochemical findings (i.e., liver enzymes), and serology point to hepatitis B. After resolution of most of his symptoms, he continues to be HBsAg-positive and anti-HBsAg antibody negative. Therefore, it can be presumed that he suffers from a persistent HBV infection and, almost certainly, there is ongoing liver damage as indicated by elevated liver-specific enzymes in his blood. He has become a carrier, and, as a food handler, he could conceivably transmit HBV to others. The likelihood of his undergoing a spontaneous cure is remote. Because HBV can be transmitted sexually, the person at highest risk is his wife, who should be vaccinated and, for the near term, monitored for possible HBV infection.

REVIEW QUESTIONS

Directions: For each of the following questions, choose the **one best** answer.

1. The reason organ and bone marrow transplant patients are susceptible to infectious agents is mostly related to
    (A) a reduction in protective antibodies in their blood
    (B) suppressed cellular immune responses
    (C) the impossibility of influencing the likelihood that the transplant donor organ will be free of adventitious agents
    (D) an ineffectiveness of antibiotics in such patients
    (E) graft-versus-host reaction

2. The most important marker for monitoring a persistent hepatitis B infection is
    (A) a group of liver enzymes
    (B) anti-HBcAg antibodies
    (C) HBeAg
    (D) anti-HBeAg antibodies
    (E) HBsAg

3. A 27-year-old man being treated for cancer with drugs that are immunosuppressive is admitted to a hospital suffering from malaise, intestinal symptoms, and jaundice. The laboratory blood tests report elevated liver enzymes and no detectable antibodies to hepatitis B surface or core antigens. Immunoglobulin G (IgG) antibodies to hepatitis A virus, herpes simplex virus 1, and cytomegalovirus are detected in a single blood specimen. It is possible to conclude that the patient is
    (A) suffering from hepatitis A
    (B) experiencing a reactivated cytomegalovirus infection
    (C) experiencing hepatitis induced by his chemotherapy
    (D) afflicted by a hepatitis but its etiology requires further diagnostic procedures

4. The most distinguishing feature of hepatitis B virus (HBV) is that it
    (A) possesses an envelope
    (B) has an icosahedral nucleocapsid
    (C) has a partially double-stranded DNA genome
    (D) is a herpesvirus
    (E) is a defective virus

5. A patient with obvious signs of active hepatitis is hospitalized and blood samples taken for analyses. During acute illness, the serum is found to contain hepatitis B surface antigen (HBsAg) and hepatitis D virus (HDV) antigen. Over a period of several weeks, the levels of these antigens remain high and no anti-HBsAg antibodies are detected. What is most likely causing this disease?
    (A) A virus with a helical nucleocapsid
    (B) Two different viruses, one of which is defective
    (C) Hepatitis B virus
    (D) A virus capable of latent infections
    (E) A virus capable of immunosuppressing its host

ANSWERS AND EXPLANATIONS

1. **The answer is B.** Immunosuppression acts primarily on the cellular immune host responses to foreign antigens (including microbes) and, in most cases, does not as dramatically affect antibody production. Therefore, option A (a reduction in protective antibodies in the blood) is incorrect. Although it is not possible to entirely eliminate the presence of adventitious agents in donor tissue, serologic and microbiologic screening tests to determine whether such donors have been infected with specific agents of concern (e.g., CMV, HBV) can influence the likelihood of transplanted infectious agents. Therefore, option C is incorrect. Option D is incorrect because antibiotics exhibit antimicrobial activity in immunosuppressed patients. Although a graft-versus-host reaction is a real phenomenon, it is not the primary reason for infections in transplant patients.

2. **The answer is E.** HBsAg in the blood is the most reliable indicator of a persistent hepatitis B infection and indicates a carrier state, persistent chronic hepatitis, or chronic active hepatitis. Elevated liver enzymes indicate hepatitis but do not provide information about its etiology; therefore, option A is incorrect. Anti-HBcAg antibodies are produced during acute and persistent hepatitis B infections and do not specifically indicate the latter. HBeAg (option C) is a form of the core antigen, and the argument above applies to it as well as to antibodies of this antigen (option D). It is true, however, that the appearance of anti-HBeAg antibodies is a favorable prognostic sign.

3. **The answer is D.** Serologic methods that would provide evidence of a particular etiologic agent include a significant elevation in antibodies between acute and convalescent sera, measurement of specific immunoglobulin M antibodies to a specific agent during or shortly after the acute phase of illness, and the isolation by culture or identification (e.g., by immunofluorescent antibody staining) of the agent in biopsied liver tissue. The presence in a single blood sample of IgG antibodies to virtually any infectious agent does not allow the differentiation between current and past infections. In fact, hepatitis A virus (HAV) antibodies against HAV of the IgG class are present in a significant percentage of adults, who usually acquire HAV as an asymptomatic infection. The same reasoning applies to any herpesvirus because all of them persist in the infected host after eliciting specific immune responses. Thus, options A and B are incorrect presumptions. Option C is a valid possibility but is unproven based on the information given; therefore, it is an incorrect answer.

4. **The answer is C.** The unique feature of all hepadnaviruses, including HBV, is their partially double-stranded DNA genome. Many different viruses, including HBV, possess an envelope and an icosahedral capsid. HBV is a member of the Hepadnavirus family and is neither a herpesvirus nor a defective virus.

5. **The answer is B.** A hepatitis patient who is positive for both HBV and HDV antigens has a case of hepatitis D, a disease caused by infection with both HBV and HDV. HDV is a defective RNA virus that requires concomitant HBV infection to form an infectious particle. Option C would be correct if there were no evidence of HDV infection. Neither HBV nor HDV possess a helical nucleocapsid. HBV and HDV are not capable of latent infections, and they do not commonly immunosuppress the host.

11 NORMAL MICROBIAL FLORA INHIBITION OF MICROBIAL PATHOGEN COLONIZATION

CHAPTER OUTLINE

Introduction to Clinical Case
Normal Microbial Flora
- Body Sites Containing Normal Flora
- Tropism of Normal Flora

Importance of the Normal Microbial Flora
- Negative Effects
- Positive Effects

Illustrative Pathogen: *Clostridium difficile*
- Biologic Characteristics
- Reservoir and Transmission
- Virulence Factors
- Pathogenesis
- Diagnosis
- Prevention and Treatment

Resolution of Clinical Case
Review Questions

INTRODUCTION TO CLINICAL CASE

A 45-year-old woman with heart problems was in the hospital for several days for a series of tests of her cardiac function. While in the hospital, she accidentally scratched her left forearm on a table in her room. Two days after this incident, the scratch appeared red. Her physician determined that there was no break in the skin and that although the scratch was undergoing a mild inflammatory reaction, there was no evidence of infection. However, to help reassure the patient, a 10-day course of oral clindamycin was prescribed. The patient left the hospital 2 days later, after her cardiac testing was completed. The next day (i.e., 3 days after the start of antibiotic treatment), the patient developed loose stools, which became a frequent, clear, watery diarrhea during the next 24 hours. By the fifth day of antibiotic therapy, she was having approximately 15 bowel movements per day, with blood visible in the toilet after most bowel movements. She informed her physician, who instructed her to stop taking the clindamycin and re-admitted her to the hospital. Physical examination was basically uninformative, but laboratory studies revealed moderate dehydration. Examination of the patient's stool revealed numerous erythrocytes and neutrophils, although routine stool culture produced no enteric pathogens. An enzyme-linked immunosorbent assay (ELISA) of the stool specimen for *Clostridium difficile* toxins was positive. The patient was given intravenous fluids and was started on metronidazole by mouth.

- What role do normal microbial flora play in the pathogenesis of this patient's illness?
- What role, if any, did the clindamycin therapy play in this illness?
- What role, if any, did the patient's presence in the hospital play in this illness?
- Is this women's illness potentially serious?

NORMAL MICROBIAL FLORA

Body Sites Containing Normal Flora

The human body essentially lacks any microbial flora at birth, but soon becomes colonized by microbes. Microorganisms normally present in the healthy body are collectively referred to as normal flora. With respect to colonization by normal flora, the healthy body maintains three types of sites:

1. *Sterile compartments.* Blood, cerebrospinal fluid, synovial fluid, and deep tissues are usually sterile. Therefore, detecting the presence of any microbes in these body sites is diagnostically significant.

2. *Body sites that normally contain low numbers of microbes.* In the absence of disease, the stomach, upper small intestine, lower respiratory tract, urinary bladder, and uterus usually contain low numbers of microbes. Therefore, finding sizable numbers of microbes (particularly sizable numbers of known pathogens) at these locations suggests disease.

3. *Body sites that are abundantly colonized in healthy individuals.* A number of body sites (Table 11-1), particularly mucosal surfaces, are routinely colonized by microbes. (Note in Table 11-1 that normal flora includes both prokaryotic and eukaryotic microbes.)

Life for normal microbial flora is not particularly easy. Each normal flora microbe encounters numerous challenges: (1) it must overcome specific and nonspecific host defense mechanisms; (2) it must find a body site that provides the right combination of environmental factors (e.g., pH, nutrients, redox potential) necessary for growth; and (3) it must find an ecologically suitable environment in which it can successfully compete against other normal microbes for nutrients and can withstand the efforts of other normal flora microbes to inhibit its growth.

Tropism of Normal Flora

Considering the limitations presented above, it is not surprising that (like most pathogens) normal flora microbes generally exhibit *tropism*, a preference for a particular body site, as shown in Table 11-1.

Why are the normal microbial flora important for medicine? As explained in the following sections, the presence of a large population of normal flora microbes in the body has a number of both positive and potentially negative consequences.

TABLE 11-1
Predominant Normal Flora in the Healthy Body

Body Site	Microbial Flora Present[a]
Conjunctiva	*Staphylococcus epidermidis*[b]
Skin	*S. epidermidis*, diphtheroids[c] *Propionibacterium* spp.[d], yeasts (e.g., *Candida* spp.)
Mouth/oropharynx	*Streptococcus viridans*[e], nonpathogenic *Neisseria* (and related gram-negative cocci), anaerobes (e.g., *Bacteroides*-like group, *Fusobacterium* spp.), yeasts (e.g., *Candida* spp.)
Nasopharynx	*S. epidermidis*, *Staphylococcus aureus*[f], *S. viridans*
Colon	Anaerobes (e.g., *Bacteroides*-like group, *Clostridium* spp., *Fusobacterium* spp., *Bifodobacterium* spp.[f], *Lactobacillus* spp.[g], coliforms[h], peptostreptococci, enterococci yeasts (e.g., *Candida* spp.)
External genitalia and anterior urethra	"Skin flora" (e.g., diphtheroids, *S. epidermidis*), anaerobes (e.g., *Bacteroides*-like group), *Lactobacillus* spp. (in women)
Vagina	*Lactobacillus* spp., "skin flora," yeasts (e.g., *Candida* spp.)

[a] Only the most common normal flora microbial species are listed; other species may also be present. Characteristics of bacteria listed here but not mentioned elsewhere in this book include: [b] gram-positive cocci; [c] gram-positive rods (nonpathogenic *Corynebacterium* spp.); [d] gram-positive rods (often grow only under anaerobic conditions); [e] gram-positive cocci (includes all alpha-hemolytic streptococci except pneumococci); [f] gram-positive rods (anaerobic); [g] gram-positive (anaerobes or facultative anaerobes); [h] *E. coli*-like bacteria (i.e., lactose-fermenting, gram-negative aerobic/facultative anaerobic rods).

IMPORTANCE OF THE NORMAL MICROBIAL FLORA

Negative Effects

Opportunistic Infections. Although normal microbial flora are often maintained in the body for many years without any ill effects, these microbes always have the potential to cause negative effects on health. Most notably, the normal microbial flora are major causes of opportunistic infections that develop under permissive conditions (e.g., conditions that result in lowered host defenses). The involvement of normal flora in opportunistic infections should not be surprising given that these microbes are present (i.e., endogenous) and adapted for growth in the body. However, it should be appreciated that not all normal flora are equally prone to cause opportunistic infections. As discussed in Chapter 2, *Bacteroides fragilis* (part of the normal colonic flora) is a more common cause of abdominal infections than would be expected simply because of the prevalence of this organism in the intestines. The major causes of endogenously acquired opportunistic infection is discussed in more detail in Chapter 28.

The ability of *B. fragilis* to cause abdominal infections illustrates another important principle concerning opportunistic infections caused by endogenous normal flora microbes. These microbes often (but not always) cause infections in body sites at or near their normal sites of colonization. As a consequence, certain normal flora species have become associated with particular types of opportunistic infections. Besides the involvement of *B. fragilis* in abdominal infections, two other examples illustrate this principle: (1) the importance of *Staphylococcus epidermidis* (present in the normal flora of the skin and elsewhere; see Table 11-1) as a cause of catheter infections, and (2) the role of *Escherichia coli* (commonly found in the large intestine and feces) as the leading cause of urinary tract infections (see Chapter 12).

Positive Effects

If the normal flora occasionally cause opportunistic infections, why does the body tolerate their presence? The short answer is that the normal flora provide several desirable effects that apparently outweigh the risk of their causing opportunistic infections.

For instance, *E. coli* and some *Bacteroides* spp. are considered important producers of vitamin K for the human host.

Effects on the Immune System. The normal flora are thought to provide at least two beneficial effects for the immune system. First, the normal flora are believed to help prime the immune system and thus contribute to the development of immune competence. In support of this view, animals raised in a germ-free environment (obtainable in special labs) exhibit a poorly developed reticuloendothelial system, produce low levels of immunoglobulins, and show other immune system deficits. Second, antibodies elicited against some normal flora microbes may cross-react with, and therefore help protect against, some pathogens.

Effects on Pathogens. Normal flora suppress the ability of pathogens to colonize or multiply in the body through two primary mechanisms. They physically block invading pathogens from adhering to and colonizing the body. Because normal flora are already present at a particular body site, there is simply no room available for pathogens (i.e., normal flora have "squatter's rights" to that body site). Also, some normal flora produce inhibitory substances such as antibiotics or bacteriocins that inhibit the ability of intruding microbes (e.g., pathogens) to colonize or multiply at body sites where these normal flora microbes reside.

The inhibitory effects of the normal flora on pathogen colonization and proliferation have been well documented, both clinically and experimentally. For example, laboratory experiments have clearly shown that administering streptomycin to mice severely disrupts the normal gastrointestinal flora of these mice. Further, the dose of *Salmonella* required to cause disease in these streptomycin-treated mice is lowered by a factor of at least 1000 (perhaps by a factor of 1,000,000) compared to the *Salmonella* dose necessary to produce disease in healthy mice carrying normal gastrointestinal flora. Experienced clinicians are also well aware of the importance of the normal flora in resisting infectious disease. Patients receiving antibiotic therapies that severely affect the normal flora are recognized as being at increased risk for infection by both exogenous and endogenous microbes. These endogenous microbes can include either normal flora organisms or pathogens present in the proper body sites at numbers insufficient to cause disease prior to initiation of antibiotic therapy. However, antibiotic treatment (often coupled with medical conditions leading to impaired immune system function) reduces competition from normal flora microbes and allows the pathogens to proliferate. For example, patients treated with antibiotics often develop yeast (e.g., *Candida* spp.) infections in the mouth or vagina. An even more compelling illustration of the importance of normal flora microbes in preventing disease is the ability of *C. difficile* to cause potentially life-threatening gastrointestinal (GI) diseases in patients that have received antibiotic therapy.

> *Not all interactions between the normal flora and the immune system necessarily benefit the host. It is believed that normal flora also may elicit immunopathologic responses in some individuals.*

> ***Bacteriocins*** *are proteins that are produced by one bacterium in order to kill or inhibit another bacterium.*

> *Healthy individuals may carry certain "pathogens" (e.g.,* Staphylococcus aureus, Streptococcus pneumoniae, *or* Neisseria meningitidis*) without ill effects because these pathogens are either present in low numbers or they are present in the wrong body site to cause disease.*

ILLUSTRATIVE PATHOGEN: *Clostridium difficile*

Biologic Characteristics

C. difficile is an anaerobic, spore-forming, gram-positive rod, which is typical of *Clostridium* spp. (see Chapter 2).

Reservoir and Transmission

Although the reservoirs and transmission of *C. difficile* have been controversial, the emerging consensus is that only a small fraction (almost certainly < 5%) of healthy adults are normally colonized by *C. difficile*. Recent studies indicate that the longer patients stay in a hospital (or nursing home), the more likely they are to be colonized by *C. difficile*, implying that *C. difficile* is usually an exogenously acquired nosocomial pathogen.

How then do hospitalized or institutionalized patients acquire *C. difficile*? Two mechanisms are thought to predominate:

> *Interestingly, many healthy neonates are colonized by fully toxigenic strains of C. difficile. Why infants are not affected by these bacteria remains unclear, but it is possible that neonates lack the proper cellular receptors necessary for intoxication by C. difficile toxins.*

- *Direct transmission.* The normal hospital environment is often heavily contaminated with *C. difficile* (particularly for their environmentally resistant spores; see Chapter 2). Fomite (or other) transmission can lead to a patient's ingesting *C. difficile* spores, which later germinate in the GI tract.
- *Indirect transmission.* Hospitalized or institutionalized patients may become colonized with *C. difficile* from the hands of personnel caring for multiple patients. Studies have shown that intensive glove use by medical personnel sharply decreases the frequency of *C. difficile*–mediated disease in hospitals.

Virulence Factors

Typical of the pathogenic clostridia, the major virulence factors of *C. difficile* are two toxins, specifically toxin A and toxin B. Although toxin A and toxin B each contain only a single polypeptide, these two proteins are the largest (> 300,000 daltons) bacterial toxins known. Besides being of similar size, these two toxins also share approximately 50% amino acid sequence identity. Consistent with this homology, recent studies have strongly suggested that toxin A and toxin B share a similar molecular action (Figure 11-1). After binding to cellular receptors and being internalized into mammalian cells, both *C. difficile* toxins A and B act by inhibiting the Rho family of mammalian proteins. This inhibition is achieved by attaching a single glucose moiety (from uridine diphosphate [UDP]–glucose) onto a specific threonine residue present in Rho proteins (i.e., toxins A and B are enzymes that have monoglucosyltransferase activity).

> The **Rho family** of protein (which includes Rho, Rac, and other proteins) are guanosine triphosphate (GTP)-binding proteins that are involved in regulating a number of essential functions in mammalian cells (e.g., assembly and disassembly of the cytoskeleton and various signal transduction pathways).

C. difficile
toxins A and B
UDP–glucose + Rho - - - - - - → Glucose–Rho + UDP
(active)   (inhibited)

◀ **FIGURE 11-1**
Molecular Mechanism of Action of Clostridium difficile *Toxins A and B.* Rho proteins act as molecular "switches" for the mammalian cell, functioning in cytoskeletal dynamics and many signal transduction pathways. Because addition of glucose to Rho results in functional inactivation of Rho, many cellular processes are disrupted by *C. difficile* toxin. UDP = uridine diphosphate.

Despite the similarity between the molecular actions of toxins A and B, toxin A is considered the stronger enterotoxin (i.e., it stimulates fluid and electrolyte losses from the intestines), whereas toxin B is considered the stronger cytotoxin (i.e., it kills mammalian cells). These different functional attributes are likely due to toxins A and B recognizing different receptors that are present only on specific types of mammalian cells. Toxins A and B appear equally important for *C. difficile* pathogenesis.

Pathogenesis

The development of *C. difficile* GI disease is dependent on at least three factors:

- *Colonization.* As mentioned above, many individuals become colonized with *C. difficile* during a hospital or nursing home stay. However, colonization of the colon by *C. difficile* is not sufficient for the development of disease because most hospital patients colonized with this bacterium remain asymptomatic.
- *Previous antibiotic therapy.* Typically, only those colonized patients receiving antibiotic therapy go on to develop *C. difficile*–mediated GI disease. The association between previous or ongoing antibiotic therapy and *C. difficile*–mediated gastrointestinal disease stems from the ability of antibiotics to alter the normal colonic flora, providing *C. difficile* with the opportunity to colonize and proliferate in the colon of these patients. Treatment with virtually any antibiotic may predispose a patient to *C. difficile*–mediated gastrointestinal disease, but clindamycin (at an especially high

rate), ampicillin, and cephalosporins are the antibiotics most frequently associated with *C. difficile*–mediated gastrointestinal illnesses. The particularly strong association between clindamycin and *C. difficile*–mediated gastrointestinal disease is understandable given that many *C. difficile* strains are resistant to clindamycin and that clindamycin is notorious for disrupting the normal colonic flora.

- *Host factors.* Host factors also play an important role in the development of *C. difficile*–mediated gastrointestinal diseases (e.g., older patients are more prone to develop these illnesses).

After successfully colonizing the antibiotic-disturbed colon, *C. difficile* proliferates (without invading into the colon) and produces toxins A and B. Through their effects on Rho-dependent cellular functions (e.g., cytoskeletal assembly/disassembly; altering signal transduction pathways), toxins A and B apparently contribute to the pathogenesis of *C. difficile*–mediated gastrointestinal disease in at least two ways. First, they can directly damage or kill colonic epithelial cells. Second, toxins A and B can provoke intense inflammation through their abilities to (1) act as chemoattractants for polymorphonuclear neutrophils (PMNs) and (2) stimulate the release of endogenous mediators of inflammation (e.g., tumor necrosis factor [TNF]) from PMNs and other inflammatory cells.

As a result of this toxin-mediated inflammation and damage to the colonic mucosa, ion and fluid secretion from the colon are stimulated. This response manifests itself clinically as diarrhea. In the most common form of *C. difficile*–mediated gastrointestinal disease, antibiotic-associated diarrhea, symptoms are generally limited to an uncomplicated diarrhea (fever or abdominal pain are present in < 25% of cases). Unfortunately, some patients develop more severe *C. difficile*–mediated colitis. A potentially life-threatening form of this colitis is referred to as *pseudomembranous colitis* because of the characteristic presence of yellowish-white plaques that contain the pseudomembrane (Figures 11-2 and 11-3) and that are visible on the colonic mucosa using endoscopy. This pseudomembrane overlies regions of the colon that have been significantly damaged by *C. difficile* toxins and is comprised of fibrin, mucus, necrotic epithelial cells, *C. difficile* cells, and leukocytes. Besides diarrhea (which varies in severity and may involve bloody feces), abdominal pain, tenesmus, and fever are other common symptoms of *C. difficile*–mediated colitis. Death can occur in patients with *C. difficile*–mediated colitis, usually from colonic perforation or systemic toxicity, which may be mediated (at least in part) by toxin-mediated inflammatory mediators (e.g., TNF, interleukin-1). *C. difficile* is considered to be responsible for approximately 25% of all cases of antibiotic-associated diarrhea and for approximately 90% of all cases of pseudomembranous colitis.

Tenesmus is the feeling of an urgent need to defecate and being unable to do so even after straining. In C. difficile-*induced gastrointestinal disease, tenesmus is probably due to an inflammatory reaction of the bowel wall.*

Diagnosis

Because symptoms of *C. difficile* gastrointestinal disease are mediated by toxins A and B, detection of these toxins in stool can be achieved using either a cell-culture cytotoxicity assay or a toxin ELISA, which is the most specific noninvasive test available for diagnosing these illnesses. Culturing stools for the presence of *C. difficile* can also provide useful information; however, positive results must be interpreted cautiously given the high background rate of asymptomatic colonized carriers in hospital settings. By demonstrating the presence of pseudomembrane-containing plaques in the colon (see Figure 11-3), endoscopy can provide useful information to assist in the diagnosis of pseudomembranous colitis.

Prevention and Treatment

Given the potential severity of *C. difficile*–mediated gastrointestinal disease and the problem of recurrences, it is obviously preferable to prevent rather than treat these illnesses. Although no vaccine is available, there are steps that can be taken to limit the occurrence and severity of *C. difficile* disease. First, patients receiving antibiotics can be closely monitored for the development of diarrhea; if diarrhea develops, antibiotic therapy should be discontinued (if medically possible) or another antibiotic (preferably one less likely to disrupt the normal colonic flora) should be substituted for the offending antibiotic. Second, rigorous changing of gloves and maintenance of strict sanitary stan-

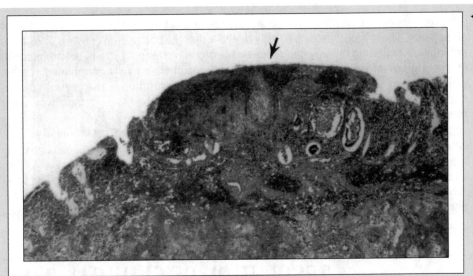

FIGURE 11-2
Histologic Appearance of Pseudomembranous Colitis. *Note the typical mushroom-like pseudomembranous lesion erupting from the mucosal surface. (Source: This figure was provided courtesy of Drs. Stuart Johnson and Dale Gerding, Medical Service, VA Lakeside Medical Center, Chicago, Illinois.)*

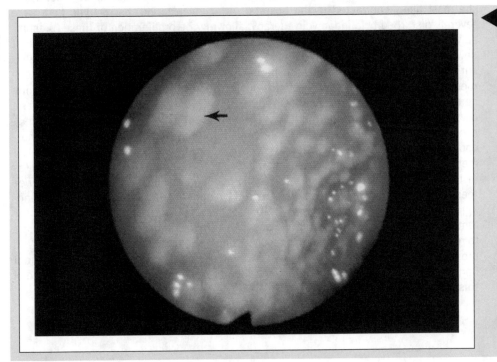

FIGURE 11-3
Plaques on the Colonic Mucosa of a Patient with Pseudomembranous Colitis Induced by Clostridium difficile. *(Source: This figure was provided courtesy of Drs. Stuart Johnson and Dale Gerding, Medical Service, VA Lakeside Medical Center, Chicago, Illinois.)*

dards in hospitals and nursing homes should be stressed to help reduce *C. difficile* colonization rates for institutionalized patients.

Simply removing the offending antibiotic (if medically possible) often resolves milder cases of *C. difficile*–mediated gastrointestinal disease. If this approach is not feasible or if the patient does not respond, the most widely used antibiotic therapies for *C. difficile*–mediated gastrointestinal diseases have traditionally been oral metronidazole or vancomycin. However, because of fears of developing further vancomycin resistance (see Chapters 4 and 5) in gram-positive bacteria (possibly including developing vancomycin resistance in *C. difficile* itself), there is current movement toward limiting the use of vancomycin to patients with severe (potentially life-threatening) *C. difficile*–mediated gastrointestinal illness. Individuals suffering from *C. difficile*–mediated gastrointestinal diseases may also require symptomatic therapy aimed at restoring fluid and electrolyte balances. Finally, agents (e.g., Lomotil) that slow intestinal motility should not be administered to patients suffering from *C. difficile*–mediated gastrointestinal diseases because these agents often worsen symptoms.

Recurrence of *C. difficile*–mediated gastrointestinal disease occurs in 5%–30% of all patients. These recurrences are likely due to either the acquisition of a new *C. difficile* strain, after antibiotic therapy had removed the original offending strain, or to a regrowth of the original infecting strain. Recurrence may result from newly germinated spores, which often are very resistant to antibiotic therapy. Re-institution of therapy with metronidazole or vancomycin almost always is effective in these cases, although a small minority of patients suffer multiple recurrences.

Nonantibiotic therapeutic regimens for *C. difficile*–mediated gastrointestinal diseases are currently under investigation. One of the more promising approaches involves the introduction of nonpathogenic microbes (e.g., the nonpathogenic yeast *Saccharomyces boulardii*) into the colon of patients suffering multiple recurrences, where it is hoped that these nonpathogenic microbes will compete against *C. difficile* for colonization of the colon.

RESOLUTION OF CLINICAL CASE

The patient in this case developed *C. difficile*–mediated gastrointestinal disease, which she most likely contracted in the hospital. After colonization, her colonic flora were severely disturbed by clindamycin therapy, allowing the proliferation of these (presumably) newly acquired *C. difficile* organisms. As a result of toxin production, this patient developed colitis, which involved more serious symptoms than *C. difficile*–mediated antibiotic-associated diarrhea. As exhibited by the patient in this case, *C. difficile*–mediated colitis typically involves tenesmus as well as fever and a diarrhea containing neutrophils (and often some blood). On colonoscopy, erosive *C. difficile* colitis produces a distinctive clinical picture termed pseudomembranous colitis. However, specific diagnosis of *C. difficile*–mediated gastrointestinal disease is usually made without colonoscopy and is based on the detection of *C. difficile* toxins in stool by one of a number of methods. When these toxins are present in feces at levels above the limit of detection (as in this case), the patient's diarrhea is almost always due to *C. difficile*. *C. difficile*–mediated gastrointestinal disease was treated by immediately discontinuing the offending antibiotic, clindamycin. An oral antibiotic that reaches a high concentration in the lumen of the colon and kills *C. difficile* was then administered along with supportive care to restore fluid and electrolyte balances. Metronidazole was used for this purpose. With proper and prompt therapy, the patient in this case recovered without any permanent harm, although the physician and patient need to be wary of the possible recurrence of this illness.

REVIEW QUESTIONS

Directions: For each of the following questions, choose the **one best** answer.

1. Which one of the following statements about *Clostridium difficile* toxins is correct?

    (A) *C. difficile* toxins A and B both inhibit polymorphonuclear (PMN) cell chemotaxis

    (B) *C. difficile* toxin A is a very large protein, whereas *C. difficile* toxin B is a polypeptide of < 30 amino acids

    (C) *C. difficile* toxins A and B both act by removing glucose residues from mammalian target proteins, which renders these proteins inactive

    (D) *C. difficile* toxins A and B both decrease the release of inflammatory mediators (e.g., tumor necrosis factor) from inflammatory cells

    (E) The mammalian target for both *C. difficile* toxins A and B are the Rho proteins

2. Which one of the following body sites contains the fewest bacteria in a healthy individual?

    (A) Urinary bladder

    (B) Stomach

    (C) Cerebrospinal fluid

    (D) Colon

    (E) Uterus

3. An elderly hospitalized woman receiving cephalosporin therapy for an infected bed sore develops a severe diarrhea (with some fecal blood and many fecal polymorphonuclear cells), cramps, and a fever. Endoscopy shows whitish-yellowish patches on her colonic wall. Which one of the following statements is true about this patient's situation?

    (A) The pathogen most likely to be causing this illness would appear as pink rods on a properly performed Gram stain of a fresh culture of this microorganism

    (B) The pathogen most likely to be causing this illness is a facultative anaerobe capable of growing in the presence or absence of oxygen

    (C) The pathogen most likely to be causing this woman's illness typically invades the colonic mucosa

    (D) The pathogen most likely to be causing this woman's illness has probably recently proliferated as a result of a cephalosporin-induced disturbance of the woman's normal colonic flora

    (E) Proper treatment for this illness involves surgical removal of the affected region of the colon

4. Which one of the following statements about the normal flora is correct?

    (A) At some body sites, the normal flora include both bacteria and fungi

    (B) Endogenous flora rarely cause opportunistic infections

    (C) Infants are born with a fully established normal flora

    (D) The composition of the normal flora is the same at virtually all normally colonized body sites

    (E) The only reason why normal flora microbes suppress the growth of pathogens is that normal flora have superior abilities to compete for nutrients

ANSWERS AND EXPLANATIONS

1. **The answer is E.** *C. difficile* toxins A and B share the same mammalian target proteins, which are the Rho proteins. Options A and D are incorrect because toxins A and B stimulate chemotaxis and the release of inflammatory mediators; both of these effects contribute to the inflammation associated with *C. difficile* pseudomembranous colitis. Option B is incorrect because both toxins A and B are exceptionally large proteins (remember also that these two toxins share some amino acid homology). Option C is incorrect because toxins A and B do not act by removing a glucose from the Rho proteins; instead, they add a glucose residue to Rho proteins, thereby causing a loss of function for this important family of mammalian proteins.

2. **The answer is C.** Cerebrospinal fluid (along with deep tissues, blood, and synovial fluids) is usually sterile (i.e., free of bacteria or other microbes) in healthy people. The urinary bladder, stomach, and uterus of normal individuals are colonized, although lightly, by microbes. The colon is perhaps the most heavily colonized body site in normal individuals.

3. **The answer is D.** This woman apparently suffers from pseudomembranous colitis. Because *Clostridium difficile* is responsible for more than 90% of all cases of pseudomembranous colitis, it is likely that *C. difficile* is the pathogen responsible for this woman's illness (however, this should be confirmed by using fecal toxin tests). *C. difficile*–mediated gastrointestinal disease (including pseudomembranous colitis) usually develops after an individual becomes colonized and antibiotic therapy has disturbed the normal colonic flora. Option A is incorrect because *C. difficile* is a gram-positive bacteria and thus should stain blue–purple on a properly performed Gram stain. Option B is incorrect because *C. difficile* is an anaerobe, not a facultative anaerobe (see Chapter 2). Option C is incorrect because in most cases of *C. difficile*–mediated gastrointestinal illness, *C. difficile* does not invade into the colonic mucosa but instead adheres to colonic epithelial cells and remains extracellular. Option E is incorrect because usual treatment of pseudomembranous colitis involves withdrawal of the offending antibiotic and treatment with vancomycin or metronidazole, not surgery.

4. **The answer is A.** The normal flora at several body locations (e.g., the vagina) do include both bacteria and fungi. Option B is incorrect because endogenous microbes are important causes of opportunistic infection (e.g., *Staphylococcus epidermidis* often causes catheter infections). Option C is incorrect because infants acquire their normal flora after birth. Option D is incorrect because many normal flora microbes exhibit tropisms (preferences) for specific body locations. Option E is incorrect because some normal flora also suppress the growth of pathogens by producing inhibitory substances (e.g., antibiotics).

12 COLONIZATION I: ADHERENCE

CHAPTER OUTLINE

Introduction of Clinical Case
Adherence
- First Step in Colonization
- Molecular Basis for Microbial Adherence
- Blocking Adherence to Prevent Infection

The Enterobacteriaceae
- Biologic Characteristics
- Differentiating the Enterobacteriaceae
- Pathogenic versus Opportunistic Enterobacteriaceae

Illustrative Pathogen: *Escherichia coli*
- Biologic Characteristics
- Reservoir and Transmission
- Virulence Factors
- Pathogenesis
- Diagnosis
- Prevention and Treatment

Illustrative Pathogen: *E. coli* O4.H5
- Biologic Characteristics
- Reservoir and Transmission
- Virulence Factors
- Pathogenesis
- Diagnosis
- Prevention and Treatment

Resolution of Clinical Case
Review Questions

INTRODUCTION OF CLINICAL CASE

A recently married 25-year-old woman who has no history of back problems presented to her family physician complaining of dull lower back pain that began the previous day. Upon questioning, she also complained of headaches, a slight fever, and painful urinary frequency and urgency. All of these symptoms occurred during the past 2 days. On physical examination, the woman appeared to be in no acute distress but complained of worsening dull back pain to the right of the midline. Her vital signs were as follows: temperature, 101°F (slightly elevated); pulse, 68 beats/min (normal); blood pressure, 118/65 mm Hg (normal); respiration 20 breaths/min (normal). The general examination was unremarkable except for pain on palpation in the right costovertebral angle (i.e., the angle formed by the spine and the lowest rib; directly over the kidney).

On questioning, the woman described a similar episode that occurred 1 month previously. She had awakened one morning while on her honeymoon with the same burning on urination, but she had no fever or back pain. She saw the staff physician at the resort. Without examining her, the staff physician prescribed a 3-day antibiotic regimen of a single second-generation penicillin. Her symptoms disappeared shortly after going on the medication.

Suspecting a urinary tract infection (UTI), the physician obtained a urine specimen from the patient and prescribed a 2-week course of the same antibiotic that the patient responded to during her first episode.

- What microbial pathogen is most likely causing these symptoms?
- What is notable about the patient's history?
- Why did the physician prescribe a 2-week regimen for the second episode?

ADHERENCE

First Step in Colonization

Previous chapters in Part II have stressed the importance of the pathogen gaining access to the human host through a variety of strategies (e.g., ingestion, sexual transmission, inhalation). Once a pathogen has gained access to the host environment, it generally must colonize that host to cause disease. Colonization is often difficult because a microbial pathogen typically must compete with commensal organisms for essential nutrients, must avoid mechanical removal by host mechanisms such as peristalsis or urinary voiding, and must resist host immune defenses.

As described in the Overview, the process of colonization generally first involves attachment by the microbial pathogen, followed by multiplication, which may or may not be followed by intracellular invasion. This chapter discusses the first step in colonization, that is, microbial adhesion to host tissues. The ability of a pathogen to adhere to host tissue is important for pathogenesis because it often defines the host range of a microbial pathogen and significantly influences the course of infection.

Adherence is implemented by specific molecules, designated adhesins, which are oriented on the surface of the microbial pathogen. These molecules have a high affinity for a receptor (or ligand) residing on the host cell surface. The interaction between the microbial adhesin and the host cell ligand can override the nonspecific defenses of the host (e.g., peristalsis or the respiratory escalator) that would normally clear microorganisms. The important role of adherence in infectious diseases is illustrated by several examples of adhesin–receptor interactions summarized in Table 12-1.

A classic example of the contribution of adherence to pathogenicity is illustrated by enterotoxigenic *Escherichia coli* involved in porcine gastrointestinal disease. Strains of *E. coli* harboring specific virulence-associated plasmids are able to cause a watery diarrhea only in pigs. These plasmids encode, among other things, a "colonization factor" (designated as K88), which is important for the attachment of bacteria to porcine intestinal mucosa. These strains also elaborate two enterotoxins, heat-labile enterotoxin (LT) and heat-stable enterotoxin (STa). These enterotoxins act on intestinal cells and cause them to secrete water, resulting in the symptoms of diarrhea (see Chapter 20). Genetically altered strains that are K88-positive but enterotoxin-negative still cause the diarrhea in pigs, albeit at greatly reduced efficiency. However, strains that are K88-negative but enterotoxin-positive are unable to cause disease. This finding underscores the multifactorial nature of the infectious process (i.e., although toxins often are required for the production of disease, bacteria must adhere to deliver these toxins efficiently to target host tissues).

▶ **TABLE 12-1**
Examples of Microbial Ligand–Host Cell Receptor Interactions

	Adhesin	Receptor	Tissue	Disease
Viral				
HIV-1	gp120	CD-4	Lymphocytic cells	AIDS
Bacterial				
Gram-negative:				
Neisseria gonorrhoeae	Type 4 pili	Carbohydrate	Urethral and cervical epithelium	Gonorrhea
Nearly all *Escherichia coli* isolates	Type 1 pili	Mannose-bearing receptor	Intestinal epithelium	Diarrhea
Uropathogenic *E. coli*	P pili (PAP)	Gal-gal disaccharide linked to a ceramide lipid	Upper urinary tract	Pyelonephritis
Bordetella pertussis	Filamentous hemagglutinin	Galactose on sulfated glycolipids	Respiratory epithelium	Whooping cough
Vibrio cholerae	Type 4 pili	Fucose and mannose carbohydrate	Intestinal epithelium	Cholera
Gram-positive:				
Streptococcus pyogenes	M-protein/ lipoteichoic acid	Fibronectin	Epithelium	Strep throat
Streptococcus mutans	Glycosyl transferase	Salivary glycoprotein	Pellicle of tooth	Dental caries
Streptococcus pneumoniae	Cell-bound protein	N-acetyl-hexosamine-galactose-disaccharide	Epithelium	Pneumonia

Note: HIV = human immunodeficiency virus; gp = glycoprotein; AIDS = acquired immunodeficiency syndrome; PAP = P blood group–associated pili.

Molecular Basis for Microbial Adherence

Adhesins are structures intimately associated with the surface of the pathogen (Figure 12-1). For example, the glycoprotein gp120 found on the surface of the human immu-

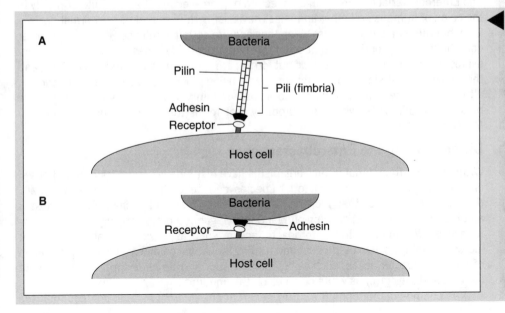

▶ **FIGURE 12-1**
Bacterial Adherence Employs Fimbrial and Afimbrial Adhesins. *(A) Demonstration of how fimbrial adhesins overcome the long-range repulsive forces between the eukaryotic and prokaryotic cell surfaces. (B) Contrast to the interactions demonstrated in A; these short-range interactions, facilitated by afimbrial adhesins, are of a surface–surface nature and often evoke a response on the part of the eukaryotic cell.*

nodeficiency virus-1 (HIV-1) facilitates the adhesion of HIV-1 to the CD4 receptor found on the surface of host lymphocytes (see Chapter 27). Among bacteria, adhesive structures are divided into fimbrial and nonfimbrial adhesins. Colonization factor K88 is actually bacterial pili (also referred to as fimbria; see Chapter 1). Bacterial pili are long, polymeric, proteinaceous appendages extending hundreds of nanometers from the bacterial cell surface. They are organized as several thousand copies of a major subunit referred to as pilin and in some cases small quantities of accessory proteins, including a specific adhesin subunit. By extending far from the bacterial cell surface, pili overcome the repulsive forces that normally exist between the bacterial cell and host cell tissues, as demonstrated in Figure 12-1. Receptors for fimbrial adhesins tend to be carbohydrates associated with glycolipid and glycoprotein molecules on the host cell surface (see Table 12-1).

Nonfimbrial bacterial adhesins also are important in the pathogenesis of infectious disease. For example, enteropathogenic *E. coli* (EPEC) initially attaches loosely to intestinal epithelial cells by means of fimbrial adhesins. These organisms also express specific outer membrane proteins that allow for a second, more intimate association between the bacteria and host cell. This second interaction may cause host cell perturbations that result in disease.

Blocking Adherence to Prevent Infection

Precisely because attachment is such a critical step for the pathogenesis of microbial infections, it presents a logical target for the prevention of disease. Antibodies specific for adhesins can block the attachment of microbial pathogens to host tissues and often are considered in the formulation of a vaccine for the prevention of a particular disease. For example, filamentous hemagglutinin (FHA), a molecule expressed on the surface of *Bordetella pertussis*, is involved in attachment of this bacterium to host cells. FHA is an important component of the vaccine used for the prevention of pertussis (see Chapter 29). In addition to antibodies, soluble receptor analogues also can function to block adhesin interactions with a cell-bound receptor. An example of this is the relationship between the host secretion of the Tamm-Horsfall protein (THP), bearing the gal-gal sugar recognized by PAP pili, and *E. coli*, causing UTI.

THE ENTEROBACTERIACEAE

Characteristics of Enterobacteriaceae
- *Gram-negative, aerobic, or facultatively aerobic rods and oxidase negative*
- *Can be isolated from feces, urine, blood, and cerebrospinal fluid*
- *Can be cultivated on media containing bile (e.g., MacConkey agar)*
- *Can be motile or nonmotile*
- *Speciation within this group relies on lactose utilization and other biochemical tests*

MacConkey agar is both a selective and differential bacterial medium. It is selective because it contains bile salts, which are detergent-like molecules similar to those found in the large intestine. Organisms that are able to survive the conditions within the human GI tract are able to grow on bile-containing media. MacConkey agar also is a differential medium because it contains neutral red and high concentrations of lactose.

Biologic Characteristics

The Enterobacteriaceae are a large collection of gram-negative bacilli found primarily in the colon of humans and other animals. They exist mainly as part of the normal healthy flora, but they can cause disease when they acquire certain virulence genes or when host conditions are appropriate. Members of this family are oxidase negative (i.e., they do not express cytochrome oxidase) and do not form spores. They are facultative anaerobes, and they grow on most simple bacteriologic media using glucose as a sole source of carbon, although some require specific amino acids, vitamins, or both. They also grow in the presence of bile salts, which is a property that forms the basis for their isolation on MacConkey agar.

Differentiating the Enterobacteriaceae

Within the enterobacterial family, organisms have historically been differentiated based on their metabolism. Enterobacterial species can be both selected for and initially differentiated based on their growth characteristics on MacConkey agar. (*P. aeruginosa* is an exception to this rule, growing on MacConkey agar and not belonging the Enterobacteriaceae.) Members of the Enterobacteriaceae, such as *E. coli*, are able to ferment lactose, forming an acid by-product and turning individual colonies pink. Other members of the Enterobacteriaceae, such as *Salmonella* spp. and *Shigella* spp., do not ferment lactose, and they grow as white colonies on this medium.

As chemo-organotrophs (i.e., they generate energy from organic compounds), the

Enterobacteriaceae employ both respiratory and fermentative metabolism. This results in the production of acid or gas, depending on the main carbon source that the organism is consuming (i.e., lactose or glucose) and the conditions under which the organism is cultured (i.e., aerobic or microaerophilic) [Table 12-2]. In addition, the Enterobacteriaceae may or may not produce hydrogen sulfide (H_2S) as part of their metabolism.

TABLE 12-2
Differentiating Selected Members of the Enterobacteriaceae

Test	Escherichia	Salmonella	Shigella	Klebsiella	Proteus	Yersinia
Glucose utilization	+	+	+	+	±	+
Lactose utilization	+	−	−	±	−	−
Sucrose utilization	±	−	±	+	±	±
Gas from glucose	+	+	−	+	±	−
H_2S (on TSI)	−	+	−	−	±	±
Motility	±	+	−	−	+	−
Urease	−	−	−	+	+	±

Note: ± indicates that variation occurs among the species but that most are positive. H_2S = hydrogen sulfide; TSI = triple sugar iron agar.

The ability to produce acid, gas, or H_2S from a certain carbon source varies among different Enterobacteriaceae and can be used for differentiating these species. Triple sugar iron (TSI) slants (Table 12-3) can be particularly useful for differentiating some common pathogenic members of the Enterobacteriaceae.

TABLE 12-3
Triple Sugar Iron Slants

Organism	Slant	Butt	Gas	Hydrogen sulfide (H_2S)
Escherichia coli	Acid	Acid	+	−
Salmonella typhimurium	Alkaline	Acid	+	+
Shigella flexneri	Alkaline	Acid	−	−
Pseudomonas aeruginosa	Alkaline	Alkaline	−	−

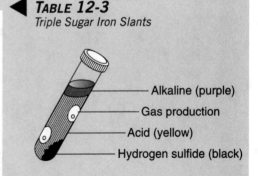

- Alkaline (purple)
- Gas production
- Acid (yellow)
- Hydrogen sulfide (black)

Pathogenic versus Opportunistic Enterobacteriaceae

Table 12-4 lists several members of the Enterobacteriaceae that are often implicated in disease. These include some *E. coli* isolates, as well as nearly all *Salmonella*, *Shigella*, and *Yersinia* isolates. Infections caused by pathogenic Enterobacteriaceae can affect

TABLE 12-4
Major Pathogenic Members of the Enterobacteriaceae

Genus	Principal Diseases
Escherichia	Diarrhea, dysentery
Shigella	Dysentery
Salmonella	Diarrhea, septicemia, enteric fevers (including typhoid fever), focal infections
Yersinia	Plague, dysentery, lymphadenitis

almost anyone but are particularly important among the very young, the very old, the malnourished, and those living in unsanitary environments. For these individuals, diarrhea represents a life-threatening disease. By contrast, opportunistic Enterobacteriaceae

(Table 12-5) usually cause infection within the hospital setting and represent a concern for the development and spread of antimicrobial resistance (see Chapter 5). In addition, all pathogenic and opportunistic Enterobacteriaceae can cause life-threatening septicemia when the immune status of the host is severely compromised.

TABLE 12-5 ▶

Major Opportunistic Members of the Enterobacteriaceae

Genus	Principal Diseases
Escherichia	Urinary tract infections, meningitis in children
Proteus	Urinary tract infections
Klebsiella	Pneumonia, septicemia, infections of compromised patients
Enterobacter	Urinary tract infections, septicemia
Serratia	Pneumonia, urinary tract infections, ophthalmic disease, wound infections
Citrobacter	Urinary tract infections, septicemia

ILLUSTRATIVE PATHOGEN: *Escherichia coli*

Biologic Characteristics

Among the Enterobacteriaceae, *E. coli* has been the object of more scientific study than any other microorganism. This organism is the major facultative anaerobe found in the normal flora of the large intestine. It is also a commonly isolated etiologic agent associated with UTIs, gastrointestinal (GI) infections, wound infections, pneumonia, meningitis, and septicemia. Biochemically, this genus and species is distinguished by its ability to produce indole, ferment glucose by mixed acid fermentation, and by a lack of H_2S production. *E. coli* isolates are commonly subdivided on the basis of their O, H, and K antigens (see Chapter 1). Recall that the O antigen is the long-chain carbohydrate repeat portion of lipopolysaccharide (LPS) that extends from the surface of the *E. coli* outer membrane. The predominance of the hydrophilic O-antigen repeat on the surface of *E. coli* allows this organism to retard detergents and to grow in the presence of bile salts. The H antigen is present as part of the flagellar structure that confers motility to those *E. coli* strains expressing flagellar organelles. *E. coli* may or may not express flagella; if they do express a flagella, a unique H serotype is associated with a specific strain. The K antigens are acidic capsular polysaccharides that coat the *E. coli* outer surface (see Chapter 18).

There are currently more than 160 recognized O types and 55 recognized H types, the combination of which creates more than 8000 possible O:H serotypes. Antisera for each of the O, H, and K antigens has been generated and given a number. In describing an *E. coli* isolate, it is the convention to write *E. coli* followed by the letter–number designation for the O:H:K antigens. Specific *E. coli* diseases often correlate with serogrouping assignments (Table 12-6). An example of this is *E. coli* O157:H11, which is often in the news because of its ability to cause a serious foodborne illness.

TABLE 12-6 ▶

Specific Diseases Associated with Escherichia Coli *Serogroups*

Serogroup	Disease
O26.H11	Enteropathogenic *E. coli* (EPEC)
O157.H7	Enterohemorrhagic *E. coli* (EHEC)
O148.H28	Enterotoxigenic *E. coli* (ETEC)
O4.H5	Urinary tract infections (UTIs)

Reservoir and Transmission

Shortly after birth, *E. coli* begin to colonize the human intestinal tract and exist as part of the commensal flora. They are passed from host to host by contamination of common vectors such as water and food. Depending on the constellation of virulence factors associated with a particular *E. coli* isolate and the status of the host, they may cause disease, or the colonizing isolate may exist simply as part of the host's normal flora.

Virulence Factors

Collectively, *E. coli* produce a number of well-described virulence factors. However, depending on the type of disease it causes, a single pathogenic *E. coli* isolate possesses only a subset of the virulence factors described below.

Fimbrial and Nonfimbrial Adhesins. Adhesins are a major contributor to *E. coli* virulence, and a diverse array of adhesins are expressed by different *E. coli* strains. These adhesins are described in unrelated designations such as colonization factor of adherence (CFA)/I, CFA/II, CFA/IV, longus, and PCFO159. More recently, a standardized nomenclature has been developed that utilizes the designation CS (for coli surface antigen) followed by a number related to the year of the adhesin's initial description. At least 21 different adhesin types have been described for pathogenic *E. coli*. Nearly all clinical *E. coli* isolates produce common (historically known as type 1) pili. These pili allow the *E. coli* to attach to mannose receptors associated with the host cell surfaces and may also allow *E. coli* to coagglutinate through bacteria–bacteria interactions. In this relationship, they are able to confront the human host as an infectious unit instead of as a single organism. Many other pilus types with unique receptor specificities are expressed by different *E. coli* isolates and are associated with specific disease states.

Iron Acquisition. The ability of a microorganism to attach to and multiply at the site of infection is critical to the process of colonization. The multiplication phase of this process requires that sufficient nutrients are available at the site of attachment. As a form of nonspecific immunity, the human host sequesters iron by binding this element with high affinity to transferrin (found in serum) or to lactoferrin (found in secretions). For a microorganism such as *E. coli* to survive in human tissues, it must be able to compete for host iron stores. To do this, *E. coli* cells produce siderophores, which are low-molecular-weight, nonproteinaceous compounds that have extremely high affinities for iron. These compounds are able to mobilize iron from host transferrin and lactoferrin and deliver this growth-essential nutrient to the bacteria, allowing it to multiply at the site of attachment. *E. coli* produce enterobactin (also referred to as enterochelin), which is encoded by chromosomal genes and produced by all clinical *E. coli* isolates. An alternative *E. coli* siderophore is aerobactin, whose biosynthetic genes can be plasmid mediated. Strains carrying this plasmid are associated with virulent *E. coli*, particularly those causing extraintestinal infections.

Toxins. Endotoxin LPS is produced as part of the outer membrane structure of all *E. coli*. This toxin is a potent exogenous pyrogen for humans and can cause endotoxic shock during disseminated disease. A hemolysin (Hly), also known as α-hemolysin, is secreted by some *E. coli* strains. This exotoxin forms pores in host cell membranes, resulting in lysis. Its role in disease is not well understood, but it apparently contributes to kidney damage during pyelonephritis caused by *E. coli*. Some *E. coli* isolates produce entero-toxins (see Chapter 20), which are often associated with plasmids or chromosomal pathogenicity islands. LT is a large oligomeric protein complex composed of one enzymatically active subunit surrounded by five identical binding subunits. The large size and complex organization of LT explains why this toxin is sensitive to denaturation by heat. The toxin binds to ganglioside GM_1 enterocyte receptors and causes an increase in cyclic adenosine monophosphate (cAMP) that results in the exclusion of fluid to the lumen of the gut, causing diarrhea. STa is a small cysteine-rich peptide with a molecular weight of approximately 3000 daltons. This short peptide has three disulfide bonds, giving rise to a compact structure that is resistant to conformational perturbations, which explains why this toxin is not inactivated by heat. STa acts by binding to a cellular receptor located on the apical surface of host cell membranes, activating guanylate cyclase, and causing an increase in cyclic guanosine monophosphate (GMP). This, in turn, leads to secretion of fluid and electrolytes, resulting in diarrhea. *E. coli* can also produce Shiga toxin (Stx), so named because it was first discovered in *Shigella* species. Stx is a large oligomeric protein complex that inactivates ribosomes, resulting in the cessation of host protein synthesis.

The term **exogenous pyrogen** refers to the property of endotoxin to induce the inflammatory cascade that results in, among other things, fever. It is distinguished from the **endogenous pyrogen** tumor necrosis factor-α, which is the cytokine that initiates this inflammatory cascade (see Chapter 21).

Pathogenicity islands are linear regions of the bacteria in which numerous virulence-associated genes are clustered (see Chapter 23).

Pathogenesis

As a pathogen, *E. coli* is known for its ability to cause intestinal diseases, UTIs, and disseminated disease. Five distinct groups of *E. coli* cause intestinal illness, including enterotoxigenic *E. coli* (ETEC), enteropathogenic *E. coli* (EPEC), enteroaggregative *E. coli* (EAEC), enteroinvasive *E. coli* (EIEC), and enterohemorrhagic *E. coli* (EHEC). As summarized in Table 12-7, each of these five groups of *E. coli* is associated with a characteristic serotype (see Table 12-6), shares a common set of individual virulence factors, and manifests distinct disease pathologies.

TABLE 12-7 ▶

Five Distinct Groups of E. coli *that Cause Intestinal Disease*

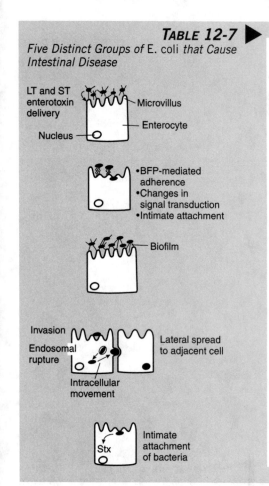

| Disease | Virulence Factors | | | |
	Adherence	Toxins	Siderophores	Invasion
Enterotoxigenic *Escherichia coli* **(ETEC)**	Colonization factors of adherence (CFAs) Type 1 pili	Endotoxin Heat-labile enterotoxin (LT) Heat-stable enterotoxin (STa)	Enterochelin	Noninvasive
Enteropathogenic *E. coli* **(EPEC)**	Bundle-forming pili (BFP) Type 1 pili Intimin	Endotoxin	Enterochelin	Poorly invasive
Enteroaggregative *E. coli* **(EAEC)**	Mucus-associated autoagglutination Type 1 pili	Endotoxin Cytotoxin (enteroaggregative ST-like toxin [EAST])	Enterochelin	Noninvasive
Enteroinvasive *E. coli* **(EIEC)**	Type 1 pili Afimbrial adhesins	Endotoxin	Enterochelin	Type III secretion system Very invasive
Enterohemorrhagic *E. coli* **(EHEC)**	Type 1 pili Afimbrial adhesins	Shiga toxin Endotoxin	Enterochelin Heme uptake system	Probably poorly invasive

ETEC. These organisms are important causes of watery diarrhea in infants and in travelers who visit regions with poor sanitation. ETEC are acquired by ingestion of contaminated food and water. The food and water vehicle of infection must be heavily contaminated with ETEC because 100 million to 10 billion organisms are required to establish disease.

As summarized in Table 12-7, ETEC colonize the small intestine using adherence factors. The fimbrial adhesins historically designated as CFA/I, CFA/II, or CFA/IV are associated with most cases of ETEC and are encoded on a plasmid. These adhesins allow the organisms to bind receptors specifically on enterocytes of the small intestine. After establishing themselves in the small intestine, ETEC organisms multiply by acquiring growth-essential nutrients that are constantly passing through the intestinal environment. They also produce STa or LT, causing fluid secretion by the host enterocyte. ETEC are noninvasive, that is, they do not gain access to the intracellular spaces of a given host cell.

Symptoms of ETEC include diarrhea without fever, which lasts for several days and may vary from minor discomfort to a severe cholera-like syndrome. Stool samples are watery and lack fecal leukocytes. The disease is generally self-limiting but can be life threatening in cases of extreme fluid loss, especially in infants. Treatment involves fluid and electrolyte replacement therapy.

Antibodies to LT can afford protection against many cases of this form of diarrhea. This explains why individuals indigenous to a region with high exposure to ETEC often are protected (i.e., their prior exposure to these bacteria have induced anti-LT antibodies). In contrast, tourists are typically more susceptible to disease from EPEC, leading to the name traveler's diarrhea. Prophylactic administration of antibiotics to tourists traveling to regions with a high incidence of traveler's diarrhea can be effective; however, it is not advised because it contributes to the development of antimicrobial-resistant strains. Antibiotics given empirically to individuals demonstrating symptoms associated with ETEC infection may shorten the course of the disease.

EPEC. These are important causes of infant diarrhea in developing countries. The hallmark of EPEC infection is attachment-and-effacing (A/E) pathology observed on biopsy. The molecular basis for this pathology is summarized in Table 12-7. It involves a three-step process: (1) localized adherence of several organisms to a specific area of the enterocyte that is mediated by a plasmid-encoded bundle-forming pilus (BFP); (2) stimulation of signal transduction pathways of the enterocyte, leading to effacement of the microvilli; and (3) intimate association of bacteria with the enterocyte mediated by an afimbrial adhesin referred to as intimin. This intimate association results in characteristic pedestal formation, which is seen on microscopy of patient biopsies.

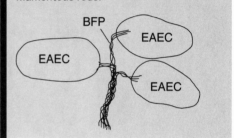

BFP are pilus filaments that have a propensity to associate with each other, in contrast to most pili that exist as single filamentous rods.

EPEC induces a watery diarrhea in the absence of a recognized toxin such as STa or LT. EPEC are only moderately invasive and induce a host inflammatory response that may lead to fever and vomiting, although no fecal leukocytes are typically found in the stool. The diarrhea and other symptoms of EPEC infections probably are caused by the intimate interaction between bacteria and host cells that interfere with normal cellular signal transduction processes.

EAEC. EAEC strains characteristically adhere to cell cultures as an aggregate of many bacteria. During natural infection they appear to enhance mucus secretion from the mucosa, trapping the bacteria in a bacteria–mucus biofilm (see Table 12-7). These strains do not secrete LT or Stx but do secrete a cytotoxin that is related to STa, which is called enteroaggregative ST-like toxin (EAST). The pathogenesis of disease produced by these organisms is not well understood. However, a growing number of studies associate these organisms with persistent diarrhea (more than 14 days in duration). The symptoms of disease caused by EAEC include watery, mucoid stool without fecal leukocytes. Low-grade fever may accompany infection; vomiting is rare. The clinical picture of EAEC infection suggests that it may result from subtle mucosal inflammation stimulated by the association of these organisms with intestinal enterocytes.

EIEC. EIEC closely resemble *Shigella* species (see Chapter 13) in their pathogenic mechanisms and the clinical illness they produce. EIEC cause disease by epithelial cell penetration, lysis of the endocytic vacuole, intracellular multiplication, directional movement through the cytoplasm, and extension to adjacent epithelial cells.

EIEC apparently lack specific fimbrial adhesins but do possess plasmid-mediated, outer-membrane afimbrial adhesins and a type III secretion system (see Chapters 8 and 13) that work in concert to facilitate invasion. They do not produce LT, STa, or Stx. EIEC penetrate and multiply within epithelial cells of the colon, causing intestinal cell destruction. The clinical presentation of EIEC infection is a watery diarrhea with occasional fecal leukocytes and blood.

EHEC. EHEC, as typified by serotype O157:H7, cause a distinct diarrheal syndrome referred to as hemorrhagic colitis (HC), which is characterized by a copious bloody stool with no fever. Pediatric diarrhea caused by EHEC may also result in acute kidney failure, a disease syndrome referred to as hemolytic uremic syndrome (HUS). EHEC is considered an emerging pathogen because its existence was first described in 1983, and cases continue to increase annually. One concern about these strains is their existence within the fecal flora of a variety of animals such as cattle, sheep, and pigs. Most cases of EHEC are transmitted by ingestion, particularly undercooked meat. In these cases, large, point source outbreaks may occur. For example, in 1992 undercooked EHEC-O157:H7-contaminated hamburgers from one restaurant chain in the northwestern United States were responsible for 732 confirmed infections, resulting in 195 hospitalizations and 4 deaths.

Point source infection originates from a common source or point rather than from person-to-person transmission. It can very effectively establish a disease outbreak.

HUS is defined by a triad of symptoms: anemia, thrombocytopenia, and renal failure. This disease is closely associated with EHEC isolates and can result in loss of kidney function and death.

The incubation period for EHEC diarrhea is usually 3–4 days postexposure. Initially, the diarrhea is not bloody, and vomiting occurs in approximately half of the patients. Within 1–2 days, the diarrhea becomes bloody, and the patient experiences increased abdominal pain. Untreated, the bloody diarrhea lasts 4–10 days. In 10% of infected individuals (particularly the young and the elderly), the disease progresses to HUS.

As shown in Table 12-7, EHEC closely associates with cells through the afimbrial adhesin intimin (the same adhesin used by EPEC isolates). EHEC are usually considered noninvasive, but this is somewhat controversial. The defining characteristic of EHEC strains is the production of a phage-encoded Stx. The Stx produced by EHEC strains is responsible for many of the GI effects of EHEC and, after absorption in the circulation, appears responsible for most of the kidney damage occurring during HUS. These strains also express hemolysin, which plays a role in the intense inflammatory response produced by EHEC strains and may also contribute to HUS. EHEC express a specialized iron transport system, which allows them to transport directly and utilize iron bound to heme; presumably, the heme is derived from eukaryotic cells that have been lysed by the hemolysin.

Urinary Tract Infection. These infections should be distinguished from hospital-acquired (nosocomial) infections that are often associated with compromised patients having obstructed or catheterized urinary tracts. UTIs are divided into those that cause cystitis, referring to infection of the lower urinary tract (including the bladder), and those that cause pyelonephritis, referring to infection of the upper urinary tract (including the kidney). A limited number of *E. coli* serogroups, all of which produce a hemolysin and at least one fimbrial adhesin, are associated with these UTIs. UTIs are among the most common bacterial infections of the human body, prompting an estimated 8 million visits a year to physicians' offices for treatment and more than 100,000 hospital admissions for serious infections. Uropathogenic *E. coli* cause 80% of community-acquired UTIs.

Disseminated Disease. *E. coli* also can gain access to the bloodstream, whereupon the production of a capsule and endotoxin play prominent roles. For example, *E. coli* ranks as a major cause of neonatal meningitis, affecting 1 in every 3000 infants. The K_1 antigen is considered the major determinant of virulence for *E. coli* strains causing neonatal meningitis. K_1, which is a homopolymer of sialic acid (see Chapter 18) that inhibits phagocytosis and complement formation, may not be the only determinant of virulence because aerobactin expression is highly correlated with these infections. Aerobactin production allows these organisms to multiply within the sterile spaces of the host. Ultimately, endotoxin induces the general features of gram-negative sepsis, such as fever, hypotension, and disseminated intravascular coagulation (see Chapter 21). Epidemiologic studies have shown that colonization by K_1-expressing *E. coli* increases during pregnancy; these strains can subsequently cause meningitis in the newborn.

Diagnosis

E. coli should be suspected when a patient presents with any of the disease states described above. Because of their relatively simple growth requirements, *E. coli* can be routinely isolated on blood agar as well as on a selective and differential media such as MacConkey agar. *E. coli* ferments lactose and forms pink-to-red colonies on this media, which distinguishes it from other enteric pathogens (e.g., *Salmonella*, *Shigella*). These organisms can be further differentiated using the TSI reaction (see Table 12-3). Differentiation between ETEC, EPEC, EAEC, EHEC, and EIEC is made on serogroup association, clinical grounds, and molecular probes (toxin tests and genetic probes).

Prevention and Treatment

Beyond encouraging proper sanitary behavior, there is no single way to prevent disease caused by *E. coli*. Treatment depends on the disease state, the site of disease, and the resistance pattern of the specific isolate responsible for the disease. For example, antibiotic therapy usually is not indicated for diarrheal disease (treatment generally relies on rehydration therapy). At the other extreme, combination antibiotic therapy is typically given parenterally in the case of *E. coli* sepsis. In the case of HUS caused by EHEC, kidney dialysis, hemofiltration, transfusion of packed erythrocytes, and platelet infusions often are used.

ILLUSTRATIVE PATHOGEN: *E. coli* 04:H5

Biologic Characteristics

The biologic characteristics of *E. coli* O4:H5 causing UTIs are similar to other *E. coli*, except for some specific virulence factors described below.

Reservoir and Transmission

In more than 80% of community-acquired UTIs, the infecting organism is *E. coli* O4:H5 (Table 12-8), usually originating from the patient's own fecal flora. To cause disease, *E. coli* O4:H5 must gain access to the human urethra. Typically, this is accomplished by transmission from feces or the perineal region into the urinary tract. Anatomically, women are much more at risk than men for contracting UTIs because of the proximity between their urethra and anal canal and because of the short length of their urinary tract leading to the bladder. Consequently, community-acquired UTIs are 14 times more common in women than men.

◀ **TABLE 12-8**
Patterns of Community-Acquired and Nosocomial Urinary Tract Infections

Community-Acquired		Nosocomial	
Escherichia coli	80%	E. coli	20%
Other pathogenic Enterobacteriaceae ⎫		Other opportunistic Enterobacteriaceae ⎫	
Staphylococcus spp. ⎬	20%	Pseudomonas spp. ⎬	80%
Enterococci		Staphylococcus spp.	
Chlamydiae ⎭		Enterococci ⎭	

Within the hospital setting, the pattern of UTIs changes dramatically (see Table 12-8). Invasive procedures, such as catheterization, place men and women at similar risk of contracting a UTI. In this setting, opportunistic Enterobacteriaceae (e.g., *Proteus, Serratia, Klebsiella* spp.) also become significant causes of UTIs, as do other bacteria (e.g., *Pseudomonas* spp., *Staphylococcus* spp., enterococci). These organisms generally are derived from the hospital environment and are likely to be antibiotic resistant. They are typically introduced into the patient as a consequence of medical intervention, underscoring the importance of sterile technique in the practice of modern medicine.

Virulence Factors

At least two adhesins are closely associated with UTIs. Type 1 pili, expressed by nearly all *E. coli* (i.e., pathogenic and those not associated with disease), bind mannose receptors that are associated with uroplakins Ia and Ib, which are two membrane proteins that line the surface of the uroepithelium. By binding these receptors, the bacteria resist being washed away by the normal voiding of urine and persist within both the lower and upper urinary tract. P pili are associated with upper UTIs. These pili are named for their ability to bind the P blood group antigen containing a D-galactose-D-galactose disaccharide that is closely associated with kidney epithelium (known as the Forssman antigen) in approximately 99% of the human population. Interestingly, UTIs are virtually never seen in the remaining 1% of the population who lack the D-galactose-D-galactose disaccharide receptor.

Multiplication of *E. coli* at the site of infection is greatly facilitated by the presence of high affinity iron-acquisition systems. Like serum, urine is an iron-restrictive environment because some breakdown products of human metabolism efficiently bind excreted iron. Thus, organisms causing UTIs must be capable of assimilating iron from urine. To accomplish this, *E. coli* causing UTIs often express both an enterochelin and aerobactin iron-uptake system.

Although attachment and multiplication are important for colonization of the urinary tract, disease is enhanced by the expression of cytotoxins. These *E. coli* produce hemolysin, which lyse many cell types, including neutrophils, monocytes, and renal tubular

P pili is also commonly referred to as ***PAP pili***, P blood group antigen–associated pili.

cells, by forming membrane pores. This leads to direct damage of bladder and kidney epithelial cells, which stimulates an inflammatory response that contributes to UTI symptoms and may precipitate kidney stone formation.

Pathogenesis

As mentioned previously, uropathogenic *E. coli* O4:H5 causes 80% of UTIs in anatomically normal, uncompromised individuals (see Table 12-8), particularly women. An important host defense mechanism for the prevention of UTIs is urine flow, which effectively clears organisms from the bladder and the urinary tract. Another host defense against UTIs is inhibition of the adherence of bacteria to the uroepithelium. Several examples of this strategy have been found for *E. coli* UTIs. For example, the most abundant protein in urine is THP, which is produced by the renal medulla and secreted into urine. Soluble THP binds to type 1 pili and blocks the ability of *E. coli* to attach to uroepithelial cells. Another example is found in cranberry juice, used as a homeopathic aid for the prevention of UTIs. Although the metabolism of cranberry juice is known to decrease the pH of urine, creating a less favorable growth environment for bacteria, it also results in the voiding of soluble carbohydrates that block the interaction between bacterial adhesin and host receptor. Finally, it should be noted that some individuals, especially young women, are prone to recurrent community-acquired UTIs. The frequency of UTIs in young women probably reflects variations in the soluble urine attachment inhibitors described above, physical activity, and the presence or quantity of specific receptors expressed on their uroepithelial surfaces.

The typical profile of a patient presenting with uncomplicated cystitis is a young, sexually active woman whose intestines have been colonized with a uropathogenic *E. coli* strain. These organisms find their way to the periurethral region and are propelled into the bladder during physical activity, particularly sexual intercourse. With the aid of type 1 pili, *E. coli* are able to attach to the mucosa of the urethra and thus withstand being swept away during the normal voiding of urine. After multiplying in the urethra, these *E. coli* then gain access to the bladder, where, through the production of toxins and the host inflammatory response, symptoms of UTI ensue (e.g., burning on urination). The bladder provides a staging area for these organisms to gain access to the kidney, for which they have a particular tissue tropism because of their production of P fimbria. Again, toxin production and the host inflammatory response result in swelling of the kidney, giving rise to fever and back pain associated with pyelonephritis. The presence of K antigens is also associated with upper UTIs, and antibody to the K antigen has been shown to afford some degree of protection in experimental infections. These capsules may promote bacterial virulence by decreasing the binding of antibody or complement to the bacterial surface.

Diagnosis

Urine secreted from the kidney is sterile but may be contaminated in the bladder with small numbers of bacteria. However, simple Gram staining and microscopic examination of urine can reveal *E. coli* when they are present in large concentrations. In general, a single bacteria found within a microscopic field is indicative of a concentration of bacteria of 1×10^5 organisms per milliliter, which is considered a high number and clinically significant. For patients with symptoms of a UTI, bacteriologic examination of uncentrifuged midstream urine demonstrating the presence of gram-negative rods can provide an immediate diagnosis. This test also is performed on patients with suspected systemic infection or fever of unknown origin. However, lower numbers of bacteria also may be associated with UTIs. In these cases, sedimentation of the urine followed by performing a Gram stain on the pellet may be useful. Also, proteinuria, which develops because of the inflammatory response associated with UTIs, is an indicator of this illness.

Quantitative culture of urine is routinely performed by spreading a defined volume of urine on blood agar. A finding of 10^5 bacteria per milliliter of urine is indicative of a UTI. The presence of fewer than 10^4 bacteria per milliliter of urine is more likely the result of contamination by the local flora. Growth of these organisms on MacConkey agar (pink-to-red colonies) as well as a TSI test and other biochemical tests establish the infecting

__Proteinuria__ refers to abnormally high levels of protein excreted in the urine. This is a marker for an inflammatory response to bacterial infection.

organism as *E. coli*. Antimicrobial resistance profiles also may be useful in designing treatment rationales. Tests for virulence factors such as adhesins, siderophores, or toxins are not routinely performed in the clinical laboratory for UTI infections.

Prevention and Treatment

UTIs, like nearly all diseases, can be mitigated by proper sanitary behavior. There is no vaccine for the prevention of UTIs, and the use of antibiotic therapy depends on the type of UTI. For example, treatment of community-acquired cystitis generally involves a short course of antimicrobial therapy (a single dose over 3 days). This is possible because antibiotics such as penicillin have a propensity to concentrate within urine. In addition, organisms causing community-acquired cystitis are generally susceptible to most anti- biotics. By contrast, treatment of pyelonephritis requires long-term therapy (weeks) because of the involvement of deeper tissues. As one might suspect, hospital-acquired UTIs of any sort (i.e., cystitis or pyelonephritis) are caused by organisms that are notoriously antibiotic resistant and are difficult to treat using antimicrobial therapy. In these cases, antimicrobial resistance patterns obtained from the diagnostic laboratory are useful for designing appropriate treatment regimens.

RESOLUTION OF CLINICAL CASE

Laboratory tests on urine demonstrated a slightly elevated white blood cell (WBC) count (10,500/μL) and an abnormally high protein content. A Gram stain of the urine indicated the presence of gram-negative rods. Urine sediment contained abnormally high numbers of WBCs, moderate numbers of red blood cells, and many structures that appeared to be bacteria. Quantitative culture of the urine demonstrated more than 10^5 organisms per milliliter that grew on both blood agar and on MacConkey agar. The colony morphology of these organisms growing on MacConkey agar were pink to red. Further workup demon- strated that organisms from these colonies were oxidase negative, indole positive, and H_2S negative, which suggested *E. coli*. Serogrouping analysis indicated that this isolate belonged to the O4:H5 serotype and was susceptible to most conventional antibiotics.

The clinical symptoms (back pain, slight fever) of this young, sexually active woman who had recently been treated for a UTI is a classic scenario. Laboratory findings providing evidence of an inflammatory response, the large numbers of bacteria isolated from her urine, and the identification of these bacteria as an *E. coli* serogroup associated with UTI were consistent with the clinical findings. It is likely that the previous infection was also caused by an *E. coli* that originated from the patient's fecal flora. For the woman's first infection, a 3-day course had been prescribed because the symptoms were typical of cystitis. In her second infection, the symptoms of fever and back pain were suggestive of pyelonephritis. Treatment for pyelonephritis requires a prolonged regimen because it involves deep tissues of the body. The selection of a single second-generation penicillin was made because most community-acquired UTIs are not antibiotic resistant. Also, this antimicrobial agent had been well tolerated by the patient during the first infectious episode. With the aid of antimicrobial treatment, this infection should resolve. However, because of the recurrent nature of bacterial UTIs, this patient may be at risk for these infections in the future.

REVIEW QUESTIONS

Directions: For each of the following questions, choose the **one best** answer.

1. A 76-year-old man is admitted to the hospital for treatment of benign prostatic hypertrophy (BPH), a condition that restricts the normal voiding of urine. He is catheterized to relieve obstruction of his lower urinary tract. Following catheterization, the patient develops back pain and a fever that does not respond to conventional antimicrobial therapy. Assuming that this patient's back pain and fever are caused by a bacterial infection, which one of the following is the most plausible explanation for his current symptoms?

   (A) Community-acquired cystitis exacerbated by patient catheterization

   (B) Hemolytic uremic syndrome resulting from ingestion of improperly cooked food

   (C) Hospital-acquired cystitis or pyelonephritis resulting from unsterile manipulation during hospitalization

   (D) Enteropathogenic *Escherichia coli* (EPEC) contamination of the catheter, causing cystitis or pyelonephritis

   (E) BPH-mediated urine obstruction resulting in "stretched ureter" syndrome and back pain; a consequence of a previous enterotoxigenic *E. coli* (ETEC) infection

2. Long-range interactions between a host cell and many pathogenic *E. coli* attempting to colonize the host cell are facilitated by

   (A) lipoteichoic acid

   (B) lipopolysaccharide (LPS)

   (C) afimbrial adhesins referred to as pili

   (D) fimbrial adhesins referred to as pili

   (E) structural homologues of M protein

3. Which of the following statements best describes the microbiologic properties of Enterobacteriaceae?

   (A) They are oxidase-positive, gram-positive rods found in feces, and they cannot be cultivated on MacConkey agar

   (B) They are oxidase-positive, gram-negative cocci that routinely colonize the urinary tract mucosa, and they can be cultivated on MacConkey agar

   (C) They are oxidase-negative, gram-negative rods that cause disease in the gastrointestinal tract, and they cannot be cultivated on MacConkey agar

   (D) They are oxidase-negative, gram-negative rods isolated from feces, urine, blood, or cerebrospinal fluid (CSF), and they can be cultivated on MacConkey agar

   (E) They are oxidase-positive, gram-negative rods isolated from feces, urine, blood, or CSF, and they cannot be cultivated on MacConkey agar

4. Depending on the virulence factors produced, *Escherichia coli* can cause pathologies that range from diarrhea to dysentery. Which one of the following statements is most accurate?

   (A) Enteropathogenic *E. coli* (EPEC) cause bloody dysentery by adhering to and aggressively invading the intestinal mucosa

   (B) Enterotoxogenic *E. coli* (ETEC) cause a watery diarrhea by adhering to the intestinal mucosa and secreting heat-labile enterotoxin (LT) and heat-stabile enterotoxin (STa)

   (C) Enteroinvasive *E. coli* (EIEC) cause a bloody diarrhea by adhering to and effacing enterocyte microvilli

   (D) Enteroaggregative *E. coli* (EAEC) cause a watery diarrhea by aggregating enterocytes at the site of bacterial attachment

   (E) Enterohemorrhagic *E. coli* (EHEC) cause a bloody diarrhea by attaching to enterocytes and secreting LT and STa

5. *Escherichia coli* can be differentiated by their serologic properties. One important *E. coli* infection that has been recently in the news is hemorrhagic colitis, which is caused by a strain designated *E. coli* O157:H7. Which one of the following statements about the basis for this serologic designation is most accurate?

   (A) The O designation refers to the O antigen of the lipopolysaccharide (LPS); the H designation refers to the flagellar type

   (B) The O designation refers to the opsoninic capsule; the H designation refers to the heterologous LPS type

   (C) The O designation refers to the O antigen of the peptidoglycan; the H designation refers to the heterologous LPS type

   (D) The O designation refers to the existence of a pilus adhesin that recognizes O-linked oligosaccharides; the H designation refers to the heavy form of lipoteichoic acid

   (E) The O designation refers to the type of disease that is associated with this *E. coli* isolate; the H designation refers to pilus specificity for a heavy species of gangliosides

ANSWERS AND EXPLANATIONS

1. **The answer is C.** The clinical scenario of a man contracting a UTI involves a hospital-acquired infection resulting from unsterile mechanical manipulation and is highly associated with an antimicrobial-resistant bacteria. Option A is incorrect because the patient developed symptoms of a bacterial infection only after being catheterized in the hospital. Although it cannot be completely excluded that this medical manipulation exacerbated a previously existing infection, the observation that the infection is not responding to antimicrobial therapy is more consistent with a hospital-acquired infection. Option B is inconsistent with the patient's history and symptoms (in particular back pain) and, thus, is unlikely. Option D is incorrect because EPEC are generally associated with pediatric diarrhea. Option E is incorrect because ETEC cause an intestinal disease and have no consequences in the urinary tract.

2. **The answer is D.** Fimbrial adhesins are pili, they exist on the surface of *E. coli*, and they help to facilitate long-range interactions between bacteria and host cells. Option A is not correct because lipoteichoic acids are associated with gram-positive organisms, not *E. coli*. Option B is not correct because LPS, although associated with the surface of *E. coli*, is not involved in long-range interactions. Option C is not correct because afimbrial adhesins are not pili. Option E is not correct because M protein is structurally distinct from the pili expressed on the surface of *E. coli*.

3. **The answer is D.** Options A, C, and E are incorrect because these organisms can be cultivated on MacConkey agar. Option B is incorrect because Enterobacteriaceae are oxidase-negative, gram-negative rods that grow on MacConkey agar.

4. **The answer is B.** ETEC cause a watery diarrhea mediated by LT and STa. Option A is incorrect because EPEC causes a watery diarrhea by attaching to and effacing microvilli of the enterocyte without actually invading these cells. Option C is not correct because the pathology described is consistent with EPEC; EIEC are associated with invasion of enterocytes without cytotoxin production. Option D is not correct because the term "aggregative" refers to aggregating bacteria, not enterocytes. Option E is not correct; EHEC are associated with the production of a shiga toxin.

5. **The answer is A.** The O designation is reserved for antisera that specifically reacts with the O antigen of LPS from this strain. Likewise, reactivity with the H antigen is based on the type of flagella expressed by this isolate. No capsular K type was given in the designation of this strain. Option B is incorrect because O reflects the LPS type, not the capsule type; H reflects the flagellar type, not the LPS type. Option C is incorrect because the O antigen has nothing to do with peptidoglycan, and the H antigen is not LPS. Option D is not correct because the O antigen does not refer to pilus specificity, and *E. coli* do not synthesize lipoteichoic acid. Option E is not correct because the O designation has nothing to do with the disease state, and the H designation has nothing to do with pilus specificity.

13

COLONIZATION II: INVASION

CHAPTER OUTLINE

Introduction of Clinical Case
Pathogen Invasion of Epithelial Surfaces
• Entry into Epithelial Cells
Pathogen Invasion of the Intestinal Epithelium
• Entry of Enteropathogenic *Yersinia* spp.
• Entry of *Shigella* spp. and *Salmonella* spp.
• Invasion Strategies: Similarities and Differences
Postinvasion Events
• Consequences for Invasive Pathogen
• Consequences for Host
Illustrative Pathogen: *Shigella* spp.
• Biologic Characteristics
• Reservoir and Transmission
• Virulence Factors
• Pathogenesis
• Diagnosis
• Prevention and Treatment
Resolution of Clinical Case
Review Questions

INTRODUCTION OF CLINICAL CASE

A 4-year-old child normally spends her daytime hours in a day care situation with 17 other children (ranging in age from 1–4 years). The child was well until 3 days ago when she had six bowel movements during a 24-hour period, each of which consisted of a large volume of brownish, watery diarrhea with little solid material. This continued until 24 hours ago, when the child began to have frequent small-volume bowel movements consisting largely of blood and mucus. In addition, she felt the need to defecate every 30–60 minutes but produced little or no stool; she strained unsuccessfully and painfully on the commode. Her temperature taken at the pediatrician's office was 101°F. The physical examination was entirely normal except for mild left lower quadrant tenderness, but it was interrupted by the child's need to defecate. A methylene-blue staining of the girl's stool revealed numerous erythrocytes and polymorphonuclear (PMN) leukocytes. A specimen was submitted for culture, and the child was started on trimethoprim-sulfamethoxazole. The girl was allowed to return home after the mother was instructed in fluid replacement and antibiotic administration.

• From what illness is this girl suffering?
• What is the causative pathogen?
• How could this girl have contracted this illness?
• What is her prognosis?

PATHOGEN INVASION OF EPITHELIAL SURFACES

Some transmission mechanisms commonly result in a pathogen being directly introduced into subepithelial tissue or internal body fluids (e.g., when the pathogen enters the body through wounds, needles, arthropod bites, or transplants). Other noninvasive transmission mechanisms (e.g., ingestion, inhalation, most sexual transmission mechanisms) typically leave a pathogen outside the epithelium. Some pathogens transmitted through one of these noninvasive routes simply attach themselves to the epithelial surface at their site of entry into the body and then cause disease directly from this location (i.e., they never penetrate the epithelium). Two examples of such noninvasive pathogens include *Vibrio cholerae* and *Corynebacterium diphtheriae*. *V. cholerae* attaches to the epithelial surface of the small intestine, where it produces cholera toxin (a toxin that acts on intestinal epithelial cells), causing the severe diarrhea associated with cholera (see Chapter 20). *C. diphtheriae* attaches to the mucosa of the pharynx, where it produces diphtheria toxin, causing the symptoms of diphtheria (see Chapter 23). These two examples illustrate a common strategy used by many (but not all) noninvasive pathogens (i.e., production of disease through toxin-mediated mechanisms).

The effectiveness of the epithelium as a barrier to most microbes is evident from the fact that normal flora microbes are usually unable to penetrate into the epithelium.

Alternatively, some pathogens must penetrate the epithelium to cause disease. For these pathogens, entering the body through a noninvasive transmission mechanism presents a challenge: unless these pathogens move themselves (translocate) across the relatively formidable host defense barrier of an intact epithelium, disease will not occur. Pathogens that contribute to their own penetration through the epithelium are referred to as *invasive pathogens*.

Some invasive pathogens simply penetrate into the epithelial cells at their site of entry and remain in this location without spreading into subepithelial tissues or spreading to other body sites. Examples of pathogens that generally confine their invasion to epithelial cells at their original site of entry or attachment are listed in Table 13-1. However, many invasive pathogens are able to continue spreading into subepithelial tissues after successfully invading epithelial cells at their site of entry. Some of these "highly invasive" pathogens can disseminate to other body sites (Table 13-2).

TABLE 13-1 ▶
Examples of Pathogens Whose Invasion Is Limited to Epithelial Cells

Body Site	Pathogens
Respiratory tract	Influenzavirus Rhinovirus
Urogenital tract	Human papillomavirus 6 *Chlamydia* spp.
Skin	Human papillomaviruses 1, 2, and 4
Intestinal tract	*Shigella* spp. Rotaviruses

Because it takes time for a pathogen to spread to a new body site and multiply there in sufficient numbers to cause disease, infections involving highly invasive (disseminating) pathogens often exhibit longer incubation periods than illnesses caused by either noninvasive pathogens or less invasive pathogens whose growth is restricted to epithelial cells at the original entry or attachment site. For example, the incubation time for shigellosis (caused by *Shigella* spp., which invade the colonic epithelium but do not multiply in subepithelial tissue) is only a few days, whereas the major symptoms of typhoid fever, a disease caused by highly invasive *Salmonella typhi* (see Chapter 24) do not develop for at least 10 days. Similarly, the symptoms of common colds and influenza, which are caused by viruses that multiply in respiratory epithelial cells, develop within days, whereas the symptoms of measles develop after 10–14 days. During that time period, the measles virus is disseminating from respiratory epithelial cells through the blood and lymph to distant sites, multiplying at these new sites, and being re-released into the blood.

Most common colds are caused by viruses such as rhinoviruses and coronaviruses, whereas influenza is caused by the influenzavirus.

TABLE 13-2
Examples of Pathogens That Invade Epithelial Cells and Spread Elsewhere in the Body

Epithelial Site of Entry	Pathogen
Gastrointestinal tract	*Salmonella typhi*
	Poliovirus
Urogenital tract	Herpes simplex virus 1 and 2
	Treponema pallidum
Respiratory tract	Measles virus
	Rubella virus
	Varicella zoster virus
	Mycobacterium tuberculosis
	Histoplasma capsulatum
Skin	*Staphylococcus aureus*

Why do some invasive pathogens remain in epithelial cells at their original site of invasion without entering further into the body? There are probably multiple explanations for this behavior. For example, rhinoviruses and coronaviruses apparently multiply in respiratory epithelial cells but not in deeper tissues because their optimum growth temperature (33°C) limits them to the cooler surface of the body (i.e., deeper tissues are simply too warm to support efficient growth of these viruses). At least two other factors are thought to explain why influenzavirus usually is limited to the respiratory epithelium of adults: (1) only cells in the respiratory epithelium may have the receptors necessary for efficient uptake of this virus, and (2) mature influenzavirus is released from the apical (external) surface of respiratory epithelial cells. Release of mature virus from basal surfaces would, obviously, be advantageous for spreading influenzavirus into sub-epithelial tissue. Finally, some pathogens may be able only to invade epithelial cells successfully because these microbes simply lack the proper virulence factors necessary for penetrating tissues (i.e., they cannot produce degradative enzymes) or overcoming (even temporarily) host defenses present in other body sites.

Entry into Epithelial Cells

What mechanisms do invasive pathogens use to enter epithelial cells? Except for some enveloped viruses that directly enter host cells by fusing their lipid envelope with the host cell's plasma membrane, most invasive pathogens penetrate into the epithelium through endocytosis. The fact that many pathogens (e.g., *V. cholerae, C. diphtheriae*) adhere to but do not enter epithelial cells indicates that the invasive pathogen must play an active role in facilitating its own uptake into epithelial cells. Consequently, the uptake of invasive pathogens into epithelial cells often represents a *pathogen-directed* (or *pathogen-stimulated)* endocytosis.

The molecular mechanisms used during pathogen-directed endocytosis are only now being explored. To date, one of the most studied systems of pathogen-directed entry into epithelial cells has been those invasive bacterial pathogens that must enter the intestinal epithelium to cause gastrointestinal disease. Although complete molecular details are not yet available, studies with several invasive enteric bacterial pathogens have become sufficiently developed to indicate that invasion of the intestinal epithelium by these pathogens commonly involves some degree of cross-talk between the host cell and bacterial cell. However, it also has recently become clear that all invasive enteric pathogens do not use the same mechanism to stimulate their uptake into intestinal epithelial cells. By extension, it would appear reasonable to expect that pathogens entering epithelial cells in other body locations also may use cross-talk strategies, but the details of this cross-talk likely vary between different pathogens.

Cross-talk refers to interactions between the pathogen and host that result in activation of signal transduction cascades in the host by pathogen-produced (or affected) factors or activation of signal transduction cascades in the pathogen by host-produced (or affected) factors.

PATHOGEN INVASION OF THE INTESTINAL EPITHELIUM

Entry of Enteropathogenic *Yersinia* spp.

The enteropathogenic *Yersinia*, which include *Y. enterocolitica* and *Y. pseudotuberculosis*, are gram-negative bacterial rods that usually are acquired by *ingestion* of contaminated food or water. Typically, both enteropathogenic *Yersinia* species cause an illness involving fever and abdominal pain, with diarrhea being more common in those infections involving *Y. enterocolitica* (this may result from *Y. enterocolitica* producing an enterotoxin that has activity similar to *Escherichia coli* heat-stable enterotoxin; see Chapter 20).

After ingestion, enteropathogenic *Yersinia* invade the epithelium of the ileum or colon to cause disease. Once through the intestinal epithelium, these bacteria penetrate into the underlying lymphoid tissue of the Peyer's patches, where they multiply both inside and (predominantly) outside host cells. Sometimes the enteropathogenic *Yersinia* drain into adjacent mesenteric lymph nodes, causing mesenteric lymphadenitis. Interestingly, while enteropathogenic *Yersinia* cells are growing in lymphoid tissue, they are able to inhibit their uptake into professional phagocytes (e.g., PMNs), which can kill internalized *Yersinia* cells. Enteropathogenic *Yersinia* inhibit their uptake into phagocytes by producing virulence factors, named *Yersinia* outer proteins (Yops), which affect phagocyte function (see below). The Yops include at least 11 different secreted or surface-localized proteins encoded by a virulence plasmid found in all pathogenic *Yersinia* spp. (including *Y. pestis*; see Chapter 8). Although it is not yet completely clear how Yops affect phagocytes, YopE is thought to cause a depolymerization of the actin cytoskeleton in phagocytes, whereas YopH is a tyrosine phosphatase that interferes with tyrosine kinase function in phagocytes (note that tyrosine kinases are important components in signal transduction pathways).

Laboratory studies have demonstrated that transferring any one of three different genes from enteropathogenic *Yersinia* spp. into a laboratory strain of *E. coli* is sufficient to allow this naturally noninvasive *E. coli* strain to enter epithelial cells. The first *Yersinia* gene capable of mediating this invasion was shown to encode an outer membrane protein named invasin. Invasin tightly binds to β_1 integrin, a protein found on the surface of some mammalian cells. As a result of these strong interactions between invasin and β_1 integrin at multiple locations on the bacterial surface, the epithelial cell membrane begins to surround the tightly adherent *Yersinia* cell. Endocytotic uptake is then completed through cytoskeletal-mediated effects triggered by signal transduction pathways that were "turned on" by the high affinity invasin–β_1 integrin binding.

Interestingly, enteropathogenic *Yersinia* spp. cannot use this uptake mechanism, which is sometimes referred to as a "zipper" entry, to move from the intestinal lumen into most of the cells present in the intestinal epithelium because most intestinal epithelial cells do not have β_1 integrins on their apical surface. How then do enteropathogenic *Yersinia* initially penetrate the intestinal epithelium? The answer appears to be that the enteropathogenic *Yersinia* invade the intestinal epithelium through specialized M cells, which do have β_1 integrins on their apical surface. Once inside these M cells, the *Yersinia* are transcytosed and released at the M cell's basal surface into the underlying lymphoid tissue of the Peyer's patches. From the Peyer's patches, enteropathogenic *Yersinia* may spread through the lymph into the mesenteric lymph nodes. The fever and pain typically associated with infection by these bacteria are likely due to inflammation induced, at least in part, by lipopolysaccharide (LPS).

Enteropathogenic *Yersinia* do not express invasin well at normal body temperature (98.6°F). At first glance, this may appear confusing, but temperature-regulated expression of invasin (and other virulence factors) actually makes good sense if the pathogenesis of enteropathogenic *Yersinia* infections is considered carefully. Enteropathogenic *Yersinia* often are acquired from foods, such as contaminated milk, that were being held at temperatures < 98.6°F before ingestion. The ability of enteropathogenic *Yersinia* to express invasin at temperatures < 98.6°F means that the newly ingested *Yersinia* already are expressing significant levels of invasin as they enter the body. With

Mesenteric lymphadenitis is inflammation of the lymph nodes to which the gastrointestinal tract drains.

M cells are highly specialized cells that overlie the Peyer's patches of the small intestine and are associated with the follicular-associated dome of rectal and colonic mucosal lymphoid structures. The function of M cells is to take up foreign particles and products and deliver these to the nearby immune cells of the Peyer's patches and rectal or colonic lymphoid structures.

Temperature is not the only host factor that can alter gene expression by enteropathogenic Yersinia; for example, host-influenced factors such as changes in calcium ion (Ca^{2+}) levels affect transcription of genes encoding Yops.

invasin already present on their surface, the newly ingested *Yersinia* are fully competent to adhere to and enter M cells. Further, once *Yersinia* cells have been present in the body for some time (e.g., during their transcytosis through host M cells), this temperature-regulated gene expression allows the *Yersinia* cell to stop making invasin and to start producing Yops (whose synthesis is specifically turned on at 98.6°F). Because enteropathogenic *Yersinia* exist primarily extracellularly in lymph tissue and can be killed if ingested by PMNs, this temperature-related expression strategy is clearly advantageous to *Yersinia*; that is, it allows an extracellular *Yersinia* cell present in subepithelial lymphoid tissue of the intestines to cease producing factors, such as invasin, that might promote its uptake into professional phagocytes and to start producing Yops that can actively inhibit its uptake into phagocytes.

It should be noted that invasin is not the only protein present on the *Yersinia* surface that can stimulate bacterial uptake into epithelial cells. As mentioned earlier, expression of at least two other *Yersinia* proteins (i.e., attachment invasion locus [Ail] and Yersinia adherence [YadA]) has also been shown to permit recombinant laboratory strains of normally noninvasive *E. coli* to enter epithelial cells. However, YadA- and Ail-mediated entry apparently occur at a significantly lower efficiency than is observed for recombinant *E. coli* expressing invasin. When these findings are combined with results from animal model studies using invasin-negative *Yersinia* mutants, it appears that other proteins like Ail and YadA may contribute to *Yersinia* entry into epithelial cells, but invasin is the major factor required for this process to operate efficiently.

Entry of *Shigella* spp. and *Salmonella* spp.

Like the enteropathogenic *Yersinia*, *Shigella* and *Salmonella* also are gram-negative bacterial rods that invade the intestinal epithelium to initiate their pathogenesis. However, the invasion mechanism used by these two bacteria is very different from that described above for the enteropathogenic *Yersinia*. These differences are evident from the number of genes required for the invasion of enteropathogenic *Yersinia* compared to that required for *Shigella* or *Salmonella* invasion. In contrast to the situation with the enteropathogenic *Yersinia*, where a single gene (encoding invasin) appears sufficient to promote efficient entry into epithelial cells, the invasiveness of *Shigella* and *Salmonella* species is a much more complicated, multifactorial process that requires at least 30 different gene products.

The reason why the *Shigella* and *Salmonella* species require so many gene products to invade the intestinal epithelium is only now becoming clear. Recent studies indicate that as the *Shigella* and *Salmonella* encounter body temperatures after being ingested, they begin to transcribe a number of different genes encoding invasion factors. In *Shigella* spp., the products of these temperature-induced genes (Figure 13-1) include both the components of the invasion plasmid antigen (Ipa) proteins and the translocon for membrane expression of Ipas, which is called the surface presentation of antigens (Mxi-Spa) translocon. After synthesis, the Mxi-Spa components assemble into an inactive translocon located on the surface of the *Shigella* cell. Meanwhile, the newly synthesized Ipa proteins continue to accumulate in the bacterial cytoplasm until the *Shigella* cell makes proper contact with the host cell surface (this process probably involves, at least in part, adherence). This host cell contact activates the Mxi-Spa translocon, leading to secretion of the preformed Ipa proteins outside the bacterium (Figure 13-2). Some or all of these secreted Ipa proteins then assemble extracellularly into a complex that interacts with the host plasma membrane to trigger signal transduction pathways in the host cell. These changes in signal transduction pathways lead to cytoskeletal changes that produce perturbations in the plasma membrane. These perturbations result in the formation of membrane projections (a process referred to as "membrane ruffling"), which results in the encirclement of the *Shigella* cell. Encirclement is then rapidly followed by endocytotic uptake of this bacterium into the host cell through macropinocytosis. With a few differences (see below), *Salmonella* appear to use a similar mechanism to enter into the intestinal epithelium.

The **Mxi-Spa translocon** refers to a specialized, entry-associated secretion apparatus in Shigella *spp. This translocon has the unusual ability to move certain proteins directly from the bacterial cytoplasm to the outside of the gram-negative bacterial cell (i.e., this process does not rely on signal peptides to move the transported protein first into the periplasm). Genes encoding the Mxi-Spa translocon (or its Salmonella equivalent, the Inv-Spa translocon) are sometimes referred to as* **type III secretion systems** *and are located on pathogenicity islands (see Section V).*

Ipa proteins *are generally encoded by genes found in* Shigella *on a large plasmid that is essential for invasiveness. Interestingly, the Ipa equivalents in Salmonella, referred to as* Salmonella *invasion proteins (Sip proteins), are chromosomally encoded.*

There is some evidence that Mxi-Spa proteins may participate in this adhesion.

FIGURE 13-1 ▶
Preinvasion Steps in the Pathogenesis of Shigella spp. Ipa = *invasion plasmid antigen*; Mxi-Spa = *membrane expression of Ipa proteins and surface presentation of antigens.*

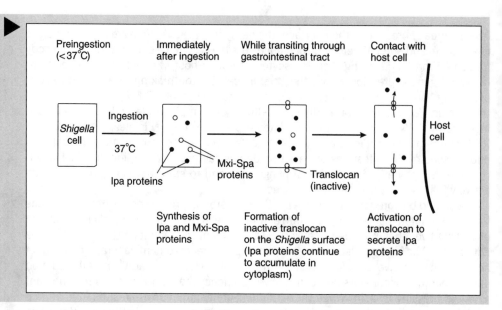

FIGURE 13-2 ▶
Early Steps in the Invasion of Shigella spp. into M Cells. Ipa = *invasion plasmid antigen*; Spa = *surface presentation of antigens.*

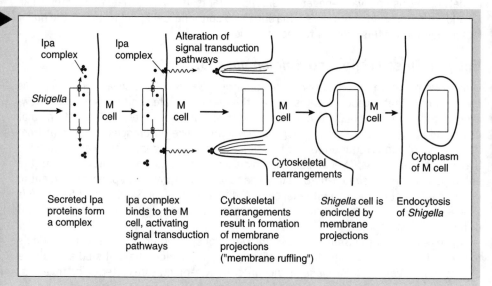

Invasion Strategies: Similarities and Differences

From the above descriptions, it is clear that there are certain shared themes in the invasive strategies used by enteropathogenic *Yersinia* spp. and the *Shigella* or *Salmonella* spp. For example, the invasion of all three of these enteric pathogens relies upon temperature-regulated bacterial gene expression and some degree of signal transduction-mediated cross-talk between the pathogen and host cell. However, there are also some obvious distinctions between the invasion strategies used by these pathogens. Besides the more genetically complicated nature of *Salmonella* and *Shigella* invasiveness compared to *Yersinia* entry, another difference is that the enteropathogenic *Yersinia* rely primarily on high-affinity binding of a single surface component (e.g., invasin) to a host protein (e.g., integrin) to trigger their uptake into epithelial cells, whereas *Shigella* or *Salmonella* spp. are thought to activate their uptake into epithelial cells primarily by using excreted proteins to induce a membrane-ruffling effect.

Although *Salmonella* shares much of the invasion strategy described above for the *Shigella*, there also are some important differences between the invasiveness of these two bacteria. First, many of the genes encoding invasiveness are plasmid encoded in *Shigella* but are chromosomal in *Salmonella*. Second, although *Shigella* spp. must initially penetrate the intestinal epithelium through M cells because these bacteria are unable to penetrate the apical surface of other intestinal epithelial cells, there is evidence that *Salmonella* spp. may be able to penetrate through the apical surfaces of other intestinal cell types in addition to M cells. Third, *Shigella* and *Salmonella* differ regarding which portions of the intestinal epithelium they primarily invade to cause disease, with *Shigella* primarily causing disease by penetrating the colonic epithelium and *Salmonella* primarily causing disease by invading the ileum. These differences regarding organ and cell-type preferences for the invasion of *Shigella* versus *Salmonella* may derive from the ability of *Salmonella* to produce additional Ipa-like invasion proteins that *Shigella* lack or the existence of differences in the regulation of secretion of Ipa-like proteins between these two bacteria. A final important difference relating to the penetration of epithelial cells by *Shigella* spp. versus *Salmonella* spp. concerns the fate of these bacteria after they enter epithelial cells. Once endocytosed, *Shigella* rapidly escape from the endosome into the cytoplasm of the epithelial cell (where they may spread cell to cell). In contrast, *Salmonella* remain enclosed in membrane-bound vesicles while they are being transcytosed to the basal surface of the epithelium, a location from which these bacteria exit into the lamina propria. These bacteria do not spread cell to cell inside the intestinal epithelium.

POSTINVASION EVENTS

Consequences for Invasive Pathogen

Once inside the epithelium, several possible fates await an invasive pathogen:

1. The pathogen may be restricted to growth in the epithelium at the site of entry (e.g., *Shigella* spp., see below).

2. The pathogen may spread from the epithelium into immediately underlying tissue without any further dissemination. The multiplication of these pathogens in sub-epithelial tissues may be either predominantly extracellular (e.g., *Y. enterocolitica*) or predominantly intracellular (e.g., nontyphoid *Salmonella* spp., which survive for some time in the macrophages of the Peyer's patches but in most cases do not disseminate beyond the lamina propria to other sites; see Chapter 24).

3. The pathogen may spread from the epithelium into more distant body locations. This spread may be facilitated in at least two ways:

   • The pathogen may produce enzymes (e.g., collagenase, hyaluronidase) that degrade constituents of the connective tissue underlying the epithelium. This degradation allows the pathogen to spread directly through connective tissue to other sites.

   • The pathogen may enter the lymph or blood to "hitch a ride" to other body sites favorable to the pathogen's proliferation. While being transported through the blood or lymph, a pathogen may be extracellular or carried inside a host cell (Table 13-3).

◀ **TABLE 13-3**
Examples of Pathogens That Are Carried in Blood

Location in Blood	Pathogen
Extracellular	Poliovirus
	Hepatitis B virus
	Streptococcus pneumoniae
	Trypanosoma spp.
Leukocytes	Measles virus
	Epstein-Barr virus
	Listeria monocytogenes
	Salmonella typhi
Erythrocytes	*Plasmodium* spp.

Pathogens entering the body without penetrating the epithelium by themselves (e.g., through wounds, needles) also may spread through the body by producing degradative enzymes or by entering the blood or lymph.

Consequences for Host

Bacterial invasion of the intestinal epithelium almost always triggers a strong inflammatory response. For gram-negative invasive pathogens, LPS clearly plays a role in eliciting this inflammatory response. Invasion-induced inflammation is important for at least two reasons. First, although inflammatory responses may be necessary for eventual resolution of infections caused by invasive pathogens, inflammation is also a major contributor to the symptomology (e.g., fever) of these illnesses. Second, invasion-induced inflammatory responses often result in the presence of elevated levels of fecal leukocytes. Therefore, microscopic examination of stool samples often provides important diagnostic information indicating that a particular patient's gastrointestinal illness involves an invasive enteric pathogen.

ILLUSTRATIVE PATHOGEN: *Shigella* spp.

Biologic Characteristics

Shigella spp., which belong to the bacterial family Enterobacteriacae, are gram-negative, facultative, anaerobic rods that do not ferment lactose in 24 hours, do not produce hydrogen sulfide, and are nonmotile. There are four recognized *Shigella* species (*S. dysenteriae*, *S. flexneri*, *S. boydii*, and *S. sonnei*), which can be differentiated on the basis of their O antigens and biochemical reactions. All four *Shigella* species can cause gastrointestinal disease (referred to as shigellosis), but the tendency is for *S. dysenteriae* and some *S. flexneri* isolates to cause the most severe cases of shigellosis and for *S. sonnei* to cause somewhat less severe cases.

Reservoir and Transmission

Interestingly, *Shigella* spp. infect only higher primates. Therefore, the primary reservoir for shigellosis is humans. Asymptomatic *Shigella* carriers have been demonstrated, particularly in Third World countries. *Shigella* spp. are typically spread by the fecal-oral route, but recent findings indicate that *S. flexneri* also can be a sexually transmitted disease among male homosexuals.

One of the most important aspects of *Shigella* transmission is the high virulence of these bacteria. In contrast to other gram-negative enteric bacterial pathogens, such as *Salmonella* spp. or *V. cholerae* (which have an oral median infective dose [ID_{50}] of 10^4–10^6 bacteria), the oral ID_{50} for *Shigella* spp. is only 100–200 bacteria. The exceptional virulence of the *Shigella* through the oral route is thought to result, at least in part, from the ability of ingested *Shigella* cells to resist death when exposed to the acidity of the stomach. *Shigella* also are reasonably resistant to other environmental stresses; this hardiness permits them to remain viable in feces or contaminated foods for significant time periods, which increases the probability of their infecting a human host.

Virulence Factors

Shigella produce an impressive array of virulence factors; the role of these in pathogenesis is described in the next section of this chapter. *Shigella* virulence factors include:

- Endotoxin (e.g., LPS), which contributes to intestinal inflammation
- Ipa proteins, which mediate invasion
- Mxi-Spa proteins, which are involved in secretion of Ipa proteins and also may be involved in the adhesion of *Shigella* to the host cell
- Proteins IcsA and IcsB, which are involved in intercellular spread of *Shigella*

- Shiga toxin, which is produced only by *S. dysenteriae* and acts by inhibiting host cell protein synthesis (see Chapter 20), an effect that is thought to contribute to the development of colonic mucosal damage during shigellosis

Pathogenesis

Ingestion of *Shigella* spp. is usually the first step leading to shigellosis. Once exposed to the warm temperature of the body, the ingested *Shigella* cells activate transcription of genes encoding Ipa proteins and Mxi-Spa proteins (see Figure 13-1). While moving through the gastrointestinal tract on their way to the colon, these *Shigella* cells produce Ipa and Mxi-Spa proteins; the newly synthesized Mxi-Spa proteins then assemble on the bacterial surface to form an (inactive) translocon. Upon initiation of proper contact between a *Shigella* cell and a host cell (presumably this contact involves, at least in part, adhesion of *Shigella* to M cells in the colon), the Mxi-Spa translocon is "turned on" and begins secreting the preformed Ipa proteins that were accumulating in the cytoplasm of the *Shigella* cell.

Once secreted outside the *Shigella* cell, at least some of these Ipa proteins assemble together into an extracellular complex. This complex then interacts with the cell membrane of the M cell to initiate changes in cell-signaling pathways (see Figure 13-2). Through a process involving the host cell cytoskeleton, these cell-signaling changes induce the formation of membrane projections (a "membrane ruffling"), causing the M cell to take up the adherent *Shigella* cell through an endocytotic process resembling macropinocytosis (see Figure 13-2). Once inside the M cell (Figure 13-3), the *Shigella*

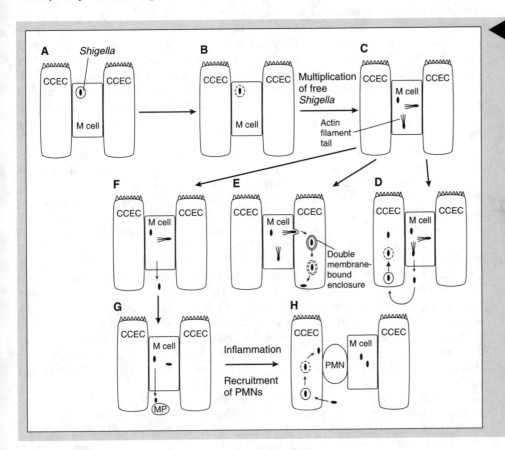

FIGURE 13-3
Events Occurring After the Uptake of Shigella into M Cells. (A) Shigella *present in endosome in M cell cytoplasm.* (B) Shigella *lyse endosome and escape free into M cell cytoplasm (see Figure 13-2).* (C) *Movement of free* Shigella *cells toward basolateral surfaces of M cells, which is propelled by polymerization of actin filaments.* (D) *Infection of CCEC from basal surface.* (E) *Intercellular spread of* Shigella. (F) Shigella *in subepithelial tissue.* (G) *Interaction between* Shigella *and macrophages (MP) in subepithelial tissue.* (H) *Entrance of* Shigella *in basal surface of CCEC after epithelium is disturbed by presence of polymorphonuclear cells (PMN). CCEC = colonic columnar epithelial cell.*

cell quickly escapes from its endosome into the cytoplasm of the M cell (this escape also apparently involves some Ipa proteins), where the free bacterium now starts multiplying. This *Shigella* (and its progeny) also begins actively moving through the cytoplasm of the infected M cell. This movement is mediated by IcsA, which promotes the attachment and polymerization of actin filaments to free shigella cells, thereby providing a propulsive force to move these bacteria through the M cell's cytoplasm. Propelled by this movement, the *Shigella* cell eventually moves to the surface of the M cell (see Figure 13-3). The next step depends on which surface of the M cell the *Shigella* cell is moving towards. If the *Shigella* moves toward (and then exits from) the basal surface of the M cell, this extracellular *Shigella* cell may then interact with the macrophages that underlie the M cell; this interaction contributes to inflammation, which is mediated by the *Shigella*'s LPS. The extracellular *Shigella* may penetrate into the basal membrane of virtually any cell in the colonic epithelium (unlike their apical membranes, the basolateral membranes of colonic columnar epithelial cells can be penetrated easily by *Shigella*), thus setting up new foci of infection. Once inside a newly infected colonic columnar epithelial cell, the *Shigella* cell again escapes into the cytoplasm using the same process as described above for M cells and begins multiplying.

Alternatively, once free in the cytoplasm of M cells (or other infected colonic epithelial cells), some *Shigella* cells move toward the portion of the M cell basolateral membrane bordering adjacent colonic columnar epithelial cells. As this surface of the M cell is approached, these *Shigella* cells become localized in a protrusion that extends from the surface of the infected host cell into the adjacent uninfected host cell (see Figure 13-3). The adjacent host cell then endocytoses this protrusion. As a result, these *Shigella* now find themselves in a double-membrane-enclosed endosome inside the adjacent host cell (i.e., intercellular spread has occurred). These *Shigella* cells then escape from this double-membrane vesicle, using IcsB, and subsequently begin multiplying in the cytoplasm of the newly infected host cell. This intercellular spread strategy has a clear advantage for *Shigella* in that it allows these bacteria to spread (at least until an effective cellular immune response can be mounted) from cell to cell in the colonic epithelium without any exposure to the exterior environment, which may contain hostile immune cells.

It has already been mentioned that some inflammation is triggered while *Shigella* cells are making their initial passage through M cells into underlying macrophages. This initial inflammation also is thought to contribute to the spread of *Shigella* through the colonic epithelium by attracting PMNs. These PMNs migrate directly into the colonic epithelium, disturbing the integrity of this epithelium. This exposes the basolateral surfaces of the colonic columnar epithelial cells to invasion by any nearby extracellular *Shigella*.

How do the processes described above result in disease? The symptoms of shigellosis are thought to result primarily from the damage to the colonic epithelium caused by *Shigella* invasion (and assisted by the production of shiga toxin, if the infecting strain is *S. dysenteriae*) and the resultant severe inflammation that ensues from this invasion. Some investigators also believe that the initial symptoms of this illness may involve an initial *Shigella* multiplication in the small intestine, but this remains controversial. Shigellosis symptoms vary from a reasonably mild, watery diarrhea to a full-blown dysentery. *Shigella* dysentery is a potentially life-threatening illness characterized by fever, cramps, tenesmus (pain and spasm when attempting to pass urine or evacuate the bowels), and frequent passage of mucoid, bloody, low-volume stools. The variation in severity of shigellosis symptoms depends both on host factors (e.g., age) and the particular *Shigella* isolate involved. As mentioned already, *S. sonnei* infections tend to cause somewhat milder disease symptoms, whereas *S. flexneri* (in the developed world) and *S. dysenteriae* (in the Third World) are more frequent causes of full-blown dysentery. In severe cases of shigellosis, death can occur (particularly in the elderly or children) due to fluid and electrolyte imbalances unless proper care is administered.

Shigella spp. are extremely important pathogens in Third World countries but they also remain significant pathogens in industrialized countries, where they cause thousands of cases of illness each year. Because of the extreme virulence of *Shigella* when entering through the fecal-oral route, shigellosis is an increasingly common problem in day care centers. Shigellosis also has been a major complication for AIDS patients.

> **Dysentery** can be defined in different ways. In this book, dysentery refers to a low-volume diarrhea that often contains blood and mucus.

Diagnosis

Microscopic examination of stool samples for the presence of elevated levels of leukocytes provides immediately helpful information for diagnosing suspected cases of shigellosis. However, a specific diagnosis of shigellosis ultimately requires laboratory culturing of *Shigella* from the stool and identification of the isolate by biochemical and serologic tests. Notable characteristics for identification include the following: *Shigella* are nonmotile, lactose-negative (they grow as clear colonies on MacConkey agar), hydrogen sulfide (H_2S)-negative, gram-negative rods.

Prevention and Treatment

Live attenuated *Shigella* vaccines are under development for use in the Third World. Good sanitary practices (e.g., adequate sewage disposal, good water treatment, frequent hand washing and wearing of gloves by personnel in day care centers) currently play the major role in preventing *Shigella* infections.

Antibiotic therapy (e.g., with a trimethoprim-sulfamethoxazole drug combination) reduces both the severity and duration of shigellosis symptoms. Supportive care often includes fluid replacement, which can be given orally in all but the most severe cases of shigellosis. Antispasmodic agents (e.g., Lomotil) are contraindicated for shigellosis and other invasive diarrheas because they tend to exacerbate symptoms.

RESOLUTION OF CLINICAL CASE

The child in this case began to improve 18 hours after visiting the pediatrician. The laboratory reported that *S. sonnei* was grown from the girl's stool.

Because *Shigella* lack intermediate animal hosts, they are acquired from human reservoirs, usually by the fecal-oral route. This transmission mechanism can include inapparent contact with feces in the day care setting (as may have occurred in this case). Day care settings present a particularly good opportunity for *Shigella* to cause disease because these bacteria can persist for hours on contaminated fingers and inanimate objects (or for weeks in foods), and *Shigella* are extremely efficient pathogens (i.e., ingestion of only a few of these bacteria can cause disease). Following an incubation period of 36–72 hours, shigellosis starts with the fairly nonspecific symptoms exhibited by the child in this case (e.g., fever, midabdominal cramps, watery diarrhea). After another 24–72 hours, when the bacteria are actively invading and multiplying in the colon, dysentery can occur. As illustrated in this case, dysentery is characterized by frequent, loose bowel movements containing blood, mucus, pus, and unformed fecal material, accompanied by tenesmus and rectal urgency. Physical examination is usually unrevealing, except for fever, but examination of the stool at this time reveals both neutrophils and blood. A Gram stain of stool is not helpful because *Shigella* cannot be differentiated from the normal flora gram-negative rods always present in feces. Patients with dysentery are treated empirically with antibiotics; trimethoprim-sulfamethoxazole or a fluoroquinolone are often used (fluoroquinolone is not used in children because it may produce an arthropathy). However, the most important aspect of therapy (particularly for children and the elderly) is the restoration of fluid and electrolyte balance disturbed by the diarrhea. With proper and prompt therapy, the outcome of shigellosis infections is usually a recovery with no long-term effects.

An **arthropathy** is a degenerative change in joints; loosely, "arthritis."

REVIEW QUESTIONS

Directions: For each of the following questions, choose the **one best** answer.

1. The direct role of Mxi-Spa proteins in *Shigella* invasion is
   (A) to permit the escape of *Shigella* from the double-membrane-bound endosome that encloses it following intercellular spread
   (B) to assemble into a translocon on the *Shigella* surface that, when activated, will secrete Ipa proteins
   (C) to affect signal transduction pathways in the host epithelial cell
   (D) to promote the polymerization of actin around free *Shigella* cells in the host cell cytoplasm
   (E) to induce membrane ruffling

2. Which one of the following statements is true about enteropathogenic *Yersinia* spp.?
   (A) These bacteria exist predominantly intracellularly in both epithelial cells and polymorphonuclear (PMN) cells
   (B) These bacteria mediate their uptake into epithelial cells primarily by secreting proteins that assemble into an extracellular complex that can interact with host cell membranes
   (C) These bacteria can enter the apical surface of most cell types present in the intestinal epithelium
   (D) These bacteria produce *Yersinia* outer proteins (Yops), which are important in invasion into epithelial cells
   (E) These bacteria produce invasin, which is a protein that binds to β_1 integrin and promotes uptake of these bacteria into invasion-susceptible cells in the intestinal epithelium

3. Differences between the invasiveness of *Salmonella* and *Shigella* correctly include which one of the following statements?
   (A) Most of the invasiveness genes for *Salmonella* are plasmid encoded, whereas none of the invasiveness genes for *Shigella* are plasmid encoded
   (B) *Salmonella* primarily invade by producing surface factors that trigger signal transduction pathways in host cells, whereas *Shigella* primarily use secreted proteins to trigger these signal transduction changes
   (C) *Salmonella* lack a translocon homologous to the Mxi-Spa translocon of *Shigella*
   (D) *Salmonella* remain inside membrane-bound vesicles after entering epithelial cells, whereas *Shigella* escape from these vesicles into the host cell cytoplasm
   (E) *Salmonella* are capable of intercellular spread in the intestinal epithelium without being exposed to the exterior environment, whereas *Shigella* cannot spread in this manner

4. Which one of the following statements regarding pathogens is true?

(A) To cause disease, pathogens either must use an entry mechanism that penetrates the epithelium or be able to penetrate the epithelium by itself

(B) Bacterial invasion into the intestinal epithelium often causes inflammation, which often results in the presence of elevated numbers of fecal leukocytes

(C) Invasive pathogens disseminate only by producing degradative enzymes that facilitate direct spread through connective tissue

(D) Invasive bacterial enteric pathogens do not produce toxins that are active on the gastrointestinal tract

(E) The epithelium is a poor protective barrier because it is permeable to virtually any microbe

ANSWERS AND EXPLANATIONS

1. **The answer is B.** After their synthesis, the Mxi-Spa proteins move to the *Shigella* surface and assemble into a translocon that, when activated by contact with a host cell, secretes Ipa proteins. IcsB mediates escape of *Shigella* from the double-membrane-bound endosome following intercellular spread. Ipa proteins affect signal transduction pathways in host cells. IcsA mediates the polymerization of actin around the *Shigella* cell, once this bacterium is free in the cytoplasm. Membrane ruffling results from the signal transduction changes in the host cell that are mediated by the Ipa proteins.

2. **The answer is E.** The enteropathogenic *Yersinia* do produce invasin, and invasin mediates uptake of these bacteria through its tight binding to β_1 integrins on the M cell surface. Enteropathogenic *Yersinia* can be killed if they are taken up into PMNs. Unlike *Shigella* or *Salmonella*, enteropathogenic *Yersinia* do not rely primarily on soluble extracellular factors to mediate their invasion. Instead, they use surface molecules like invasin. The only cells in the intestinal epithelium that *Yersinia* can enter from the apical surface are M cells (only M cells have the β_1 integrins necessary to interact with invasin). Although it is true that these bacteria produce Yops, Yops are not involved in invasion of epithelial cells (they actually function to inhibit uptake of *Yersinia* into immune cells).

3. **The answer is D.** *Salmonella* remain inside membrane-bound vesicles when transcytosing through M cells and other intestinal epithelial cells, whereas *Shigella* rapidly escape from the endosome into the cytoplasm of both M cells (during the initial infection) or other intestinal cells (following entry of *Shigella* through the basolateral membranes of epithelial cells). Many genes necessary for *Salmonella* invasion are chromosomally encoded, whereas many genes necessary for *Shigella* invasion are plasmid encoded. Both *Salmonella* and *Shigella* use secreted proteins to induce the signal transduction changes in the host cell that are necessary for their invasion (it is enteropathogenic *Yersinia* that use surface factors for initiating signal transduction changes in the host cell). *Salmonella* do have a translocon (named Inv-Spa translocon) that is homologous to the Mxi-Spa translocon of *Shigella*. The *Shigella* (not *Salmonella*) are capable of intercellular spread through the intestinal epithelium without being exposed to the environment outside the epithelial host cell.

4. **The answer is B.** Invasion does cause inflammation, and this correlates with higher levels of fecal leukocytes. A number of pathogens (e.g., *Vibrio cholerae*) are noninvasive and simply remain on the epithelial surface during disease. Although producing degradative enzymes to spread through connective tissue is one strategy used by pathogens to disseminate, other dissemination strategies also exist (e.g., being transported through lymph or blood). At least some invasive bacterial enteric pathogens (e.g., *Shigella dysenteriae*, which produces Shiga toxin) can produce toxins active on the gastrointestinal tract. It is clear that normal flora microbes and noninvasive pathogens normally do not penetrate the epithelium.

PART III: MICROBIAL SUBVERSION OF HOST DEFENSES

OVERVIEW

INTRODUCTION

Under ideal conditions, pathogenic microorganisms such as *Escherichia coli* have a generation time of approximately 20 minutes. When compared with the average human generation time of approximately 20 years, it is quite remarkable that we, as a fertile breeding ground for microbes, are not overcome by the shear mass of microbes growing within us. Instead, the host immune system provides a formidable barrier against microbial infection. How the host immune system prevents us from being overwhelmed by the vast quantity and diverse array of microbial pathogens encountered every day is a subject addressed by the fascinating science of immunology. Given the purpose of this text (see Preface), many of the molecular details of immunology have been left for another book. However, the role of the host immune response to infection by microbial pathogens is inextricably tied to the process of infectious diseases and cannot be ignored. Therefore, the student should possess a minimal appreciation for how a healthy human immune system prevents us from being overrun by these aggressive microbial pathogens.

INNATE AND SPECIFIC IMMUNITY

In general the host immune system is best viewed as a two-armed barrier, involving both innate and specific immune strategies to prevent infection by microbial pathogens. *Innate immunity* utilizes an elaborate system of constitutively expressed physical and chemical obstacles to prevent infection. In terms of sheer surface area covering a human, the major physical obstacle to bacterial infection contracted from the environment is the skin, which prevents the free passage of microbial pathogens into the sterile spaces of the human host. In addition, the normal physiology of the skin promotes the removal of these microbial pathogens by the exfoliation of cells (desquamation). The alternative to entry of microbial pathogens through the skin is entry through the moist mucosal surfaces of the human host. Cells comprising mucosal surfaces are often highly differentiated and are able to undergo a number of different processes that discourage microbial pathogens from establishing infection. These include peristalsis by cells of the gastrointestinal tract, mucocilliary movement by cells in the respiratory tract, and the flushing of mucosal surfaces with liquids (e.g., flow of tears within the eye). Innate chemical obstacles to infection by microbial pathogens complement these physical barriers. Examples of these chemical obstacles include the antimicrobial action of organic acids found in sweat, the low pH environment that exists within the stomach, and proteins such as lysozyme and lactoferrin that are associated with secretions and lysosomal granules. By itself, the innate immune system provides a formidable challenge for the establishment of infectious diseases that were stressed in Part II.

Compounding this challenge is *specific immunity*, the second arm of immunity that protects the human host from infection by microbial pathogens. This involves the production of antibodies and T-lymphocytes that "specifically" recognize the invading microbial pathogen. Conceptually, this is a much more efficient means of warding off microbial pathogens and therefore represents a significant advantage over the innate immunity arm. However, specific immunity is an educational process and, as such, requires prior exposure to the microbial pathogen. It also presumes that a specific response can discriminate between the microbial pathogen and the host. So, how does a microbial pathogen evade this formidable host immunity? In the "war" between microbial pathogens and the human host, several remarkably sophisticated strategies have evolved to subvert specific components of the host defenses. Each of these strategies has a single goal—to overcome the gauntlet of defense mechanisms imposed by the healthy human host by weakening one or a few of the many mechanisms of innate or specific immunity. Thus, subversion of the host response to infection is the common theme emphasized in Part III. The common strategies used by microbial pathogens to subvert host defenses are summarized below and are expanded in Chapters 14 through 19.

COMMON SURVIVAL STRATEGIES

Surviving the Chemical and Physical Defenses of the Host

In this scenario the adage that "the best defense is a great offense" seems appropriate. It is amazing that we ingest millions, if not billions, of microorganisms every day without being infected by them. In large part this is accomplished by "filtering" these organisms through the stomach, which, as part of the host system of innate immunity, discourages the passage through, or colonization of, this highly acidic environment. Therefore, only those bacteria strong enough to survive these harsh conditions are able to cause disease. The pathogenesis of *Helicobacter pylori* represents an excellent paradigm. Chapter 14 describes how *H. pylori* survives within the acidic conditions of the stomach and how this organism colonizes the lower portion of the stomach, ultimately giving rise to ulcers.

Intracellular Survival

This strategy involves the invasion, survival, and growth within eukaryotic cells. Viral pathogens do this as part of their natural biology, but some bacterial and parasitic pathogens also employ this strategy. Obligate and intracellular microbial pathogens have been highlighted throughout this text, and Chapter 15 reinforces the importance of these pathogens in medical microbiology. *Legionella pneumophila*, *Lysteria monocytogenes*, and *Plasmodium* spp. are used to illustrate this concept. Intracellular survival strategy effectively removes these microbial pathogens from the extracellular host defenses; they then must survive the intracellular environment, which can be quite harsh. The mechanisms by which these three pathogens survive within the host environment are contrasted in this chapter.

Molecular Mimicry

Molecular mimicry is the ability of a microbial pathogen to effectively cloak itself in the costume of the host. This results in two outcomes, which are described in Chapters 16 and 18. In the first outcome, the specific arm of the immune response is unable to recognize the microbial pathogen because the formation of such a response would cross-react with host tissues. This is the case for *Neisseria meningitidis*, one of the illustrative pathogens in Chapter 18. This is largely the result of the production of a poorly immunogenic carbohydrate capsule that surrounds not only this bacterial pathogen, but also many others. This poorly immunogenic capsule allows *N. meningitidis* to invade the bloodstream or the cerebral spinal fluid of the host, without detection by the host immune system, and cause severe disease. In the second outcome, an immune response is engendered to the microbial antigen, resulting in an immune response that cross-reacts with host tissues. In doing so, an immunopathologic response that is deleterious to the host results. An example of this is rheumatic fever that results from a *Streptococcus pyogenes* infection, as described in Chapter 16.

Antigenic Variation

A number of microbial pathogens vary their surface antigens so that an immune response formed against one set of antigens does not recognize the organism when it expresses another set of antigens. This allows pathogenic viruses, bacteria, and parasites to evade the specific immune response to infection. Antigenic variability may have additional advantages by conferring the ability to attach or detach from specific cell types. Three pathogens known for their antigenic variability—influenzavirus, *Neisseria gonorrhoeae*, and the malarial pathogens—are described in Chapter 17.

Surface and Secreted Factors

Surface components such as Protein A, expressed by *Staphylococcus aureus*, and lipo-polysaccharide (LPS), expressed by all gram-negative bacterial pathogens, can have profound effects for subverting the immune defenses of the human host. Likewise, secreted enzymes (e.g., proteases secreted by *Pseudomonas aeruginosa*) and bacterial toxins skirt host defenses and contribute to the pathogenesis of a variety of organisms. In Chapter 19, *S. aureus* is presented as an illustrative pathogen that relies heavily upon surface and secreted factors to cause disease.

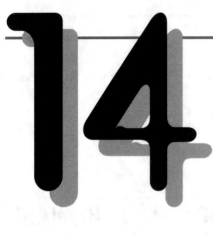

OVERCOMING THE PHYSICAL AND CHEMICAL DEFENSES OF THE HUMAN BODY

CHAPTER OUTLINE

Introduction of Clinical Case
Overcoming the Physical and Chemical Defenses of the Human Body
- Skin
- Conjunctiva
- Respiratory Tract
- Urogenital Tract
- Gastrointestinal Tract

Combating Exposure to Stomach Acidity
- Surviving Transit through the Stomach
- Microbial Growth in the Stomach

Illustrative Pathogen: *Helicobacter pylori*
- Biologic Characteristics
- Reservoir and Transmission
- Virulence Factors
- Pathogenesis
- Diagnosis
- Prevention and Treatment

Resolution of Clinical Case
Review Questions

INTRODUCTION OF CLINICAL CASE

A 56-year-old business executive presented to his family physician because of an intense pain in his stomach. This pain had been present for 4 days and seemed to be getting steadily worse. There was no accompanying nausea, vomiting, or diarrhea, but the pain was not relieved by the ingestion of acetominophen or antacids. The patient had experienced approximately six episodes of similar, but less intense, pain during the past 2 years. These previous episodes were at least partially relieved by the ingestion of antacids. His vital signs were normal. There was point tenderness high in the mid-epigastrium. There was no rebound tenderness or organomegaly. The patient was started on clarithromycin, amoxicillin, and omeprazole, and arrangements were made for the patient to undergo upper gastrointestinal endoscopy the following day. Endoscopy revealed an active duodenal ulcer, as well as a moderately intense inflammatory gastritis.

> **Point tenderness** *refers to the elicitation of pain on palpation with a single finger, as opposed to pain spread over a wide area.*

- What relationship, if any, might exist between this man's duodenal ulcer and infectious disease?
- Why is this man being given antimicrobial agents?
- Is this therapy likely to relieve the man's ulcer? If so, will he likely suffer a later relapse?

OVERCOMING THE PHYSICAL AND CHEMICAL DEFENSES OF THE HUMAN BODY

A number of physical and chemical defenses help protect the human host against microbial pathogens. Many of the body's physical defenses are aimed at preventing pathogen entry (e.g., the ability of intact skin to act as a potent barrier to infection) or promoting pathogen clearance (e.g., ciliary action). In contrast, the body's chemical defenses are primarily directed at killing or inhibiting the growth of microorganisms (e.g., gastric acid has potent antimicrobial properties). Not surprisingly, successful pathogens have devised strategies to overcome the physical and chemical defense mechanisms of the human body. For example, many pathogens overcome the barrier function of intact skin by entering the body through more vulnerable epithelial surfaces than the skin (e.g., through the gastrointestinal epithelium) or by entering the body through damaged skin (e.g., through wounds).

This section of the chapter briefly reviews the physical and chemical defenses present at major locations of the body (many of these defenses have already been introduced in Part II of this book) along with specific strategies used by successful pathogens to circumvent these defenses.

Skin

A few pathogens (e.g., S. aureus) are able to grow on the skin.

Although all epithelial surfaces provide some degree of protection against pathogen entry into internal tissues, the intact skin is the most effective epithelial barrier against infection. The skin also provides an unfavorable growth environment for most microorganisms because of: (1) the constant desquamation of dead epithelial cells from the skin, which removes microorganisms adhering to these epithelial cells, (2) the dryness and low pH of the skin, which inhibits microbial growth, and (3) the skin being rich in fatty acids (produced by the sebaceous glands) that possess antimicrobial properties.

A few parasites (e.g., schistosomes and hookworms) are thought to penetrate directly into intact skin.

Most pathogens find it difficult or impossible to overcome the intact skin's effectiveness as an entry barrier. Consequently, some pathogens depend on a physical break in the integrity of the skin (e.g., a wound, surgical incision, burn) to enter the body. Another strategy for bypassing the barrier imposed by intact skin is for a pathogen to be introduced into subcutaneous tissue by the bite or scratch of an animal or by an arthropod bite. In the latter case, pathogens typically reside inside an arthropod vector until they are subcutaneously injected during the biting process (i.e., the arthropod vector serves as a "flying syringe" for the pathogen; see Chapter 8).

Conjunctiva

*As introduced in Chapter 1, **lysozyme** is a host enzyme that cleaves the covalent bond between the N-acetylglucosamine and N-acetylmuramic acid of peptidoglycan. This action can result in lysis of susceptible bacterial cells. As introduced in Chapters 1 and 2, **lactoferrin** is a host protein that binds iron tightly. Because iron is essential for bacterial, fungal, and parasitic growth, these pathogens must devise some strategy for gaining iron that has been sequestered by transferrin and lactoferrin in the human host.*

The conjunctiva is physically protected by both the mechanical action of blinking and the washing action of tears. Tears also contain a number of antimicrobial substances, including lysozyme, lactoferrin, and immunoglobulin A (IgA). Despite these defenses, the conjunctiva represents a fairly common site of infection, especially for viral infections. This susceptibility is partially explained by the fact that viruses are not susceptible to the antibacterial effects of the lactoferrin and lysozyme found in tears. However, some prokaryotes (e.g., *Chlamydia trachomatis*) are able to infect the conjunctiva. Typically these prokaryotes resist the clearing action of tears or blinking by adhering tightly to the conjunctiva. Further, many (but not all) of these prokaryotes are opportunists that cause a secondary infection after the physical and chemical defenses of the conjunctiva have been damaged by a viral infection.

Respiratory Tract

As introduced previously (see Chapter 7), the respiratory tract also is protected by several physical and chemical defenses. For example, respiratory tract mucus (often assisted by IgA) is an effective trap for many inhaled microorganisms. Once entrapped in mucus, these microbes often are removed from the respiratory tract by ciliary action. Additionally, mucus of the respiratory tract is rich in antimicrobial substances such as defensins (which are cationic antimicrobial peptides), lactoferrin, and lysozyme.

Although the physical and chemical defenses of the respiratory tract are very potent (causing a number of inhalation-acquired pathogens to infect people preferentially with compromised physical or chemical respiratory defenses), pathogens have developed several strategies to help overcome these defenses. For example, many respiratory pathogens resist the potent clearing action of the cilia by producing adhesins (see Chapter 12) that facilitate tight adherence to respiratory epithelial cells. Many respiratory pathogens also produce inhibitory substances that inhibit ciliary action, further reducing microbial clearance from the respiratory tract. Successful respiratory pathogens typically are resistant to the biochemical defenses of the respiratory tract. As mentioned above, inhalation-acquired viruses are insensitive to both lysozyme and lactoferrin; even many of the bacteria causing respiratory infections are relatively resistant to lysozyme and lactoferrin. For example, the outer membrane provides a shield against lysozyme for gram-negative bacteria. Similarly, many gram-positive bacteria causing respiratory disease produce capsules or other external surface layers that reduce the accessibility of their cell walls to lysozyme. Bacterial strategies for overcoming lactoferrin-mediated (and transferrin-mediated) iron restriction include producing high-affinity, iron-chelating compounds named siderophores to remove iron from host iron-binding compounds and removing iron from host lactoferrin that has been directly bound to the bacterial surface (see Chapter 1 for more details).

> Remember that the peptidoglycan target of lysozyme is located in the periplasmic space in gram-negative bacteria.

Urogenital Tract

Considering that little or no normal flora is present in the urinary tract to inhibit pathogen growth and there is only limited deployment of the immune system in the lower urinary tract, physical and chemical defenses obviously play a particularly important role in protecting the lower urinary tract from infection. Among the most important of the physical and chemical defenses of the urinary tract is the flow of urine through the urethra. Urine flow provides a physical cleansing action that removes many microorganisms from the urinary tract before they can enter the bladder or kidneys. In fact, one reason why women are more prone than men to urinary tract infections is that the shorter length of the female urethra makes it easier for pathogens to reach the kidneys or bladder of a woman before being displaced by urination. The sphincter action of the urethral opening provides a physical barrier to pathogen entry into the bladder or kidneys. The urinary tract also is protected by chemical defenses. These most notably include the potent antimicrobial effects exerted by both the high concentration of urea (a breakdown product of proteins) and the typically low pH of urine.

Pathogens resist the physical/chemical defenses of the urinary tract by employing several strategies. First, urinary tract pathogens resist being flushed from the body during urination by producing adhesins that allow them to bind tightly to the urinary epithelium. For example, *Escherichia coli* strains causing urinary tract infections often produce P blood group antigen-associated pili (PAP pili; see Chapter 12). The presence of PAP pili allows these *E. coli* strains to adhere to the epithelium of the urinary tract. Additionally, some common bacterial urinary tract pathogens (e.g., many *Proteus* species) produce urease, an enzyme that decreases the concentration of urea and raises the pH of the microenvironment surrounding these bacteria. This allows these bacteria to grow even when bathed in the low pH of urine.

The mucosa of the human genital tract is also protected by physical and chemical defense mechanisms. In men, spermine (and other substances in sperm) possess antimicrobial properties that may help protect the testicles from infection. In women, the vagina not only receives protection from normal flora (see Chapter 11) but also typically presents an unfavorable environment for pathogen growth due to its normally low pH.

During childbearing years, estrogen promotes the secretion of large amounts of glycogen into the vagina. *Lactobaccilus* spp. (part of the normal vaginal flora) then metabolize this glycogen to lactic acid, which decreases the normal vaginal pH to 5. The importance of maintaining a low pH as a vaginal defense mechanism is illustrated by the increased rates of vaginal infections following metabolic or hormonal changes that alter glycogen secretion. Likewise, douching disturbs the *Lactobacillus* spp. found in normal healthy vaginal flora and sometimes triggers bacterial vaginosis by allowing the establishment in the vagina of unhealthy bacteria such as *Gardnerella vaginalis*.

Despite these physical and chemical defenses, the male and female genital tracts are susceptible to infection, particularly by pathogens adapted for sexual transmission (see Chapter 9). A major explanation for why sexually transmitted pathogens are so efficient at establishing infection is that pathogen colonization and invasion is facilitated by the creation of "microabrasions" in the urogenital tract during sexual intercourse.

Gastrointestinal Tract

Extensive physical and chemical defenses against infection are also deployed in the human gastrointestinal tract. Immediately after ingestion, microorganisms encounter the acidic conditions of the stomach. Further, extensive physical and chemical defenses are also present in the intestines, including:

- Peristalsis, which helps remove nonadherent microorganisms from the gastrointestinal tract
- The frequent turnover of small intestinal epithelial cells, which helps remove adherent pathogens from the intestinal epithelium
- Bile and digestive enzymes (e.g., trypsin, chymotrypsin), which inhibit or kill many microorganisms
- Mucus, which (like the mucus of the respiratory tract) shields the gastrointestinal epithelium against some microorganisms and also promotes the clearance of non-adherent microorganisms

The large number of intestinal pathogens described in this book confirms that many microorganisms have developed strategies to overcome the physical and chemical defenses of the intestines. For example, like respiratory and urinary tract pathogens, most intestinal pathogens resist the clearing actions of mucus and peristalsis by adhering tightly to the gastrointestinal epithelium. Further, a number of successful intestinal pathogens are innately resistant to bile and digestive enzymes (e.g., the long "O" antigen side chains of the lipopolysaccharide found in most gram-negative enteric pathogens keeps bile away from the otherwise sensitive lipid bilayers of the outer and cytoplasmic membranes of these bacteria).

COMBATING EXPOSURE TO STOMACH ACIDITY

Understanding how ingestion-acquired pathogens resist killing by the low pH of the stomach provides an excellent illustration of how pathogens can overcome even the most potent physical and chemical defenses of the body. However, before discussing this subject, it should be appreciated that two very different situations exist whereby a pathogen has to resist the low pH of the stomach: ingestion-acquired pathogens causing disease in the intestines (or other regions of the body) need to survive only a short-term exposure to gastric acid, whereas *Helicobacter pylori*, which actually multiplies and causes disease in the stomach, must be able to persist for long periods in the hostile stomach environment.

Surviving Transit Through the Stomach

Microorganisms (particularly bacteria) are often quite sensitive to acidic conditions. Therefore, surviving a temporary exposure to the low pH of the stomach until their release into the intestines (and chance to cause disease) represents a significant challenge for most ingestion-acquired pathogens. Strategies used to overcome their short-term exposure to gastric acid include:

- Relying upon being ingested in large numbers (ingesting a large dose of a pathogen increases the probability that at least some of these ingested microorganisms will survive long enough to escape from the stomach into the "more favorable" environment present in the intestines)
- Relying upon being ingested inside food particles (which physically shields pathogens from stomach acid)
- Relying upon being ingested in foods (e.g., milk) that have buffering capacity
- Developing strong innate resistance to acid (e.g., *Shigella* spp. are highly acid resistant, although the precise biochemical mechanism of this bacterium's pH resistance is not yet clear)

Microbial Growth in the Stomach

Considering how challenging many ingestion-acquired pathogens find surviving even a short-term exposure to stomach acidity, *H. pylori* is quite remarkable. Once present in the stomach, this bacterium not only survives but also multiplies (and causes disease) in the hostile environment of this organ.

H. pylori uses at least two strategies to overcome the hostile, low-pH environment of the stomach (Figure 14-1). First, this bacterium is motile, which enables it to enter into

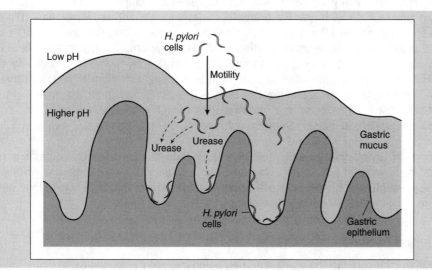

◀ **FIGURE 14-1**
Strategies Used by* Helicobacter pylori *to Survive and Grow in the Stomach. *To escape the low pH of the stomach, H. pylori uses its motility to enter the gastric mucus, where a more favorable pH exists. Once present in the gastric mucus, it produces urease, which converts urea to ammonia (NH_3), as well as water and carbon dioxide, thereby raising the pH of the local microenvironment. Some H. pylori cells may move through the mucus and adhere to the gastric epithelium.*

the gastric mucus (sometimes *H. pylori* even traverses through the gastric mucus to the underlying gastric epithelium). Entering into the gastric mucus is favorable for *H. pylori* survival because the pH of gastric mucus (and the underlying gastric epithelium) is much higher than the pH present in the lumen of the stomach. A second low-pH survival mechanism used by *H. pylori* involves production of an extremely potent urease (Figure 14-2). The ammonia end product of urease action raises the pH of the microenvironment surrounding the *H. pylori* cell, further facilitating survival and growth of this bacterium in the normally hostile environment of the stomach.

The normal physiologic role of gastric mucus is to protect the gastric epithelium from gastric acid. The effectiveness of this protection is illustrated by the fact that the lumen of the stomach normally has a pH of 1–2, whereas the pH on the epithelial side of the mucus layer is nearly physiologic (pH = 7.0).

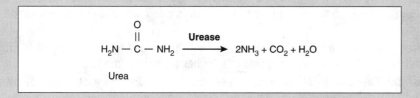

◀ **FIGURE 14-2**
Enzymatic Action of Urease. *When urease breaks down urea, ammonia (NH_3) forms, and it is highly basic. This formation of ammonia raises the pH of the surrounding microenvironment.*

ILLUSTRATIVE PATHOGEN: *Helicobacter pylori*

Biologic Characteristics

H. pylori is a spiral-shaped, oxidase-positive, gram-negative bacterium that shares many characteristics with *Campylobacter* spp. (in fact, *H. pylori* was originally classified as *C. pylori*). Like *Campylobacter* spp., *H. pylori* is fastidious and microaerophilic. Because of these similarities, the same medium (i.e., Skirrow's medium) and growth conditions can be used for isolation of both *Campylobacter* spp. and *H. pylori*, although *H. pylori* tends to grow slower than most *Campylobacter* isolates. *H. pylori* also resembles *Campylobacter* spp. by its motility. However, one important distinguishing feature between *H. pylori* and the *Campylobacter* spp. is that *H. pylori* produces an extremely potent urease.

Reservoir and Transmission

Although the transmission and reservoirs for *H. pylori* are not completely understood, this bacterium is believed to have a human reservoir (note that other *Helicobacter* spp. specifically infect other animal species). *H. pylori* infections often occur in intrafamilial clusters, supporting the person-to-person spread of *H. pylori*. This person-to-person transmission of *H. pylori* is thought to involve oral–oral spread (*H. pylori* can be found in dental plaque) or fecal–oral spread.

In countries with good sanitation facilities, stomach colonization by *H. pylori* increases substantially with age. For example, in developed countries, fewer than 10% of children younger than 10 years are colonized by *H. pylori*, whereas more than 50% of individuals older than 60 years are colonized by this bacterium. In contrast, the rate of *H. pylori* colonization of both children and adults is significantly higher in less developed societies, with colonization rates of more than 80% being common for adults in these areas. These higher *H. pylori* colonization rates in less developed countries are thought to result, at least in large part, from overcrowding (which probably facilitates oral–oral spread of *H. pylori*) and poor sanitation (which probably facilitates fecal–oral spread of *H. pylori*).

Once *H. pylori* colonizes the stomach of an individual, it probably remains present for many years, if not for life. However, many colonized people remain asymptomatic, suggesting that host factors are important for progression to *H. pylori*-mediated disease.

Virulence Factors

Molecules implicated in the virulence of *H. pylori* include the following.

Cytotoxin. This toxin, whose mechanism of action remains unknown, contributes to damage of gastric (and possibly duodenal) epithelial cells.

Lipopolysaccharide (LPS). Although the endotoxic activity of *H. pylori* LPS is relatively weak, it still may contribute to inflammation.

Urease. This enzyme may contribute to pathogenesis in three ways: (1) it facilitates survival in the stomach by raising the pH of the *H. pylori* microenvironment, (2) it provides access to nitrogenous nutrients needed for growth of *H. pylori*, and (3) the NH_4^+ end product of urease action may contribute to *H. pylori*-induced epithelial cell damage and inflammation in the stomach and duodenum.

Mucinase. This enzyme, which is a protease, degrades gastric mucus and exposes the underlying gastric epithelium to gastric acid (this can contribute to inflammation and ulceration).

Flagella. These structures give *H. pylori* the motility needed to enter the gastric mucus, thus allowing this bacterium to reside in a higher pH environment.

Adhesin(s). These allow *H. pylori* cells penetrating through the gastric mucus layer to attach to the gastric epithelium. This may assist long-term stomach colonization.

Pathogenesis

Once *H. pylori* has entered the stomach, it survives gastric acid, using mechanisms introduced earlier in this chapter; that is, by producing a potent urease that increases the pH of the bacterium's microenvironment and by translocating itself into the gastric mucus.

Once stomach colonization has been achieved, *H. pylori* often remains present for many years without causing illness. However, in certain colonized individuals with incompletely understood risk factors, disease develops. The hallmark of *H. pylori* disease is gastric inflammation, which is often accompanied by epithelial cell destruction. At least two pathogenic processes appear to be involved in *H. pylori*-induced damage. First, *H. pylori* directly damages the gastric (and sometimes duodenal) epithelium, which is achieved by any of the following mechanisms: (1) *H. pylori* can produce a toxin that induces vacuolization in gastric (and possibly duodenal) epithelial cells, which can lead to inflammation and damage mucus production; (2) *H. pylori* can cause the production of NH_3 (from the urease-induced cleavage of urea; see Figure 14-2), which also can be toxic to the gastric epithelium and lead to decreased mucus production; and (3) *H. pylori* can produce mucinase, which can degrade the gastric mucus layer. This exposes the underlying epithelium to gastric acid-induced damage, which contributes to inflammation and ulceration. Second, the presence of *H. pylori* in the stomach also can trigger a strong inflammatory response that results in immunopathologic damage and also may trigger increased acid production in the stomach (which further contributes to gastric and duodenal damage).

> *H. pylori* are not believed to invade the gastric epithelium.

The most common consequence of *H. pylori*-induced damage is gastritis. However, if *H. pylori*-induced damage becomes severe enough, peptic ulcer disease develops. Symptoms of *H. pylori*-induced gastritis or peptic ulcers commonly include nausea, anorexia, vomiting, and epigastric pain. Although still poorly understood, a link also has been established between *H. pylori* colonization and stomach cancer, with *H. pylori* colonization increasing the risk of a person developing stomach cancer by approximately sixfold (see Chapter 26).

> Peptic ulcers are ulcers of the stomach, duodenum, or lower end of the esophagus.

Diagnosis

Both noninvasive and invasive tests are available for the diagnosis of *H. pylori*-induced disease. Noninvasive tests include serologic tests that detect the presence of serum antibodies to *H. pylori*. Although these tests are accurate, they are not useful for confirming whether antimicrobial therapy has been successful at eliminating *H. pylori* from the stomach (because *H. pylori* antibodies persist in the serum long after the organism has been cleared from the stomach). Another noninvasive test for *H. pylori* infection is the urease breath test, which involves the patient ingesting a labeled urea as a substrate for *H. pylori* urease.

> **Urease breath test**
> The patient usually drinks a liquid containing ^{13}C-labeled urea (which is not radioactive) and breathes into a container. The exhaled breath is then analyzed with a mass spectrophotometer to detect $^{13}CO_2$, which is formed when urease from H. pylori hydrolyzes the labeled urea given to the patient. A radioactive version of this test is also available.

The gold standard for diagnosis of *H. pylori* infection is biopsy of the stomach via gastroscopy. The biopsied specimen then can be cultured for *H. pylori*. This sample also can be subjected to a urease test for rapid presumptive diagnosis of *H. pylori* infection by placing a small piece of the biopsied material directly into urea-containing medium. If *H. pylori* are present in this specimen, the pH of the urea-containing medium rapidly rises and changes the color of a pH indicator included in the urea test medium. Provided that appropriate stains are used (e.g., Giemsa stain), histologic analysis of biopsied specimens also is useful for confirming the presence of *H. pylori*.

Despite improvements in noninvasive tests for diagnosis of *H. pylori* infections, many physicians still run direct histologic analyses of biopsied specimens because this approach provides a direct evaluation of the extent of damage present in the patient's stomach and also allows the physician to rule out the possibility of carcinoma.

Prevention and Treatment

Because many people remain asymptomatically colonized by *H. pylori* for long periods, therapy should be administered only upon the development of illness. Despite ongoing research, no *H. pylori* vaccine is currently available.

The recent recognition that *H. pylori* is a major cause of gastritis and peptic ulcers

Omeprazole is one member of a class of compounds that inhibits gastric acid secretion by specific inhibition of the acid (proton) pump.

has dramatically changed the treatment of these illnesses. Treatment for these *H. pylori*-induced diseases typically involves the administration of several antimicrobial agents (e.g., metronidazole, bismuth salts, clarithromycin, tetracycline, amoxicillin) in combination with omeprazole. Multiple types of antimicrobial agents are used in these therapeutic regimens because of the common development of antimicrobial resistance in *H. pylori*. Multiple antimicrobial therapy approaches commonly achieve cure rates of 80%–95% for *H. pylori*-mediated disease, and relapse rates for *H. pylori*-induced ulcers are much lower (~2%) than the 75% relapse rates previously noted using only therapeutic agents aimed at inhibiting acid production.

RESOLUTION OF CLINICAL CASE

Biopsies of this patient's stomach revealed an inflammatory infiltrate that contained gram-negative bacteria having a morphology consistent with *H. pylori*. Following introduction of clarithromycin, amoxicillin, and omeprazole, the patient's pain abated within 3 days. Therapy with the specified antibiotics was continued for 2 weeks, and omeprazole therapy continued for a total of 4 weeks. It is likely that this therapy has cured this patient of *H. pylori*, and it is unlikely that there will be a relapse (for reasons which are not yet clear, reinfection and recurrence of clinical disease are uncommon after eradication of *H. pylori*).

The most common consequence of *H. pylori* infection is a chronic superficial gastritis, which may produce a nonspecific gastroenteritis characterized by nausea, vomiting, epigastric pain, and fever of 3–14 days duration. However, the most important clinical role of this bacterium is the production of peptic ulcer disease. Approximately 50%–80% of peptic ulcers and 95% of duodenal ulcers that are not caused by the ingestion of nonsteroidal anti-inflammatory drugs (NSAIDs) have been associated with *H. pylori*. Until recently, testing for active *H. pylori* infection required upper gastrointestinal endoscopy and biopsies; noninvasive tests are now available for detecting *H. pylori* infection. However, given the overwhelming involvement of *H. pylori* in peptic ulcers not caused by NSAIDs, a strong case can be made for not performing any test to diagnose *H. pylori* infection in patients with previously diagnosed duodenal ulcers who have no history of ingesting NSAIDs, no symptoms or signs of a hypersecretory state, and no history of treatment with antimicrobial agents that might have cured an *H. pylori* infection.

H. pylori readily becomes resistant to metronidazole and, to a lesser extent, clarithromycin, if either agent is given alone (*H. pylori* does not usually become resistant to luminally active agents such as bismuth, tetracycline, and amoxicillin). Consequently, combinations of two or three agents are used to treat *H. pylori*-induced disease. The therapeutic regimen specifically used for this patient is reported to be highly (perhaps >90%) effective. Addition of metronidazole or amoxicillin to clarithromycin and omeprazole during the first 2 weeks of therapy raises the rate of eradication of *H. pylori* from the stomach to 90% or higher.

REVIEW QUESTIONS

Directions: For each of the following questions, choose the **one best** answer.

1. Which one of the following statements about the body's chemical and physical defenses is correct?

    (A) Lysozyme has potent antiviral properties

    (B) The skin is relatively ineffective as a barrier to microbial entry into deeper tissues

    (C) The high pH of the vagina inhibits microbial growth

    (D) The protective effects of mucus are limited to the respiratory tract

    (E) The sebaceous glands of the skin produce fatty acids that have antimicrobial properties

2. *Helicobacter pylori* is best described by which one of the following statements?

    (A) It stains blue on properly performed Gram stains

    (B) It is a strict anaerobe

    (C) It produces lipopolysaccharide

    (D) It is highly invasive

    (E) It does not produce exotoxins

3. Which one of the following statements is true about peptic ulcers?

    (A) The relapse rate for *H. pylori*-induced peptic ulcers is similar in patients treated with antimicrobials plus omeprazole as for patients treated with omeprazole alone

    (B) Most peptic ulcers not caused by ingestion of nonsteroidal anti-inflammatory drugs (NSAIDs) are caused by *H. pylori* infection

    (C) Everyone infected with *H. pylori* eventually develops peptic ulcers

    (D) Only a small percentage of the United States population ever becomes infected with *H. pylori*

    (E) The rate of *H. pylori* infection is similar in the United States and in Third World countries

4. *H. pylori*-induced disease is best characterized by which one of the following statements?

    (A) It most commonly presents as gastritis

    (B) It does not involve inflammation

    (C) It responds well to therapy with a single antimicrobial agent

    (D) It rarely involves the duodenum

5. *H. pylori* can multiply in the stomach, at least in part, because of which one of the following actions?

    (A) It directly produces urease, which lowers the pH of the bacterium's microenvironment

    (B) It invades deep into the gastric epithelium, where it is sheltered from acid

    (C) It exists in the gastric lumen, where the pH is higher than in other parts of the stomach

    (D) It is highly motile, so it can enter into the relative safety of the gastric mucus layer

    (E) It directly produces highly basic compounds that raise the pH of the microenvironment

ANSWERS AND EXPLANATIONS

1. **The answer is E.** Lysozyme's target is peptidoglycan, so it has only antibacterial activity because peptidoglycan is found only in bacteria. The skin is a highly effective barrier to infection; only a few pathogens can penetrate healthy intact skin. The low pH of the vagina inhibits microbial growth. Mucus in the gastrointestinal tract also offers protection against microbial infection.

2. **The answer is C.** *H. pylori* does produce lipopolysaccharide (LPS), although its LPS has relatively weak endotoxic activity. *H. pylori* is gram negative, so it should Gram stain red or pink. Further, this bacterium is microaerophilic, not anaerobic (see Chapter 2 for the difference between a microaerophile and an anaerobe). There is currently no evidence for extensive *H. pylori* invasion of the gastric epithelium. Finally, *H. pylori* does produce an exotoxin, which creates vacuoles in the gastric epithelium.

3. **The answer is B.** Inclusion of antimicrobials has greatly lowered the relapse rate for *H. pylori*-induced peptic ulcers. Current thinking is that many people colonized by *H. pylori* remain asymptomatic. In the United States, *H. pylori* stomach colonization rates increase steadily with age, such that a majority of the elderly carry this bacterium. There is a much higher rate of *H. pylori* colonization (particularly in the young) in Third World countries compared to industrialized societies.

4. **The answer is A.** Inflammation is an important contributor to the symptoms of *H. pylori* disease. Because *H. pylori* often develops antibiotic resistance, therapy against this bacterium usually involves multiple types of antimicrobial agents. Through still incompletely understood mechanisms, *H. pylori* infection does commonly cause duodenal ulcers to develop.

5. **The answer is D.** *H. pylori* does produce urease, but urease action raises the pH of the microenvironment. *H. pylori* is not thought to be invasive. *H. pylori* exists in the gastric mucus (or under this layer on the gastric epithelium), not in the lumen, which has a very low pH. *H. pylori* raises the pH of its local microenvironment by producing urease, which in turn produces basic end products.

15 IMMUNE SURVIVAL STRATEGIES OF INTRACELLULAR PROKARYOTIC AND EUKARYOTIC PATHOGENS

CHAPTER OUTLINE

Introduction of Clinical Case
Intracellular Survival
• Medical Microbiology and Intracellular Invasion and Survival
Illustrative Pathogen: *Legionella pneumophila*
• Biologic Characteristics
• Reservoir and Transmission
• Virulence Factors
• Pathogenesis
• Diagnosis
• Prevention and Treatment
Illustrative Pathogen: *Listeria monocytogenes*
• Biologic Characteristics
• Reservoir and Transmission
• Virulence Factors
• Pathogenesis
• Diagnosis
• Prevention and Treatment
Illustrative Pathogen: *Plasmodium* spp.
• Biologic Characteristics
• Reservoir and Transmission
• Virulence Factors
• Pathogenesis
• Diagnosis
• Prevention and Treatment
Resolution of Clinical Case
Review Questions

INTRODUCTION OF CLINICAL CASE

A 54-year-old salesman was admitted to the hospital because of fever, shaking chills, and a nonproductive cough, all of which had begun abruptly 4 days previously. The patient had seen a physician 2 days prior to his admission and had been started on oral cephalothin (a first-generation cephalosporin). There was now pain in the left anterior and lateral chest associated with the coughing. Examination revealed a temperature of 101.7°F, a pulse rate of 72 beats/min, and a respiratory rate of 35 breaths/min. Rales were heard over the left and right lower chest posteriorly, but there were no signs of consolidation or pleural effusion. The white blood cell (WBC) count was mildly elevated (11,000 cells/mm³), and the liver function tests were modestly elevated. The chest roentgenograph showed hazy infiltrates of the left lower lobe and of the right lower and middle lobes.

Further history revealed that no other family member was ill. The patient had had no contact with birds. Four days before the onset of the illness, the patient had gone on a company-sponsored trip to Pittsburgh, Pennsylvania. One of the features of the trip was a dinner and evening cruise on a small tour boat down the Ohio River and back. The patient remarked that while standing on the bow, the spray from the boat swept over him, dampened his clothes, and he became chilled.

The patient was started on cefuroxime (a second-generation cephalosporin), erythromycin, and rifampin, all intravenously. A Gram stain of his sputum did not indicate any abnormalities, and culture of the sputum was negative after 2 days of culture. A chest x-ray taken the day after admission showed denser infiltrates and spread to the left lingula.

- From what disease is this patient suffering?
- Does the lack of a positive Gram stain indicate that this is a viral infection?
- Why was antimicrobial therapy initiated?
- Why is a history of no bird exposure and an Ohio River cruise in Pittsburgh relevant to this case?

INTRACELLULAR SURVIVAL

Prokaryotic and eukaryotic pathogens have dimensions that are measured in micrometers and thus are generally much smaller than the host cells with which they interact (see Chapter 1). This size disparity allows selected microbial pathogens to exist within the confines of larger host cells, provided they can traverse the plasma membrane and survive within the intracellular spaces of the host cell. In fact as described in Part I, Overview, microbial pathogens are often conveniently categorized as those that absolutely must invade and replicate within a host cell (obligate intracellular pathogens), those that can invade and exist within the intracellular host environment but can also survive extracellularly (facultative intracellular pathogens), and those that live an exclusively extracellular existence (extracellular pathogens).

This chapter focuses on the general concept of host cell invasion and intracellular survival by microbial pathogens. In doing so it contrasts the molecular strategies of parasite-directed endocytosis, as illustrated by *Listeria monocytogenes* and *Plasmodium* spp., with host-directed phagocytosis, as illustrated by *L. pneumophila*. In the end, the student should appreciate that these two strategies are merely two different means toward the same goal, that is, intracellular invasion and survival.

Medical Microbiology and Intracellular Invasion and Survival

The ability of a microbial pathogen to invade and survive within a host cell appears to afford two significant advantages: (1) the intracellular environment protects it from host immune surveillance, and (2) the intracellular environment should be flush with preformed biologic nutrients such as adenosine triphosphate (ATP), amino acids, and nucleotides. While these advantages intuitively favor the intracellular multiplication of most or all microbial pathogens, this notion presumes a friendly intracellular environment. While this presumption may be true for an epithelial or endothelial cell that is not specifically designed for microbial killing, it is much less true for a phagocyte that is well equipped to kill and degrade intracellular microbial pathogens. Thus, the advantages of intracellular invasion and survival depend to some extent on the type of cell that is invaded.

The invasion of any host cell by a microbial pathogen is an obvious first step in the process of intracellular survival. In many cases invasion is a directed property, meaning that proteins (generally referred to by several terms including *internalins* and *invasins*) are produced by the microbial pathogen to facilitate this process. This type of invasion has been referred to as parasite-directed endocytosis and is generally accomplished by the specific interaction of a microbial surface structure with a eukaryotic cytoskeletal protein. (Note that in this context the term *parasite* refers to prokaryotic and eukaryotic pathogens alike.) Some well-characterized examples of microbial pathogens, invasins, and the mechanisms by which they invade cells are described in Table 15-1. Many of these, as well as additional examples, have been discussed previously (see Chapters 8, 9, 12, and 13) or are described later (see Chapters 16–18, and 28) in this text.

◀ **TABLE 15-1**
Well-Characterized Examples of Microbial Pathogen Invasion Utilizing Parasite-Directed Endocytosis

Microbial Pathogen	Invasin/Cellular Target[a]	Mechanism of Invasion
Yersinia pseudotuberculosis	Inv protein/$\beta 1$ chain integrin YadA protein/$\beta 1$ chain integrin	Entry is promoted by a "zipper" mechanism which involves invasin binding to multiple integrin receptors on the host cell plasma membrane (see Chapters 8 and 13).
Shigella flexneri	Ipa proteins/Cellular target unknown	An Ipa complex induces cytoskeleton rearrangements in the host cells (see Chapter 13).
Listeria monocytogenes	Internalin/E-cadherin	E-cadherin is preferentially expressed in epithelial tissues at the basolateral membrane of enterocytes, allowing *L. monocytogenes* to gain access within the intestine.
Salmonella typhimurium	Sip proteins/Cellular target unknown	Interaction of Sip proteins with a cellular receptor induces membrane ruffling, major cytoskeletal rearrangements, and macropinocytosis of *S. typhimurium* (see Chapters 13 and 24).
Toxoplasma gondii	Invasin unknown/Cellular target unknown	*T. gondii* invades cells by an actin-dependent mechanism (see Chapter 28).

[a] Cellular target refers to the structure on the surface of the host cell that the invasin binds or perturbs to facilitate invasion.

In contrast to parasite-directed endocytosis, host-directed phagocytosis refers to the ability of highly differentiated host cells, such as macrophages, to phagocytize microbial pathogens. Generally this process involves opsonins, which are molecules that facilitate the uptake of microbial pathogens by macrophages. Antibodies are prime examples of opsonins; they specifically bind the pathogen through an antigen-combining site, facilitating the uptake of the microbial pathogen by a surface Fc receptor on the phagocyte cell surface. Another common opsonin is the complement component C3b, which is commonly deposited on the surface of microbial pathogens and for which phagocytes also encode a surface receptor. Like parasite-directed endocytosis, host-directed phagocytosis allows microbial pathogens access to intracellular spaces; the difference is that the gauntlet of antimicrobial activity associated within a macrophage makes it very difficult for most microbial pathogens to survive this environment. Those that do survive within a macrophage must possess mechanisms that subvert its formidable intracellular killing mechanisms. Some well-characterized examples of microbial pathogens that invade macrophages by host-directed phagocytosis and the mechanisms by which they survive intracellular killing are described in Table 15-2.

Gaining access to the confines of the host cell is only the first step in the process of intracellular survival (Figure 15-1). For those organisms that invade nonprofessional phagocytes (such as the malarial pathogens), this is less of a problem than for those that invade phagocytes, because the gauntlet of intracellular antimicrobial defenses are at a much higher level in professional phagocytes. Survival within phagocytes is accom-

TABLE 15-2 ▶

Well-Characterized Examples of Microbial Pathogen Survival Utilizing Host-Directed Phagocytosis

Microbial Pathogen	Mechanism of Survival
Mycobacterium spp.	Inhibit endosome-lysosome fusion.
Legionella pneumophila	Mip outer membrane protein interacts with the complement C3b. Using C3b receptors, phagocytes take up *L. pneumophila*. Uptake via this pathway decreases exposure to toxic oxygen compounds. *L. pneumophila* also inhibits phagosome-lysosome fusion.
Rickettsia spp.	Dissolve the endosomal membrane prior to fusion with the lysosome.

plished by a number of strategies. These include the resistance of the invading microbial pathogen to the antimicrobial processes that occur within the fused endosome-lysosome. The production of catalase by invasive pathogens serves to break down toxic hydrogen peroxide that is produced within a fused endosome-lysosome and is thus another mechanism that facilitates the intracellular survival of these pathogens. Another means to accomplish intracellular survival is by inhibiting endosome fusion with lysosomal granules. A final strategy used for intracellular survival is to escape from the endosome prior to the endosome fusing with the lysosome.

FIGURE 15-1 ▶

Journey of a Bacterium through a Macrophage. The deposition of human proteins such as the complement protein C3b or specific antibody on a bacterial cell surface facilitates the uptake of bacteria because macrophages have C3b and Fc receptors (Step 1). This results in engulfing the microorganism into an endosome (Step 2). The endosome-trapped bacterium in turn fuses with lysosomal granules (Step 3) and puts into play the process of endosome-lysosome killing (Step 4). This chemical and enzymatic onslaught employs both oxidative and nonoxidative strategies to kill and digest the trapped bacterium. Breaking down the bacterium into progressively smaller components such as peptides is referred to as processing in immunologic terms. These digested peptides are presented by the major histocompatibility complex (MHC) [Step 5] to other immune cells and stimulate an effective cellular immune response that is specific for, and usually results in the clearance of, the microbial pathogen. Those microbial pathogens that exist within professional phagocytes as an integral part of their pathogenic life style must overcome the gauntlet of antimicrobial defenses. Inhibition of endosome-lysosome fusion and escape into the cytosol by digestion of the endosomal membrane are two ways that a bacterium can subvert this formidable defense.

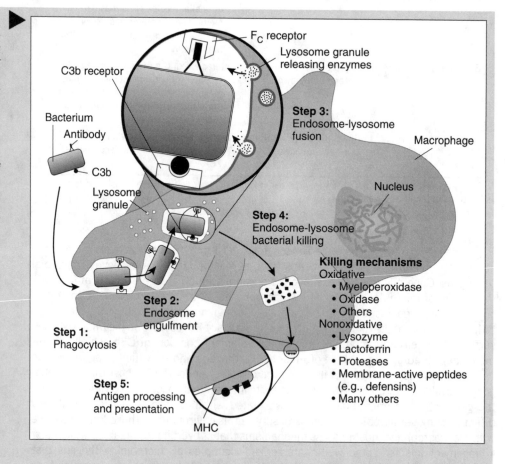

ILLUSTRATIVE PATHOGEN: *Legionella pneumophila*

Biologic Characteristics

L. pneumophila causes pneumonia and other systemic complications (legionellosis) that are commonly (although not always) associated with the immunocompromised host. This organism is an example of an emerging pathogen. It was only first recognized in 1976 when a fulminant pneumonia occurred in 221 persons attending an American Legion convention in Philadelphia, Pennsylvania (hence, the name *Legionella*). The etiologic agent causing this disease was a bacterium that was not related to any other pathogen described at the time. Retrospective analysis of undiagnosed epidemic respiratory illness that occurred prior to 1976 revealed that several outbreaks were attributable to *Legionella* spp., indicating that this organism caused disease prior to its identification in 1976. For example, a 1968 outbreak in Pontiac, Michigan (referred to as Pontiac Fever), was subsequently ascribed to *Legionella*. Since the initial description of this pathogen in 1976, nearly 40 different species of *Legionella* have been described. Because of their unique biologic features these organisms have been taxonomically grouped within a family that is designated the Legionellaceae.

Of the Legionellaceae, *L. pneumophila* serotype 1 is the organism responsible for nearly all cases of legionellosis and is typical of this family. *L. pneumophila* is a small, slow-growing, motile, gram-negative rod that is difficult to culture because it requires very specific growth conditions. Further complicating this, cultured *L. pneumophila* Gram stains poorly. Culture of *L. pneumophila* is accomplished using complex media such as buffered charcoal-yeast extract agar supplemented with α-ketoglutarate. Optimal growth conditions require a temperature of 35°C and a humidity level of 90%. When cultivated under these conditions small visible colonies can be seen on agar media only 3 days postinoculation. It seems odd that the Legionellaceae would have these fastidious growth requirements in light of the fact that in nature this bacterium can survive and multiply in simple tap water for periods lasting more than a year.

> The Legionellaceae are small, slow-growing, motile, gram-negative rods with fastidious growth requirements. As a result, culturing these organisms challenges most clinical laboratories.

Reservoir and Transmission

In nature, *Legionella* survives principally in water and, to a lesser extent, in soil. Human disease is acquired primarily by inhalation of aerosols contaminated with bacteria; person-to-person transmission has not been documented. Contaminated (particularly warm) water systems have been responsible for both community-acquired and hospital-acquired outbreaks of Legionnaires' disease. The disease has been traced to contaminated water used for drinking, bathing, and whirlpools. Community-acquired *Legionella* pneumonia occurs more frequently in the summer, the season when the overall incidence of pneumonia is the lowest. Presumably, this is because of increased exposure to contaminated aerosols. The attack rate is higher in persons with certain underlying conditions, including persons over 50 years of age, smokers, and patients with chronic lung disease, neoplastic disease, organ transplants, renal failure, and those immunosuppressed by cytotoxic chemotherapy or corticosteroids. The period from exposure to disease is typically 2–10 days.

Virulence Factors

L. pneumophila expresses an endotoxin and two exotoxins, a hemolysin, and a cytotoxin. However, any role for these toxins in legionellosis is not well defined. This pathogen also expresses several extracellular proteases that have been shown to degrade interleukin 2 (IL-2) and CD4 molecules from human cells, suggesting that this protease may interfere with T-cell activation. A genetic locus designated as *Mip* (macrophage infectivity potentiator) encodes a surface protein that enhances the ability of *L. pneumophila* to invade human macrophages. In the presence of complement, Mip promotes the phagocytosis of these organisms. One other factor that has been described is a phosphatase that blocks superoxide anion production by stimulated neutrophils, facilitating the survival of these organisms within an endosome. The resistance of all *L. pneumophila* to β-lactam anti-

> **Virulence Factors of L. pneumophila**
> Endotoxin
> Hemolysin
> Cytotoxin
> Extracellular proteases
> Mip
> Intracellular phosphatase
> Penicillin resistance

biotics is also a factor in the progression of these infections because they present as pneumonia, and most (but not all) pneumonias can be treated by the administration of a β-lactam antibiotic.

Pathogenesis

Upon gaining access to the lower respiratory tract, alveolar macrophages, which are the primary defense against pulmonary infection, phagocytose the *L. pneumophila*. This host-directed phagocytosis is augmented by the interaction between Mip and complement. After uptake, these pathogens survive the hostile intracellular environment of the macrophage by blocking phagosome fusion with lysosomal granules. This protects *L. pneumophila* from exposure to the gauntlet of antimicrobial substances housed within the alveolar macrophage. The prevention of endosome-lysosome fusion is critical to the pathogenesis of legionellosis because, by subverting this event, the alveolar macrophage is converted from a formidable soldier of the host immune system into the functional equivalent of a *Legionella* incubator.

L. pneumophila replicates only within nonactivated phagocytes. This property accounts for its association with immunocompromised individuals. The unimpeded multiplication of *L. pneumophila* within nonactivated phagocytes leads to death and subsequent lysis of the host cell. This in turn leads to the release of a new generation of organisms that can infect other alveolar macrophages. In addition, the process of macrophage lysis culminates in the "spilling" of host cytokines. This then results in an influx of monocytes and polymorphonuclear neutrophils into the colonized area of the body. This immunopathologic response gives rise either to a destructive pneumonia that compromises respiratory function or, less frequently, to systemic disease symptoms (Figure 15-2).

FIGURE 15-2 ▶

Legionella pneumophila *Uptake and Replication in Nonstimulated Macrophages.* L. pneumophila *are efficiently taken up by macrophages. This is facilitated either by deposition of complement on the cell surface, which is encouraged by a macrophage infectivity potentiator (Mip), or by the binding of specific antibody. Upon establishing an endosomal existence, the bacterium prevents endosome-lysosome fusion. These microbial pathogens efficiently replicate in nonactivated macrophages associated with an unhealthy host. In contrast, they do not replicate well in activated macrophages associated with a healthy host. This explains why individuals whose immune systems are compromised are more susceptible to legionellosis than those individuals who have healthy immune systems.*

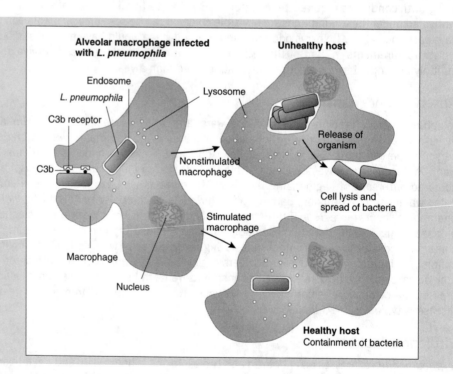

Diagnosis

Sporadic *Legionella* pneumonia cannot be epidemiologically or clinically differentiated from the other, more common community-acquired pneumonias. Early in the illness, *Legionella* resembles an atypical pneumonia, such as that caused by *Mycoplasma* or *Chlamydia*, in that the cough is not productive and the chest x-ray shows only an interstitial or patchy infiltrate. As the infection progresses, the cough may become productive and frank consolidation is seen on the chest film. Nonpneumonic clinical features, such as obtundation (confusion) or toxic encephalopathy (seen in 30%–40% of all cases), abdominal pain, vomiting, diarrhea (33% of all cases), and relative bradycardia (a heart rate lower than would be expected from the height of the fever) are also seen with equal frequency in other community-acquired pneumonias. Likewise, abnormal laboratory tests, including hyponatremia (low sodium levels), hypophosphatemia (low phosphate levels), abnormal liver function tests, proteinuria and microscopic hematuria, and other elevated protein chemistries are seen with equal frequency in *Legionella* and other pneumonias. Instead, one of the best clues to the diagnosis of Legionnaires' disease is the spread of the pneumonia and clinical deterioration while the patient is being treated with a β-lactam antibiotic, which (as mentioned) is not active against *L. pneumophila*.

If a sputum sample is available, a Gram stain showing neutrophils but no bacteria (legionellae do not Gram stain in clinical specimens) is typical of *Legionella* pneumonia. A definitive diagnosis is made by isolation of legionellae from sputum, or bronchial washings, using the appropriate media. Unfortunately, the sensitivity of culture is low because Legionellaceae are slow-growing, and their growth is easily masked by the rapidly growing normal flora associated with the culture specimen. Therefore, it is more practical to examine these respiratory specimens either by direct fluorescent antibody (DFA) staining or by using nucleic acid probes. For DFA, a fluorescently labeled antibody is added to the sputum sample, and legionellae associated with this sample are located by fluorescence microscopy. For probing with nucleic acid probes, a complementary piece of DNA that is unique to the *L. pneumophila* genome is tagged with a specific reporter molecule and used to hybridize to the patient specimen. Both of these tests require specialized equipment. Because of this, the DFA and DNA tests are very labor intensive and time-consuming and thus are not routinely performed except in highly specialized laboratories. *Legionella* antigen may also be detected in the urine by an antibody-based assay. The reagent currently available for this test is specific to *L. pneumophila* serogroup 1, which covers about 85% of all human legionellosis. This urinary antigen test has good diagnostic sensitivity. Again, this test requires a highly specialized laboratory.

Prevention and Treatment

In confined settings that are frequented by immunocompromised individuals, which include health care centers, prevention of legionellosis is accomplished by bacteriologic monitoring of water supplies and by appropriate water treatment. These efforts are generally monitored by infection control personnel within the hospital or by public health officials in settings outside of the hospital.

Currently, there is no definitive consensus on the best course of antimicrobial therapy for human legionellosis. Some studies indicate that patients who were given erythromycin fared better than patients treated with β-lactams, which is not surprising given that *L. pneumophila* is generally resistant to the penicillins. Other antibiotics that appear to be clinically effective include the fluoroquinolones (ciprofloxacin, ofloxacin), the azoles (clarithromycin, azithromycin), and trimethoprim-sulfamethoxazole.

ILLUSTRATIVE PATHOGEN: *Listeria monocytogenes*

Like legionellosis, disease caused by *L. monocytogenes* (listeriosis) is also an infectious disease of emerging importance. In part this is because past diagnoses were missed due to the inability to find this organism within clinical specimens. However, the more likely contributor for the increase in listeriosis cases is the increased number of immunocompromised individuals within the population. In the past, these individuals may not have survived their primary illness (which resulted in immunosuppression) long enough to become infected with *L. monocytogenes*. However, with improved standard of care for immunosuppressive illness, secondary infection by *Listeria* is now becoming more common. For example, over 70% of listeriosis cases occur in immunosuppressed individuals, particularly those suffering from cancer; in fact, this organism is the leading cause of meningitis in cancer patients.

When ingested in sufficient numbers, *L. monocytogenes* is a food-borne pathogen that causes an infrequent but serious infection that is associated with a high mortality rate. The primary manifestations of listeriosis include sepsis, meningitis, or both.

Biologic Characteristics

L. monocytogenes is a gram-positive bacillus that is a non-spore-forming, catalase-positive, motile, facultative anaerobe. This pathogen grows at temperature, pH, and salt extremes—it can even grow at 4°C—which explains why it has the propensity to contaminate refrigerated foods. *L. monocytogenes* can be routinely cultivated on blood agar plates and may demonstrate limited β-hemolysis (see Appendix 1) when cultivated under these conditions.

Reservoir and Transmission

L. monocytogenes is found in soil, sewage, stream water, plants, processed foods, and the intestinal tract of mammals. Both sporadic and point-source outbreaks of listeriosis are the result of food contamination. Outbreaks have been linked to dairy products (e.g., contaminated milk or cheese), undercooked chicken, and refrigerated foods stored for prolonged periods. The overall morbidity of listeriosis is relatively low, with only 0.7 cases reported annually per 100,000 population. Despite its relatively low morbidity, listeriosis concerns public health officials because this disease is associated with a high mortality rate. As stated above, listeriosis typically occurs in immunocompromised persons such as the elderly, pregnant women, patients with defects in cell-mediated immunity, cancer patients, transplant patients receiving high doses of corticosteroids, and patients with acquired immunodeficiency syndrome (AIDS).

> *Sporadic food poisoning refers to a variety of food products being sporadically contaminated with an infectious agent. This is different from point-source food poisoning in which the infectious agent is spread from one specific source.*

Virulence Factors

> **Virulence Factors of L. monocytogenes**
> *Inls*
> *LLO*
> *ActA*
> *Competition for intracellular and extra-cellular iron*
> *Phospholipases*

Parasite-directed endocytosis of *L. monocytogenes* is facilitated by surface-associated proteins referred to as internalins (Inls). InlA specifically recognizes E-cadherin, which is a calcium-dependent, cell–cell adhesion molecule that is found on epithelial cells. Expression of InlA alone is enough to facilitate the uptake of a bacterium by an epithelial cell. Another Inl, designated InlB, is specific for hepatocyte uptake. The Inls bear structural similarity to the streptococcal M protein (see Chapter 16) and functional homology with the *Shigella* Ipa proteins (see Chapter 13). *L. monocytogenes* secrete a hemolytic cytolysin designated listeriolysin O (LLO). This pore-forming toxin is similar in structure and activity to streptolysin O and pneumococcal pneumolysin. LLO is critical for the escape of *L. monocytogenes* from the endosome and into the cytosol. In addition, two phospholipases participate in this movement by digesting membrane lipids. A lysterial surface protein, designated ActA, reorganizes host cell actin into a tail that facilitates the translocation of organisms into adjacent host cells. Listeria are able to mobilize iron from extracellular and intracellular host sources, which facilitates intra-endosomal and cytosolic multiplication.

Pathogenesis

L. monocytogenes attaches to and invades undifferentiated epithelial cells, M cells, intestinal crypt cells, and macrophages using the internalins described above. Ingested *L. monocytogenes* are thought to be taken up by M cells associated with the intestinal epithelium. Invading organisms enter these cells within an endosome and rapidly escape this endosome by the actions of LLO and the phospholipases (unlike *L. pneumophila*, which prevents the fusion between the endosome and lysosome and replicates within the endosome). Once inside the cytosol, *L. monocytogenes* rapidly multiply and stimulate, through the activity of ActA, the reorganization of host cell actin. This parasite-directed actin reorganization stimulates actin filament assembly, resulting in the formation of a cytoskeletal tail. New actin monomers are added at the interface between the bacterium and the actin filament tail, and this tail progressively lengthens. This lengthening actin filament propels the bacterium through the cytoplasm and against the host plasma membrane, where philopodia are formed. The double membrane between the two adjacent eukaryotic cells is digested by the activity of LLO and the phospholipases, and the bacteria are transferred to adjacent cells. This allows *L. monocytogenes* to spread from cell to cell without directly contacting the extracellular environment (Figure 15-3).

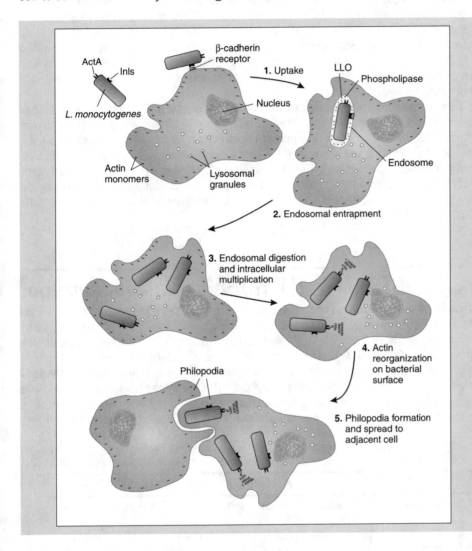

◀ FIGURE 15-3
Progression of Infection by **Listeria mono-cytogenes.** *(1) Upon ingestion of* L. mono-cytogenes, *these organisms direct their uptake into a number of different eukaryotic cell types via the expression of internalins (Inls) oriented on their cell surface. (2) Upon being entrapped within an endosome, protein products such as listeriolysin O (LLO) and phospholipases break down the endosome, (3) enabling* L. monocytogenes *access to the cytosol, where these pathogens readily replicate. (4) A listerial surface protein, ActA, facilitates cellular actin reorganization that in turn (5) propels the bacterial pathogen into an adjacent cell. This process results in* L. monocytogenes *avoiding the gauntlet of intracellular antimicrobial activity as well as the host humoral immune response. Because of this, control of this pathogen is largely the result of the cellular immune response. This explains why those individuals with specific deficits in their cellular immunity are at risk for listerial infection.*

Disease is typically the result of the spread of *Listeria* throughout the human host, giving rise to meningitis. Because of this intracellular life style, a functional cell-mediated immune system is important for limiting the spread of *L. monocytogenes* within the body. Consequently, individuals with reduced immune function are particularly susceptible to listerial infections. For example, pregnant mothers may be transiently infected by *L. monocytogenes*, transplacentally exposing the fetus. This can result in perinatal human listeriosis that presents as meningitis. These cases are associated with a high mortality rate even when appropriate antibiotic treatment is administered. Adults, particularly those that are immunocompromised, develop listerial meningoencephalitis. In these cases, the mortality rate is also extremely high, and those who survive often have permanent neurologic damage.

Diagnosis

In an immunocompromised host, treatment of listeriosis should be initiated pending laboratory diagnosis. *L. monocytogenes* can be readily cultured on blood agar from infected body fluids. Microscopic examination of these cultured organisms reveals a characteristic tumbling motility that is indicative of these organisms. Gram stain of cerebrospinal fluid (CSF) or meconium fluid showing gram-positive rods is strongly suggestive of transplacental infection with *L. monocytogenes*.

Prevention and Treatment

Because of the low morbidity of listeriosis associated with healthy individuals, and the fact that it most often strikes immunocompromised individuals, a vaccine is not indicated for this disease. Furthermore, it is not possible to eliminate the ubiquitous reservoir of *L. monocytogenes* found within our environment. Prevention of disease can best be accomplished by instructing patients at risk how to minimize the multiplication of *L. monocytogenes* in food and how to kill the organisms within potentially contaminated foods. For example, people at risk need to avoid unsterilized dairy products, undercooked meats, and prepared foods that have been refrigerated but not sterilized by high-temperature reheating.

Development of effective treatment modalities for listeriosis has been limited because of the low morbidity of this disease. High dose β-lactams are the recommended antimicrobial therapy. In immunosuppressed patients, relapse has been reported after 2 weeks of penicillin therapy because of the hosts' impaired ability to clear infected cells, thereby allowing *L. monocytogenes* to persist for prolonged periods in a protected, intracellular environment. Because of this trimethoprim-sulfamethoxazole may also be considered for the treatment of *Listeria*. This drug combination readily enters host cells and is bactericidal for these bacteria.

ILLUSTRATIVE PATHOGEN: *Plasmodium* spp.

Malaria is caused by a closely related family of eukaryotic blood sporozans (see Table 15-3). These are highly specialized, pigment producing, ameboid intracellular parasites of vertebrates that cyclically inhabit RBCs and other (generally liver) cells. In all cases transmission to humans is accomplished by the bite of a mosquito.

Malaria is a disease caused by protozoal pathogens of the *Plasmodium* spp., with *P. vivax*, *P. falciparum*, *P. malariae*, and *P. ovale* representing the four major species. The type of malaria and some of the defining characteristics associated with each species are summarized in Table 15-3. Characteristic symptoms of malaria are anemia, pigmentation of infected organs, and hypertrophy (enlargement) of the liver and spleen. Anemia is the result of direct destruction of red blood cells (RBCs) by the invading parasite. The removal of infected RBCs by the spleen also contributes to the anemia. The disease is also characterized by repeated episodes of a shaking chill followed by a fever that returns

TABLE 15-3 ▶

Characteristics of Plasmodium *spp.* Malaria

	P. vivax	P. falciparum	P. malariae	P. ovale
Type of malaria	Benign tertian malaria	Malignant tertian malaria	Quartan malaria	Ovale malaria
Level of usual maximum parasitemia	Up to 30,000 parasites/μL of blood	Can exceed 200,000 parasites/μL of blood	Fewer than 10,000 parasites/μL of blood	Fewer than 10,000 parasites/μL of blood
Length of pre-erythrocytic cycle in humans	8 days	6 days	16 days	9 days
Length of asexual cycle in humans	48 hours	36–48 hours	72 hours	48 hours
Continual reproduction in the liver	Yes	No	No	Yes
Episodes of fever and chills	48-hour intervals	Usually continuous	72-hour intervals	48-hour intervals
Anemia	Yes	Yes	Yes	Yes
Severe clinical manifestations	No	Yes (brain and kidney)	No	No

to normal after several hours. *P. falciparum* infection is more dangerous than those of the other three species because it is often accompanied by very long periods of extremely high fever, convulsion, coma, and cardiac failure.

Biologic Characteristics

In the complex classification of eukaryotic pathogens, the plasmodia are designated as blood sporozoa because the disease that they cause is transiently associated with the invasion of RBCs. *Plasmodium* spp. are single-cell protozoa that exhibit alternating sexual (occurring within the mosquito) and asexual (occurring within humans) expansion as part of their life cycle. The sexual and asexual components of their life cycle are summarized diagrammatically in Figure 15-4. This complex life cycle provides a formidable challenge to the human immune system to clear these organisms. One reason for this is that the antigenic composition of the organism changes with the many morphologies it assumes throughout the malarial life cycle. Most importantly, *Plasmodium* spp. are highly invasive pathogens and thus escape extracellular immune recognition.

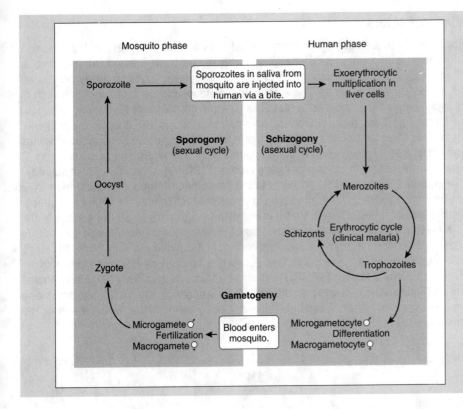

FIGURE 15-4
General View of the Life Cycle of Malarial Parasites. *Human infection is initiated with the bite of a mosquito, starting the asexual component of this life cycle. The exoerythrocytic component occurs within the liver and produces merozoites. These invade RBCs and differentiate into trophozoites and then into schizonts, which reinfect RBCs as part of the erythrocytic cycle. The erythrocytic cycle gives rise to the characteristic cyclical pattern of fever and chills within human infectees. The other two phases, gametogeny and sporogony, require a mosquito vector to proceed.*

Plasmodium spp. can be cultivated in fluid medium containing serum, erythrocytes, inorganic salts, and other growth factors. However, only those forms that comprise the schizogony phase of the malaria life cycle are found. Within RBCs, malaria parasites convert hemoglobin to globin and hematin. The hematin component becomes modified, which gives rise to the characteristic malarial pigment.

Reservoir and Transmission

Malaria is a human disease, transmitted between individuals by the bite of a female anopheles mosquito. In the First World, malaria has a relatively low rate of occurrence and therefore may not be a perceived problem. However, it should be appreciated that an estimated 60 million cases of malaria occur annually worldwide. Furthermore, the number of malaria cases is on the rise throughout the tropics, especially on the Indian subcontinent. This is significant because within the United States cases of malaria are generally imported, being associated with an individual traveling from an area endemic for malaria. For example, in 1992 there were 910 cases of malaria reported in the United

States, and all but 7 were acquired outside of the United States. Cases of malaria originating within the United States are rare, and when they do occur they result not from spread by an insect bite but more likely from a blood transfusion.

Each *Plasmodium* spp. has its own unique geographic distribution and prevalence pattern. *P. vivax* is the most widely distributed throughout the world; it is also the second most prevalent cause of the disease. *P. falciparum* is as prevalent as *P. vivax* in subtropical and tropical regions, but fails to establish itself in areas with long, cold seasons. This species is responsible for the greatest number of cases worldwide. *P. malariae* is limited to tropical and subtropical areas and is considerably less prevalent than *P. falciparum* and *P. vivax*. *P. ovale* is the least prevalent cause of malaria. It is reported sporadically in regions of Africa, South America, and Asia.

Transmission by a mosquito is required for the complex life cycle demonstrated by *Plasmodium* spp. This form of transmission is quite efficient because the mosquito acts as a "flying syringe," capable of penetrating the host barriers and introducing this pathogen into the sterile spaces of the human host. In developed countries malaria is prevented by mosquito control programs.

Virulence Factors

The primary virulence strategy employed by all the malarial pathogens is invasion and multiplication within nonprofessional phagocytes of the body. Beyond this the precise mechanism by which these pathogens invade hepatocytes or erythrocytes is not understood at the molecular level. One interesting molecular aspect of virulence factors employed by malarial pathogens is that *P. falciparum* demonstrates antigenic variation. In an interesting twist distinct from organisms described in the chapter on antigenic variation (see Chapter 17), the variant antigens of *P. falciparum* are organized as knobs on the surface of infected erythrocytes (Figure 15-5). These antigens are known as *P. falciparum* infected erythrocyte membrane protein 1 (PfEMP-1) and function by modifying the infected RBC so that it attaches to the vascular endothelium, resulting in their retention in vascular beds. This allows infected cells to avoid clearance within the spleen. The down side of this strategy is that it presents a foreign antigen on the surface of the infected erythrocyte, negating some advantages of intracellular invasion and survival. To mitigate this disadvantage, a complex mechanism of antigenic variation of the PfEMP-1 protein that involves at least 50 variant genes is employed by *P. falciparum*. Further confusing this, the different PfEMP-1 variant genes attach to different host endothelial receptors (Figure 15-5). Aside from the PfEMP-1 component, the molecules facilitating the pathogenesis of *Plasmodium* spp. have not been defined, due in large part to the complexity of the plasmodial life cycle.

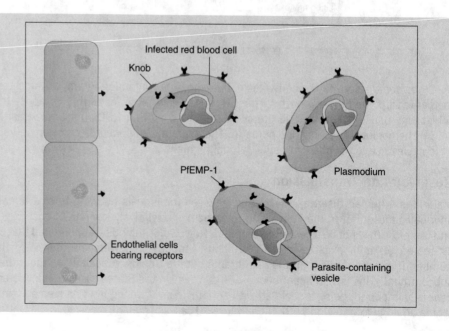

FIGURE 15-5 ▶

PfEMP-1 Expression on the Infected Erythrocyte Cell Surface. *This diagram depicts a plasmodium within a vacuole on the inside of an infected erythrocyte. From this endosomal vacuole P. falciparum secretes PfEMP-1, which is assembled on a knob of the red blood cell (RBC) surface. In this molecular organization, the PfEMP-1 binds to specific receptors on the surface of endothelial cells. This allows an infected RBC to attach to the endothelial vasculature and avoid destruction by the spleen. It also attracts the attention of the host immune system. Because of this a sophisticated mechanism of PfEMP-1 variation is exercised by this pathogen. PfEMP-1 = P. falciparum infected erythrocyte membrane protein 1.*

Infected red blood cell

Knob

PfEMP-1

Plasmodium

Endothelial cells bearing receptors

Parasite-containing vesicle

Pathogenesis

A person becomes inoculated with malarial sporozoites upon deposition of this pathogen into their blood through the bite of a mosquito. This leads to a pre-erythrocytic, an exo-erythrocytic, and an erythrocytic existence. In the context of this chapter it should be noted that this life cycle avoids any interaction with phagocytic cells as a strategy to avoid host clearance. In the pre-erythrocytic stage, the sporozoites immediately invade the intracellular spaces of hepatocytes, where they can multiply and differentiate into trophozoites. In the exo-erythrocytic stage, these trophozoites enlarge en masse and divide into thousands of nuclei. During this stage the parasite is referred to as a *schizont*. A cytoplasm and plasma membrane surrounds each of these nuclei to form a merozoite, after which the host cell ruptures and releases the merozoites to the erythrocytic stage. This stage involves the invasion of a RBC by the merozoite and its differentiation into an immature trophozoite. This trophozoite continues to mature and divides into multiple nuclear masses (schizogony). After a membrane surrounds each nucleus, this form is again referred to as a merozoite. Eventually, the RBC ruptures and releases the merozoites into the circulation, where they can invade additional RBCs. After one or more cycles of asexual reproduction in the RBCs, some of the immature trophozoites form male gametocytes (microgametocytes) and female gametocytes (macrogametocytes) [gametogony]. These are terminally differentiated sexual forms of the organism that are required for the transmission to another mosquito vector. These forms degenerate within 6–12 hours unless ingested by a mosquito. Recurrent cycles of schizogony in the erythrocyte continue to generate a population of gametocytes, which are essential for the transmission of the parasite to mosquitoes and the initiation of their sexual phase (sporogony).

The repeated periods of chills, fever, and sweating characteristic of malarial infection are induced by the lysis of erythrocytes, which in turn stimulates the release of tumor necrosis factor α (TNF-α). Recurrent erythrocytic stage attacks result in a significant anemia, particularly in children younger than 5 years of age. Untreated, attacks may continue for 3–6 weeks, after which the parasites appear to be cleared from systemic compartments. Relapses are common for a year or more, suggesting that *Plasmodium* spp. can exist in a pre- or exo-erythrocytic stage. After 1–2 years, the organisms are generally cleared and, if not reinfected, the individual may be permanently cured of the disease.

Diagnosis

Laboratory findings include anemia, leukopenia, thrombocytopenia, hyperbilirubinemia, and laboratory test abnormalities that reflect specific organ involvement. A confirmatory diagnosis depends on the recognition of parasites in Giemsa-stained smears of peripheral blood. DNA probes, polymerase chain reaction (PCR) tests, and antigen-capture assays are also available for the rapid diagnosis of *P. falciparum* infections. Immune-based serologic tests for *Plasmodium* spp. have limited diagnostic value because they do not discriminate between active and past infection.

Prevention and Treatment

In the United States, the most effective method of controlling malaria is to identify and treat infected persons to render them noninfective. Worldwide, the elimination of the mosquito vector is the most important mechanism for limiting the spread of malaria. No vaccine is currently available for the prevention of this disease.

Acute attacks associated with all *Plasmodium* spp., except *P. falciparum*, are usually treated with oral chloroquine. Other antiparasitic drugs used to treat malaria include primaquine, quinine sulfate, and pyrimethamine. Chloriquine resistance is common among *P. falciparum*. For drug-resistant cases of *P. falciparum*, combination therapy using quinine sulfate and pyrimethamine is recommended. Because of increasing resistance to current drugs, new agents are being investigated for the treatment of malaria.

RESOLUTION OF CLINICAL CASE

The day after admission, the test result on the patient's urine for *Legionella* antigen was positive. Treatment was continued with erythromycin and rifampin, and the patient slowly recovered.

The finding of a *Legionella* antigen-positive urine explains many of the findings described in this case. The fact that the patient did not respond to cephalosporin treatment is consistent with the fact that these organisms are resistant to this class of antibiotics. The inability of the organism to be seen on Gram stain and to grow after only 2 days on culture medium is also characteristic of this pathogen. The exposure of this individual to water that *L. pneumophila* normally inhabits was the most likely source of infection. *Chlamydia psitisci* is another cause of pneumonia but is generally associated with the inhalation of bird droppings. This is why the patient was asked about bird exposure. The patient recovered because he was placed on an appropriate antibiotic course and because he had a generally intact immune response. One of the reasons the elderly or hospitalized patients do not recover from this disease, even after appropriate antimicrobial treatment, is that they lack an effective cellular immune response.

REVIEW QUESTIONS

Directions: For each of the following questions, choose the **one best** answer.

1. In mid-summer, an elderly man attending a convention in a highly air-conditioned hotel comes down with a severe pneumonia. He is immediately treated with a first-generation cephalosporin but fails to get better. A Gram stain of his sputum reveals only polymorphonuclear neutrophils (PMNs) and not bacteria. Which one of the following is most correct concerning this patient's condition?

   (A) The inability to Gram stain or to cultivate organisms from the patient's sputum can be taken as evidence that this is a viral infection

   (B) The ineffectiveness of the antibiotic administered to the patient should be taken as evidence that this is a viral infection

   (C) The treatment of the patient with a cephalosporin may have selected for an antibiotic-resistant bacterium in this patient that is responsible for his infection

   (D) The apparent resistance of this infection to antibiotic therapy is consistent with infection caused by *Listeria monocytogenes*

   (E) The circumstances and the lack of response to cephalosporin therapy are consistent with infection caused by *Legionella pneumophila*

2. A 65-year-old patient suffering from the end stages of cancer comes down with meningitis after ingesting a meal that included some refrigerated, uninspected cheese that was processed in Mexico. The most likely microbial pathogen causing this meningitis is

   (A) *Legionella pneumophila*

   (B) *Listeria monocytogenes*

   (C) *Neisseria meningitidis*

   (D) *Haemophilus influenzae*

   (E) *Clostridium perfringens*

3. Which one of the following statements is most true about the four organisms associated with malaria?

   (A) *Plasmodium falciparum* is the most common cause of malaria and also causes the most severe symptoms of this disease

   (B) *Plasmodium vivax* is the least common cause of malaria but causes the most severe symptoms of this disease

   (C) *Plasmodium falciparum* causes only sporadic cases of malaria, and these cases only occur in North America

   (D) *Plasmodium malariae* is the most common cause of malaria but causes the least severe symptoms of this disease

   (E) *Plasmodium ovale* is the most common cause of malaria but causes the most severe symptoms of this disease

4. Both *Listeria monocytogenes* and *Legionella pneumophila* are intracellular pathogens. Which one of the following statements about how either of these organisms invades and/or survives the intracellular environment is most true?

    (A) *L. monocytogenes* uses an outer membrane protein that is designated as macrophage infectivity potentiator (Mip) that, in the presence of complement components, facilitates the uptake of this organism into macrophages

    (B) *L. pneumophila* survives the intracellular defenses by expressing listeriolysin O (LLO) and phospholipases that digest the endosomal membrane, preventing fusion with lysosomal granules and allowing these organisms to grow uninhibited within the cytosol

    (C) *L. monocytogenes* expresses an outer membrane protein that is designated as PfEMP-1 that prevents fusion between the endosome and the lysosomal granules within a macrophage, thereby allowing these organisms to survive within the macrophage

    (D) *L. pneumophila* invades all cell types by a mechanism that is facilitated by an outer membrane protein referred to as internalin A (InlA)

    (E) *L. monocytogenes* expresses an outer membrane protein that is designated as InlA that facilitates the invasion of enterocytes; this organism then prevents fusion between the endosome and the lysosomal granules within these cells by the expression of LLO and phospholipases that dissolve the endosomal membrane and allows the organism access to the cytosol

5. Malarial pathogens all demonstrate a characteristic life cycle. Which one of the following statements about this life cycle is most correct?

    (A) The sexual phase of the plasmodial life cycle can occur in either humans or in the mosquito

    (B) Schizogony occurs only during human infection

    (C) Sporogony occurs only during human infection

    (D) The characteristic cycle of chills followed by fever of clinical malaria is the result of waves of exoerythrocytic parasite multiplication within the liver

    (E) Anemia associated with malaria is the result of *Plasmodium* spp. shutdown of spleen and liver function

ANSWERS AND EXPLANATIONS

1. **The answer is E.** This patient acquired his pneumonia in the middle of summer, and his lung infection is not responding to cephalosporin treatment. These are characteristics of pneumonia caused by *L. pneumophila*. Option A is incorrect because *L. pneumophila* does not stain using Gram stain; therefore, it would not be prudent to simply conclude that this is a viral infection. Option B is incorrect because the lack of a response to a given antimicrobial agent, even if it is broadly active, cannot be taken as evidence that the infection is viral because of the occurrence of antibiotic-resistant organisms. Option C is not correct because selection for an antibiotic-resistant bacterial strain that continued to cause disease within this individual is unlikely. It is more likely that the organism causing this infection was resistant to the antimicrobial agent prior to causing disease. Option D is not correct because *L. monocytogenes* is not associated with pulmonary infections.

2. **The answer is B.** *L. monocytogenes* is a leading cause of meningitis among cancer patients. Option A is incorrect because *L. pneumophila* is not generally associated with meningitis. Option C is incorrect because meningitis caused by *N. meningitidis* is associated with infants and adolescents. Option D is incorrect because *H. influenzae* is tightly associated with meningitis in infants but not with meningitis associated with cancer patients. Option E is incorrect because *C. perfringens* is more typically associated with gastrointestinal disease or histotoxic infections, not meningitis among cancer patients.

3. **The answer is A.** *P. falciparum* is the most common cause of malaria, and it causes the most severe form of this disease. Option B is incorrect because *P. vivax* may be the most widely distributed form of malaria throughout the world; however, it is second to *P. falciparum* in malarial morbidity. Furthermore, *P. vivax* does not exhibit the severity of disease caused by *P. falciparum*. Option C is incorrect because *P. falciparum* does not cause sporadic cases in North America, rather this pathogen causes endemic disease in the warm climates of the tropics and the subtropics. Option D is incorrect because *P. malariae* is much less prevalent than *P. vivax* and *P. falciparum*. It does, however, produce symptoms that are much less severe than those caused by *P. falciparum*. Option E is incorrect because *P. ovale* causes only sporadic cases of malaria, and the symptoms associated with infection by this pathogen are much less severe than those caused by *P. falciparum*.

4. **The answer is E.** *L. monocytogenes* expresses an outer membrane protein, designated as InlA, that facilitates the invasion of enterocytes. Option A is incorrect because Mip is an outer membrane protein that is associated with the surface of *L. pneumophila*. It is true that Mip, in the presence of complement components, facilitates the uptake of *L. pneumophila* by macrophages. What is not true is that a similar protein exists for *L. monocytogenes*. Option B is incorrect because *L. monocytogenes*, not *L. pneumophila*, survive the intracellular defenses by expressing LLO and phospholipases that digest the endosomal membrane and prevent endosome-lysosome fusion. Option C is incorrect because *P. falciparum*, not *L. monocytogenes*, expresses PfEMP-1 on the surface of the erythrocytes that they invade. Option D is incorrect because *L. monocytogenes*, not *L. pneumophila*, expresses the internalin that is designated as InlA and which facilitates the invasion of *L. monocytogenes* into enterocytes. This organism then prevents fusion between the endosome and the lysosomal granules by the expression of LLO and phospholipases that dissolve the endosomal membrane.

5. **The answer is B.** Schizogony (the asexual phase of the plasmodial life cycle) occurs only during human infection. Option A is not correct because the sexual phase of the plasmodial life cycle occurs in humans and not in mosquitos. Option C is not correct because sporogony occurs only during the parasite's existence within the mosquito. Option D is not correct because the characteristic cycle of chills followed by fever of clinical malaria is the result of waves of erythrocytic parasite multiplication within the bloodstream, not exoerythrocytic multiplication within the liver. Option E is incorrect because anemia associated with malaria is the result of *Plasmodium* spp. destruction of RBCs and the clearance of infected RBCs by the spleen.

16

IMMUNE EVASION STRATEGIES: MOLECULAR MIMICRY

CHAPTER OUTLINE

Introduction of Clinical Case
Molecular Mimicry
Illustrative Pathogen: *Neisseria meningitidis*
• Biologic Characteristics
• Reservoir and Transmission
• Virulence Factors
• Pathogenesis
• Diagnosis
• Prevention and Treatment
Illustrative Pathogen: Group A streptococci
• Biologic Characteristics
• Reservoir and Transmission
• Virulence Factors
• Pathogenesis
• Diagnosis
• Prevention and Treatment
Resolution of Clinical Case
Review Questions

INTRODUCTION OF CLINICAL CASE

An 8-year-old boy was brought to his pediatrician's office because of a sore throat that had persisted for 4 days; no other persons in his immediate family had reported any illnesses during this time. It was difficult for the patient to swallow, and he had been ingesting only liquids for 3 days; however, his temperature was normal. An examination of the boy's throat revealed intense inflammation of the tonsils and pharynx. The tonsils were symmetrically enlarged. Numerous 1- to 2-centimeter lymph nodes were palpable in both anterior cervical chains. There was no rash, and the remainder of the examination was noncontributory. During the child's visit, a rapid enzyme immunoassay was used to determine that the child was positive for group A streptococci. A swab was also taken for confirmatory culture. The child was given a single dose of benzathine penicillin G in the office. The following day, laboratory analysis of the culture confirmed the presence of group A streptococci.

The child's sore throat resolved over the next 4 days. Six days after the visit to the physician's office, the boy mentioned to his mother that his urine had become dark (cola-colored). The boy was seen the next day by the pediatrician. Examination was notable only for 2+ (moderate) edema of both feet and ankles, extending about one-third of the way up toward the knee. Urinalysis revealed a large amount of protein and erythrocytes too numerous to count. No leukocytes were seen on microscopic examination. The mother was reassured that her son's condition was not unusual and that no therapy was necessary.

- To what was the sore throat due?
- What is the nature of the urinary tract illness? Is there any relationship between the pharyngitis and the urinary problem?

MOLECULAR MIMICRY

Molecular mimicry *results in two disease outcomes:*

1. Lack of an immune response, allowing microbial pathogens to avoid any significant host immune response and grow to sufficient numbers that results in disease

2. Induction of an immune response that cross-reacts with host tissues, resulting in disease pathology

Molecular mimicry refers to the production of bacterial, parasitic, or viral antigens that the human immune system cannot discriminate from its own antigens. As a result, two outcomes ensue: (1) an inadequate immune response is developed by the host, allowing the microbial pathogen to proliferate to the point of causing disease; or (2) an immune response is induced that results in cross-reactivity with host tissues, leading to pathologic destruction. The outcome of either form of molecular mimicry is human disease.

To illustrate how often molecular mimicry is used by microbial pathogens, several representative examples of this strategy are summarized in Table 16-1. This nonexhaustive list also emphasizes that molecular mimicry is used by a variety of microbial pathogens. In this chapter, two important examples of molecular mimicry, illustrated by *Neisseria meningitidis* and by group A streptococci, are described.

TABLE 16-1 ▶
Specific Examples of Molecular Mimicry among Diverse Microbial Pathogens

Organism	Disease	Mechanism of Molecular Mimicry
Neisseria meningitidis	Meningococcemia Meningococcal meningitis	Poorly immunogenic polysialic acid capsule that is antigenically identical to human neuronal tissues
Escherichia coli K1	Bacterial meningitis	Poorly immunogenic polysialic acid capsule that is antigenically identical to human neuronal tissues
Staphylococcus aureus	Cutaneous infection Systemic infection	Surface-associated protein A binds human immunoglobulin through the Fc region, rendering the immunoglobulin nonfunctional and coating the organism in protein of human origin
Streptococcus pyogenes	Pyogenic disease Toxogenic disease Immunologic sequelae	Nonimmunogenic hyaluronic acid capsule that is antigenically identical to the ground substance from human tissues Induction of antibodies that cross-react with human tissues

ILLUSTRATIVE PATHOGEN: *Neisseria meningitidis*

N. meningitidis causes bacterial sepsis (meningococcemia) and bacterial (meningococcal) meningitis.

Members of the genus *Neisseria* are gram-negative, oxidase-positive diplococci that exist only as part of the human flora. The genus can be divided into pathogenic members and nonpathogenic members (Table 16-2). The nonpathogenic (commensal) members of this genus exist as normal flora of a healthy human host and are only rarely associated with disease. The two pathogenic members of this genus are *Neisseria gonorrhoeae* (see Chapter 17) and *N. meningitidis*, and both are commonly associated with human disease. Bacterial sepsis and meningitis caused by *N. meningitidis* result from a hematogenous dissemination of organisms that have previously colonized the nasopharynx.

Biologic Characteristics

N. meningitidis is commonly referred to as the meningococcus.

The growth of *N. meningitidis*, like that of the gonococcus, can be selected by propagation on Thayer-Martin or Martin-Lewis agar media; nonpathogenic *Neisseria* and bacteria other than pathogenic *Neisseria* spp. generally do not grow on these two media. Clini-

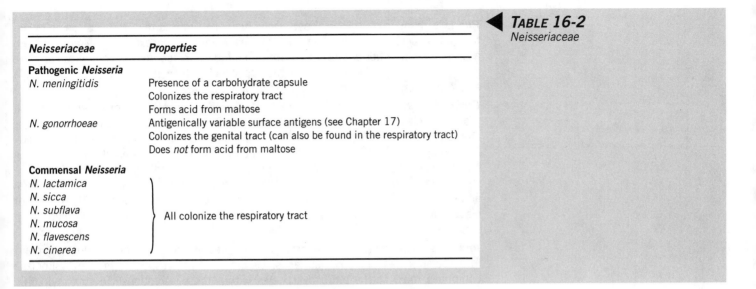

TABLE 16-2
Neisseriaceae

Neisseriaceae	Properties
Pathogenic Neisseria	
N. meningitidis	Presence of a carbohydrate capsule
	Colonizes the respiratory tract
	Forms acid from maltose
N. gonorrhoeae	Antigenically variable surface antigens (see Chapter 17)
	Colonizes the genital tract (can also be found in the respiratory tract)
	Does not form acid from maltose
Commensal Neisseria	
N. lactamica	
N. sicca	
N. subflava	All colonize the respiratory tract
N. mucosa	
N. flavescens	
N. cinerea	

cally, the meningococcus is differentiated from the gonococcus on the basis of their ability to produce acid when grown in the presence of maltose as a carbohydrate source. With regard to the production of virulence factors, meningococci are differentiated from gonococci by their association with a characteristic carbohydrate capsule. *N. gonorrhoeae* does not produce a similar capsule but rather avoids the host immune response by a sophisticated system of antigenic variation (see Chapter 17).

Reservoir and Transmission

Meningococcal sepsis and meningitis are exclusively human diseases. Meningococci typically colonize the nasopharynx without causing disease (asymptomatic infection). This is referred to as the carrier state and may last for a few days or for several months. On average, about 20% of all individuals are colonized by meningococci at any one time in their lives; the carrier state is highest in young adults and is associated with certain geographic regions. In spite of the high carriage rate within the human population, persons coming in contact with meningococci experience systemic disease less than 1% of the time.

Carrier state refers to a person or an animal with asymptomatic infection that can be transmitted to another susceptible person or animal.

*In certain areas of the world, meningococcal disease is prevalent across regions defined by latitude. These regions are referred to as **meningococcal belts**.*

Virulence Factors

Meningococci use the strategy of molecular mimicry by coating themselves in a poorly immunogenic, antiphagocytic carbohydrate capsule. Other virulence factors allow these organisms to attach to host tissues, multiply within the human host, and cause disease pathology. Meningococcal virulence factors are described individually below.

Capsule. The importance of a carbohydrate capsule in meningococcal disease is illustrated by the observation that antibodies specific to this capsule allow for the efficient clearance of these organisms by phagocytic leukocytes. The chemical composition of capsular types separates meningococci into at least nine serogroups. Of these serogroups, purified capsular vaccines have been prepared from A, C, Y, and W-135 capsular types, which are the predominant serogroups associated with disease. One additional serogroup, designated serogroup B, is poorly immunogenic. The structure of the serogroup B capsule is a form of polysialic acid, and antibodies elicited to this immunogen are cross-reactive with polysialosylglycopeptides of human fetal brain tissue. Thus, meningococcal infection caused by serogroup B represents a paradigm for molecular mimicry because the capsular antigen appears to be identical with carbohydrate structures that are expressed by the human host and are nonimmunogenic, allowing these organisms to evade the human immune response to infection. Analogously, a structurally identical capsule is found in a strain of *Escherichia coli* that is designated K1, which, like the meningococcus, can cause bacterial meningitis.

Virulence Factors Associated with N. meningitidis
- *Capsule production*
- *Pili*
- *Outer membrane proteins*
- *IgA protease*
- *High-affinity iron acquisition mechanisms*
- *Endotoxin*

Meningococcal serogroups are determined by their capsular polysaccharide. These serogroups are designated A, B, C, D, X, Y, Z, W-135, and 29E.

E. coli K1 is associated with bacterial meningitis in neonates. This strain produces a capsular polysaccharide that is structurally identical to N. meningitidis serogroup B.

Pili. Like many other bacterial pathogens described in this text, the expression of pili facilitates bacterial attachment to host tissues. Meningococci express type 4 pili that are associated with other pathogenic bacteria, including *Pseudomonas aeruginosa* and the gonococcus. Unlike the gonococcus, meningococcal pili are not as antigenically variable as those observed for *N. gonorrhoeae* (see Chapter 17).

Outer Membrane Proteins. Five species (referred to as classes) of outer membrane proteins have been implicated in meningococcal virulence. Class 2 and class 3 outer membrane proteins are porins (see Chapter 1); either one of these porins is expressed by all meningococcal strains. Class 5 outer membrane proteins are highly variable—they may or may not be expressed at all, and if they are expressed, they demonstrate significant antigenic variability. Proteins of this class are thought to function as afimbrial adhesins, similar to the gonococcal Opa family of proteins (see Chapter 17). The role of class 1 and class 4 outer membrane proteins in the pathogenesis of meningococcal infection has yet to be resolved.

Immunoglobulin A1 (IgA1) Protease. IgA is the predominant immunoglobulin type found in association with mucosal surfaces. Of the total IgA response, the IgA1 subclass comprises most of the antibody species within these secretions. To survive in this environment, meningococci actively secrete an IgA1 protease. This protease attacks the hinge region of IgA1, creating Fab and Fc fragments and inactivating IgA1 antibodies. An IgA1 protease is also produced by *N. gonorrhoeae, Streptococcus pneumoniae, Haemophilus influenzae,* and *Ureaplasma urealyticum* (see Chapter 19)—all pathogenic species that colonize mucous membranes.

Iron Acquisition System. The ability of meningococci to multiply within the human host is correlated with the ability of these pathogens to obtain iron efficiently from the host environment. Meningococci are able to accomplish this by directly binding to human transferrin, using a specific receptor referred to as the transferrin-binding protein (Tbp). In addition to binding human transferrin, a mechanism for the removal and uptake of iron must also be expressed. This iron acquisition system is not found in nonpathogenic *Neisseria* spp. and is thought to facilitate the expansion of meningococci within the human host.

Endotoxin. The outer membrane of *N. meningitidis* is composed, in part, of a potent form of lipopolysaccharide (LPS). This molecule is also referred to as lipooligosaccharide (LOS) because it lacks the highly repeated O-antigen portion of the LPS described for the Enterobacteriaceae (see Chapter 1). Meningococcal endotoxin is thought to be an important contributor to disease, particularly in meningococcal sepsis.

Pathogenesis

In order for *N. meningitidis* to cause systemic infection, it must attach to mucosal epithelium, avoid local defense mechanisms, penetrate the mucosal barrier, and survive and multiply in the intravascular space, where it can induce a significant inflammatory response by the production of endotoxin. Pili facilitate meningococcal attachment to nonciliated epithelial cells, and cellular invasion may be facilitated by meningococcal outer membrane proteins through intimate surface association with the host cell. Meningococcal secretion of an IgA1 protease is thought to facilitate infection by disabling IgA1 as a major mucosal defense mechanism. Endocytosis and the intracellular transport of meningococcal-containing phagosomes appear to mediate the passage of these organisms to the submucosa. To cause disease, the meningococci must also evade the nonspecific and specific humoral and complement-mediated immune defenses and invade the host submucosa, gaining access to the systemic circulation or the cerebrospinal fluid (CSF). The high bacterial load results in the production of large quantities of endotoxin, which in turn results in an inflammatory response that is symptomatic of meningococcemia or meningococcal meningitis. Meningococcal infection is primarily a disease of infants and young children. In large part this can be attributed to a combination of the immaturity of their immune system and the poorly immunogenic nature of bacterial capsules as described in Chapter 18. Immunity is acquired with increasing age, probably as a result of asymptomatic nasopharyngyl meningococcal colonization.

The bactericidal activity of the complement system is important in preventing primary and recurrent invasive neisserial infections. There is a strong correlation between individuals who are complement deficient and meningococcal infection: individuals with inherited, terminal complement deficiencies (e.g., a deficiency of the C5, C6, C7, C8, or C9 components of the complement system) are uniquely susceptible to invasive neisserial disease, with rates of meningococcal infection that are 1000-fold higher than in the general population. About half of all individuals with terminal complement deficiencies experience at least one episode of meningococcal infection.

Individuals with deficiencies in their terminal complement components (C5–C9) are very susceptible to meningococcemia and gonococcemia (see Chapter 17).

Diagnosis

In the differential diagnosis of meningococcemia, a characteristic skin rash, referred to as petichiae or purpura, is often (but not always) an associated symptom. This rash can be distributed over all parts of the body except for the face and may progress from a few ill-defined lesions to a generalized rash within hours. The differential diagnosis is difficult: the symptoms of meningococcal meningitis are so similar to those of other forms of acute bacterial meningitis that it is difficult to identify the causative bacterial agent without laboratory tests that require days to obtain results.

*Petechiae (minute hemorrhagic spots in the skin) or **purpura** (hemorrhages into the skin) occur from the first to the third day of illness in half of meningococcal disease cases, whether or not meningitis is involved. Petechiae or purpura tend to occur more frequently in areas of the skin that are subjected to pressure, such as at the folds, the beltline, or areas of the back.*

For suspected meningococcal disease, specimens from the blood, CSF, and nasopharynx should ideally be collected before any antimicrobial agents are given, since this may decrease the chances of finding these organisms. Blood and CSF specimens should be Gram stained for the presence of *N. meningitidis* associated with white blood cells (Figure 16-1). These specimens should also be cultured overnight at 37°C on chocolate or blood agar (containing supplements) for the presence of bacteria (in healthy individuals, specimens of blood and CSF should be sterile). Nasopharyngeal samples are contaminated by the complex local flora of the throat. For these specimens, Gram staining is not informative; rather, these specimens require propagation on selective media. The identification of oxidase-positive colonies that contain organisms staining as gram-negative diplococci provides a presumptive diagnosis of disease mediated by *N. meningitidis*. The production of acid from glucose and maltose results in a confirmatory diagnosis of *N. meningitidis* as the causative agent. If necessary, the meningococcal isolate can be serogrouped and further typed based on the antigenic specificity for the meningococcal outer membrane proteins.

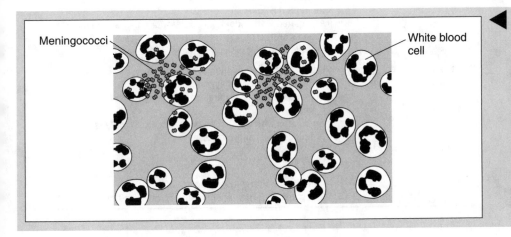

Meningococci

White blood cell

◄ **FIGURE 16-1**
Artist's Rendering of a Diplococcus Associated with a White Blood Cell. This is indicative of what would be seen upon examination of a Gram stain from a sedimented cerebrospinal fluid sample of a patient with meningococcal meningitis.

Prevention and Treatment

The reduction of personal contacts within a population with a high carrier state of *N. meningitidis* is the most significant means of controlling this disease. This can be achieved by quarantine. Prophylatic antibiotics given to persons closely associated with colonized individuals (household, day care) can reduce the carrier state. For adults going into a closed setting such as a military barracks, an effective capsular vaccine is available for most meningococcal serogroups, with the exception of group B meningococci.

Because of the rapid onset of symptoms and the delay in obtaining culture results, antimicrobial therapy for meningococcal infection should be initiated as soon as the disease is suspected. The standard regimen for adults with meningococcemia or meningococcal meningitis is high-dose penicillin. Unlike the gonococcus (see Chapter 17), β-lactamase production is not a significant problem for the treatment of meningococcal disease.

ILLUSTRATIVE PATHOGEN: Group A streptococci

The streptococci are gram-positive, nonmotile, non–spore-forming, catalase-negative cocci that are arranged either in pairs or in chains. Like *Neisseria*, the genus *Streptococcus* comprises a broad range of nonpathogenic and pathogenic species. The nonpathogenic species are often associated with the normal flora in humans, and the pathogenic species are associated with local and systemic disease. Within humans, streptococci typically colonize the mucosal surfaces of the mouth, nares, and pharynx. Under certain circumstances they may also be associated with skin, heart, or muscle tissue. Also like *Neisseria*, select streptococcal species employ strategies of molecular mimicry during the production of disease.

TABLE 16-3 ▶

Pathogenic Streptococci

Streptococcal Strain	Properties
S. pyogenes	Group A streptococci β-Hemolytic Inhabits the throat and skin Associated with pharyngitis, impetigo, rheumatic fever, scarlet fever, glomerulonephritis
S. agalactiae	Group B streptococci Generally β-hemolytic Inhabits the female genital tract Associated with neonatal sepsis and meningitis
Enterococcus faecalis	Group D streptococci α-Hemolytic or γ-hemolytic Inhabits the colon Associated with abdominal abscess, urinary tract infection, endocarditis Emerging antimicrobial resistance
Viridans streptococci (many species)	Usually not typed by the Lancefield system α-Hemolytic or γ-hemolytic Inhabits the upper respiratory tract, colon, and female genital tract Associated with dental caries (especially *S. mutans*), endocarditis, and abscesses
S. pneumoniae	Not typed by the Lancefield system α-Hemolytic Inhabits the upper respiratory tract Associated with pneumonia, endocarditis, and meningitis

Hemolytic Patterns of Streptococci on Blood Agar
α-Hemolysis describes a colony surrounded by a partial zone of hemolysis with a greenish discoloration.
β-Hemolysis describes a colony surrounded by a cleared zone of complete hemolysis.
γ-Hemolysis describes no zone of hemolysis surrounding colony.

Streptococci generally have very fastidious growth requirements and therefore are typically cultivated on blood agar. The growth of streptococci on blood agar can give rise to three distinctive patterns, referred to as α, β, or γ hemolysis. These patterns of hemolysis are useful for differentiating the streptococci (Figure 16-2). Streptococcal pathogens are more specifically classified into Lancefield serogroups according to carbohydrate antigens that are associated with their cell walls. Lancefield serogroups of human significance include group A streptococci (largely *S. pyogenes*), group B streptococci (largely *S. agalactiae*), and group D streptococci (*Enterococcus faecalis*, formerly *Streptococcus faecalis*). At least two species that do not have a Lancefield-type, *S. pneumoniae* and *viridans* streptococci, are also significant human pathogens. Of the

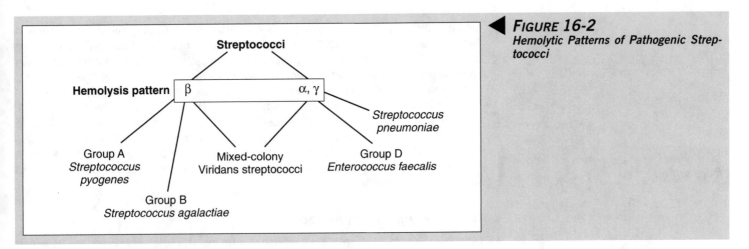

FIGURE 16-2
Hemolytic Patterns of Pathogenic Streptococci

streptococci, *S. pyogenes* is the most common agent responsible for disease, causing an estimated 25 million infections a year in the United States alone. It is this pathogen that is responsible for the case described at the beginning of this chapter.

Biologic Characteristics

The general structure of *S. pyogenes* is demonstrated in Figure 16-3. *S. pyogenes* is often recognized in the laboratory by the β-hemolysis pattern produced by most isolates. However, these criteria alone are not definitive since up to 4% of *S. pyogenes* may be nonhemolytic, and there are non–*S. pyogenes* that are also β-hemolytic (e.g., many *S. agalactiae* isolates). A definitive identification of *S. pyogenes* uses serology-based Lance-

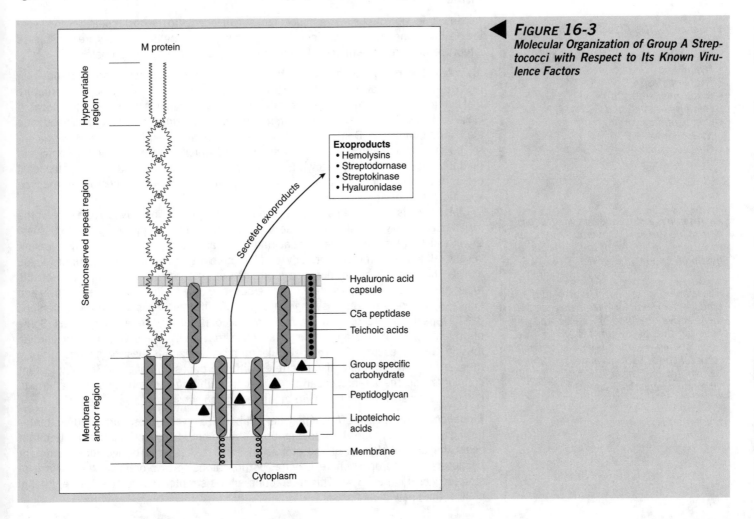

FIGURE 16-3
Molecular Organization of Group A Streptococci with Respect to Its Known Virulence Factors

field groupings specific for a group-specific carbohydrate (a polymer of rhamnose and N-acetylglucosamine) associated with group A streptococci. Additionally, bacitracin is used to differentiate β-hemolytic streptococci; almost all S. pyogenes are inhibited by low concentrations of this antibiotic, whereas other streptococci are generally resistant. Another test used to differentiate between the streptococci is the PYR test, which assays for the hydrolysis of L-pyrrolidonyl-2-naphylamide (PYR). Of the streptococci, only S. pyogenes and enterococci are PYR-positive. Finally, S. pyogenes may be subdivided based on serologic reactivity to the major surface protein designated M protein (see Figure 16-3). This division is important since a subset of S. pyogenes with specific M protein (see below) serotypes are strongly correlated with certain streptococcal diseases such as acute glomerulonephritis.

> **S. pyogenes** *is bacitracin-sensitive and PYR positive.*

Reservoir and Transmission

Disease caused by S. pyogenes is confined to humans. It is spread between individuals by aerosols, by contaminated objects (fomites), or by direct contact, either from asymptomatic carriers or from patients with symptomatic pharyngitis. Both the carrier state and the incidence of disease are highest in late winter and early spring and in school children. Disease typically results from the acquisition of a new strain that is allowed to colonize as a consequence of an alteration within the normal bacterial flora. Uncommonly, S. pyogenes gain access to the bloodstream from the pharynx. Bacteremia is more often a consequence of a skin or soft-tissue infection due to group A streptococci. Bacteremia caused by S. pyogenes can in turn give rise to pneumonia, bone and joint infections, meningitis, and endocarditis.

Virulence Factors

To cause infection, group A streptococci must gain access to the host, colonize, and avoid the host immune response. Molecules involved in promoting this process are considered streptococcal virulence factors. These virulence factors are described below.

> **Virulence Factors Associated with S. pyogenes**
> - M protein
> - Hyaluronic acid capsule
> - Hyaluronidase
> - Pyrotoxins (superantigens)
> - Hemolysins (SLS and SLO)
> - C5a peptidase
> - Streptokinase
> - Streptodornase

M Protein. Figure 16-3 demonstrates the basic structure of M protein and its association with the streptococcal cell envelope. Structurally, M protein is a rod-like, coiled structure that extends 60 nm from the streptococcal cell surface. Domains of the M protein located close to the cell surface are involved in membrane anchoring, are highly conserved, and are nonimmunogenic. Domains in the middle of the M protein sequence are semiconserved and tandemly repeated linear sequences, which are weakly immunogenic and bind lipoteichoic acid (see below). Portions of the M protein distal to the streptococcal cell surface are immunogenic and antigenically variable and are responsible for the type specificity of these organisms.

> *An **opsonin** is a molecule that when deposited on the surface of a microbial pathogen facilitates the uptake of this pathogen by host professional phagocytes.*

> *Researchers have shown that M protein binds factor H. Factor H regulates complement activity by binding to C3b and enhancing the decay of C3 convertase. Sequestering Factor H near the streptococcal surface affords a measure of protection by preventing activation of the alternate complement pathway.*

M protein is a major constituent of group A streptococci and serves a role both in the resistance to phagocytosis and in the attachment of these organisms to host tissues. Organisms that lack this protein are avirulent and are readily opsonized by complement via the alternate pathway. Antibody to M protein can overcome this antiphagocytic activity; however, these antibodies are directed at an antigenic variable portion of this molecule. Anti-M antibodies are protective because they facilitate the phagocytosis and killing of S. pyogenes. Because there are over 80 different types of M protein, persons can be repeatedly infected with group A streptococci bearing different M proteins. Some M-protein types induce an antibody response that cross-reacts with human cardiac muscle; this represents a form of molecular mimicry that allows these organisms to cause rheumatic fever. M protein also interferes with the deposition of the C3b complement component on the streptococcal cell surface, inhibiting the activity of the alternate complement pathway and host C3b-mediated phagocytosis.

Lipoteichoic Acid (LTA). LTA is a polymer of about 25 glycerophosphate subunits terminating with a lipid group. This lipid group is able to bind fibronectin, a host protein that coats the epithelial cells of the oropharynx. LTA serves as a bridge for attachment because the glycerophosphate polymer portion binds to M protein on the surface of streptococci (Figure 16-4). This interaction allows streptococci to attach to epithelial cells of the pharyngeal tissues.

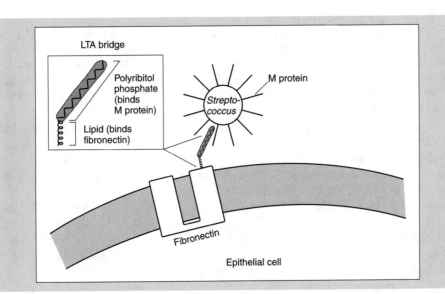

FIGURE 16-4
M Protein, Lipoteichoic Acid (LTA), and Fibronectin Interactions That Allow for Attachment to Human Epithelium

Cell Wall Components. The injection of purified group A streptococcal peptidoglycan into laboratory rabbits causes symptoms that are similar to those of endocarditis. On the basis of this finding, the presumption is that this antigen evokes the principle of molecular mimicry during local infection, contributing to rheumatic fever. Less well-defined molecules suspected to be involved in molecular mimicry are those associated with the lipid/protein protoplast membrane that evokes a host immune response, cross-reacting with cardiac muscle.

Similar to the staphylococci, the group A streptococci have proteins associated with their cell wall that bind immunoglobulins through their Fc regions. Binding these molecules in this fashion serves a similar purpose as the IgA1 protease described earlier in this chapter for *N. meningitidis* because it effectively uncouples the effector region of an antibody from its specificity-determining regions. This strategy has the added advantage of contributing to the molecular mimicry associated with streptococci by coating this foreign cell surface with a predominant host-derived protein, immunoglobulin.

Hyaluronic Acid Capsule. Like other bacterial capsules, the group A streptococcal hyaluronic acid capsule interferes with the phagocytosis of streptococci. Hyaluronic acid is also a component of ground material (connective tissue) of the host. As such, it is only a weak immunogen and represents yet another example of molecular mimicry. By virtue of its chemical composition, this capsule may also encourage adherence to connective tissue, such as heart valves.

Hyaluronidase. Perhaps as a result of producing a hyaluronic acid capsule, hyaluronidase activity has also been described for group A streptococci. While this enzyme may function in the polymerization and depolymerization of the streptococcal hyaluronic acid capsule, it also has the detrimental effect of breaking down host tissues. This facilitates the spread of *S. pyogenes* through these tissues. This enzyme is almost certainly associated with the cutaneous diseases (e.g., impetigo) caused by group A streptococci.

C5a Peptidase. This peptidase cleaves six amino acids from the carboxy-terminus of C5a, the principal chemotactic factor generated by the complement cascade. This represents an enzymatic contributor to the subversion of the host immune response to streptococcal infection inhibiting C5a function as an opsonin.

Pyrogenic Exotoxins. Phage-encoded streptococcal pyrogenic exotoxins (SPEs) act as superantigens by nonspecifically stimulating a cellular immune response that leads to a detrimental release of host cytokines, which in turn results in a pathologic condition in the host. These toxins are associated with scarlet fever and a disease that is similar to staphylococcal toxic shock syndrome.

Hemolysins. Streptolysin O (SLO) and streptolysin S (SLS) not only cause red blood cells (RBCs) to lyse but also inhibit the normal function of other cells during the course of natural infection. SLO is oxygen-labile, meaning that in the presence of oxygen, its hemolytic activity is inhibited. SLO is antigenic, and antiSLO titers rise after infection.

SLS is oxygen-stable, is a small peptide, and is nonantigenic. SLS is responsible for the β-hemolytic activity observed for group A streptococci streaked on the surface (oxidizing conditions) of blood agar; SLO activity is associated with β-hemolytic activity associated with organisms "stabbed" into the agar (reducing conditions). While both SLO and SLS detrimentally affect cells other than RBCs, they are referred to as hemolysins simply because this is a convenient means to assay for their activity.

Nucleases. Streptodornase is the name given to a group of streptococcal enzymes that degrade DNA. These enzymes break the viscous DNA that is the result of lysis of host leukocytes that, if not degraded, would limit the diffusion of these nonmotile bacteria. As a result, streptodornase is thought to facilitate the spread of streptococci, allowing these organisms to diffuse freely within host tissues.

Streptokinase. This enzyme promotes the dissolution of fibrin blood clots by catalyzing the conversion of plasminogen (an inactive plasma component) to plasmin (an active plasma protease). This plasmin is bound to streptococci in an active form, streptokinase, and is thought to facilitate the invasion of group A streptococci by allowing them to hydrolyze connective tissue and basement membrane components.

Streptokinase is used therapeutically to treat heart attacks.

Diseases Caused by S. pyogenes

Pyogenic disease
- *Pharyngitis*
- *Pyoderma (impetigo)*

Toxogenic disease
- *Scarlet fever*
- *Toxic shock syndrome*

Immunologic disease
- *Rheumatic fever*
- *Acute glomerulonephritis*

Pathogenesis

Any of three clinical manifestations ensue as a consequence of streptococcal disease: pyogenic infection, toxogenic infection, or immunologic sequelae.

Pyogenic Infection. The most common pyogenic infection is pharyngitis. In these infections, attachment to host tissues is mediated by way of M protein and LTA interactions that target host fibronectin. Upon attachment and multiplication, *S. pyogenes* elaborates many virulence factors (described above) that account for its ability to produce tissue damage and inflammation. This tissue damage in turn facilitates the rapid spread of streptococci to other tissues. Among the virulence factors associated with tissue damage are the hemolysins and streptokinase, both factors that promote clot dissolution (fibrinolysis) and consequently allow streptococci to spread to other host tissues. Contributing to this spread is hyaluronidase, known as spreading factor because of its ability to digest the hyaluronic acid of connective tissue. The symptoms of group A streptococcal pharyngitis are not distinctive; nothing differentiates these bacterial diseases from those associated with viruses and mycoplasma. This disease is for the most part self-limited, and the duration of the illness is generally not affected by antibiotic therapy. However, group A streptococcal pyogenic infection can give rise to serious sequelae of either an infectious (suppurative) or a noninfectious (nonsuppurative) nature. Because of this, immediate antimicrobial therapy is indicated.

Streptococci also cause pyoderma (impetigo), which is a local infection of the superficial layers of the skin. Recently, the bacteria causing these types of infections have been referred to as flesh-eating bacteria. This disease presents as superficial blisters that eventually burst, forming a sore that is filled with pus and forms a crust. If left untreated, the sore may increase in size. If these organisms infect skin wounds, more widespread infection can occur and can progress to cellulitis. Streptococcal pyoderma is associated with certain M protein types and may precede acute glomerulonephritis but does not typically lead to rheumatic fever.

Toxogenic Infection. Another way in which group A streptococci cause disease is by elaboration of pyrogenic (also called erythrogenic) toxins. These are exotoxins that are responsible for scarlet fever and streptococcal toxic shock syndrome. In this disease, pharyngeal infection results in the SPEs entering the circulation, where they act as superantigens and damage small blood vessels. This activity results in the rash that is characteristic of scarlet fever as well as in disease that is very similar to toxic shock syndrome.

Noninfectious Immunologic Sequelae. The two serious noninfectious sequelae (also referred to as nonsuppurative sequelae) that can result from group A streptococcal pharyngitis are rheumatic fever and acute glomerulonephritis.

Acute rheumatic fever is largely a disease of children and teenagers, the age groups in which group A streptococcal carriage and symptomatic pharyngitis are most prevalent. When, rarely, rheumatic fever occurs in adults, it is usually manifested only by polyarthritis, and endocarditis seldom occurs. Early therapy of diagnosed pharyngitis with an antibiotic active against *S. pyogenes* prevents rheumatic fever. However, less than one-half of pharyngitis cases are symptomatic, and these infections can still progress to rheumatic fever.

Rheumatic fever occurs approximately 18 days following either symptomatic or asymptomatic pharyngitis and is characterized as a multisystem, immune-mediated disease. The manifestations of acute rheumatic fever are listed in Table 16-4. If supported by evidence of a preceding group A streptococcal infection, then the presence of one major and two minor manifestations listed in the table indicates a high probability of acute rheumatic fever.

◄ **TABLE 16-4**
Manifestations of Acute Rheumatic Fever

Clinical Diseases	Symptoms/Diagnostic Tests
Major manifestations	
Carditis	Pericarditis, myocarditis, and endocarditis
Polyarthritis	Migratory; large joints of extremities
Chorea	Purposeless, involuntary movements
Erythema marginatum	Asymptomatic, evanescent rash
Subcutaneous nodules	Granulomas; extensor joint surfaces
Minor manifestations	
Arthralgia	Fever and pain on movement
Fever	Laboratory findings: elevated acute phase reactants, increased erythrocyte sedimentation rate
	Supporting evidence of antecedent group A streptococcal infection
	Previous history of a sore throat
	Positive throat culture or rapid streptococcal antigen test
	Elevated or rising ASO, antihyaluronidase, antistreptokinase, or streptozyme slide test

Note: ASO = antistreptolysin O.

The molecular basis of rheumatic fever is not known. It is believed to result from molecular mimicry between streptococcal antigens and human tissue, particularly cardiac tissues. Although acute rheumatic fever is a self-limited illness, damage to the heart valves can result in permanent cardiac disease and eventually lead to congestive heart failure. Subsequent group A streptococcal infections engender additional immunologic damage to the heart valves. Therefore, when rheumatic fever is diagnosed, the patient is given long-term prophylaxis to prevent group A streptococcal infections, usually in the form of monthly injections of a depot form of penicillin (benzathine penicillin G).

The other nonsuppurative sequela of group A streptococcal infection is acute post-streptococcal glomerulonephritis. The pathogenesis of poststreptococcal glomerulo-nephritis is more completely understood than that of rheumatic fever. This disease appears to result from the deposition of streptococcal antigen–antibody complexes on the basement membrane of the glomeruli, followed by association with complement. Only 15 of the 80 group A streptococci M protein types are nephritogenic. Acute glomerulonephritis can follow either streptococcal pharyngitis or infections of the skin and soft tissue. The latent period between the acute infection and glomerulonephritis is much shorter (10 days) than the incubation period preceding rheumatic fever (21 days). This may explain why even prompt, appropriate therapy for group A streptococcal infection does not prevent glomerulonephritis, as it does acute rheumatic fever.

The clinical manifestations of poststreptococcal glomerulonephritis vary from asymptomatic hematuria and mild proteinuria to a full-blown nephritic syndrome, which consists of gross hematuria (cola-colored urine), proteinuria, oliguria, edema, hypertension, and renal insufficiency. Serum complement levels are usually low because they are being consumed during this disease. Anti-SLO and particularly antistreptodornase titers are elevated. As might be expected from its pathogenesis, there is no specific therapy for poststreptococcal glomerulonephritis. Luckily, the course is almost always benign, with all symptoms and signs resolving in weeks to months. Poststreptococcal glomerulo-nephritis does not recur following subsequent group A streptococcal infections, so there is no need for prophylactic antibiotic therapy.

Diagnosis

The nature of the specimen examined depends on the specific streptococcal infection. Microscopic examination of smears from pus often shows single cocci or pairs rather than the chains observed on a stained laboratory culture specimen. Also, a Gram stain of material obtained from a throat swab is not informative because S. viridans is normal oral flora and stains similarly to group A streptococci. Specimens suspected to contain streptococci are typically cultured at 37°C overnight on blood agar in a 10% carbon dioxide environment. The characteristic zone of β-hemolysis is generally observed as soon as colonies are observed. A bacitracin-containing disk is routinely placed on the blood agar plate at innoculation so that sensitivity to this antibiotic will be known the next day. Organisms from colonies suspected of being group A streptococci can be tested for a positive PYR test result and for their sensitivity to bacitracin.

As an alternative to culture, rapid (minutes to hours depending on the test) antigen detection kits that test for group A–specific substances directly from a swab are in current use. This allows for the identification of antigen while the patient is still in the physician's office. These tests are 60% to 90% as sensitive as bacterial culture and are very specific and cost effective.

Serologic analysis of patients for antibodies to streptococcal virulence factors are useful, especially for demonstrating previous exposure to group A streptococci. The antibodies most commonly used in this determination are anti-SLO, antistreptodornase, and antihyaluronidase.

Prevention and Treatment

Human carriers are the sole source of group A streptococci, and control procedures are aimed primarily at this source. The disease is controlled by early detection and anti-microbial therapy of pharyngeal or skin disease. All group A streptococci are sensitive to penicillin G; however, high levels of this antibiotic must be maintained for 10 days to prevent the suppurative sequelae. For persons who have suffered rheumatic fever, large-dose (depot) injections of benzanthine penicillin G every 3 to 4 weeks are required. This practice is referred to as chemoprophylaxis and is important because individuals that have suffered an initial episode of rheumatic fever are susceptible to subsequent bouts of this disease. Because of the antigenic variability of group A streptococci (associated with the M protein), immunity to the strain causing the infection will not prevent reinfection. In rheumatic fever patients, chemoprophylaxis must be carried out for up to 2 years.

RESOLUTION OF CLINICAL CASE

The culture results from this case indicated that the child most likely suffered from pharyngitis due to group A streptococci. The fact that the boy did not show signs of a rash, characteristic of scarlet fever, can be simply explained by the fact that the strain of group A streptococci causing the pharyngitis was not producing any SPEs or that these toxins were not a factor in this disease.

Recall that high levels of antibiotic must be achieved for the treatment for pharyngitis to prevent the progression of strep throat to a suppurative or a nonsuppurative sequelae. Thus, the appropriate antimicrobial treatment was given to the patient. The patient is currently suffering from acute glomerulonephritis which is responsible for the edema in his extremities and his cola-colored urine, the result of the presence of high protein and RBC levels. The physician was correct not to prescribe an antimicrobial regimen for acute glomerulonephritis because antimicrobial therapy will not cure a disease that is attributable to the immune response to group A streptococci being cleared from the host.

REVIEW QUESTIONS

Directions: For each of the following questions, choose the **one best** answer.

1. A child returns from school irritable, feverish, and complaining of a sore throat. He is taken to a clinic, where a throat culture is performed. The laboratory reports the growth of β-hemolytic colonies on blood agar. The Gram stain of this culture indicates that the organisms are gram-positive cocci occurring in chains that are catalase-negative and bacitracin-sensitive. The organism responsible for this disease uses which molecule as a form of molecular mimicry to cause the child's symptoms?

    (A) M protein, which is similar to host tissue antigens, results in an autoimmune response to the host pharyngeal tissues and causes a sore throat.

    (B) Streptodornase converts the DNA from lysed host cells into a nucleic acid capsule that cannot be recognized by the host response.

    (C) A polysialic acid capsule is immunologically identical to a carbohydrate found on fetal neuronal tissues and is poorly immunogenic.

    (D) Lipoteichoic acid is identical to the lipooligosaccharide (LPS) associated with members of the normal human bacterial flora and does not induce an immune response.

    (E) A hyaluronic acid capsule is immunologically similar to the hyaluronic polymer found in host connective tissues and is poorly immunogenic.

2. Group A streptococci typically are characterized by which of the following?

    (A) A clear zone of complete hemolysis around an isolated colony on blood agar

    (B) An incomplete zone of hemolysis around an isolated colony on blood agar

    (C) A clear zone of complete hemolysis around an isolated colony on chocolate agar

    (D) An incomplete zone of hemolysis around an isolated colony on MacConkey agar

    (E) No hemolysis around an isolated colony on blood agar.

3. A high school student returns from school with a severe headache, a fever, and a runny nose. He is taken to a clinic, where a throat culture is performed. The laboratory reports the growth of colonies on Thayer-Martin media. The Gram stain indicates that the organisms constituting these colonies are gram-negative diplococci. These organisms are also oxidase positive. The organism causing the child's symptoms would most likely have which one of the following virulence factors?

    (A) A polysialic acid capsule that is immunologically identical to a carbohydrate found on fetal neuronal tissues

    (B) Lipoteichoic acid (LTA) that is nonimmunogenic and allows the organism to evade the host immune response in the bloodstream and the cerebrospinal fluid

    (C) A hyaluronic acid capsule that is immunologically similar to the hyaluronic polymer found in host connective tissues and that is poorly immunogenic

    (D) M protein, which is critical for the attachment of this organism to host tissues

    (E) The elaboration of erythrotoxins that are responsible for the teenager's fever

4. Which one of the following statements about rheumatic fever is correct?

(A) It is an autoimmune syndrome that can be caused by a variety of gram-positive and gram-negative bacteria

(B) It is easily treatable with short-course antimicrobial therapy

(C) It results in cardiac damage as a result of group A streptococci generating antibodies that cross-react with this tissue

(D) It is primarily the result of the combined toxicity of streptolysin O (SLO) and streptolysin S (SLS) for cardiac tissue

(E) It is especially associated with patients who have a benign group A streptococcal pyodermal infection

ANSWERS AND EXPLANATIONS

1. **The answer is E.** The poorly immunogenic hyaluronic acid capsule is structurally similar to hyaluronic acid found within host connective tissue. The description of the child's symptoms and the microbiologic workup of his disease are most consistent with a diagnosis of group A streptococci. Option A is incorrect because the child has symptoms of pharyngitis, which is caused by tissue destruction and inflammation and is not an autoimmune-mediated disease. Option B is incorrect because streptodornase breaks down DNA and does not polymerize this DNA into an immunologically cryptic capsule. Option C is incorrect because a polysialic acid capsule is a characteristic of group B meningococci and *Escherichia coli* K1, not group A streptococci. Option D is incorrect because lipoteichoic acid (LTA) shares no extensive structural similarity with LPS.

2. **The answer is A.** A classic characteristic of group A streptococci is that they are β-hemolytic. Option B is incorrect because this describes the phenomenon of α-hemolysis. Option C is incorrect because chocolate agar is already completely hemolysed. Option D is incorrect because group A streptococci do not grow on bile-containing MacConkey agar. Option E is incorrect because β-hemolysis is defined by a clear zone of inhibition around an isolated colony.

3. **The answer is A.** The description of the symptoms and the microbiologic workup of the disease are consistent with a diagnosis of meningococcal disease. Meningococci produce a polysialic acid capsule that is nonimmunogenic. Other serogroups of meningococci produce structurally different capsular polysaccharides and are poorly immunogenic. Option B is incorrect because LTA is not produced by the gram-negative meningococcus. Option C is incorrect because a hyaluronic acid capsule is not a characteristic of meningococci; rather, it is a characteristic of group A streptococci. Likewise, option D is incorrect because M protein is a *S. pyogenes* virulence factor, not a meningococcal virulence factor. Option E is incorrect because the meningococcus does not produce erythrotoxins.

4. **The answer is C.** There appears to be an autoimmune response, induced by several streptococcal components that cross-react with heart tissue. Option A is incorrect because rheumatic fever is generally associated only with group A streptococci. Option B is incorrect because patients with diagnosed rheumatic fever have to receive long-term antimicrobial prophylaxis. Option D is incorrect because SLO and SLS activity are not directly linked to rheumatic fever. Option E is incorrect because group A streptococcal pyoderma may result in acute glomerulonephritis but rarely progresses to rheumatic fever.

17 IMMUNE EVASION STRATEGIES: ANTIGENIC VARIATION

CHAPTER OUTLINE

Introduction of Clinical Case
Phenotypic and Antigenic Variation
- Genetic Mechanisms of Antigenic Variation: Point Mutation, Recombination, and Reassortment

Illustrative Pathogen: The Gonococcus
- Biologic Characteristics
- Reservoir and Transmission
- Virulence Factors
- Pathogenesis
- Diagnosis
- Prevention and Treatment

Illustrative Pathogen: Influenzavirus
- Biologic Characteristics
- Reservoir and Transmission
- Virulence Factors
- Pathogenesis
- Diagnosis
- Prevention and Treatment

Resolution of Clinical Case
Review Questions

INTRODUCTION OF CLINICAL CASE

In January, a 48-year-old male schoolteacher presented to his physician complaining of a 5-day history of fever, headache, nonproductive cough, nausea, vomiting, and lack of energy. He also complained of a lack of appetite, myalgia, nasal congestion, and short-ness of breath. He noted that several of his students recently missed class with similar symptoms, although not quite as severe. The patient stated that he had a history of smoking and that he received a "flu" vaccine 1 year previously. Physical examination of the patient revealed a temperature of 102.2°F and an increased respiratory rate of 35 breaths/min. He was dehydrated, and rales were heard at the base of his right lung. Laboratory tests were normal except that the analysis of arterial blood gases showed mild hypoxia and respiratory alkalosis. A chest x-ray revealed an infiltrate in his right lower lobe. An induced sputum sample was obtained and sent to the laboratory for routine bacterial and viral culture. A Gram stain of the sputum was unremarkable. The patient was admitted to the hospital and given supplemental oxygen and intravenous hydration. Oral erythromycin therapy was begun while sputum culture results were pending. He was also given antipyretics to limit fever. During the next 3 days, steady improvement was noted, and the patient was discharged.

- What microbial pathogen is causing these symptoms?
- Is the patient's vaccination history relevant?
- Is the patient responding to the antibiotic or simply resolving the infection on his own?

PHENOTYPIC AND ANTIGENIC VARIATION

One common strategy microbial pathogens use to overcome host defenses is to vary their molecular composition. This is referred to as phenotypic variation, and this type of variation has at least two possible outcomes for the pathogen: (1) it can alter its immunologic presentation to the host, subverting the host immune response from clearing the pathogen, or (2) it may confer some nonimmunologic, pathogenic advantage (e.g., attachment to or release from the host cell). The advantage conferred by this property is a selective one and depends on the circumstance in which the organism finds itself. For example, a selective advantage may favor a microbial pathogen that expresses a variant surface protein versus one that expresses the original surface protein because antibodies elicited to the original surface protein would result in clearance of the pathogen. The same is true outside of an immunologic context. During colonization, it may be favorable for an organism to express a certain adhesin, whereas the contrary may be true during the transmission phase of infection, when the release of organisms from host tissues may be favored. From the microbial pathogen's vantage point, the propensity for genetic variability confers an increased ability to adjust to adverse and unstable elements of the host environment. As will become apparent below, the "mind set" of some microbial pathogens is such that "it is better to have changed (phenotypic variation) and failed, than never to have changed at all."

> **Genomic plasticity** refers to the property of a microbial pathogen to retain genetic information critical to replication while at the same time varying genetic information that is functionally dispensable.

Phenotypic variation can be used synonymously with antigenic variation because antibodies historically have been used to monitor antigenic changes in the microbial composition and are referred to as such in this chapter. Antigenic variation is possible because microbial pathogens have short generation times and exhibit a high degree of genomic plasticity. The phenomenon of antigenic variation occurs among all classes of microbial pathogens—viruses, bacteria, fungi, and parasites (Table 17-1).

Genetic Mechanisms of Antigenic Variation: Point Mutation, Recombination, and Reassortment

There is no single genetic mechanism that microbial pathogens use to generate antigenic variation; in fact, some microbial pathogens use a combination of several mechanisms.

Viruses. Viruses generate diversity by at least three classic mechanisms (Table 17-2). Point mutation, the most common of these means, is used by RNA viruses because the viral RNA replicases that make new viral genomes lack the proofreading properties of DNA replicases. Because viruses replicate at a very high rate, they are able to generate a large number of variants (i.e., point mutations) during infection within a host. Recombination results in rearrangement of the viral genome and can lead to deletions or duplications of viral genes as well as to the acquisition of foreign genetic material. Recombination is more prevalent in DNA viruses because host recombination machinery exists for DNA but not for RNA. A third mechanism is a type of recombination involving reassortment of genomic fragments. Segmented RNA viruses possess discrete genomic segments independent of one another, much like chromosomes. If more than one virus strain infects the same cell, these segments may reassort during replication, producing progeny virions with divergent phenotypes. An excellent example of viral reassortment is provided by influenzavirus (see Chapter 3, Figure 3-10), one of the illustrative pathogens described in this chapter.

TABLE 17-1
Selected Examples of Antigenic Variation Among Viruses, Bacteria, Fungi, and Parasites

Microbial Pathogen	Variable Antigen	Pathogenic Function
Viruses		
Influenzavirus	Neuraminidase	Sialic acid cleavage
	Hemagglutinin	Attachment
Retroviruses	Surface unit (gp120)	Attachment
Bacteria		
Neisseria gonorrhoeae	Pilin	Fimbrial adhesin
	Opa	Afimbrial adhesin
	LOS	Endotoxin
Streptococcus pyogenes	M protein	Phagocytosis inhibition; binding of fibrinogen and albumin
Fungi		
Candida albicans	PEP1, others yet to be characterized	Determination of colony morphology, other virulence factors
Parasites		
Plasmodium falciparum	PfEMP-1	Surface adhesin
African trypanosomes	VSG	Phagocytosis inhibition

Note. PEP1 = pepsinogen 1; PfEMP-1 = Plasmodium falciparum infected erythrocyte membrane protein 1; VSG = variable surface glycoprotein.

TABLE 17-2
Mechanisms of Viral Genetic Diversity

Mechanism	Viral Genome
Point mutation	RNA or DNA*
Reassortment	Segmented RNAs
Recombination	DNA (commonly), RNA (rarely)

* DNA synthesis involves proofreading; RNA synthesis does not.

Bacteria. Bacteria generate antigenic diversity using mechanisms associated with their transcription, translation, and recombination machinery (Figure 17-1). Like viruses, these mechanisms include point mutations that can alter the antigenic properties of surface proteins or the susceptibility of microbial targets of antibiotics. Antigenic variation of bacteria can also involve genomic rearrangements. In classically understood genomic rearrangements, DNA is lost; this has important consequences for bacteria that are haploid and cannot afford to lose essential genetic information. Therefore, if genomic rearrangements do occur in bacteria, the rearranged genetic information must be preserved by some additional strategy. A third mechanism of generating antigenic diversity is gene conversion. This involves recombination between a variant gene and a homologous region of a recipient gene such that no genetic information is lost, as is the case for genomic rearrangements. During gene conversion, the incoming genetic material is placed in an expression (or recipient) locus, and the outgoing genetic material is placed in an unexpressed (or donor) genetic loci. This mechanism is the basis by which many pathogens undergo phase variation (see Chapter 1), a property that can result in the turning on or the turning off of the expression of bacterial pili and bacterial motility. The paradigm for this strategy is gonococcal pilin variation, which is described below. A fourth mechanism is translational regulation. In this form of regulation, a gene is constitutively transcribed, but the production of messenger RNA (mRNA) expressing a functional gene product is compromised by base substitutions or deletions made by the DNA polymerase that place the gene in the correct open reading frame (resulting in a functional gene product) or in one of the other two incorrect reading frames (resulting in a nonfunctional gene product). One common way that this occurs is by slipped-strand mispairing at hypermutable sites during bacterial replication.

Slipped-strand DNA synthesis can occur in segments of highly repetitive DNA. These regions are hypersusceptible to DNA endonucleases that nick the DNA and cause partial nuclease digestion in this region. The region is repaired but is deleted or repeated in one of the daughter cells, resulting in a frameshift mutation.

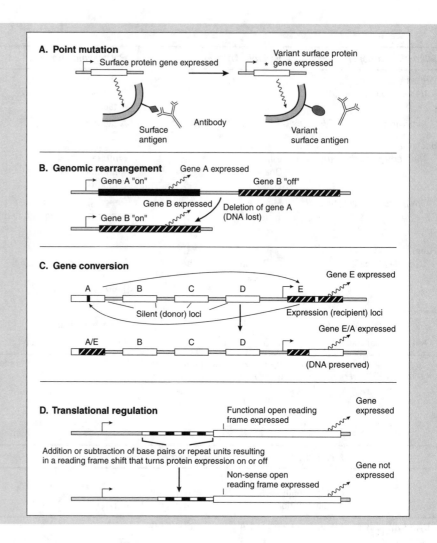

FIGURE 17-1 ▶

Mechanisms of Bacterial and Parasitic Antigenic Variation. Panel A illustrates point mutation variation of surface antigens and how this may allow a pathogen to evade the immune response. Note that the original antibody to the surface antigen no longer reacts with the variant surface antigen. Panel B illustrates what generally occurs during the course of genomic rearrangement, when DNA is typically lost from the chromosome. Panel C illustrates the mechanism of gene conversion in which a protein, typically expressed from a single locus (referred to as the recipient locus), is converted by genetic exchange with a variant, unexpressed (silent or donor) locus. Under these conditions, DNA is preserved. It is also possible for an entire gene to be replaced. Panel D demonstrates translational regulation that allows for expression or nonexpression of a protein depending on whether an alteration in the protein reading frame occurs.

Fungi and Parasites. Fungi and parasites exhibit even more sophisticated mechanisms of antigenic variation than do bacterial and viral pathogens. These mechanisms operate in a eukaryotic (diploid) background so that dispensable elements can be stored on the second copy of the chromosome. The parasitic paradigm for antigenic variation is *Trypanosoma brucei*, the causative agent of African sleeping sickness, which switches forms of its variable surface glycoprotein (VSG). In the absence of antibody specific for a given VSG, the organism proliferates, resulting in a parasitemia, until an appropriate immune response is evoked. Once an appropriate immune response is evoked, parasites expressing the specific VSG are cleared. However, variant *T. brucei* expressing different VSGs still remain and can subsequently proliferate. Consequently, *T. brucei* produces rising and falling waves of parasitemia by generating subpopulations of antigenically distinct VSGs that repeatedly challenge the immune response.

Antigenic variation can result from random mutagenic events that occur at equal frequency throughout the genome of the microbial pathogen (e.g., random point mutations of the influenzavirus genome) or they may be targeted to particular loci (e.g., gene conversion of the pilin loci of *Neisseria gonorrhoeae*). In the case of the latter, hypermutability is generally confined to a minority of nucleotide sequences within a genome. These hypermutable regions are referred to as contingency loci and encode many of the virulence factors described throughout this text. The advantage of having contingency loci is that microbial pathogens can produce a repertoire of variant molecules that modulate such properties as antigenicity, motility, chemotaxis, attachment to host cells, acquisition of nutrients, and sensitivity to antibiotics, while avoiding the deleterious effects that high mutation rates would have on loci encoding housekeeping functions (e.g., DNA synthesis, protein synthesis, respiration).

ILLUSTRATIVE PATHOGEN: The Gonococcus

Biologic Characteristics

N. gonorrhoeae is the etiologic agent of gonorrhea, which ranks among the most common sexually transmitted diseases (see Chapter 9). It is caused by a catalase-positive, oxidase-positive, gram-negative diplococcus that is one of two well-characterized pathogenic members of the genus *Neisseria*, the other being *Neisseria meningitidis*, the meningococcus (see Chapter 16 for a description of this genus). Pathogenic *Neisseria* spp., and the gonococcus in particular, have fastidious growth requirements that include a temperature optimum of 37°C, an atmosphere of 5% CO_2, and a media rich in preformed nutrients (e.g., blood or chocolate agar). Thayer-Martin or Martin-Lewis media are rich agar media containing antimicrobial compounds selective for the isolation of pathogenic *Neisseria* spp. from specimens contaminated with other microbial flora (e.g., vaginal or throat samples).

The gonococcal and meningococcal genomes are approximately 80% related. These two pathogens have been distinguished historically based on sugar fermentation patterns; the major difference is that meningococci can ferment maltose and the gonococcus cannot. From the point of view of how these organisms cause disease, the major difference between these two species is that gonococci are associated with genital tract infections and are extremely antigenically variable, whereas the meningococci are associated with meningitis and produce a characteristic capsule that is relatively antigenically stable (see Chapter 16).

Reservoir and Transmission

Gonorrhea is a disease that is exclusively confined to humans; there is no other animal or environmental reservoir. It is epidemic in many undeveloped countries and is endemic within the United States. Gonorrhea is a disease of high morbidity but of relatively low mortality. Between 1990 and 1995, an average of 500,000 cases of gonorrhea were reported in the United States yearly by the Centers for Disease Control and Prevention, with a fatality rate of less than 0.01%. In the past several years, the overall incidence has progressively declined, although the disease remains endemic and, in fact, may be on the rise in many geographic regions of the United States.

Gonococcal infection occurs almost exclusively by sexual intercourse and is transmitted most efficiently from men to women (90% per episode of intercourse), although both men and women are generally exposed to a large inoculum (10^6 organisms) during intercourse. Because of the differences in the anatomy and physiology between the male urinary tract and the female reproductive tract, the manifestations of disease in men and women are significantly different (Figure 17-2). What is common to gonococcal infection

> **N. gonorrhoeae** *(referred to as the gonococcus) is an oxidase-positive, catalase-positive, gram-negative diplococcus with a characteristic kidney bean shape.*

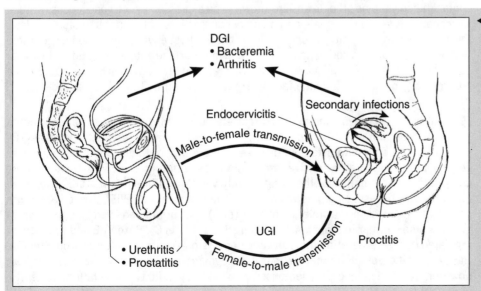

◄ **FIGURE 17-2**
Diversity of Gonococcal Diseases. DGI = *disseminated gonococcal infection;* UGI = *uncomplicated gonococcal infection.*

in both men and women is that *N. gonorrhoeae* flourishes on the genital mucosa of either gender.

In men, gonorrhea presents most often (> 90% of cases) as a self-limited urethral inflammation that results in burning on urination and a purulent yellow discharge. In approximately 10% of infected males, the disease is asymptomatic. By contrast, gonococcal disease in females is characterized by a spectrum of symptoms that include asymptomatic infection, mild endocervical inflammation, and upper genital tract disease. Of particular concern is the asymptomatic carriage of this organism by roughly one-third of all infected women. Asymptomatic infection of men and women is the reservoir that allows gonococci to be maintained within the human population.

Localized infections confined to the genital mucosa are referred to as uncomplicated gonococcal infection (UGI). In approximately 15% of untreated women, gonococcal infection progresses from the lower genital tract to the upper genital tract and involves infection of the fallopian tubes, resulting in pelvic inflammatory disease (PID). This can lead to scarring of the tubes and result in the potentially life-threatening condition of ectopic pregnancy (see Chapter 9) and infertility.

In approximately 1% of all gonococcal infections, and more frequently in women than men, gonococci gain access to the lymphatics, and a bacteremia ensues. This is particularly true for individuals with complement deficiencies. These types of infections are referred to as disseminated gonococcal infection (DGI). Left untreated, DGI involves the joints, and gonococcal arthritis is a common outcome. An increased DGI rate is associated with human immunodeficiency virus type 1 (HIV-1) infected individuals, and this population may become an increasingly important reservoir of gonococcal infection. Other gonococcal syndromes that occur in adults include pharyngitis and proctitis. In children, a common manifestation of gonococcal disease is ophthalmia neonatorum. This disease is transmitted from infected mother to child during delivery and can cause blindness in the infant. In the United States, this disease has been mitigated by the prophylactic treatment of infants at birth with 0.1% silver nitrate or an equally effective antimicrobial solution.

One hallmark of gonorrhea is the recurrence of infections in the same individual, often by the same gonococcal strain. Recurrent gonococcal infection has been attributed to limitations of the host immune response at the genital mucosa and the ability of gonococci to evade host defenses through the rapid variation of their surface antigens. Consequently, many of the virulence factors attributed to the gonococcus are antigenically variable surface antigens.

Virulence Factors

Gonococci are notable for their lack of toxin production. Aside from endotoxin and a contact hemolysin, no other toxins are known to be expressed by the gonococcus. Rather, the capacity to avoid the innate and memory components of the immune system allows these pathogens to multiply successfully within the host environment. Gonococci avoid immune detection by a sophisticated mechanism of surface antigen variation. The major surface antigens of the gonococcus are diagramatically shown in Figure 17-3. The recognized gonococcal virulence factors are summarized in Table 17-3 and described below.

Pili. Expression of pili is unambiguously correlated with virulence. In studies of human infection, 10^6 nonpiliated gonococci were required to cause infection, whereas 10^2 piliated gonococci could establish disease. Pili are fimbrial adhesins associated with gonococci that undergo extensive intrastrain phase and antigenic variation. They are composed predominantly of the antigenically variable pilin subunit, PilE, and small amounts of a tip associated adhesin, PilC. The variability of PilE is associated with gene conversion from multiple silent loci (*pilS*) that are encoded in the gonococcal chromosome (similar to that shown in Figure 17-1, Panel C). Both PilE and PilC can be regulated by phase variation through gene conversion events or by translational regulation. A specific host cell receptor that is recognized by PilC has yet to be identified; however, piliated gonococci demonstrate a high specificity for binding to genitoepithelial cells.

Most Common Diseases Associated with N. gonorrhoeae:
UGIs
  Urethritis
  Prostatitis
  Endocervitis
  Pharyngitis
  Proctitis
  Ophthalmia neotatorum (conjunctivitis)
Secondary infections
  Acute salpingitis
DGIs
  Bacteremia
  Arthritis

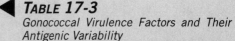

Virulence Factor	Mechanism of Variation	Effect of Variation	Result of Variation
Pilus	Gene conversion of a silent pilus locus into the expression locus	Antigenic variation	Evasion of the immune system
	Phase variation	Pilin expression turned on or off	Evasion of the immune system; attachment or release from a host cell
Opacity-associated proteins (Opas)	Phase variation	Opa expression turned on or off	Evasion of the immune system; attachment or release from a host cell
Porin	Intrastrain heterogeneity	Strain-to-strain heterogeneity	Lack of memory response to reinfection
Transferrin-binding proteins	Intrastrain heterogeneity	Strain-to-strain heterogeneity	Lack of memory response to reinfection
Lipooligosaccharide	Interstrain heterogeneity	Variation of surface carbohydrates	Evasion of the immune system
IgA1 protease	Antigenically stable	None	None

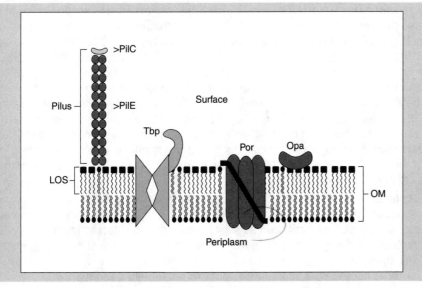

FIGURE 17-3
Surface Antigens of N. gonorrhoeae Associated with Antigenic Variation. LOS = lipooligosaccharide; Tbp = transferrin-binding protein; Por = porin; Opa = opacity-associated protein; OM = outer membrane.

Opa. The term Opa (for opaque) refers to the colony morphology of gonococci propagated on agar and viewed through a dissecting microscope. Colonies that appear opaque are correlated with the expression of a family of surface-associated, afimbrial adhesins referred to as opacity-associated (Opa) proteins, whereas transparent colonies are comprised of gonococci that do not express Opa proteins. As many as nine different Opa genes can be carried by any given gonococcal strain. Each of these Opa genes can be turned on and off by translational regulation (similar to that shown in Figure 17-1, Panel D). In addition, antigenic diversity can be generated by recombination between the Opa loci.

When expressed, Opa proteins are major components of the gonococcal cell surface. Polymorphoneutrophils (PMNs) function as afimbrial adhesins and allow gonococci to adhere intimately to host cells. Depending on the Opa variant expressed, gonococci preferentially adhere to different cell types (e.g., uroepithelial cells) and also may promote gonococcal invasion of host cells. Opa variability may explain how the gonococcus can exist in such diverse environments as the male urethra, the female cervix, the bloodstream, and synovial fluids.

Por. The most abundant protein in the gonococcal outer membrane is Por. This protein functions as a porin (see Chapter 1), allowing for the diffusion of small, hydrophilic compounds across the outer membrane. It is genetically stable within a given gonococcal isolate and forms the basis for the serogrouping of gonococcal strains. The role of Por in the pathogenesis of gonococcal infection is significant; it is known that intimate juxta-positioning of the gonococcal membrane with the eukaryotic cell membrane allows for transfer of Por to the host cell, resulting in alterations in ionic permeability of the plasma membrane. Por variants also may confer low-level antimicrobial resistance to gonococcal isolates by limiting the diffusion of certain antibiotics (e.g., penicillins) across the outer membrane.

Tbps. Transferrin sequesters free extracellular iron within the human host. In turn, pathogenic bacteria must be able to compete with this iron source for growth. Pathogenic *Neisseria* spp. do not secrete siderophores to compete for host iron. Rather, these organisms bind human transferrin to their surface and directly remove iron from this molecule, subverting the need for a siderophore. This is accomplished by the bacterium's transferrin-binding proteins (Tbps). The surface-associated extraction of transferrin-bound iron by the gonococcus is one of the reasons why gonococci flourish (i.e., multiply) on the mucosal surfaces of the human host. Like Por, strain-to-strain variation among the Tbps exists. This variation must reside in structurally dispensable regions of the Tbps and not in those residues that function in the binding and removal of iron from transferrin.

LOS. The gonococcal equivalent of gram-negative lipopolysaccharide (LPS) is lipo-oligosaccharide (LOS). As described in Chapter 1, this designation is given to distinguish LOS, which lacks the highly repeated O antigen, from LPS, which is characterized by this highly repeated O antigen. Gonococcal LOS has the identical endotoxic properties of LPS because the lipid A (toxic) components of either structure are virtually identical. The sugars that makeup the hydrophilic portion of the gonococcal LOS can vary depending on the expression of enzymes that encode its synthesis. The expression of these enzymes is under translational regulation (see Figure 17-1). LOS composition also may be influenced by the natural transformation (see Chapter 4) and genomic recombination of genes from heterologous gonococcal strains. Finally, LOS may be varied by the covalent attachment of a host-derived sialic acid residue to a terminal LOS galactose, a process referred to as sialylation. This modification effectively results in molecular mimicry (see Chapter 16) by rendering the sugars on the gonococcal surface similar in chemical composition to that of the host glycosylation patterns. It also hinders the capacity of complement to lyse these organisms.

IgA1 Protease. Like the meningococcus (see Chapter 16), the gonococcus produces an IgA1 protease that is thought to play a role in subverting the host immune response to gonococcal infection. Recent studies suggest that the gonococcal immunoglobulin A (IgA) protease also may play a role in modulating the intracellular survival of gonococci. The IgA1 protease distinguishes itself from the other gonococcal virulence factors described above because this protein does not exhibit antigenic variation.

Natural Transformation. The ability of pathogenic *Neisseria* to take up naked DNA efficiently from a lysed organism of the same species and to genetically recombine this DNA into their genome further contributes to the antigenic diversity of these organisms. Because transformation contributes to pilin and Opa antigenic variation, it is also considered to be a virulence factor.

Pathogenesis

Gonococci are considered facultative intracellular pathogens because their pathogenesis entails extracellular multiplication, attachment, endocytosis, transport, and exocytosis of gonococci by epithelial cells and neutrophils. The mechanism by which these organisms cause UGI is summarized in Figure 17-4. Upon gaining access to the cervix or urethra by sexual contact, these organisms subvert the humoral immune response by

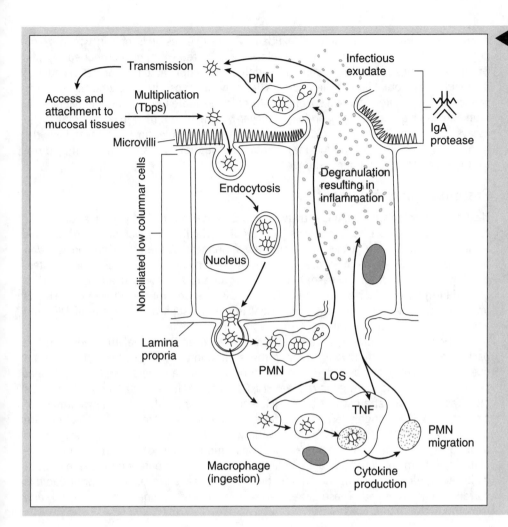

FIGURE 17-4
Summary of the Mechanism by which the Gonococcus Causes Disease on the Mucosal Surface. In this drawing, the prominent gonococcal virulence factors are emphasized. PMN = polymorphonuclear cell; Tbps = transferrin-binding proteins; LOS = lipooligosaccharide; TNF = tumor necrosis factor.

antigenic variation of surface molecules or by the production of IgA1 protease. Piliated *N. gonorrhoeae* then attach to nonciliated, low-columnar epithelial cells at or near the site of inoculation. Subsequently, intimate association between the gonococcal outer membrane and the epithelial plasma cell membrane occurs. This interaction may be mediated by nonfimbrial adhesins such as Opa proteins. Invasion of epithelial cells by gonococci results from the retraction of microvili to which gonococci are bound, which effectively encompasses the organism and creates a membrane-bound endocytic vesicle. Host-cell killing of bacteria within these vesicles is inhibited, perhaps by the membrane perturbing activity of Por. Next, the membrane-bound vesicles, containing multiple organisms, migrate close to the cytoplasmic face of the basal surface of the epithelial cell. Thus, vesicles are transported from the apical to the basal aspect of the cell, accompanied by multiplication of single organisms within vesicles or the coalescence and fusion of several vesicles. Fusion of the basal plasma and vesicular membranes ensues, followed by exocytosis of gonococci onto the basement membrane and lamina propria of the subepithelial space, where they may multiply in a sterile environment devoid of competing commensal organisms. Multiplication is aided by the ability of gonococci to obtain iron bound to host transferrin by the Tbps. In this location, a host inflammatory response, perhaps in response to LOS, causes the symptoms of UGI. Being in proximity to local lymphatics and blood vessels, the organism has the opportunity to gain access to systemic circulation and cause DGI (in approximately 1% of gonorrhea cases).

Diagnosis

A history of recent sexual activity, including the sexual activity of the patient's most recent contact, is useful for the diagnosis of gonococcal infections. In men, immediate laboratory diagnosis of gonococcal infection can be based on clinical symptoms and a direct Gram stain of their urethral exudate. A positive result is one in which gram-negative diplococci are found within or closely associated with polymorphoneutrophils. Gram staining of exudates from women is much more complicated to interpret because of the resident microbial flora of the vagina. A definitive diagnosis is established by isolating gonococci from male or female specimens (urethral exudate from males, a cervical swab from females) on selective agar (e.g., Thayer-Martin medium). Molecular diagnostic assays for antigen or nucleic acid detection are also available; however, these have the disadvantage of not allowing for antimicrobial susceptibility testing, which may prove useful in designing treatment regimens.

Prevention and Treatment

Next to abstaining from sexual activity, use of a barrier method of contraception (e.g., condoms) is the most effective means for preventing the transmission of gonorrhea. Like all sexually transmitted diseases, maintaining a monogamous relationship and knowing the sexual history of partners are also preventative measures. In the United States, gonorrhea is a reportable disease, meaning that all cases of gonorrhea diagnosed by a physician must be reported to the Centers for Disease Control and Prevention. This is important for tracking trends of gonococcal infection, such as outbreaks of DGI and antimicrobial resistant organisms.

Gonococcal infection generally responds well to antimicrobial treatment. In the past, penicillin was effective for treating these infections. However, the indiscriminate use of this antibiotic has led to the selection for resistant organisms, in particular penicillinase-producing *N. gonorrhoeae* (PPNG). In some United States communities, as many as 2% of all strains may be PPNG. Another consideration for the treatment of gonorrhea is that roughly 50% of all infected individuals are also coinfected with *Chlamydia* (see Chapter 9). Therefore, antimicrobial therapy is generally designed to treat both gonococcal and chlamydial infections simultaneously. Standards for the treatment of all forms of gonorrhea are regularly reported by the Centers for Disease Control and Prevention. For uncomplicated infections of mucosal surfaces, oral ciprofloxacin is currently recommended. These cases also respond to ceftriaxone, spectinomycin, and trimethoprim-sulfamethoxazole.

ILLUSTRATIVE PATHOGEN: Influenzavirus

Biologic Characteristics

The Orthomyxoviridae family is comprised of influenzavirus types A, B, and C. This family is characterized by spherical, enveloped virus particles possessing a genome consisting of eight single-strand RNA (ssRNA) molecules of negative polarity (seven ssRNA molecules in the case of influenzavirus type C) within a helical nucleocapsid (Figure 17-5). With two exceptions (i.e., matrix [M_1] and nonstructural [NS] RNA segments), each ssRNA encodes a single gene product. Bound to each viral RNA is a virus-encoded, RNA-dependent RNA transcriptase complex made up of three proteins (each of which are encoded on a separate ssRNA): PB_1 (initiates transcription), PB_2 (binds the caps of mRNAs), and PA (polymerizes nucleotide strands). The protein capsid is formed by the viral nucleoprotein (NP). M_1, the most abundant virion protein, forms a matrix between the nucleocapsid and the viral envelope. The influenzavirus envelope contains three viral proteins, the hemagglutinin (HA), neuraminidase (NA), and ion channel (M_2) proteins. HA is an envelope glycoprotein organized in trimers to form a stalk-like structure on the surface of the influenza virion. Smaller quantities of the tetrameric NA have a similar structure. Because of their exposure on the outer surface of the envelope, HA and NA are subject to, and correspondingly exhibit a higher level of, antigenic variation as a consequence of immune selection. The integral membrane ion channel protein designated M_2 is present in smaller quantities, apparently is less exposed, and presumably is not subject to this immunologic pressure.

Influenzavirus types A, B, and C are classified based on antigenic differences

> Instead of separate HA and NA proteins, the type C influenzavirus particle contains a protein, **HE**, that has combined hemagglutinatin and esterase activities and acts as the attachment protein of the virus.

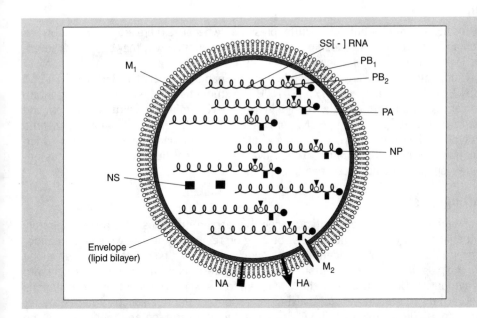

FIGURE 17-5
Composition of the Mature Influenzavirus Virion. The helical nucleocapsids are composed of eight segments. Each segment contains one ss[−]RNA molecule, nucleoproteins (NP), and polymerase proteins (PA, PB$_1$, PB$_2$). ss[−]RNA = single-stranded RNA with a negative polarity; HA = hemagglutinin; NA = neuraminidase; M$_2$ = ion channel protein.

between their NP and M proteins. Type A influenzaviruses are further divided into subtypes based on their HA and NA proteins. Among the human type A influenzaviruses, there are three different HA serotypes (H1, H2, or H3) and two NA serotypes (N1, or N2).

Reservoir and Transmission

Type A influenzaviruses can infect a variety of animals, including birds, horses, pigs, and man. They are responsible for most cases of human influenza. Aquatic birds act as the most important reservoir for type A influenzaviruses, and new viral strains probably evolve in these animals. These strains can then infect man directly or via other reservoirs (e.g., swine). In contrast, the only known reservoir for type B and type C influenzaviruses is humans. Influenzaviruses are transmitted from infected to uninfected persons by respiratory aerosols, making influenza a highly communicable disease.

Virulence Factors

The single most important determinant of influenzavirus virulence is the HA protein. The HA protein functions as an adhesin, binding to sialic acid (*N*-acetylneuraminic acid) residues that are commonly found on eukaryotic cell membrane proteins. This promotes virus entry into the cell. Interestingly, the HA of newly synthesized virions are glycoproteins containing sialic acid and thus are vulnerable to self-agglutination by the HA. However, as its name implies, NA enzymatically removes neuraminic (sialic) acid residues from these carbohydrates. Therefore, NA probably acts on the sialyl components of the HA glycoprotein to prevent influenzavirus autoagglutination and to facilitate the release of virus particles from the infected cell.

Another dimension adding to the capacity of influenzaviruses (particularly type A viruses) to cause disease is their ability to undergo antigenic variation. Antigenic drift (see Chapter 3), which is a direct consequence of point mutations in the HA gene (and the NA gene to a lesser degree), results in gradual changes in the antigenicity of the HA and NA proteins. This permits newly emerging strains to escape the protective antibodies formed in response to previous influenzavirus infections. Antigenic drift occurs yearly, from one flu season to the next. In contrast, it is theorized (and demonstrable in vitro) that a dramatically different type A serotype can arise abruptly when two type A viruses infect a common host cell (e.g., an aquatic bird or domesticated swine) and exchange RNA segments by genetic reassortment (antigenic shift). If the reassortant virus contains a novel HA (or NA gene), and this virus is transmitted to a human in whom it can replicate, virions will be produced that share few, if any, of the important surface antigenic epitopes of past influenzaviruses. Consequently, previous influenzavirus exposures offer no protection against this new virus serotype. Antigenic shifts among type A viruses seem to occur every 10–20 years. In nature, types B and C

In 1997, four people in Hong Kong died of influenza caused by a H5N1 serotype. This virus normally only infects fowl and was somehow contracted by at least 17 people. Fortunately, human-to-human transmission proved to be very inefficient.

viruses do not undergo antigenic shifts, presumably because there are no virus subtypes circulating in animal reservoirs. In part, this may account for why they cause less severe and less frequent human disease.

Antigenic shifts were responsible for the pandemics of 1918 (H1N1), 1957 (H2N2), 1968 (H3N2), and 1977 (H1N1). The student should recognize the signature of an antigenic shift; that is, the change in the H or N numbers of a virus strain from one year to another (e.g., H1N1 to H2N2, or H2N2 to H3N2). Rarely does an influenzavirus serotype that is infectious for an animal other than humans infect a human. Such infections are ominous because, like a novel reassortment human strain, previous immune responses are not protective.

Pathogenesis

Upon spread from an infected to a susceptible person, the virus adsorbs to respiratory epithelial cells by adhering to a sialyl-bearing protein receptor. The virus is then endocytosed into the cell. Acidification of the endosome causes fusion of the viral envelope with the plasma endosomal membrane, uncoating the nucleocapsid and releasing it into the cytoplasm. During this time, the M_2 protein forms an ion channel that allows protons to enter into the nucleocapsid, causing alterations in the nucleocapsid necessary for gene expression. Unlike most RNA viruses, active transcription and replication of the influenzavirus genome occurs in the nucleus.

The clinical symptoms of disease occur several days after infection. The patient experiences a form of tracheobronchitis characterized by malaise, sore throat, fever, myalgia, and an initially unproductive cough. The respiratory symptoms result from virus-induced damage to respiratory epithelium. Influenzaviruses can replicate and involve the lower respiratory tract as well. In severe cases, which often appear in neonates or the elderly, a primary influenzavirus pneumonia develops that can be fatal. In individuals suffering from other respiratory diseases (e.g., asthma, emphysema, cancer), influenza may foster a fatal secondary bacterial pneumonia. *Staphylococcus*, *Streptococcus*, and *Haemophilus* species are the most common bacterial copathogens. For example, the mortality rate of influenza complicated by staphylococcal pneumonia is 40%. Characteristically, influenzavirus epidemics always cause excess mortality from acute respiratory syndromes. Major determinants of disease outcome rest on previous immunologic experience with related influenzaviruses (i.e., the presence of at least partially protective antibodies in body fluids) and the general health of the infected individual.

Diagnosis

Influenza is diagnosed primarily by clinical symptoms associated with a febrile acute respiratory disease and epidemiologic considerations. The "flu" is a seasonal disease restricted to the winter months in northern climates. Typically, in the northern United States, flu peaks in December or January. Virus isolation, usually in chick embryo cells, is performed primarily for epidemiologic information. A variety of immunologic tests (e.g., complement fixation, inhibition of viral hemagglutination [HI] of chicken red blood cells) can be employed to detect an increase in serum immunoglobulin G (IgG) antibodies over the course of disease, but such tests are not routinely used in hospitals.

Prevention and Treatment

By far, the most practical and effective approach to influenza control is through yearly vaccination using a virus subunit preparation consisting of the HA and NA proteins. This vaccine is prepared from purified virus grown in embryonic eggs. Government public health laboratories, in conjunction with worldwide influenzavirus surveillance, permit the manufacture each year of a vaccine containing the envelope proteins of the virus strains most likely to be encountered. In the United States (Table 17-4), the vaccine is administered in October and November to those most vulnerable to influenza morbidity and mortality. These include the elderly, healthcare professionals, and those suffering from any condition that predisposes them to virus infections.

TABLE 17-4
Recent Changes in Influenzavirus Vaccines in the United States as a Result of Antigenic Drift

Virus Type	Virus Subtype	1995–1996	1996–1997	1997–1998
A	H3N2	A/Johannesburg/33/94[a]	A/Wuhan/359/95	A/Nanchang/993/95
A	H1N1	A/Texas/36/91	A/Texas/36/91	A/Johannesburg/82/96
B	—[b]	B/Beijing/184/93	B/Beijing/184/93	B/Harbin/07/94

[a] Strains are designated by the geographic site of isolation, the culture number, and the year of isolation.
[b] Type B viruses do not undergo antigenic shift, so a subtype is not designated.

Alternatively, amantadine and rimantadine are two relatively nontoxic drugs licensed for prevention or treatment of only type A influenzavirus. The target of these drugs is the M_2 envelope protein, which functions as an ion channel in the viral envelope. Amantadine and rimantadine (see Chapter 3, Figure 3-10) block the function of this channel and ultimately interfere with viral gene expression. Both drugs are most effective if administered before virus exposure. In people who are immunocompromised or allergic to egg proteins (which are present in the subunit vaccine because the virus is propagated in eggs), either drug can be used to prevent or treat influenza. Generally, the drugs are approximately 50% effective in preventing infection and approximately 70% effective in ameliorating disease.

RESOLUTION OF CLINICAL CASE

On the sixth day after discharge, the laboratory reported a positive influenzavirus culture. At this point, the patient's symptoms had resolved, and he was able to return to work.

The symptoms associated with this patient are typical of an influenzavirus pneumonia. The disease is seasonal, occurring in the winter months, and generally resolves on its own. Why this individual had such severe symptoms is not clear; it may be related to the strain of virus or to the individual's immune status. With this patient's history of smoking (predisposing him to infection) and his contact with diverse members of the community (teaching school), he is at risk for contracting a community-acquired respiratory infection. The fact that vaccination with the previous year's influenzavirus vaccine did not protect him from the current year's "flu" is not surprising because of year-to-year antigenic drift. In high-risk populations, vaccination for the prevention of influenza should be performed yearly, prior to the winter season.

REVIEW QUESTIONS

Directions: For each of the following questions, choose the **one best** answer.

1. In the pathogenesis of influenzavirus, the viral hemagglutinin (HA) is the most important virulence factor because it is
    (A) the transcriptase responsible for viral gene expression
    (B) the adhesin that binds to cell receptors
    (C) subject to a greater rate of mutation than other viral proteins
    (D) responsible for the cytopathic effects of the virus on infected cells
    (E) an RNA-binding protein that is part of the viral nucleocapsid

2. In the United States, during the fall and winter of 1996–1997, people at risk received a vaccine containing the HA and NA proteins of A/Wuhan/359/95 (H3N2), A/Texas/36/91 (H1N1), and B/Beijing/184/93. During that "flu" season," a virus strain—A/HongKong/35/97 (H2N1)—was isolated from a confirmed influenza patient. Which one of the following statements is correct?
    (A) The new virus isolate resulted from antigenic shift
    (B) The new virus isolate arose from antigenic drift
    (C) One is unable to distinguish between drift and shift as an explanation for how this new virus arose
    (D) This isolate must be a nonhuman influenzavirus strain that infected a human
    (E) The virus is a type A influenzavirus, so the 1996–1997 vaccine would provide adequate protective immunity

3. Which one of the following observations best describes why individuals who have had an initial gonococcal infection are often reinfected?
    (A) Gonococcal isolates are extremely virulent and can cause disease much more rapidly than a protective immune response can prevent infection
    (B) Gonococci are extremely antigenically variable, such that challenging an individual with the same gonococcal isolate that caused the initial infection results in a reinfection
    (C) Production of an IgA1 protease effectively neutralizes any previously established humoral immune response to gonococcal infection
    (D) The nonimmunogenic nature of the capsular polysaccharide expressed on the surface of gonococci results in a limited immune response to this organism
    (E) Gonococci infect a high proportion of HIV-1 infected individuals that cannot mount an immune response to an initial gonococcal infection

4. Gonococci and meningococci are 80% related at the level of their genomic DNA. Which one of the following virulence properties pertain to gonococci, but not to meningococci?
    (A) Expression of an IgA protease
    (B) Production of a polysaccharide capsule
    (C) Expression of highly variable cell surface proteins
    (D) Production of adhesin factors such as pili
    (E) The production of catalase and oxidase

5. Which one of the following statements is most true about the mechanisms of antigenic variation among viral pathogens?

    (A) All RNA viruses use genetic reassortment as their primary means of antigenic variation

    (B) The frequency of point mutations is much higher in an RNA virus with a segmented genome than a virus with a single RNA molecule

    (C) Reassortment of DNA molecules is a commonly used mechanism among DNA viruses

    (D) The frequency of point mutations leading to phenotypic changes is much higher in RNA viruses than in DNA viruses

    (E) Genetic recombination does not occur among DNA viruses

ANSWERS AND EXPLANATIONS

1. **The answer is B.** The purpose of this question is to test knowledge of the biology of influenzavirus as described in this chapter. The hemagglutinin, an envelope protein, possesses neither polymerase activity (option A) nor RNA-binding activity (option E). All viral genes are subject to approximately the same rate of random mutation, so option C is incorrect. There is no evidence that the HA protein is directly responsible for viral-induced cytopathology, so option D is incorrect.

2. **The answer is A.** Whenever a novel HA or NA subtype arises, it signals a reassortant virus (i.e., an antigenic shift). Shifts introduce unique antigenic changes, so a vaccine would not be effective (option E). Option B is wrong because antigenic drift refers to point mutations that do not alter the subtype (i.e., the HA and NA numbers stay the same). Option C is invalid because specific antibodies are routinely used to subtype influenzaviruses to determine if antigenic shift or drift occurred. Option D is wrong because HA subtypes 1–3 and NA subtypes 1–2 are human viruses; an animal-specific virus infecting humans, such as occurred late in 1997, would have a unique HA or HA subtype (e.g., H5N1).

3. **The answer is B.** Antigenic variation plays a major role in gonococcal reinfection. Option A is incorrect because gonococci produce few toxins and cause disease over the course of days. During this time, an immune response to stable gonococcal antigens should result in preventing the infection. Option C is not correct because although the IgA1 protease is produced, IgA1 is not the only antibody isotype produced during infection. IgA1 protease may contribute to reinfection, but it is much less important than antigenic variation. Option D is not correct because gonococci do not produce a capsular polysaccharide. Option E is not correct because even individuals free of HIV-1 experience gonococcal reinfection.

4. **The answer is C.** Antigenic variation is a major factor in gonococcal infection. Option A is incorrect because both gonococci and meningococci express IgA1 protease. Option B is incorrect because only meningococcal strains produce a polysaccharide capsule. Options D and E are incorrect because both meningococci and gonococci produce pili and are catalase-positive and oxidase-positive.

5. **The answer is D.** Unlike DNA synthesis, RNA synthesis does not entail proofreading functions that limit mutation frequencies. Option A is not correct because reassortment occurs only in viruses with a segmented genome. Option B is incorrect because mutation frequency is not affected by the configuration (segmentation) of a viral genome. Option C is incorrect because DNA viruses do not have segmented genomes that allow for reassortment. Option E is incorrect because genetic recombination occurs for all kinds of replicating DNA molecules, viral or nonviral.

18 IMMUNE EVASION STRATEGIES: CAPSULES

CHAPTER OUTLINE

Introduction of Clinical Case
Microbial Capsules
- Cellular Location
- Chemical Composition

Capsules as Virulence Factors
- Inhibition of Phagocytosis
- Immune Response to Encapsulated Pathogens

Illustrative Pathogen: *Streptococcus pneumoniae*
- Biologic Characteristics
- Reservoir and Transmission
- Virulence Factors
- Pathogenesis
- Diagnosis
- Prevention and Treatment

Resolution of Clinical Case
Review Questions

INTRODUCTION OF CLINICAL CASE

A 67-year-old man was essentially in good health until 6 days earlier, when he developed flu-like symptoms consisting of fever, headache, muscle aches, a stuffy nose, and a nonproductive cough. This upper respiratory infection appeared to be resolving until the previous evening, when the cough intensified, became productive, and was accompanied by stabbing right posterolateral chest pain. When the patient developed a shaking chill, he was brought to the emergency department by his wife.

The man's temperature was 103.2°F. There was dullness to percussion, and decreased breath sounds were heard at the right lung base posteriorly. Rales were heard two-thirds of the way up the right posterior and lateral lung. The leukocyte count was 12,340/mm³, with a differential of 78% polymorphonuclear leukocytes and 16% band forms. Chest x-ray showed a dense, alveolar infiltrate in essentially all of the right lower lobe, and a

Dullness to percussion is caused by fluid in the pleural spaces (i.e., pleural effusion, which is usually due to pneumonia). Decreased breath sounds are heard when the air spaces of the lung are filled with fluid (i.e., edema). Pneumonia and heart failure are frequent causes of this physical finding.

This is an elevated white blood cell count with an increased fraction of neutrophils and above-normal numbers of immature neutrophils (bands). This pattern is indicative of the host's response to systemic infection.

small right pleural effusion. A Gram stain of the sputum showed numerous polymorphonuclear leukocytes and mixed flora, primarily gram-positive cocci. A sputum culture and two blood cultures were obtained, the patient was given antibiotics, and he was admitted to the hospital.

- From what illness is this man suffering?
- What pathogen is responsible for this man's illness?
- What is the most important virulence factor of this pathogen, and how does this virulence factor contribute to pathogenesis?

MICROBIAL CAPSULES

Internalization into professional phagocytes is usually lethal for extracellular pathogens and those intracellular pathogens specialized for infecting nonphagocytic cells; consequently, these pathogens typically employ one or more strategies to avoid being engulfed by phagocytes (see Overviews, Parts I and III). One of the most common and most important of such antiphagocytic strategies is the production of an extracellular capsule.

Examples of some medically important encapsulated pathogens are given in Table 18-1. Notice from Table 18-1 that most encapsulated microorganisms are bacteria. However, there is at least one medically important encapsulated fungus, *Cryptococcus neoformans*, which is a very important opportunistic pathogen that commonly causes meningitis in human immunodeficiency virus (HIV)–positive individuals (see Chapter 28).

TABLE 18-1 ▶
Examples of Medically Important Encapsulated Microorganisms

Microorganism	Capsule
Streptococcus pneumoniae	Polysaccharide (approximately 90 types known)
Streptococcus pyogenes	Hylauronic acid
Bacillus anthracis	Polypeptide (polyglutamic acid)
Haemophilus influenzae type b	Polyribosylribitol phosphate (PRP or PRRP)
Neisseria meningitidis	Polysaccharides (capsule of each group has a different polysaccharide composition—note that the group B capsule contains sialic acid)
Salmonella typhi	Polysaccharide (called Vi antigen)
Klebsiella pneumoniae	Polysaccharide (referred to as K antigen)
Pseudomonas aeruginosa	Polysaccharide (called alginate)
Cryptococcus neoformans	Polysaccharide
Escherichia coli	K polysaccharides (over 80 different *E. coli* capsular polysaccharides have been identified; these polysaccharides are referred to as K antigens, e.g., the K1 antigen is a sialic acid polymer)

Cellular Location

When present, capsules are located on the outer microbial surface (see Chapter 1), an excellent location for capsules to carry out their antiphagocytic, antidessication, and adherence functions.

The presence of a capsule can be demonstrated microscopically by suspending an encapsulated microorganism in India ink. As shown in Figure 18-1, capsules repel the India ink particles; consequently, encapsulated microorganisms appear to be surrounded by a clear halo against a dark background. This India ink stain, which is sometimes referred to as a capsule stain, can be diagnostically useful. For example, if India ink staining demonstrates the presence of encapsulated yeast cells in cerebrospinal fluid (CSF), this provides evidence that a patient with meningitis is infected with *C. neoformans* (see below).

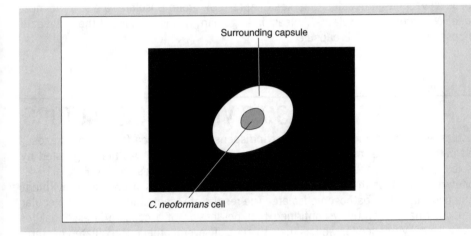

◀ **FIGURE 18-1**
*Microscopic Appearance of an Encapsulated Microorganism, **Cryptococcus neoformans**, after India Ink Staining (1000 × magnification)*

Chemical Composition

Microbial capsules are typically composed of polysaccharides (the major exception to this generalization is the capsule of *Bacillus anthracis*, which is a polypeptide composed of glutamic acid; see Table 18-1). Capsules usually, but not always, contain a single type of polysaccharide, which typically differs between microbial species. However, a few taxonomically unrelated pathogens produce chemically identical capsular polysaccharides. Most notably, the group B *Neisseria meningitidis* capsular polysaccharide and the capsular polysaccharide found in *Escherichia coli* K1 are composed of the same polysaccharide.

Conversely, the chemical composition of the capsular polysaccharide often varies among different isolates belonging to the same microbial species. Such intraspecies variations in capsular polysaccharide composition typically result in antigenic differences that can be exploited for classification purposes. For example, antigenic differences between capsular polysaccharides are used to classify *N. meningitidis* isolates into several serogroups (see Chapter 16). Furthermore, over 80 serologically different types of capsules (referred to as K antigens) have been identified for *E. coli* (see Chapter 12). However, the best-studied example of capsular diversity within a single microbial species is the pneumococcus (*Streptococcus pneumoniae*). Each clinical pneumococcal isolate can be assigned to one of approximately 90 serotypes, depending on the antigenic reactivity of its capsule. These antigenic differences reflect intraspecies variations in the chemical composition of the pneumococcal capsular polysaccharide, which consists of repeating units of 2–8 monosaccharides linked into branched or unbranched polymers (Table 18-2). The polysaccharide composition of a pneumococcal capsule can also influence the thickness of the capsular layer. For example, type 3 pneumococci typically produce a thick capsule.

As shown in Table 18-1, both N. meningitidis *group B and* E. coli *K1 produce a **sialic acid capsule**. This capsule inhibits phagocytosis but is poorly immunogenic (sialic acid is not recognized as a foreign molecule by the immune system, since the human body produces many sialic acid–containing proteins and lipids). The similar composition of their capsules gives group B* N. meningitidis *and* E. coli *K1 similar protection against phagocytosis and helps to explain why* E. coli *K1 and group B* N. meningitidis *are both important causes of meningitis.*

Many Enterobacteriaceae *besides* E. coli *produce K antigens, which are typically capsular polysaccharides of varying composition.*

Serotype 3 pneumococci are highly virulent, suggesting that capsule thickness may also influence virulence.

◀ **TABLE 18-2**
Chemical Composition of Some Representative Pneumococcal Capsules

Capsular Serotype	Constituent Monosaccharides
2	Rhamnose, glucose, and glucuronic acid
3	Glucose and glucuronic acid
6	Galactose, glucose, and rhamnose
14	Galactose, glucose, and *N*-acetylglucosamine

Besides their usefulness for classification and epidemiologic purposes, intraspecies differences in capsule composition (and thickness) are also important, since they can influence virulence. For example, fewer than 25 of the approximately 90 known serotypes of *S. pneumoniae* are responsible for more than 90% of cases of pneumococcal pneumonia in unvaccinated people. Similarly, even when the protective effects of meningococcal vaccines are factored in (see Chapter 16), group B isolates are still the most virulent *N. meningitidis* isolates. At least in large part, this is because of the sialic acid composition of the group B capsule.

CAPSULES AS VIRULENCE FACTORS

The experiments by Griffith are perhaps the single most important study in biology as they uncovered the principle of transformation (see Chapters 1 and 5). Attempts to discover the chemical nature of the "transforming factor" behind Griffith's results eventually led to the identification of DNA as the hereditary molecule.

While Griffith's results are highly suggestive (and were very sophisticated for their time), they did not rule out the possibility that some unrecognized gene, co-transferred with capsule production, was responsible for the conversion of avirulent to virulent pneumococci. As indicated in the text, the importance of the pneumococcal capsule for virulence has now been unambiguously demonstrated by molecular biology techniques.

Capsules are generally important, if not indispensable, virulence factors for encapsulated pathogens. The importance of capsules in pathogenesis was first suggested by classic experiments conducted in the 1920s by Griffith. Griffith's results (Figure 18-2) strongly suggest that the acquisition of a capsule can convert a previously avirulent pneumococcus into a pathogenic isolate. The results of recent studies using molecular approaches have definitively confirmed that possession of a capsule is essential for pneumococcal virulence (as well as the virulence of several other encapsulated bacteria such as *B. anthracis*). The importance of capsules for virulence also receives support from clinical observations indicating that natural recovery (i.e., recovery without antimicrobial therapy) from pneumococcal pneumonia, for example, usually correlates with the patient's development of anticapsular antibodies.

Capsules contribute to microbial virulence in several ways. First, they can facilitate disease transmission by preventing desiccation (drying) of the encapsulated pathogen. This helps to explain why so many inhalation-acquired pathogens (which might otherwise be killed by desiccation during airborne transmission) are encapsulated. Capsules can also promote colonization of both mucosal surfaces and inanimate objects. The ability of capsules to adhere to inanimate objects helps explain why, for example, encapsulated pathogens are common causes of nosocomial infections in people with indwelling catheters (see Chapter 28).

Inhibition of Phagocytosis

While capsules also help pathogens adhere and resist dessication, the major pathogenic function of capsules is to exert a potent antiphagocytic effect, which contributes to pathogen survival in vivo. The antiphagocytic properties of capsules have been apparent for many years, as established by experiments such as those shown in Table 18-3.

TABLE 18-3 ▶

Evidence That the Hyaluronic Acid Capsule of Group A Streptococci Has Potent Antiphagocytic Properties

Treatment of Group A Streptococci	Capsule Present	Percent of Group A Phagocytosed
None (control)	+	3
Hyaluronidase	−	49

What has not yet been fully elucidated is the molecular basis by which capsules exert their antiphagocytic effects. Evidence suggests that the antiphagocytic properties of capsules may involve some or all of the following:

1. Capsules can physically interfere with phagocytosis. The presence of a surface capsule makes it more difficult for a phagocyte to attach to and engulf an encapsulated microorganism. At least two physical properties of capsules probably contribute to this effect:

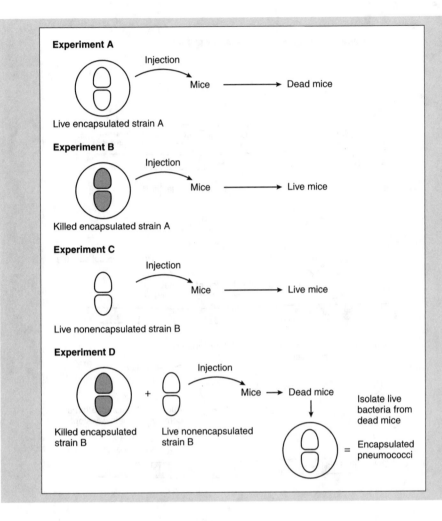

◀ **FIGURE 18-2**
Griffith Experiment: Evidence That the Pneumococcal Capsule Is Important for Virulence. *In a series of experiments, mice were injected with live or killed pneumococci, as indicated, and later inspected for viability. Besides providing key support for the importance of the capsule for pneumococcal virulence, experiment D also illustrates the principle of transformation.*

- Most capsules are composed of "slimy" polysaccharides, making a capsule-encoated microbe "slippery" to the phagocyte.
- There are usually charge repulsions between the capsule and phagocyte.

2. Capsules interfere with activation of the alternate complement cascade. Since the alternate complement cascade promotes opsonization of pathogens (and lysis of some gram-negative pathogens) in the period before an antibody response develops, this is a very important host defense mechanism. Capsules can interfere with activation of the alternate complement pathway in several ways:

- The presence of a capsule can interfere with the access of alternate complement pathway components to underlying microbial molecules that would otherwise be very reactive with these alternate complement pathway factors. For example, the pneumococcal capsule is thought to block access of factor B to any C3b fragments deposited on pneumococcal molecules underlying the capsule (Figure 18-3); this stops further activation of the alternate complement pathway.
- Some capsules bind serum factors that inhibit activation of the alternate complement pathway. Coating the microbial surface with these inhibitory factors blocks activation of the alternate complement cascade. For example, the sialic acid–rich capsule of group B streptococci binds serum factor H, which inhibits C3b deposition on group B streptococci (Figure 18-3).
- Some capsules contain embedded enzymes that can block or inactivate components of the alternate complement pathway. For example, group B streptococci make a C5a-degrading enzyme, which blocks C5a-induced PMN chemotaxis to the site of infection.

Note that capsules of group B streptococci can interfere with phagocytosis in several ways.

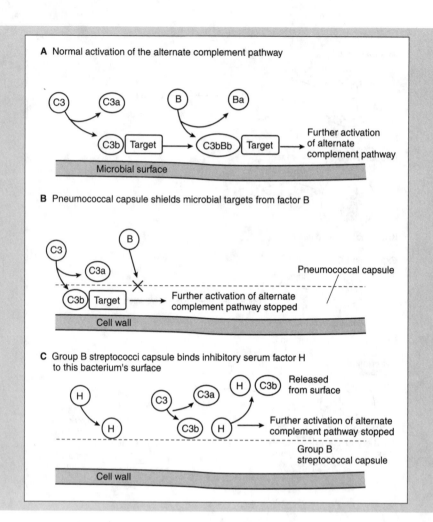

FIGURE 18-3 ▶

How Capsules May Interfere with Activation of the Alternate Complement Pathway. (A) Early steps in the activation of the alternate complement pathway. C3 is converted to C3b, which binds to a target on the microbial surface. Factor B of the alternate complement pathway is then cleaved and the Bb cleavage product binds to C3b deposited on the microbial surface, forming BbC3b convertase. This leads to further activation of the alternate complement pathway (including production of C5a, which is chemotactic for phagocytes, and continued deposition of more C3b, which is an opsonin, on the microbial surface). (B) The pneumococcal capsule inhibits the access of factor B to the microbial surface, thus inhibiting further activation of the alternate complement pathway. (C) The capsule of group B streptococci binds serum factor H to the microbial surface. Serum factor H is a natural inhibitor of alternate complement pathway activation that acts by binding and removing C3b from the microbial surface.

A Normal activation of the alternate complement pathway

B Pneumococcal capsule shields microbial targets from factor B

C Group B streptococci capsule binds inhibitory serum factor H to this bacterium's surface

IMMUNE RESPONSES TO ENCAPSULATED PATHOGENS

Because capsules are so effective at interfering with phagocytosis, using the mechanisms just described, infections involving encapsulated pathogens often have a fatal outcome unless effective antimicrobial therapy is administered. If recovery from an infection with an encapsulated pathogen does occur in the absence of antimicrobial therapy, it generally requires that the patient develop a strong antibody response directed against the capsule. Once present, these anticapsular antibodies promote efficient opsonization of the encapsulated pathogen.

The polysaccharide composition of most microbial capsules has important consequences for the formation of capsular antibodies. Since polysaccharide antigens usually generate only a T-cell–independent humoral immune response, and young children and the elderly (see Part VII) have considerable difficulties in mounting strong T-cell–independent humoral immune responses, it is not surprising that encapsulated microorganisms are particularly important causes of infection in children (e.g., *N. meningitidis*, *Haemophilus influenzae* type b, *S. pneumoniae*) and the elderly (e.g., *S. pneumoniae*).

ILLUSTRATIVE PATHOGEN: *Streptococcus pneumoniae*

Biologic Characteristics

S. pneumoniae, also known as the pneumococcus, is a gram-positive, lancet-shaped coccus that commonly grows in pairs, referred to as diplococci (Figure 18-4). The pneumococcus is assigned to the genus *Streptococcus* because of its morphology (gram-positive cocci), energy metabolism (like other streptococci, the pneumococcus obtains its energy exclusively through fermentation), and failure to produce catalase. As mentioned earlier in this chapter, the pneumococci readily undergo natural transformation (see Chapter 5), which contributes to the spread of pneumococcal antibiotic resistance and may also help maintain virulence factor diversity within the *S. pneumoniae* population.

> Because of its arrangement in diplococci, the pneumococcus was once named Diplococcus pneumoniae.

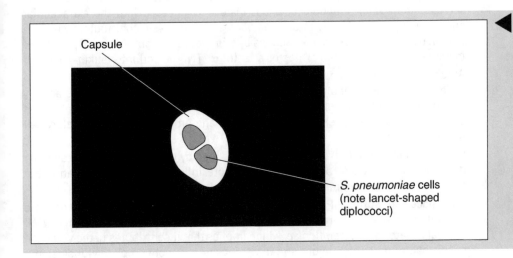

Capsule

S. pneumoniae cells (note lancet-shaped diplococci)

FIGURE 18-4
Microscopic Appearance of **Streptococcus pneumoniae** *under India Ink Staining (1000 × magnification).* Note the presence of the capsule and the arrangement of these bacteria as diplococci.

Most strains of *S. pneumoniae* grow best when incubated in a 5% to 10% carbon dioxide–containing atmosphere. The pneumococci are α-hemolytic but can be readily differentiated from other α-hemolytic streptococci (e.g., *Streptococcus viridans*). First, pneumococcal growth is inhibited by optochin, while this chemical has no effect on the growth of viridans streptococci. Second, the addition of bile or deoxycholate to a culture promotes the lysis of pneumococci but does not affect viridans streptococci. Note that the pneumococci are prone to low levels of spontaneous lysis even in the absence of bile or deoxycholate. This "autolysis" (self-lysis) results from *S. pneumoniae* producing autolytic enzymes (referred to as autolysins) that can be activated to break down the peptidoglycan component of the pneumococcal cell wall. Because of their autolytic tendencies, pneumococci are relatively challenging to Gram stain accurately (older cells can easily stain gram-negative, as their cell wall is degraded).

Reservoir and Transmission

The pneumococcus is only a human pathogen. This bacterium is typically spread person-to-person via the inhalation of aerosols. Interestingly, *S. pneumoniae* is transiently present in the nasopharynx of about 25% of the healthy human population, which provides an important reservoir for this bacterium.

The presence of *S. pneumoniae* in many healthy people indicates that there is an opportunistic component to pneumococcal disease. This view is supported by clinical observations indicating that the frequency of pneumococcal pneumonia increases with age (as immune function declines) and often follows a viral illness (which can impair the function of the mucociliary escalator). Virtually anything (e.g., age, immunodeficiencies, alcoholism, malnutrition) that impairs host defenses increases the risk of pneumococcal disease. The highest incidence of pneumococcal infections occurs during the winter and early spring, in part because the transmission of pneumococci is facilitated by people spending more time in crowded indoor environments at that time of year.

Virulence Factors

Capsule. The importance of the polysaccharide capsule as the major virulence factor of the pneumococci has already been stressed in this chapter. Recall that each pneumococcal isolate produces one of approximately 90 serologically distinct types of capsule and that certain capsular serotypes appear to function better as virulence factors than others.

Noncapsular Factors. These have also been implicated in the virulence of *S. pneumoniae*, including the following.

Pneumolysin. Pneumolysin is a membrane-active toxin that belongs to the sulfhydryl-activated toxin family (see Chapter 20). Interestingly, pneumolysin is not secreted from viable pneumococci but instead is released into the extracellular environment upon autolysis of *S. pneumoniae*. Pneumolysin contributes to inflammation during pneumococcal infections by stimulating the production of proinflammatory cytokines (e.g., tumor necrosis factor-α [TNF-α] and interleukin-1 [IL-1]).

Autolysin. As mentioned above, *S. pneumoniae* produces enzymes (referred to collectively as autolysins) that break down peptidoglycan. This enzymatic activity results in lysis of the pneumococci (see Chapter 1). Lysis of the cell wall contributes directly to virulence by releasing pneumolysin and producing proinflammatory cell wall fragments.

Cell Wall Fragments. Cell wall fragments produced by the autolysin-induced breakdown of pneumococcal peptidoglycan promote inflammation by stimulating the production of proinflammatory cytokines such as IL-1 and TNF-α.

Pneumococcal Surface Protein A (PspA). PspA shows structural and antigenic variability between different pneumococcal strains. PspA is found in nearly all clinical isolates of *S. pneumoniae*, which implies that it contributes to the virulence of this bacterium. The role of PspA in pathogenesis is not completely understood, but it may help interfere with complement activation.

Immunoglobulin A (IgA) Protease. Like several other inhalation-acquired pathogens (see Chapters 7 and 19), the pneumococcus produces an IgA protease that may facilitate colonization by promoting fabulation (see Chapters 7 and 19), thereby inhibiting opsonization. IgA protease also promotes colonization by interfering with the clearance of pneumococci by the mucociliary escalator (see Chapters 7 and 19).

Neuraminidase and Surface Protein Adhesins. The mechanisms by which *S. pneumoniae* cells adhere to the respiratory epithelium remain controversial, but some evidence suggests that this adherence may involve the pneumococci's ability to produce neuraminidase and still unidentified surface protein adhesins.

> *Neuraminidase removes sialic acids from mammalian glycoproteins and thus may alter the surface of the respiratory epithelium so it becomes more favorable for pneumococcal adhesion.*

Pathogenesis

In order to initiate pathogenesis, *S. pneumoniae* must first enter the body (often this occurs via inhalation) and then colonize a favorable location (typically, the initial colonization site is the nasopharynx). While the specific virulence factors contributing to this initial colonization remain controversial, likely candidates include adhesins, neuraminidase, and IgA protease. Once present in the nasopharynx, pneumococci may then be aspirated deeper into the respiratory tract. Under conditions where host defenses are suboptimal (e.g., in an elderly or alcoholic person), the aspirated *S. pneumococci* can sufficiently evade the clearance mechanisms and immune defenses of the lower respiratory tract so that colonization of the lower respiratory tract occurs. Several strategies are used by pneumococci to survive in, and colonize, the lower respiratory tract:

- Production of H_2O_2, which inhibits the function of ciliated cells and thus reduces clearance of *S. pneumoniae* by mucociliary clearance mechanisms (see Chapter 7)
- Production of IgA protease, which probably helps prevent the clearance of pneumococci via the mucociliary escalator and inhibits opsonization
- Production of pneumolysin, which also inhibits the function of ciliated cells and phagocytic cells
- Production of a polysaccharide capsule, which (as discussed) has potent antiphagocytic activity

Once *S. pneumoniae* has successfully colonized and multiplied in the lungs, a powerful inflammatory response is evoked, resulting in the symptoms of pneumococcal pneumonia (see below). Pneumococcal factors important in eliciting this inflammation include pneumolysin and cell wall fragments, which, as mentioned previously, trigger the production and release of potent proinflammatory cytokines such as TNF-α and IL-1.

Induction of an inflammatory response during pneumococcal pneumonia has several important pathologic consequences:

- It causes a significant accumulation of fluid (referred to as edema) in the lungs. This edema interferes with gas exchange (which can lead to death by suffocation) and facilitates the spread of pneumococci throughout the lung.
- It results in fever and shock (mediated by cytokines such as TNF-α and IL-1).
- It facilitates the entrance of *S. pneumoniae* into the bloodstream. This explains why bacteremia is such a common consequence of pneumococcal infection. Once present in blood, *S. pneumoniae* can infect many body sites outside the respiratory tract (e.g., pneumococci can cause endocarditis and peritonitis). However, *S. pneumoniae* is notorious for its ability to cause meningitis. Presumably, the entrance of pneumococci across the blood–brain barrier into the meninges is facilitated by the same inflammatory processes used to gain entrance into the blood.

Despite the availability of a pneumococcal vaccine (see below), pneumococcal pneumonia remains the leading cause of bacterial pneumonia. Furthermore, even with antimicrobial therapy, pneumococcal pneumonia has a mortality rate of 5% to 10%. Clinically, pneumococcal pneumonia is characterized by a sudden onset, usually beginning with a shaking chill and high fever. Commonly, the patient has a cough, producing "rusty" sputum (which derives its red color from red blood cells), and pleuritic pain. Without therapy, patients who recover continue these symptoms for 5 to 10 days until a "crisis" occurs. During this crisis, there is a sudden drop in temperature and a general improvement in the patient's symptoms. This recovery correlates with the patient's development of effective levels of opsoninizing anticapsular antibodies. Since pneumococcal pneumonia does not cause permanent damage to the lungs, no long-term respiratory problems are present if the patient survives.

Pneumococcal meningitis affects all ages, but it has been the leading cause of bacterial meningitis in adults. Pneumococcal meningitis typically follows pneumococcal pneumonia but can also develop after pneumococcal infections at other body sites and sometimes occurs even in previously asymptomatic patients. Because of the intense inflammation induced during pneumococcal meningitis, untreated cases of this meningitis have higher rates of neurologic sequelae than meningitis caused by *H. influenzae* type b or *N. meningitidis*. Fortunately, the introduction of combined treatment with antimicrobials and dexamethasone has lessened the incidence of neurologic problems in patients surviving pneumococcal meningitis.

S. pneumoniae is also one of the most important causes of otitis media and sinusitis. Pneumococcal otitis media is particularly common in young children recovering from a viral infection. This infection is becoming increasingly difficult to treat because of the recent increase in antibiotic resistance in the *S. pneumoniae* population.

Cell wall breakdown products also contribute to the inflammation during other illnesses (e.g., pertussis; see Chapter 29).

Before the introduction of antimicrobial therapy, pneumococcal pneumonia was fatal in at least one-third of infected patients.

Although S. pneumoniae *has, until recently, been very sensitive to β-lactam antibiotics, the use of β-lactam agents to treat pneumococcal meningitis once presented problems. The reason was that β-lactam antibiotics induce lysis of the pneumococci, which releases pneumolysin and cell wall fragments, increasing inflammation and leading to further swelling of the brain. However, by the use of dexamethasone, an anti-inflammatory corticosteroid, along with β-lactams (or other effective antibiotics), the mortality rate of pneumococcal meningitis has been reduced from 40% to 5%, and the frequency of neurologic sequelae in survivors has also been dramatically reduced.*

Pneumococcal otitis media and sinusitis typically result from pneumococci in the nasopharynx entering into the eustachian tube or sinuses.

Diagnosis

Because its onset and symptoms are relatively distinct, pneumococcal pneumonia can often be suspected on clinical grounds (note that it is uncommon to see more than two or three of these characteristics in a single patient):

Preceded by upper respiratory tract infection	Productive cough, "rusty" sputum
Abrupt onset	Pleuritic pain
True rigor	Tachypnea and dyspnea
Rapid rise in temperature	Lobar infiltrate

Rigor is a "total-body" shaking chill. Pleuritic pain is pain in the chest area arising from the pleura. It is usually worse when one takes a deep breath or coughs. Tachypnea is increased frequency of breathing. Dyspnea is the subjective feeling of not being able to get enough air.

Because S. pneumoniae colonization of the nasopharynx is relatively common, it is important that the sputum sample be mucus from the lungs, not saliva.

Since S. pneumoniae is relatively fastidious, this bacterium cannot always be cultured from an individual with pneumococcal pneumonia (i.e., a negative culture does not necessarily eliminate a possible diagnosis of pneumococcal pneumonia).

Quellung is German for "swelling." This assay involves mixing a specimen (e.g., sputum or CSF) with antibodies to pneumococcal capsular polysaccharides. In the presence of the proper antibody, the capsule will appear swollen under the microscope. The quellung reaction can be performed with a polyvalent antiserum against many pneumococcal capsular serotypes, or with antiserum specific for one capsular serotype (this approach can be used to identify the particular serotype of pneumococci involved in the infection).

Since these clinical features do not clearly differentiate pneumococcal pneumonia from other bacterial pneumonias, laboratory confirmation of this clinical suspicion is also important. Usually this involves Gram staining a sputum sample in a search for the presence of gram-positive "lancet-shaped" diplococci and neutrophils; when more than 10 of these gram-positive diplococci are present per oil immersion field, it is highly probable that the patient has pneumococcal pneumonia. Culture of an appropriately collected sputum specimen on blood agar can provide final laboratory confirmation of this diagnosis. On culture, pneumococcal isolates should be catalase-negative, optochin-sensitive, bile-soluble, α-hemolytic, gram-positive diplococci. *S. pneumoniae* can also be identified by the *quellung reaction*, which involves mixing a specimen with antibodies to pneumococcal capsules in a search for "swelling" in pneumococci.

Microscopic examination of Gram-stained CSF is essential for diagnosing pneumococcal meningitis. Blood or CSF cultures may also help diagnose cases of this meningitis, as well as pneumococcal bacteremia. If cultures are negative, serologic tests (e.g., latex agglutination tests) specific for detecting the presence of pneumococcal capsules in CSF or blood may be used.

Prevention and Treatment

When an effective antibiotic is administered during a case of pneumococcal pneumonia, the response can be impressive. Symptoms, such as fever and cough, sometimes noticeably abate within as little as 12 to 24 hours of antimicrobial treatment. Pneumococcal infections have traditionally been responsive to pencillins. Unfortunately, this pathogen is now developing considerable resistance to β-lactams and other antibiotics (Table 18-4; see Resolution of Clinical Case). The increasing resistance of pneumococci to β-lactam antibiotics is thought to result, at least in part, from pneumococci producing altered transpeptidases (see Chapters 4 and 5) that no longer strongly bind β-lactam antibiotics.

The increasing problem of pneumococcal antibiotic resistance makes vaccination against pneumococcal diseases ever more attractive. As this book is being written, the licensed pneumococcal vaccine consists of a mix of the 23 different pneumococcal capsular polysaccharides responsible for most (approximately 90%) pneumococcal in-

TABLE 18-4 ▶

Antibiotic Resistance of Pneumococci

- For many years, all isolates of *Streptococcus pneumoniae* were penicillin-susceptible. Until 1965, most isolates were susceptible to less than 0.04 µg/mL, and all strains had minimum inhibitory concentrations (MICs) of less than 0.1 µg/mL.

- From 1987 to 1992, the proportion of *S. pneumoniae* strains highly resistant to penicillin (MIC > 1.0 µg/mL) increased from 0.02% to 1.3%.

- In a survey of invasive pneumococcal disease in the United States (1993), antibiotic-resistant organisms caused 19.4% of the cases: relative penicillin resistance (MIC > 0.1 to < 1.0 µg/mL) was found in 7.6%, and high-level penicillin resistance occurred in 1.4%; 11% of strains were resistant to other antibiotics.

- Strains of pneumococci that are more resistant to penicillin are often resistant to other antibiotics that would logically be used as alternates to treat pneumococcal disease, including first- and second-generation cephalosporins, erythromycin and other macrolides, quinolones, clindamycin, and trimethoprim-sulfamethoxazole.

- Because of the high levels of antibiotic that can be achieved, the treatment of pneumococcal pneumonia with or without bacteremia has not changed. Penicillin or another equally active β-lactam antibiotic is administered. If high-level penicillin resistance is found for the patient's isolate, vancomycin or imipenem or an extended-spectrum cephalosporin (if the MIC is 8 µg/mL or less) is substituted.

- Since the penetration of penicillin into the central nervous system is poor, in the case of pneumococcal meningitis, an extended-spectrum cephalosporin with good penetration (e.g., cefotaxime or ceftriaxone) is given. In areas with high rates of pneumococcal resistance to extended-spectrum cephalosporins, vancomycin plus cefotaxime or ceftriaxone may be given from the beginning of therapy.

fections. The current vaccine is administered to members of high-risk groups, such as elderly or immunocompromised individuals. However, the effectiveness of this vaccine (particularly for children; see Part VII) can undoubtedly be improved by conjugating the constituent capsular polysaccharides to protein carriers. Preliminary studies with such pneumococcal conjugate vaccines have been very promising. When these pneumococcal conjugate vaccines become available, they should be particularly useful for immunizing young children, who are at particular risk for pneumococcal infections but mount poor immune responses to the unconjugated polysaccharides present in the current pneumococcal vaccine.

RESOLUTION OF CLINICAL CASE

The patient was given intravenous cefuroxime and erythromycin. He became afebrile in 48 hours, and his cough and pleuritic pain remitted during this time. The sputum culture grew only normal oropharyngeal flora. Blood drawn at the time of admission and cultured grew pneumococci, which proved to be susceptible to penicillin. On the third day, the patient was discharged from the hospital to complete 10 days of oral cefuroxime at home. He made a full recovery.

This case involves a community-acquired pneumonia (CAP), which is one of the most common serious infections among adults. As in this case, most patients are quite well until the onset of CAP. However, immunocompromised hosts are at increased risk for CAP, as they are for most infections. About 75% of CAP is due to "typical" bacteria, with *S. pneumoniae* causing most (20%–60%) cases. Other typical pathogens causing CAP include *H. influenzae*, including type b (which commonly affects children) and non–type b (which commonly affects adults with chronic obstructive pulmonary disease), *S. aureus*, and gram-negative bacilli, such as *Klebsiella*. The so-called atypical CAPs are due to *Mycoplasma pneumoniae* and *Chlamydia pneumoniae*. In general, the typical bacterial pneumonias produce fever, with or without chills; pleuritic chest pain, with or without pleural effusion; and dense, alveolar, lobar infiltrates on chest x-ray.

> M. pneumoniae *and* C. pneumoniae *are atypical organisms, since they cannot be seen when the Gram stain is used.*

Although there is considerable overlap in the clinical picture between the typical and atypical pneumonias, the latter are more likely to manifest with a dry (nonproductive) cough, little or no pleuritic pain, and a patchy, bronchopneumonic (i.e., nonlobar: not involving an entire lobe) infiltrate. However, *Legionella* pneumonia, in particular, presents features of both typical and atypical CAP, with legionellosis resembling an atypical pneumonia early and then evolving toward the features of a typical bacterial pneumonia later in the disease course.

Etiologic diagnosis is difficult in CAP. The yield of *S. pneumoniae* on culture of sputum from bacteremic patients is only about 50%. Sputum culture is unreliable because the sputum passes through the oropharynx and may be contaminated with bacteria, such as pneumococci and *H. influenzae*, which may be carried in the pharynx of normal individuals, as well as being a potential cause of CAP. A positive blood culture makes a definitive diagnosis, but the sensitivity of blood culture is only 20% in pneumococcal pneumonia and is probably lower with other pathogens. *Legionella* is difficult to culture from sputum, although there are tests for the presence of *Legionella* antigen or nucleic acid, which are quite specific (see Chapter 15). *Mycoplasma* and *Chlamydia* are difficult to grow in the lab. A retrospective diagnosis of CAP involving these two agents is usually made by serologic tests, but it may be weeks before a significant increase in titer to these agents occurs. For all these reasons, empiric antibiotic therapy is administered while diagnostic tests are still underway. A common regimen for treating CAP is a second-generation cephalosporin that has good activity against *H. influenzae* (e.g., cefuroxime) and pneumococci, combined with erythromycin or another macrolide (azithromycin, clarithromycin) that has good activity against *Mycoplasma, Chlamydia,* and *Legionella*. Unfortunately, the therapy of CAP may soon be complicated by the fact that pneumococci are rapidly becoming resistant to penicillins, cephalosporins, and other antibiotics.

REVIEW QUESTIONS

Directions: For each of the following questions, choose the **one best** answer.

1. A bacterium with a polypeptide capsule is isolated from a patient suffering from pneumonia. Based upon this information, which one of the following can be considered a likely cause of this infection?

   (A) *Streptococcus pneumoniae*, serotype 3

   (B) *Salmonella typhi*

   (C) Group B *Neisseria meningitidis*

   (D) *Streptococcus pyogenes*

   (E) *Bacillus anthracis*

2. Which one of the following statements about capsules is true?

   (A) The hyaluronic acid capsule of group A streptococci is an important virulence factor because it promotes phagocytosis

   (B) The capsule of pneumococci is a potent virulence factor, at least in part, because it promotes the binding of factor Bb, a component in the alternate complement cascade

   (C) The capsule of group B streptococci is a potent virulence factor, at least in part, because it promotes the binding of serum factor H to the surface of group B streptococci

   (D) The capsules of all pneumococci are composed only of glucose or rhamnose

   (E) Capsules are generally less important virulence factors for extracellular pathogens than for the intracellular pathogens able to survive inside professional phagocytes

3. An elderly man, who is a heavy smoker, is hospitalized to receive chemotherapy for small cell lung cancer. Several weeks later he suddenly becomes ill with chills, pleuritic pain, and a fever of 103.5°F. Gram staining of this man's rusty sputum shows the presence of many gram-positive, lancet-shaped diplococci. The laboratory reports substantial leucocytosis. Considering this information, which one of the following statements about the pathogen most likely to be causing this infection is true?

   (A) It has a zoonotic reservoir

   (B) It is β-hemolytic

   (C) It is catalase-negative

   (D) It is nonencapsulated

   (E) It is a facultative intracellular pathogen

4. Pneumolysin has which of the following characteristics?

   (A) It inhibits inflammation

   (B) It has no homology with any other bacterial toxins

   (C) It is an exotoxin that is secreted from viable pneumococci

   (D) It may promote colonization by interfering with mucociliary clearance

   (E) It has no effect on tumor necrosis factor-α (TNF-α) or interleukin-1 (IL-1) production

5. Which one of the following statements concerning pneumococcal pneumonia is correct?

   (A) Pneumococcal pneumonia has been virtually eliminated because of the use of the existing pneumococcal vaccine

   (B) Many deaths from pneumococcal pneumonia result from suffocation caused by inflammation-induced edema in the lungs

   (C) *Streptococcus pneumoniae* rarely causes bacteremia

   (D) Pneumococcal pneumonia is highly contagious for healthy, young, immunocompetent adults

ANSWERS AND EXPLANATIONS

1. **The answer is E.** *B. anthracis* is the only one of the listed bacteria that has a polypeptide capsule. *S. pneumoniae, S. typhi*, group B *N. meningitidis*, and *S. pyogenes* all have polysaccharide capsules.

2. **The answer is C.** The hyaluronic acid capsule of group A streptococci is a potent virulence factor because it inhibits phagocytosis (group A streptococci are extracellular pathogens that do not want to be phagocytosed). The pneumococcal capsule inhibits the interaction of complement factor B with the pneumococcal surface (this interaction is important for the full activation of the alternate complement pathway). The capsular polysaccharides that are present in various serotypes of pneumococci are chemically different. Because the most important function of capsules is to inhibit phagocytosis, capsules are generally more important virulence factors for extracellular pathogens than for intracellular pathogens able to survive in phagocytes (i.e., uptake into a phagocyte typically means death for an extracellular pathogen).

3. **The answer is C.** This infection is most likely pneumococcal pneumonia. *Streptococcus pneumoniae* pathogens are catalase-negative, α-hemolytic, encapsulated, and extracellular. Pneumococci have a human reservoir, not an animal reservoir.

4. **The answer is D.** Pneumolysin can impair the function of ciliary cells, which inhibits microbial clearance by the mucociliary escalator and thus promotes colonization. Pneumolysin also promotes inflammation by stimulating production of TNF-α and IL-1. Pneumolysin shares homology with other members of the sulfhydryl-activated family of bacterial toxins. This toxin is not secreted by viable pneumococci but, instead, is released when autolysins induce lysis of the pneumococcal cell.

5. **The answer is B.** Edema is a major contributor to the death of many victims of pneumococcal pneumonia. Although a pneumococcal vaccine is available, this disease is still very common and still claims many lives. About 25% of patients with pneumococcal pneumonia also suffer bacteremia. Because there is an opportunistic component to pneumococcal pneumonia, this infection is not considered to be very contagious for healthy, young, immunocompetent adults.

19

IMMUNE EVASION STRATEGIES OF BACTERIA: NONCAPSULAR SURFACE FACTORS AND SECRETED FACTORS

CHAPTER OUTLINE

Introduction of Clinical Case
Noncapsular Surface Factors
- Proteins
- Polysaccharides

Secreted Factors
- Enzymes
- Toxins

Illustrative Pathogen: *Staphylococcus aureus*
- Biologic Characteristics
- Reservoir and Transmission
- Virulence Factors
- Pathogenesis
- Diagnosis
- Prevention and Treatment

Resolution of Clinical Case
Review Questions

INTRODUCTION OF CLINICAL CASE

A 19-year-old woman with no recent medical problems noticed the onset of fever, sore throat, and myalgia on the third day of an otherwise unremarkable menstrual period. Her temperature soon reached 103.3°F. Over the next 12 hours she felt increasingly tired and went to bed. She experienced nausea and vomited twice. This was followed by diarrhea. During one of her trips to the bathroom, she fainted. Her roommate called 911.

In the emergency department her temperature was 104.2°F, and her blood pressure was 65 mm Hg systolic. The patient was arousable but was disoriented as to place and time. There was a confluent erythematous macular (not raised) rash diffused over the face, trunk, arms, and legs. The remainder of the general physical examination was noncontributory. Two intravenous lines were established, and isotonic solutions were instilled at a high rate. When the blood pressure had risen to 80/40 mm Hg, a pelvic examination was performed. The tampon that was in place was removed and cultured, as were the sanguineous vaginal contents. The vaginal wall appeared hyperemic. Except for a trickle of blood coming from the cervical os, the other physical findings were unremarkable. Two blood cultures were obtained, and the patient was given nafcillin (a staphylococcal β-lactamase–resistant penicillin) intravenously.

The leukocyte count was 10,300/mm³ with a differential of 68% polymorphonuclear leukocytes and 4% band forms. The platelet count was 96,000/mm³ (normal: 150–350,000/mm³). The total bilirubin was 2.4 mg/dL, the aspartate aminotransferase (AST) was 63 U/L, the alanine aminotransferase (ALT) was 75 U/L, and the γ-glutamyl transpeptidase (GTP) was 250 U/L (all elevated values). The creatine kinase level was 280 U/L (normal: 40–150 U/L).

- What illness is this woman suffering from?
- Is it relevant that this woman was menstruating at the onset of illness?
- Do only women get sick with this illness?
- What pathogen causes this illness?

NONCAPSULAR SURFACE FACTORS

This chapter focuses on several bacterial immune evasion mechanisms, involving noncapsular surface factors and secreted proteins (such as toxins and enzymes), that have not yet been discussed in Part III. The pathogenic role of several of these noncapsular surface factors and secreted factors are then illustrated using *Staphylococcus aureus*, an important bacterial pathogen.

While capsule production is the single most important pathogenic mechanism for bacterial immune evasion, other factors on the bacterial surface can also contribute to immune evasion. The most important of these noncapsular surface factors are discussed here.

Proteins

Protein A and Protein G. Protein A, which is located on the surface of the bacterium *S. aureus*, binds immunoglobulin G (IgG) via the Fc region (Figure 19-1). This protein A–bound IgG no longer functions as an opsonin because its Fc region is blocked from interacting with the Fc receptor on phagocytes. Consequently, phagocytosis of the *S. aureus* cell is inhibited (at least until the appearance of protein A–specific IgG, which can promote phagocytosis by binding to protein A via its Fab region). Additionally, protein A–mediated binding of IgG via Fc regions results in a coating of the *S. aureus* surface with antibodies, making it more difficult for the immune system to recognize the infecting bacterium as foreign.

FIGURE 19-1 ▶
Antiopsonic/Antiphagocytic Effects of* Staphylococcus aureus *Protein A. *(A) This figure shows the normal interaction between a bacterium and immunoglobulin G (IgG). (B) This figure shows the interaction between protein A–producing* S. aureus *and IgG. Protein G of* S. pyogenes *brings about the same effect. Fab = antigen-binding fragment; Fc = constant antibody fragment.*

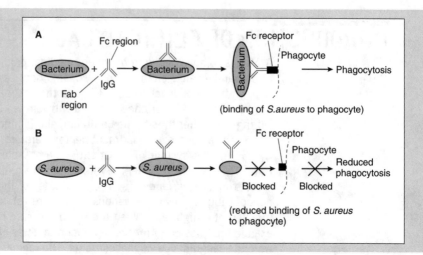

Streptococcus pyogenes produces protein G, which is a functional equivalent of protein A (i.e., since protein G also binds the Fc region of antibodies, it affords *S. pyogenes* protection from opsonization and phagocytosis).

M Protein. The contribution of M protein to the pathogenesis of *S. pyogenes* infections has already been discussed in Chapter 16, where it was mentioned that M protein promotes the adherence of *S. pyogenes* to mammalian tissue and can also induce an immunopathologic response against heart muscle because of shared epitopes between M protein and some heart muscle proteins. However, for this chapter, it is worth reemphasizing that M protein has three properties relevant to immune evasion: (1) the M protein found on different *S. pyogenes* isolates can be antigenically variable, (2) M protein binds large amounts of mammalian proteins, such as fibrin, to the *S. pyogenes* surface (which effectively masks this bacterium from the immune system), and (3) M protein interferes with opsonization and phagocytosis, which results, at least in part, from the ability of M protein to bind high concentrations of serum factor H to the *S. pyogenes* surface. Since binding of factor H to the bacterial surface inhibits activation of the alternate complement cascade (see Chapter 18), an *S. pyogenes* cell coated with factor H is protected from opsonization and phagocytosis, at least until an antibody response to M protein develops.

Pili. In addition to being antigenically variable (see Chapter 17), the pili of *Neisseria gonorrhoeae* also contribute to immune evasion through their antiphagocytic properties; the mechanism by which these pili exert their antiphagocytic effects is not clear.

Enzymes. The surface of some bacteria has enzymes that interfere with, or degrade, complement factors. For example, a C5a-degrading enzyme is embedded in the polysaccharide capsule of group B streptococci. The activity of this enzyme inhibits PMN chemotaxis to the site of infection.

> *The functional similarities between protein A of S. aureus and protein G of S. pyogenes represent only one of several shared pathogenic strategies used by these two gram-positive cocci. Another example is the ability of both these bacteria to produce superantigenic toxins. Considering their shared virulence strategies, it is not surprising that these two pathogens cause several similar diseases (e.g., both S. aureus and S. pyogenes can cause toxic shock syndrome–like illnesses).*

Polysaccharides

Lipopolysaccharide (LPS). Surface proteins, or protein-containing surface structures such as pili, are not the only noncapsular surface factors that pathogens use to evade the immune system. Gram-negative bacteria with short O-antigen side chains in their LPS (see Chapter 1) are very susceptible to complement-induced killing because membrane attack complex (MAC) forms directly on the outer membrane of these bacteria and induces membrane lysis.

In contrast, many pathogenic gram-negative bacteria (e.g., *Salmonella* spp.) are not killed by complement; therefore, they are termed serum-resistant. One of the most important mechanisms by which gram-negative bacteria become serum-resistant is by producing long O-antigen side chains on their LPS. When these long O side chains are present on the bacterial surface, they protect the bacterium because MAC formation occurs too far away from the lipid bilayer of the outer membrane to induce outer membrane lysis.

Lipooligosaccharide (LOS). Some strains of *N. gonorrhoeae* are also serum-resistant, but they achieve this effect by a slightly different mechanism from that described above for gram-negative bacteria such as *Salmonella* spp. *N. gonorrhoeae* removes sialic acid from the blood and adds this carbohydrate onto galactose residues present in its LOS (see Chapter 1). The addition of sialic acid onto LOS impedes the access of MAC to the outer membrane of the gonococcus, thus protecting the bacterium from MAC-mediated lysis. Further, since sialic acid is present on many host glycoproteins/glycolipids, this sialic acid modification of LOS also interferes with the ability of the immune system to see the *N. gonorrhoeae* cell as foreign.

SECRETED FACTORS

Pathogenic bacteria secrete many proteins that contribute to immune evasion. Generally, these secreted proteins have enzymatic or toxic properties.

> *Since many (although not all) toxins have been shown to possess enzymatic properties, the terms toxins and enzymes are becoming somewhat blurred.*

Enzymes

One of the simplest ways a bacterium evades the immune system is by secreting an extracellular protease that inactivates complement factors or antibodies. This strategy is used by the gram-negative bacterium *Pseudomonas aeruginosa*, which produces an enzyme named elastase. Elastase is a protease with a broad substrate specificity: it can inactivate complement components C3b and C5a, as well as IgG. Therefore, it is not surprising that elastase is an effective virulence factor that acts by diminishing the opsonization/phagocytosis of *P. aeruginosa* cells.

Some gram-positive bacteria also secrete enzymes that can inhibit opsonization/phagocytosis. For example, *S. pyogenes* produces a C5a peptidase that (as implied by its name) degrades complement factor C5a. This action of C5a peptidase interferes with effective immune responses to *S. pyogenes* by inhibiting the chemotaxis of phagocytes to the site of infection.

The ability of several pathogenic bacteria (particularly inhalation-acquired bacterial pathogens) to produce IgA protease (IgAse) has already been mentioned several times in this book (see Chapters 7, 17, and 18). As described previously, one of the contributions of these IgAses to pathogenesis is their ability to cause fabulation (i.e., coating of the microbial surface with nonopsonizing Fab fragments). Fabulation inhibits phagocytosis and helps mask the IgAse-producing pathogen from the immune system.

Toxins

Many bacterial toxins affect phagocytes (Table 19-1). Generally, these toxins can actually kill phagocytes at high concentration. However, even low concentrations of these toxins can affect phagocytosis, since these low toxin levels are sufficient to impair phagocyte function (e.g., they impair phagocyte-mediated killing of internalized pathogens or inhibit chemotaxis of phagocytes to the site of infection). Several toxins possessing activity against phagocytes have even been named for this property: they are referred to as leukocidins. However, it is important to appreciate that many toxins without the formal name *leukocidin* can also affect phagocytes. For example, although streptolysin O and staphylococcal α toxin are commonly thought of as hemolysins because they lyse erthrocytes, both of these toxins also have considerable activity against the membranes of phagocytes. In fact, the antiphagocytic effects of these two toxins are arguably even more important for pathogenesis than their hemolytic effects.

TABLE 19-1 ▶
Examples of Toxins That Affect Phagocytes

Toxin[a]	Source
Streptolysin O	*Streptococcus pyogenes*
Leukocidin	*Staphylococcus aureus*
α toxin	*S. aureus*
Anthrax toxin	*Bacillus anthracis*
Perfringolysin O	*Clostridium perfringens*
α toxin	*C. perfringens*
Exotoxin A	*Pseudomonas aeruginosa*
Leukocidin	*P. aeruginosa*
Adenylate cyclase	*Bordetella pertussis*

[a] Although *S. aureus* and *P. aeruginosa* both produce leukocidins, these are different proteins. Similarly, the α toxins of *S. aureus* and *C. perfringens* share a similar name but are different proteins.

Superantigenic toxins (e.g., toxic shock syndrome toxin-1, to be discussed further below) also deserve mention as a class of toxins that may potentially help bacteria evade the immune system. This might seem paradoxical, since a major response of the immune system to superantigens is a massive cytokine release that heightens inflammation. However, exposure to superantigens may also lead to immunosuppression (this occurs, at least in part, because superantigens can cause anergy and apoptosis of stimulated T cells). This superantigen-induced immunosuppression may contribute to the pathogenesis of some infections involving superantigen-producing bacteria.

ILLUSTRATIVE PATHOGEN: *Staphylococcus aureus*

Biologic Characteristics

The staphylococci are gram-positive cocci that typically are arranged in grape-like clusters. They are catalase-positive, a characteristic that readily differentiates the staphylococci from the catalase-negative streptococci. Staphylococci are facultative anaerobes that obtain their energy from fermentations. They grow readily on most non-selective bacterial media—that is, they are not fastidious and are more resistant to environmental stresses, such as drying and osmotic extremes, than most other bacteria. The hardiness and relatively simple nutritional needs of these bacteria make it very difficult to eliminate staphylococci from the human environment, which helps explain why staphylococcal infections are so common.

On the basis of their ability to produce the enzyme coagulase, the staphylococci can be classified as either coagulase-positive (*S. aureus*) or coagulase-negative (e.g., *S. epidermidis* and *S. saphrophyticus*). *S. aureus* is considered more virulent than other staphylococci and is clearly a major human pathogen. At one time, the medical importance of coagulase-negative staphylococci was debatable, but it is now recognized that the coagulase-negative staphylococci, which are normally present in the commensal flora of the skin, nares, and ear canal, are increasingly important opportunistic pathogens responsible for many nosocomial infections and infections in immunocompromised individuals (see Chapter 28).

> Some investigators believe that catalase may be a virulence factor, since it converts toxic H_2O_2 produced by phagocytes to water and oxygen.

Reservoir and Transmission

Humans represent the major reservoir for *S. aureus*. About 30% of healthy people carry *S. aureus* in their anterior nares. This includes many health care workers, who often carry antibiotic-resistant strains. *S. aureus* can also be transiently found as skin flora. Because of its hardiness, *S. aureus* often persists on inanimate objects for extensive periods (this "survivability" contributes to the difficulty of removing *S. aureus* from the hospital environment).

S. aureus causes a remarkable variety of infectious diseases, ranging from food-borne intoxications to localized pyogenic infections to systemic infections. In the community, *S. aureus* pyogenic infections are often autoinfections caused by *S. aureus* present in the nares or skin of the infected person. Nosocomial infections involving *S. aureus* are very common, and are increasingly troubling because of their high levels of antibiotic resistance. Nosocomial infections involving *S. aureus* can be spread person-to-person through a patient population, either by fomites or by the contaminated hands of medical personnel. Staphylococcal food poisoning often develops when *S. aureus* is present on the skin of a food worker or preparer and contaminates the food.

> *Pyogenic* means "pus-producing." S. aureus and S. pyogenes *are often referred to as gram-positive pyogenic cocci because their infections often involve pus production.*

Virulence Factors

S. aureus produces an extensive array of virulence factors. Consistent with the theme of this chapter, several of these virulence factors are noncapsular surface factors or secreted factors that act, at least in part, by interfering with the immune system's response to *S. aureus* infection.

Coagulase. This staphylococcal enzyme promotes the clotting of plasma. One consequence of coagulase action may be the inhibition of phagocyte access to the site of infection (i.e., phagocytes have a difficult time penetrating the fibrin clots promoted by coagulase). Additionally, coagulase causes the deposition of fibrin on the surface of *S. aureus*, which may help hide this bacterium from the immune system.

Protein A. The antiopsonic/antiphagocytic protection that protein A affords *S. aureus* by binding to the Fc region of IgG has already been discussed in this chapter.

Capsule. Like many other bacteria (see Chapter 18), *S. aureus* produces a polysaccharide capsule with antiphagocytic properties.

Teichoic Acid. Because of teichoic acid's ability to bind mammalian fibronectin, this bacterial surface factor probably promotes the adherence of the *S. aureus* cell to mammalian tissue.

Peptidoglycan Fragments. These fragments contribute to inflammation during *S. aureus* infection by triggering the alternate complement pathway.

Degradative Enzymes. *S. aureus* produces many enzymes, such as hyaluronidase, nucleases, and proteases, that probably contribute to the spread of these bacteria through mammalian tissue during invasive infections.

Hemolysins. *S. aureus* produces several toxins with hemolytic properties, the most important of which is α toxin, a membrane-active toxin (see Chapter 20). In addition to affecting erythrocytes, these hemolysins are also potent antiphagocytic factors because of their ability to inhibit or kill phagocytes (as explained earlier in this chapter). As a consequence of their effects on phagocytes, some of these hemolysins (e.g., α toxin) also trigger a massive cytokine release that may contribute to the shock, fever, and other symptoms associated with some *S. aureus* infections. These toxins also kill other mammalian cells and thus are important contributors to necrosis.

Leukocidin. This is another membrane-active toxin that kills phagocytes and inhibits their functions.

Pyrogenic Exotoxins. Many strains of *S. aureus* can produce pyrogenic exotoxins with a superantigenic action similar to that of the pyrogenic exotoxins of *S. pyogenes* (see Chapters 20 and 16). The staphylococcal superantigens cause inflammatory effects such as shock and fever by affecting cytokine production/release (see Chapter 21). These superantigens may also cause immunosuppression, which could contribute to some *S. aureus* infections. *S. aureus* produces two major types of pyrogenic exotoxins (superantigenic toxins):

1. *Staphylococcal enterotoxin* (serotypes A–F) are responsible for the vomiting and, to a lesser extent, the diarrhea of staphylococcal food poisoning. The emetic action of these heat-stable enterotoxins is probably due to their effects on neural receptors in the gut (the exact mechanism behind this effect is unclear, but it probably does not directly involve the superantigenic properties of these enterotoxins). The staphylococcal enterotoxins are also thought to be produced in some nonenteric infections (e.g., occasional cases of toxic shock syndrome), where their superantigenic properties probably contribute to inflammation and may contribute to immunosuppression.

2. *Toxic shock syndrome toxin (TSST-1)* is considered the major virulence factor in most cases of staphylococcal toxic shock syndrome. Its superantigenic properties are responsible for the inflammatory response that leads to the fever, hypotension, and shock associated with toxic shock syndrome, and it may also contribute to immunosuppression.

Exfoliatin. This virulence factor causes (by an unknown biochemical action) the splitting of the epidermis between the stratum spinosum and stratum granulosum. This effect leads to significant epithelial desquamation, which is often clinically visible. Exfoliatin is a particularly important virulence factor in staphylococcal scalded skin syndrome (see below).

AgrC and AgrA. The AgrC and AgrA proteins are the sensor and regulator, respectively, of a two-component regulatory system (see Chapter 24) present in *S. aureus*. Activation of this regulatory system leads to increased expression of toxins but decreased expression of some surface factors.

Pathogenesis

Given the impressive array of virulence factors produced by *S. aureus*, it is not surprising that this bacterium causes a diverse spectrum of diseases. The skin is a common site of *S. aureus* infection. *S. aureus* is an important cause of impetigo, which is a spreading skin infection limited to the epidermis. Staphylococcal impetigo, primarily a disease of children, is characterized by bullous lesions and the development of a "crusty" appearance on the infected skin. *S. aureus* also commonly causes skin abscesses. These skin abscesses usually start when *S. aureus* infects a hair follicle; the resultant localized abscess is referred to as a furuncle or boil. If infection spreads beyond the original hair follicle to adjacent subcutaneous tissue, it is referred to as a carbuncle.

Sometimes *S. aureus* cells escape from a localized skin abscess and enter the blood (this can even occur from abscesses too small to be noticed). Usually, these bloodborne *S. aureus* cells are controlled by the immune system before they cause serious illness, but life-threatening disease may develop if a person's immune system is not functioning optimally. If not controlled by the immune system, bloodborne *S. aureus* can cause bacteremia, pneumonia, or deep infections of bones (causing osteomyelitis), joints (about 50% of the cases of bacterial arthritis are caused by *S. aureus*), and internal organs including the brain and heart (e.g., endocarditis). These deep infections often result in the formation of abscesses that seriously impair organ function.

S. aureus does not necessarily need to disseminate beyond its original site of infection in order to affect distant body sites. Several *S. aureus*–mediated diseases involve the absorption of toxins from the original site of infection into the bloodstream, which results in transport of the toxin throughout the body. One such toxin-mediated *S. aureus* disease is scalded skin syndrome, which primarily occurs in children but also occurs in immunocompromised adults. Scalded skin syndrome is characterized by extensive desquamation of skin; this desquamation often occurs beyond the actual site of *S. aureus* infection as a result of exfoliatin (see Virulence Factors, above) being absorbed into the circulation. Another toxin-mediated disease caused by *S. aureus* is toxic shock syndrome (TSS). This illness was originally recognized in menstruating women who used highly absorbent tampons, but TSS can also develop from surgical or skin infections involving *S. aureus*, so that men and children too can get TSS. The pathogenesis of staphylococcal TSS typically involves the absorption of TSST-1, or occasionally one of the staphylococcal enterotoxins, which also have superantigenic activity (see Virulence Factors), from the vagina or other localized site of infection into the bloodstream. The superantigenic activity of this circulating TSST-1, or staphylococcal enterototoxin, then triggers a massive release of proinflammatory cytokines, such as tumor necrosis factor-α and interleukin-1, which causes the high fever, shock, hypotension, vomiting, pain, and diarrhea associated with TSS (see Chapter 21). Skin rashes and desquamation of the skin also develop during TSS, although the precise toxins causing these epidermal effects are not yet clear. Both TSS and scalded skin syndrome can be life-threatening illnesses.

Besides causing illnesses involving the dissemination of toxin from localized sites of infection, *S. aureus* can also cause true intoxications: disease in the absence of infection. Many cases of staphylococcal food poisoning are true intoxications that occur when food containing a heat-stable staphylococcal enterotoxin is consumed. As described previously (see Chapter 6), staphylococcal food poisoning is a fast-developing illness characterized by vomiting and some diarrhea.

Diagnosis

In addition to clinical signs, which can be quite distinct in diseases such as scalded skin syndrome, laboratory results often prove helpful for diagnosing *S. aureus* infections. Abscesses generally contain large numbers of *S. aureus* cells (along with polymorphonuclear leukocytes), which can be visualized by Gram staining a specimen of pyogenic material withdrawn from the lesion. This specimen can also be cultured (as can blood, which may reveal whether bacteremia has occurred) on selective agar such as CNA (see Appendix 1), and biochemical tests (e.g., the coagulase test) can be performed on isolates to confirm that an infection involves *S. aureus*.

S. aureus food poisoning is usually diagnosed on the basis of clinical signs. However, if some suspect food remains, it can be tested for the presence of staphylococcal enterotoxins using serologic tests (e.g., latex agglutination tests). Since staphylococcal food poisoning can be an intoxication, culturing the feces of food poisoning patients is not usually helpful, as this illness often develops in the absence of any viable *S. aureus* in the body.

Bullous lesions *have a blister-like appearance.*

S. pyogenes *also causes a TSS-like illness, which is not surprising, since* S. pyogenes *also produces pyrogenic exotoxins with superantigenic activity.*

Prevention and Treatment

Simple *S. aureus* abscesses of the skin can often be treated by drainage alone. However, if a skin abscess is severe or the patient develops a fever, antimicrobials are usually administered. Treatment of *S. aureus* abscesses in other body locations usually requires both surgical drainage and antimicrobial therapy. Antimicrobial therapy is essential for controlling systemic *S. aureus* infections such as bacteremia. (The resolution of this chapter's clinical case discusses of the treatment for TSS.)

Unfortunately, the increasing antibiotic resistance of clinical *S. aureus* isolates makes antimicrobial to a wide range of antimicrobial agents makes therapy of *S. aureus* infections ever more difficult. For example, *S. aureus* clinical isolates are often resistant to most β-lactam antimicrobials, with approximately 90% of *S. aureus* clinical isolates producing β-lactamase and many of these clinical isolates also producing altered penicillin-binding proteins (e.g., transpeptidases; see Chapter 5) that make them resistant even to β-lactamase–resistant penicillins and cephalosporins, such as methicillin. Until recently, vancomycin was always a reliable agent of last resort for treating *S. aureus* infections. However, vancomycin-resistant *S. aureus* isolates are now being reported in the United States, raising the frightening specter that some *S. aureus* infections may soon be totally unresponsive to antimicrobial therapy.

Because of the high levels of antibiotic resistance now being reported for *S. aureus* clinical isolates, it is particularly important to determine the antimicrobial susceptibility patterns of these isolates to identify the most efficacious available agent and thus limit the further spread of antimicrobial resistance through the *S. aureus* population.

Given these emerging difficulties in treating *S. aureus* infections with antimicrobials and the lack of any effective vaccine, the best way to reduce the occurrence of these infections is to reduce the presence of *S. aureus* in the human environment, particularly in hospitals. Good hygienic practices, such as the frequent use of disposable gloves by health care workers and regular cleaning of the hospital environment, are essential for limiting nosocomial infections involving *S. aureus*. Unfortunately, the hardiness of *S. aureus*, as mentioned earlier, makes reducing the presence of this bacterium in the hospital—or any other—environment a tough challenge.

> **MRSA** *is a commonly used term for methicillin-resistant* Staphylococcus aureus.

> *Antibiotic-resistant* S. aureus *is present in most operating rooms, hospital nurseries, and patients' rooms.*

RESOLUTION OF CLINICAL CASE

The young woman was suffering from staphylococcal TSS. The blood cultures were negative. The woman responded to the nafcillin therapy and recovered.

As mentioned earlier, staphylococcal TSS is a toxin-mediated disease whose manifestations are attributable to one or more toxins produced by proliferating *S. aureus*, particularly TSST-1. Usually, the toxin arises from the proliferation of staphylococci on tampons used by women during menstruation; only 10% of cases are related to other staphylococcal infections. Hundreds of cases occurred each year in the United States until the withdrawal of superabsorbent tampons from the market in 1981. Currently, less than 100 cases are reported each year; 71% are associated with menstruation.

The onset of this illness commonly occurs on the third or fourth day of menstruation. The toxin involves numerous organ systems, producing the signs and symptoms shown in Table 19-2. Unexplained marked hypocalcemia is also often observed with TSS. Cultures of the vaginal fluid, tampon, or other site of infection may be positive for *S. aureus*, which can be tested in the lab for TSST-1 production. Blood cultures show no growth in most cases.

The management of TSS consists of immediate treatment of hypotension and shock by vigorous fluid replacement and the administration of catecholamines, if necessary. Removal of a tampon or drainage of the site of *S. aureus* infection should be accomplished promptly. Systemic therapy with a β-lactamase–resistant penicillin or cephalosporin should be given to prevent the further formation of toxin.

The mortality rate from TSS is on the order of 5% to 10% because irreversible shock often occurs before medical attention is obtained. When resuscitation is successful, the prognosis is excellent.

Fever ≥ 102°F

Rash (diffuse macular erythroderma)

Desquamation (1–2 weeks after onset)

Hypotension or orthostatic dizziness

Involvement of three or more organ systems
    Gastrointestinal: nausea, vomiting, diarrhea
    Muscular: myalgia, elevated serum creatine kinase, rhabdomyalysis
    Mucous membrane: hyperemia of conjunctiva, pharynx, vagina
    Renal: azotemia, pyuria in the absence of infection
    Hepatic: elevated bilirubin and liver function test results
    Hematologic: thrombocytopenia
    Central nervous system: encephalopathy

TABLE 19-2
Clinical Criteria for Defining Toxic Shock Syndrome

REVIEW QUESTIONS

Directions: For each of the following questions, choose the **one best** answer.

1. A 20-year-old college football player injures his knee and requires knee surgery. Several days later he develops a significant fever, severe pain, and swelling in the surgically repaired knee. *Staphylococcus aureus* is isolated from the infected knee. Which one of the following statements is correct about this situation?

    (A) This infection should respond to therapy with almost any β-lactam anti-microbial agent

    (B) This infection involves a catalase-negative bacterium

    (C) This infection is unlikely to involve pus formation

    (D) This infection involves an encapsulated bacterium

    (E) This infection is uncommon in surgical patients

2. Which one of the following statements about antiphagocytic/antiopsonic virulence factors is correct?

    (A) M protein decreases the binding of serum factor H to the surface of *Streptococcus pyogenes*

    (B) Protein G interferes with the binding of the Fc region of IgG to the Fc receptor on phagocytes

    (C) Possessing short O-antigen side chains is advantageous for the virulence of gram-negative bacteria

    (D) Streptolysin O does not affect phagocytosis if present at less than lethal concentrations

    (E) *Pseudomonas aeruginosa* elastase interferes with antibody-mediated opsonization but not with opsonization via the alternative complement cascade

3. A 35-year-old menstruating woman develops a high fever and rash. The microbiology laboratory reports that the cause of her infection is coagulase-positive cocci that are arranged in grape-like clusters. This bacterium stains blue on properly performed Gram stains. Considering this information, which one of the following statements is true about the pathogen responsible for this infection?

    (A) This bacterium produces M protein

    (B) This bacterium produces protein A, which acts by binding serum factor H to the bacterial surface

    (C) Adherence of this bacterium is mediated by pili

    (D) Leukocidin is the only antiphagocytic protein secreted by this bacterium

    (E) This bacterium produces a large number of enzymes that facilitate its spread through tissue

4. Furuncles have which of the following characteristics?

    (A) They usually form at hair follicles

    (B) They do not involve abscess formation

    (C) They result from a carbuncle

    (D) They cannot give rise to bacteremia

    (E) They usually do not involve any pus formation

5. Scalded skin syndrome is best described by which of the following statements?

   (A) It is a true staphylococcal intoxication, not an infection

   (B) It is uncommon in children

   (C) It involves exfoliatin

   (D) It rarely involves toxin absorption into the bloodstream

   (E) It manifests symptoms only at the original site of *Staphylococcus aureus* infection

ANSWERS AND EXPLANATIONS

1. **The answer is D.** This young man apparently has developed *S. aureus* infection from his recent knee surgery. Option A is incorrect because *S. aureus* (particularly nosocomial isolates) are resistant to many β-lactam antimicrobials. Option B is incorrect because *S. aureus* (and all staphylococci) are catalase-positive, which distinguishes them from the catalase-negative streptococci. Option C is incorrect because *S. aureus* is notoriously pyogenic (i.e., many of its infections involve pus formation). Option E is incorrect because *S. aureus* is a very common cause of postsurgical infection.

2. **The answer is B.** Protein G is the *S. pyogenes* equivalent of protein A and acts, at least in part, by binding the Fc region of IgG, which denies this Fc region access to the Fc receptor on phagocytes and therefore inhibits phagocytosis. Option A is incorrect because M protein acts, at least in part, by increasing the binding of serum factor H to the *S. pyogenes* surface (factor H is an inhibitor of activation of the alternate complement pathway). Option C is incorrect because having long O-antigen side chains is favorable for virulence, as these long side chains protect the bacterial outer membrane by keeping MAC away. Option D is incorrect because streptolysin O inhibits phagocyte function even at sublethal concentrations. Option E is incorrect because elastase of *P. aeruginosa* can degrade several complement components (as well as antibodies), thus interfering with the activation and function of both the alternate and classical complement pathways.

3. **The answer is E.** This woman is suffering from a *Staphylococcus aureus* infection (possibly TSS). Option A is incorrect because *S. aureus* does not produce M protein; M protein is made only by *Streptococcus pyogenes*. Option B is incorrect because protein A binds the Fc region of IgG, not factor H. Option C is incorrect because adherence of *S. aureus* involves teichoic acid, not pili. Option D is incorrect because staphylococcal hemolysins, such as α toxin, also have antiphagocytic activity.

4. **The answer is A.** Options B and E are incorrect because furuncles do involve abscess formation with pus. Option C is incorrect because carbuncles develop from furuncles, not the other way around. Option D is incorrect because furuncles (and carbuncles) can give rise to bacteremia.

5. **The answer is C.** The skin symptoms of scalded skin syndrome are thought to involve exfoliatin. Option A is incorrect because scalded skin syndrome is not an intoxication—viable *S. aureus* cells must be present in the body for scalded skin syndrome to develop. Option B is incorrect because scalded skin syndrome is most common in children. Options D and E are incorrect because severe cases often involve toxin absorption into the bloodstream, which can result in the manifestation of symptoms far from the site of *S. aureus* infection.

PART IV: MECHANISMS BY WHICH PATHOGENS DAMAGE THE HOST

OVERVIEW

Parts II and III of this book have described how microbial pathogens successfully establish themselves in the human body and subvert the immune system. Occasionally,

*When pathogens establish themselves in the body without causing disease, this is termed a **subclinical infection**.*

a pathogen establishes itself in the body without making the human host ill. However, the presence of a pathogen or its products in the human body often results in significant damage, causing illness. Part IV explores the most important mechanisms by which pathogens or their products cause damage to the host. These mechanisms generally fall into two broad categories: (1) direct host damage caused by pathogens or their products and (2) indirect host damage resulting from inflammatory responses to pathogens or their products.

DIRECT HOST DAMAGE

Many microbial pathogens or their products are directly toxic for the host, that is, they do not act through the host's inflammatory response. In fact, several infectious diseases (e.g., foodborne botulism, see Chapter 20) are typically intoxications, which are diseases caused by toxins in the absence of viable pathogens in the body.

Bacterial Products

While many bacterial products cause direct damage to the host, the most notorious of these toxic factors are the exotoxins. The bacterial exotoxins, which are generally proteins or polypeptides, include the most toxic molecules known to exist in nature (e.g., 1 g of botulinum toxin can kill 10^{10} mice!). Some bacterial exotoxins actually kill host cells (these toxins are termed cytotoxic toxins), while other bacterial exotoxins alter host cell function without causing cell death (these toxins are termed cytotonic toxins). The molecular action and pathogenic role of the most important bacterial exotoxins are discussed in Chapter 20.

Instead of producing classic exotoxins, some pathogens (e.g., *Yersinia* species) produce highly toxic molecules termed effector proteins. Unlike classic exotoxins, these effector molecules (which include several Yops, see Chapter 15) are not usually toxic when applied externally to host cells, that is, effector proteins cannot directly bind to receptors or penetrate the host cell plasma membrane. Instead, type III secretion systems (see Chapter 13) deliver these toxic effectors into the host cell cytoplasm, where they exert their toxic effects.

Apoptosis *is programmed host cell death.*

Some intracellular bacterial pathogens produce toxic molecules when growing inside host cells. For example, *Shigella flexneri* produces IpaB (see Chapter 13), which binds to interleukin-1-converting enzyme (ICE) that is present in the cytoplasm of macrophages. This binding activates ICE, which then triggers apoptosis and leads to the death of mammalian cells.

Fungal Products

Some fungi (e.g. poisonous mushrooms) cause potentially lethal foodborne intoxications. Symptoms of such fungal intoxications are induced by mycotoxins. Mycotoxins are unusually structured organic molecules that cause organ damage or, in the case of aflatoxin, liver cancer. Mycotoxins apparently do not contribute to systemic mycoses; the symptoms of mycoses primarily result from inflammation and immunopathology.

Viral Products

A **syncytium** *is a multinucleated cell created by the fusion of adjacent cells to one another, so that their nuclei share a common cytoplasm. Syncytia-producing viruses always possess an envelope fusion proteins that mediates this process.*

Many, but not all, human viruses exert a cytopathic effect (CPE) on cells. This CPE can take the form of cell lysis (polioviruses, see Chapter 29), disruption of cytoskeletal components (adenovirus, see Chapter 7; herpes simplex virus [HSV], see Chapter 9), chromatin margination (HSV), membrane permeability changes (rotavirus, see Chapter 6; human immunodeficiency virus [HIV], see Chapter 27), viral-induced fusion of infected cells with other infected or noninfected cells to form syncytia (herpesviruses, paramyxoviruses such as respiratory syncytial virus, HIV), or the hypertrophy of normal cells (human papillomaviruses [HPV], see Chapter 26). One example of a viral product that mediates damage to the host is the rotavirus nonstructural protein, which increases intracellular calcium levels and thus causes fluid and electrolyte loss from the gastrointestinal tract. Additionally, a region of the HIV gp120 glycoprotein is capable of binding calmodulin, which enables it to alter host membrane permeability. A final example of viral products that damage the host are the two nonstructural proteins expressed from the HPV genome; these two HPV proteins induce hypertrophy or transformation of infected epithelial cells (see Chapter 26).

A nonstructural protein is encoded by, and expressed from, a viral genome, but is not present in the mature virus itself.

There is keen interest in the idea that many virus infections (e.g., adenovirus) trigger apoptosis. Further, it is believed that viruses (e.g., HSV) capable of persistent infections succeed because they synthesize one or more viral products that block apoptosis. This enables these viruses to establish a latent infection that allows the virus to persist for the life of the host.

Viruses can also damage the host cell by altering or usurping the host cell macromolecular machinery. For example, human cytomegalovirus (CMV, see Chapter 10) stimulates host cell macromolecular synthesis to replicate; this stimulatory effect contributes to the CPE observed during lytic infection. HSV not only encodes enzymes that stimulate the synthesis of nucleotide pools in quiescent nondividing cells to replicate, but also synthesizes proteins that regulate the splicing and transport of both viral and some cellular RNAs (see Chapter 9). The Rev protein of HIV performs a similar function to regulate the preferential transport of some viral messages (see Chapter 27).

INDIRECT HOST DAMAGE: INFLAMMATORY RESPONSES

As a consequence of activation of the alternate or classical complement pathways, the body typically mounts an inflammatory response early in the course of infection. Inflammation typically results in the release of mediators (e.g., interleukin-1 [IL-1], tumor necrosis factor [TNF], histamine, kinins, prostaglandins, serotonin) that induce the classic features of inflammation, including swelling, vasodilation, local or systemic elevation in temperature, and pain. Inflammation also helps control infections (see Chapters 21 and 22); for example, inflammation causes an increased flow to the lymphatics (which facilitates development of specific immune defenses), increases migration of phagocytes to the site of infection, and promotes formation of fibrin clots that help isolate the site of infection.

Unfortunately, inflammation sometimes has serious deleterious effects for the host. As discussed in Chapter 21, septic shock is a severe (often lethal) inflammatory response that results in high fever, shock, and intravascular coagulation. The large number of microbial factors (e.g., endotoxin, peptidoglycan breakdown products, bacterial and viral superantigens) known to induce septic shock are described in Chapter 21.

In addition to septic shock, inflammation can have several other potential immunopathologic consequences, which are discussed in Chapter 22. One clinically important immunopathologic consequence of inflammation discussed in Chapter 22 is immune complex disease. An example of immune complex disease is the glomerulonephritis that sometimes develops as a postinfection sequela of group A streptococcal infection. This condition results from the formation of immune complexes between antibodies and group A streptococcal antigens. When these immune complexes are deposited in the glomeruli of the kidney, localized inflammation and renal damage result. Infections involving group A streptococci can also trigger another serious immunopathologic response, the formation of antibodies that cross-react with human tissue. Rheumatic fever, one of the most important postinfection sequelae of group A streptococcal infection, is believed to result from formation of antibodies elicited against certain epitopes of the M protein of group A streptococci (see Chapter 16). In some cases, these M protein antibodies cross-react with epitopes found in cardiac tissue. This cross-reactivity results in severe cardiac inflammation that is clinically manifested as rheumatic fever, a disease that can lead to heart failure. The last immunopathologic response discussed in Chapter 22 is granuloma formation. Some infections, particularly those involving intracellular bacterial or eukaryotic pathogens, trigger potent cell-mediated immune (CMI) responses. While CMI responses are necessary to control these infections, they can also result in the formation of a granuloma, particularly in more chronic infections. As explained in Chapter 22, granulomas help localize infections; unfortunately, they also result in localized destruction of host tissue.

CMI responses to virus infections can also result in inflammatory responses that are deleterious to the human host. For example, the CMI response to recurrent episodes of reactivated HSV leads to the destruction of stromal fibroblasts within the eye, resulting in corneal opacity and ultimately blindness.

Viruses can also influence (positively or negatively) the host inflammatory response by encoding molecules with cytokine activity or by producing factors that elicit or antagonize the host immune response to infection. For example, viruses such as human CMV (see Chapter 10) and vaccinia synthesize molecules that are similar in structure to host receptors that bind specific cytokines (interferon-γ [IFN-γ], IL-1, interleukin-6 [IL-6], and TNF) or chemokines involved in the host inflammatory response to virus infection. Epstein-Barr virus (EBV), a human herpesvirus, encodes a homolog of the cellular cytokine interleukin-10 (IL-10), which inhibits the synthesis of inflammatory cytokines such as IFN-γ, IL-1, and TNF. In contrast, the HIV TAT gene product (see Chapter 27) activates the expression of cellular cytokines such as transforming growth factor-β (TGF-β), interleukin-2 (IL-2), IL-6, and TNF, thereby augmenting the host response to HIV-infected cells.

Recent studies suggest that M protein shares some epitopes with myosin, which is an abundant protein in cardiac tissue.

20 BACTERIAL EXOTOXINS

CHAPTER OUTLINE

Introduction of Clinical Case
Microbial Toxins
Molecular Action of Bacterial Exotoxins
- Protein Synthesis–Inhibiting Toxins
- Enterotoxins
- Membrane-Active Toxins
- Bacterial Exotoxins That Induce Pathologic Immune Responses
- Neurotoxins
Illustrative Pathogen: *Clostridium botulinum*
- Biologic Characteristics
- Reservoir and Transmission
- Virulence Factors
- Pathogenesis
- Diagnosis
- Treatment and Prevention
Resolution of Clinical Case
Review Questions

INTRODUCTION OF CLINICAL CASE

A 42-year-old oil company executive visited his company's oil drilling operations in Alaska. While there, he was invited to a traditional Native American–Eskimo dinner prepared by local oil field workers. At that dinner he enjoyed many traditional foods, including home-smoked fish. The next day he developed diplopia, swallowing difficulties, and diarrhea, followed later by constipation. The man was admitted to

Diplopia is "double vision," or blurred vision.

the local clinic, where blood studies showed normal levels of leukocytes. Urinalysis and chest x-ray appeared normal, and the man's blood pressure was 120/80 mm Hg. That same day, three other people who had attended the same dinner were admitted with similar symptoms.

In the hospital, the executive developed a progressively more severe flaccid paralysis. Thirty-two hours after admission, he suffered a cardiac arrest but was resuscitated. However, despite repeated efforts, spontaneous respiration could not be maintained, and the patient was placed on a respirator.

- Does this illness have a microbial origin? If so, is this an infection or an intoxication?
- What virulence factor(s) is responsible for these symptoms?
- How should this illness be treated?

MICROBIAL TOXINS

It has recently been suggested that rotaviruses produce an enterotoxin.

The incredible potency of some microbial
toxins is illustrated by experiments demonstrating that, on a molar basis, botulinum and tetanus toxins are approximately 10^{11} times more lethal for mice
than is sodium cyanide.

One example of a recently emerging toxin-
producing pathogen is E. coli O157:H7,
which causes hemorrhagic colitis and hemolytic uremic syndrome.

A protective immune response can be generated against tetanus toxin by injecting a
patient with large amounts of tetanus toxoid, which is an inactivated tetanus toxin
preparation that retains antigenicity.

Nevertheless, so much endotoxin is often
present in the body during a massive gram-
negative septicemic infection that death
occurs.

Many pathogenic microorganisms, including bacteria, fungi, algae, protozoa, and (possibly) viruses, produce toxins, which can be defined as molecules that kill or injure the host
when administered in small quantities. By definition, the symptoms of microbial intoxications (e.g., most cases of foodborne botulism and staphylococcal food poisoning)
always involve toxins. However, toxins also cause or contribute to the symptoms of many
bacterial infections. Historically, toxin-mediated infections such as cholera, diphtheria,
and tetanus have ranked as major medical problems. While these traditional toxin-
mediated illnesses remain major public health concerns, particularly in underdeveloped
countries, new infections involving toxin-producing pathogens continue to emerge.

Toxin production represents an effective strategy for inducing host damage, particularly because microbial toxins are often potent enough to kill or injure a host before the
immune system has had an opportunity to respond. Some toxins (e.g., tetanus toxin and
botulinum neurotoxin) are so potent that only minuscule doses are needed to cause
disease symptoms. For example, during tetanus, such small amounts of tetanus toxin are
present in a patient's body that a protective antitoxin immune response is never generated!

Because toxins play their most important role in bacterial diseases, this chapter
focuses on bacterial toxins. Bacterial toxins can be described in several ways. Sometimes
these toxins are described by their site of action in the host: enterotoxins affect the
gastrointestinal tract, while neurotoxins affect the nervous system. Alternatively, bacterial toxins are sometimes described on the basis of their location with respect to the
bacterial cell. Toxins secreted outside the bacterial cell, referred to as exotoxins, are
usually very potent and almost always proteinaceous in composition. The pathogenesis of
most illnesses caused by gram-positive pathogens involves exotoxin production; this is
not surprising, since it is relatively straightforward for these bacteria to secrete a protein
across their single membrane (see Chapter 1). However, despite the challenge of secreting proteins across two membranes (see Chapter 1), many gram-negative pathogens also
produce exotoxins that play an important role in their pathogenesis (e.g., *Vibrio cholerae*
produces cholera toxin, which is responsible for the severe diarrhea of epidemic cholera;
see Chapter 23). Although any toxin located within a bacterial cell could technically be
termed an endotoxin, this term is usually reserved for the lipid A component of lipopolysaccharide, which is found in the outer membrane of gram-negative bacteria (see
Chapter 1). Relative to most exotoxins, endotoxin is more heat-stable but less potent on a
molar basis. The action and involvement of endotoxin in gram-negative bacterial infections are considered in Chapter 21.

MOLECULAR ACTION OF BACTERIAL EXOTOXINS

Many pathogenic bacteria produce exotoxins; the most medically important bacterial
exotoxins are listed in Table 20-1. The mechanisms by which these medically important
exotoxins damage the host are then briefly discussed.

Protein Synthesis–Inhibiting Toxins

When initially produced by the gram-positive bacterium *Corynebacterium diphtheriae*
(see Chapter 23), diphtheria toxin is a single polypeptide. However, soon after its
synthesis and secretion, the diphtheria toxin polypeptide is nicked into two fragments
(fragment A and fragment B), which remain connected by a disulfide bond (Figure 20-1).
Fragment A possesses the toxic activity of diphtheria toxin, while fragment B mediates
the binding and internalization of this toxin.

As shown in Figure 20-2, the initial step in diphtheria toxin action is binding of the
nicked toxin to a receptor present on the surface of human cells. The bound toxin is then
internalized in an endocytic vesicle, which subsequently undergoes acidification. Exposure to this low-pH environment inside the endocytic vesicle induces a conformational

The receptor for diphtheria toxin has recently been identified as an epidermal
growth-factor-like protein.

◀ **TABLE 20-1**
Medically Important Bacterial Toxins

Bacterium	Toxin	Toxin Action
Bacillus anthracis	Anthrax toxin complex (consists of protective antigen, edema factor, and lethal factor)	Edema factor: activates mammalian adenylate cyclase Lethal factor: kills cells (may be a protease)
Bacillus cereus	Emetic toxin (heat-stable)	?
	Diarrheal toxin (heat-labile)	?
Bordetella pertussis	Adenylate cyclase	A bacterial adenylate cyclase that increases cAMP levels in host cells
	Pertussis toxin	ADP-ribosylates the Gi regulatory protein of the mammalian adenylate cyclase system, increasing cAMP levels in host cells
Clostridium botulinum	Botulinum neurotoxin (seven serologically distinguishable types)	Causes flaccid paralysis by blocking acetylcholine release through its protease activity aimed at host proteins involved in synaptic vesicle docking
Clostridium difficile	Toxin A Toxin B	Both toxin A and toxin B are monoglucosyltransferases that add a single glucose residue onto the Rho host protein; this causes cytoskeletal and signal transduction disruptions
Clostridium perfringens	α Toxin[a]	Phospholipase C (damages host cell membranes)
	Enterotoxin	Damages brush border membranes, leading to fluid and electrolyte loss
Clostridium tetani	Tetanus neurotoxin (also known as tetanospasmin)	Blocks release of inhibitory neurotransmitters by its protease activity, which interferes with the docking of synaptic vesicles; causes spastic paralysis
Corynebacterium diphtheriae	Diphtheria toxin	ADP-ribosylates elongation factor 2, shutting off host protein synthesis
Escherichia coli	Heat-labile enterotoxin	ADP-ribosylates the Gs regulatory protein of mammalian adenylate cyclase system, increasing intestinal cAMP levels; this leads to intestinal electrolyte and fluid secretion
	STa (heat-stable enterotoxin active against humans)	Binds to and activates intestinal guanylate cyclase; this increases intestinal cGMP levels and leads to intestinal fluid and electrolyte secretion
	Shiga toxin (several serotypes)	Inactivates host ribosomes by cleaving a glycosidic bond in an rRNA; this shuts down host protein synthesis
Listeria monocytogenes	α Hemolysin	Forms pores in host cell membranes
	Listeriolysin	Forms pores in host cell membranes
Pseudomonas aeruginosa	Exotoxin A	ADP-ribosylates elongation factor 2, shutting off host protein synthesis
Shigella dysenteriae	Shiga toxin	Inactivates host ribosomes by cleaving a glycosidic bond in an rRNA; this shuts down host protein synthesis
Staphylococcus aureus	α Toxin[a]	Forms pores in host cell membranes
	Enterotoxins (six serotypes)	Cause vomiting and diarrhea during staphylococcal food poisoning; mechanism unclear Also: these toxins are superantigens that sometimes contribute to systemic S. aureus infections by promoting fever and shock
	Toxic shock syndrome toxin-1	Superantigen that contributes to staphylococcal toxic shock syndrome by promoting fever and shock
	Exfoliatin	Causes desquamation associated with some staphylococcal infections (e.g., scalded skin syndrome)
Streptococcus pneumoniae	Pneumolysin	Forms pores in host cell membranes
Streptococcus pyogenes	Streptolysin O	Forms pores in host cell membranes
	Pyrogenic exotoxins A and C (also known as erthyrogenic exotoxins A and C)	Superantigens that contribute to fever and other symptoms associated with some S. pyogenes infections (e.g., scarlet fever)
Vibrio cholerae	Cholera toxin	ADP-ribosylates the Gs regulatory protein of the mammalian adenylate cyclase system, increasing intestinal cAMP levels; this leads to intestinal electrolyte and fluid secretion

Note. cAMP = cyclic adenosine monophosphate; ADP = adenosine diphosphate; cGMP = cyclic guanosine monophosphate.
[a] *C. perfringens* α toxin and *S. aureus* α toxin are not the same protein: they do not share any homology at the amino acid level, and they have different actions.

FIGURE 20-1 ▶

Proteolytic Nicking of Diphtheria Toxin.
After synthesis by Corynebacterium diphtheriae, *the single ~60 kDa diphtheria*
toxin polypeptide is nicked, forming frag-
ment A (study hint: remember A for activ-
ity) and fragment B (study hint: remember
B for binding and internalization). Follow-
ing nicking, fragments A and B remain
connected by a disulfide bond (shown by
dashed line).

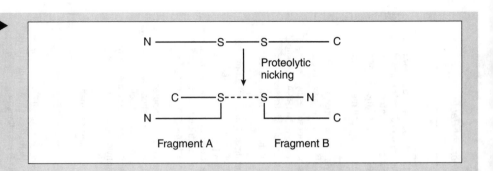

FIGURE 20-2 ▶

Mechanism of Action of Diphtheria Toxin.
(1) Diphtheria toxin binds to a surface re-
ceptor and is then (2) internalized inside
an endocytic vesicle. (3) Acidification of
this diphtheria toxin-containing endosome
then causes the insertion of fragment B
into the endosomal membrane. This in-
sertion promotes the entry of fragment A
(but not fragment B) into the cytoplasm,
where (4) fragment A exerts its NAD-
dependent, ADP-ribosyltransferase activ-
ity on elongation factor 2 (EF-2), resulting
in (5) cell death. NAD = nicotinamide ad-
enine dinucleotide, ADP = adenosine
diphosphate.

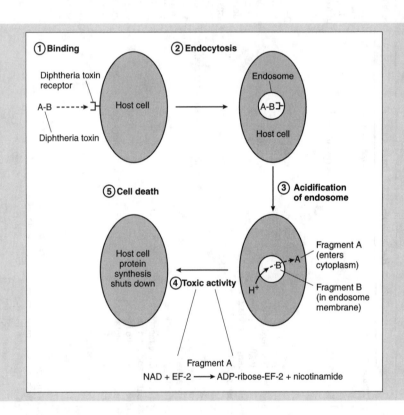

The presence of a single molecule of diph-
theria toxin fragment A in the cytoplasm of
a mammalian cell is sufficient to kill that
cell.

The ADP-ribosylation of EF-2 by fragment
A is very specific, that is, other host pro-
teins are not ADP-ribosylated by fragment
A. This specificity is due to the fact that
fragment A adds an ADP-ribose onto a
modified histidine residue (called diph-
thamide) that is only present in EF-2.

The shiga toxin produced by EHEC was
once referred to as shiga-like toxin; this
toxin is still termed Verotoxin by some in-
vestigators.

change in the B fragment of diphtheria toxin, facilitating the insertion of this conforma-
tionally altered B fragment into the membrane of the endosome. The presence of this
fragment B in the endosomal membrane then somehow facilitates the entrance of
fragment A into the cytoplasm. Once inside the cytoplasm, fragment A exerts its toxic
activity, which involves catalyzing the addition of an adenosine diphosphate (ADP)-ribose
onto elongation factor 2 (EF-2) of the mammalian protein synthesis system (i.e., diphtheria toxin fragment A is an enzyme with nicotinamide adenine dinucleotide [NAD]–
dependent, ADP-ribosyltransferase activity). Because EF-2 is indispensable for protein
synthesis, the intoxicated host cell soon dies.

Diphtheria toxin is not the only bacterial toxin that catalyzes an ADP-ribosylation of
EF-2. Exotoxin A, produced by *Pseudomonas aeruginosa*, shares this same enzymatic
action. Despite their shared enzymatic activity, diphtheria toxin and exotoxin A exhibit
relatively little amino acid sequence homology. Further, the binding and internalization
of these two toxins differ considerably (e.g., exotoxin A recognizes a different receptor
from diphtheria toxin, and unlike diphtheria toxin, exotoxin A is nicked into fragments
after it enters endosomes).

Bacterial toxins can also use mechanisms other than ADP-ribosylation of EF-2 to
inhibit host protein synthesis. Shiga toxin, produced by some strains of *Shigella dysenteriae* (see Chapter 13) and EHEC strains of *Escherichia coli* (see Chapter 12), belong to
the 5B:1A subunit family of enterotoxins (Figure 20-3). After binding, internalization,

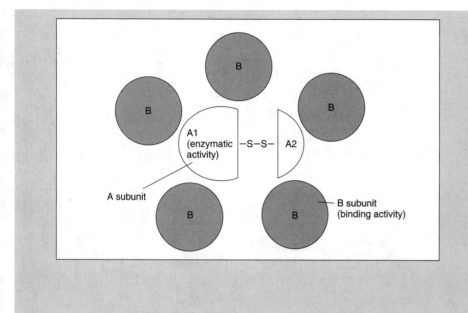

FIGURE 20-3
Composition of the Five B Subunit: One A Subunit Enterotoxin Family. *Many enterotoxins (e.g., shiga toxin, cholera toxin) made by gram-negative bacteria are composed of five identical B subunits and one centrally located A subunit, which is usually composed of single A1 and A2 fragments held together by a disulfide bond. The five B subunits mediate binding (typically to host cell glycolipids), while the A subunit (specifically the A1 fragment) contains the enzymatic activity of the toxin. Although similar in subunit composition, members of the 5B:1A subunit enterotoxin family are not necessarily homologous at the amino acid sequence level: while cholera toxin and E. coli heat-labile enterotoxins share homology, their amino acid sequences differ from that of shiga toxin. These differences in amino acid sequence explain why 5B:1A subunits do not all share the same enzymatic action.*

and entry of the A-1 fragment of shiga toxin into the cytoplasm of a mammalian cell, the host ribosome becomes inactivated, and protein synthesis soon stops. The A-1 fragment inactivates ribosomes by specifically cleaving a glycosidic bond present in one of the rRNA constituents of the 60S ribosomal subunit.

Enterotoxins

Bacteria usually induce intestinal fluid and electrolyte loss by one of two mechanisms: (1) by invading the gastrointestinal (GI) tract, which induces a strong inflammatory response (see Chapter 13), or (2) by producing enterotoxins. Enterotoxins induce their GI effects either by inducing gross histopathologic damage to the intestines, thereby altering the ability of the intestines to regulate the absorption and secretion of fluids and electrolytes, or by altering intestinal secretory pathways without causing histopathologic damage.

Two medically important enterotoxins that induce intestinal fluid and electrolyte secretion without causing gross intestinal damage are cholera toxin and *E. coli* LT heat-labile enterotoxin (LT) [see Chapter 12]. Cholera toxin and LT both belong to the 5B:1A subunit enterotoxin family introduced previously (see Figure 20-3) and also share significant homology at the amino acid sequence level. Therefore, it is not surprising that, after utilizing generally similar binding and internalization processes, these two enterotoxins exert identical enzymatic actions. Specifically, once the A1 fragment of either cholera toxin or LT enters the cytoplasm of an enterocyte, it ADP-ribosylates the Gs regulatory protein of the mammalian adenylate cyclase system (Figure 20-4). The addition of an ADP-ribose moiety onto Gs blocks the hydrolysis and release of bound guanosine triphosphate (GTP). Consequently, the ADP-ribosylated Gs subunit is constantly "activated" to stimulate adenylate cyclase. (Interestingly, this activation can be further stimulated by host proteins called ADP-ribosylation factors [ARFs]; ARFs can interact with the A1 subunit to increase its ADP-ribosyltransferase activity.) This effect leads to an overaccumulation of cAMP in cholera-toxin treated intestinal epithelial cells, which triggers a metabolic cascade culminating in hypersecretion of fluid and ions from the small intestine.

Besides LT, enterotoxigenic *E. coli* can also produce small polypeptide enterotoxins referred to as heat-stable enterotoxins. These heat-stable enterotoxins differ in their species specificity and action; the *E. coli* heat-stable enterotoxin involved in most or all human gastrointestinal disease is termed STa (stable toxin a). Like cholera toxin and LT, STa affects intestinal secretion without inducing histopathologic damage. However, in

The only apparent difference between the early steps in the action of cholera toxin versus LT is that cholera toxin recognizes only a single receptor (the ganglioside GM1), while LT apparently can bind to either GM1 or an intestinal glycoprotein.

FIGURE 20-4 ▶

Mammalian Adenylate Cyclase Enzyme System. (A) The mammalian adenylate cyclase enzyme system is composed of adenylate cyclase, which converts adenosine triphosphate (ATP) to cyclic adenosine monophosphate (cAMP); a Gs protein which, when activated, stimulates adenylate cyclase activity; and a Gi protein which, when activated, inhibits adenylate cyclase activity. Note that cholera and Escherichia coli heat-labile enterotoxins affect the Gs protein. (B) Activation of the Gs regulatory protein by guanosine triphosphate (GTP) binding; this Gs activation is normally relieved by guanosine triphosphatase (GTPase) activity present in Gs. Note that the adenosine diphosphate (GDP) ribosylation of Gs catalyzed by cholera toxin and Escherichia coli heat-labile enterotoxin blocks the cleavage of Gs-bound GTP, leaving Gs constantly activated.

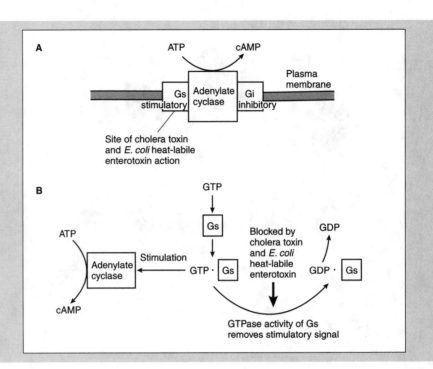

C. difficile *toxins A and B also have strong proinflammatory properties that (indirectly) contribute to colonic cell death.*

Amino Acid Sequence of One STa

Asn-Thr-Phe-Tyr-Cys-Cys-Glu-

Leu-Cys-Asn-Pro-Ala-Cys-Ala-

Gly-Cys-Tyr

Note the presence of several cysteine (Cys) residues in this sequence; these residues give some structure to this peptide, helping it resist inactivation by heat. Other STa's have slight variations from this sequence (although they are also usually rich in Cys), but they still act by increasing intestinal cyclic guanosine monophosphate (cGMP) levels. Asn = asparigine; Thr = threonine; Phe = phenylalanine; Tyr = tyrosine; Glu = glutamic acid; Leu = leucine; Pro = proline; Ala = alanine.

contrast to the accumulation of intestinal cAMP promoted by cholera toxin or LT, STa acts by inducing an increase in intestinal cyclic guanosine monophosphate (cGMP) levels. STa exerts this effect by directly binding to a guanylate cyclase present on the surface of intestinal epithelial cells. Through incompletely understood mechanisms, this binding causes the intestinal guanylate cyclase to produce high levels of cGMP. Several other gram-negative bacteria (e.g., *Yersinia enterocolitica*) also produce heat-stable enterotoxins similar to STa, although the importance of these other heat-stable enterotoxins in pathogenesis remains controversial.

Enterotoxins that act, at least in part, by causing histopathologic damage to the intestines include *Clostridium difficile* toxins A and B, shiga toxin, and *Clostridium perfringens* enterotoxin. These enterotoxins induce damage to the intestines, at least in part, because, unlike cholera toxin, LT, and STa, they are cytotoxic and kill intestinal cells. This enterotoxin-induced death of large numbers of intestinal epithelial cells causes dysfunctional intestinal secretion and absorption.

It is not surprising that shiga toxin is able to kill host cells, since, as discussed earlier, this toxin shuts off host cell protein synthesis. *C. perfringens* enterotoxin is a membrane-active toxin that alters the membrane permeability properties of intestinal epithelial cells; these alterations in membrane permeability then lead to host cell death by either cell lysis or a shut-down of vital metabolic processes. As previously explained in Chapter 11, *C. difficile* toxins A and B are glucosyltransferases that catalyze the addition of glucose onto the host Rho protein. Since Rho is a critical regulator of cytoskeletal assembly/disassembly and signal transduction processes, the modification of Rho induced by toxin A and toxin B apparently has cytotoxic consequences.

Adenylate Cyclase System. Because of its importance in signal transduction processes, the activity of the mammalian adenylate cyclase system is under exquisitely fine control. This system involves adenylate cyclase (which actually is responsible for converting ATP to cAMP), whose activity is controlled by two regulatory proteins, Gs and Gi (see Figure 20-4). When activated by GTP binding, Gs stimulates adenylate cyclase to produce more cAMP. However, since cAMP is a critical intracellular messenger, this stimulation of adenylate cyclase must be transient. The cell normally relieves stimulation of Gs by cleaving the bound GTP to GDP using GTPase activity present in Gs (see Figure 20-4). In contrast, when GTP binds to Gi, this causes an inhibition of cAMP production; this can be relieved by the GTPase activity present in Gi.

Another bacterial toxin, pertussis toxin, ADP-ribosylates the Gi regulatory protein of the adenylate cyclase system present in respiratory epithelial cells and immune cells.

This ADP-ribosylation interferes with the ability of Gi to dampen adenylate cyclase's activity and results in increased cAMP levels in these cells. This effect contributes to the symptoms of pertussis.

Although these cAMP-mediated effects are apparently the primary mechanism by which cholera toxin and *E. coli* heat-labile toxins induce intestinal fluid and electrolyte secretion, reports suggest that cholera enterotoxin may also affect intestinal secretion by increasing (through incompletely understood mechanisms) the release of prostaglandins into the intestinal lumen.

Membrane-Active Toxins

Another major target site of bacterial toxin action is the host plasma membrane. Some membrane-active bacterial toxins are enzymes that degrade important membrane constituents. For example, as previously described in Chapter 2, *C. perfringens* α toxin is a phospholipase C, with activity against phosphotidylcholine (lecithin) and sphingomyelin.

Alternatively, many membrane-active toxins lack enzymatic activity but act by physically disrupting the permeability properties of the host cell's plasma membrane. Often these "physical" toxins (e.g., staphylococcal α toxin) alter membrane permeability properties by forming pores (Figure 20-5). This toxin-induced pore formation typically results in a net influx of ions and water into the host cell; at high concentrations, pore-forming toxins can cause cell death by osmotic lysis. However, even at low concentrations, pore-forming toxins can cause changes in intracellular ion concentrations that significantly impair cell function.

> Because membrane-active toxins do not have to undergo endocytosis to exert their effects, they often kill or damage a host cell very quickly.

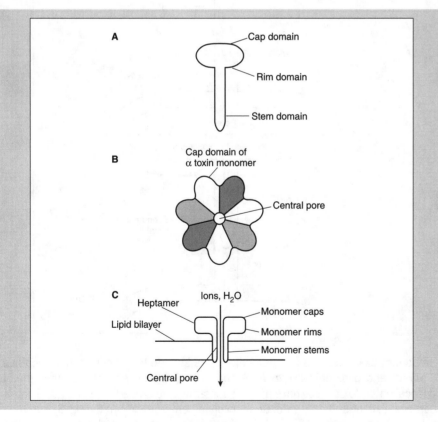

◀ *Figure 20-5*
***Pore Formation by* Staphylococcus aureus α Toxin.** *(A) Side view of a monomer of S. aureus α toxin, consisting of cap, rim, and stem domains. (B) Once bound to a host cell plasma membrane, seven identical α-toxin monomers self-assemble into a heptameric pore structure. Also shown is a top view of the α-toxin heptamer; note the presence of an opening (a pore) in the center of the heptamer. (C) Side view of the heptamer when present in host plasma membranes (note the mushroom-like shape). The cap region of each individual α-toxin monomer is located on the exterior surface (i.e., away from the host cell's cytoplasm) of the heptamer, while the rim region of the monomers lies on or near the surface of the membrane. The portion of the central pore that extends through the membrane lipid bilayer is formed from a combination of stem regions of all seven monomers present in the heptamer. It is through this central pore that fluid and ions enter the host cell, which can cause cell lysis and affect cellular metabolism.*

Many membrane-active toxins affect a broad range of host cells (e.g., many of these toxins are referred to as hemolysins because they lyse red blood cells). However, one of the most important targets of most membrane-active toxins appears to be phagocytic cells. As explained in Chapter 19, membrane-active toxins often contribute to the ability of a pathogen to evade the immune system by killing or impairing phagocytes. Sometimes this causes phagocytes to release cytokines, such as tumor necrosis factor-α (TNF-α), that can have immunopathologic effects.

Bacterial Exotoxins That Induce Pathologic Host Immune Responses

As will be described in Chapters 21 and 22, the symptoms of many infectious diseases result primarily from immunopathologic responses. For infections involving gram-negative bacteria, endotoxin often plays a key role in inducing these immunopathologic responses. Although they lack endotoxin, some gram-positive pathogens (e.g., *Staphylococcus aureus* and *Streptococcus pyogenes*) are still very adept at triggering strong immunopathologic responses. Often these gram-positive bacteria induce shock, fever, and related symptoms, at least in part by producing protein exotoxins that interact with immune cells.

Probably the most important group of exotoxins involved in triggering strong immunopathologic responses is made up of the superantigenic toxins. As shown in Figures 20-6 and 20-7, superantigenic toxins can induce a massive T-cell proliferation, which leads to a large release of cytokines, such as TNF, that cause the shock and fever associated with some diseases (e.g., toxic shock syndrome) involving gram-positive bacteria. As mentioned in Chapter 19, longer-term exposure to superantigens may induce anergy and apoptosis of T cells, which could help superantigen-producing bacteria evade the immune system during chronic infections.

FIGURE 20-6 ▶

Molecular Interactions of T-Cell Stimulation by Conventional Antigens versus Superantigenic Toxins. (A) Stimulation by conventional antigens is highly specific (i.e., only a small number [<0.01%] of T cells express a T-cell receptor [TCR] capable of recognizing the processed antigen presented in the peptide-binding groove of the major histocompatibility complex [MHC] class II of macrophages or other antigen-presenting cells). (B) However, after binding to MHC II, superantigenic toxins form a trimolecular complex by binding to the variable (V) domain of the TCR β chain. Since this binding occurs outside the portion of the β chain that is involved in antigen recognition, virtually all T cells with a particular Vβ domain are stimulated (some superantigenic toxins can even recognize and bind to more than one type of Vβ domain). Therefore, superantigenic toxins typically induce a massive T-cell proliferation; depending on the particular superantigenic toxin involved, 8%–40% of a host's T-cell population can be stimulated.

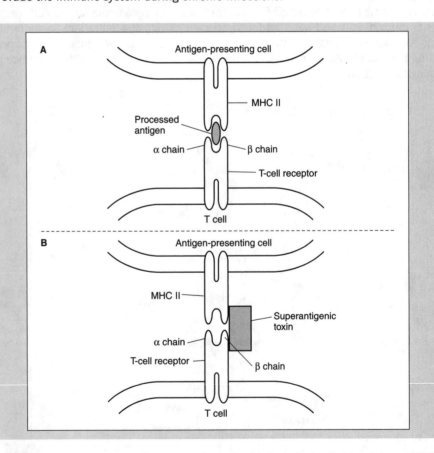

B. anthracis *produces a tripartite toxin. Protective antigen has no known toxic activity but serves as the binding subunit for the other two components of anthrax toxin, lethal toxin and edema factor (see Table 20-1).*

Important examples of superantigenic toxins include toxic shock syndrome toxin 1 of *S. aureus* and pyrogenic exotoxins A and C of *S. pyogenes*. Interestingly, the staphylococcal enterotoxins also have potent superantigenic properties, which contribute to the pathogenesis of systemic infections involving enterotoxin-producing *S. aureus* isolates. However, the superantigenic properties of the staphylococcal enterotoxins do not seem to explain their ability to cause vomiting and diarrhea during staphylococcal food poisoning.

Although very important, superantigens are not the only toxins of gram-positive bacteria that can induce immunopathologic effects. For example, the lethal toxin of *Bacillus anthracis* kills macrophages, causing a large release of cytokines such as TNF-α. It is believed that this effect is responsible for most or all of the shock and fever associated with the disease anthrax.

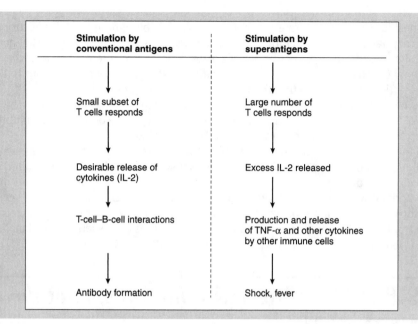

FIGURE 20-7

Immunopathologic Consequences of T-Cell Stimulation by Conventional Antigens versus Superantigenic Toxins. *The stimulation of a limited number of T cells by a conventional antigen generally has beneficial effects, such as the stimulation of antibody formation. In contrast, the large-scale proliferation of T cells induced by superantigenic toxins often has immunopathologic consequences because it eventually results in the release of large amounts of tumor necrosis factor-α (TNF-α) and other cytokines into the circulation. Release of these cytokines can then induce shock, fever, and other symptoms. IL-2 = interleukin-2.*

Neurotoxins

Interestingly, the two most potent bacterial toxins, tetanus toxin and the botulinum neurotoxins, are neurotoxins that induce opposite types of paralytic effects. Tetanus toxin induces spastic paralysis by interfering with the release of inhibitory neurotransmitters (e.g., glycine or γ-isobutyric acid) at synapses in the central nervous system (CNS). In contrast, botulinum neurotoxins induce flaccid paralysis by interfering with the release of stimulatory neurotransmitters (e.g., aceteylcholine) at cholinergic synapses located at neuromuscular junctions and in the autonomic nervous system (Figure 20-8).

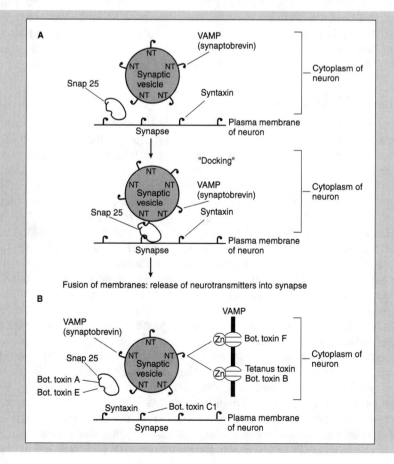

FIGURE 20-8

Molecular Actions of Tetanus and Botulinum Toxins. *(A) Normal exocytosis of neurotransmitters in the absence of a clostridial neurotoxin, that is, a synaptic vesicle filled with neurotransmitters (NT) docks with the inner surface of the plasma membrane of a neuron. This docking, which involves several proteins (including VAMP, Snap-25, and Syntaxin), facilitates the fusion of the synaptic vesicle membrane with the plasma membrane, thereby resulting in the release of NT into the synapse. (B) Sites where tetanus toxin and the various botulinum neurotoxins proteolytically cleave their targets, that is, various docking proteins involved in neuro-exocytosis. Note in this figure the specificity of cleavage for each neurotoxin. Once cleaved, the docking proteins no longer support synaptic vesicles docking; consequently, neurotransmitters are not released into the synapse from the neuro-toxin-treated neuron. VAMP = vesical associated membrane protein; Snap = synaptosomal associated protein; Zn = zinc.*

Like diphtheria toxin, both tetanus and botulinum toxins are nicked after synthesis and then held together by a disulfide bond, that is, these neurotoxins belong to the A-B family of toxins. In the case of tetanus and the botulinum neurotoxins, the A fragment is referred to as the light chain and the B fragment as the heavy chain. The light chain of the clostridial neurotoxins has the toxic (enzymatic) activity, while the heavy chain mediates binding and internalization. Only a single serologic type of tetanus toxin has been identified, but there are several serologically distinguishable types of botulinum neurotoxin. All of them induce flaccid paralysis.

Considering the very different physiologic effects of botulinum and tetanus toxins, it was somewhat surprising when recent studies revealed that these two clostridial neurotoxins share very similar molecular actions. After binding and internalization of their "A fragment" (referred to as the light chain) into the cytoplasm of neurons, both tetanus toxin and the botulinum neurotoxins specifically cleave proteins involved in the exocytosis of synaptic vesicles (i.e., these toxins are highly specific proteases). The net effect of this neurotoxin-induced proteolysis of neuronal docking proteins is an inhibition of neurotransmitter release into the synapse (see Figure 20-8).

If the botulinum toxins and tetanus toxin share similar enzymatic properties, why do they induce opposite paralytic effects? The answer seems to be that they are bound and internalized by different kinds of neurons, with tetanus toxin being bound and internalized primarily by inhibitory neurons located in the CNS (i.e., to neurons that secrete inhibitory neurotransmitters), while the botulinum neurotoxins are bound and internalized primarily by cholinergic neurons (i.e., to neurons that secrete acetylcholine).

ILLUSTRATIVE PATHOGEN: *Clostridium botulinum*

Biologic Characteristics

Like all species of the genus *Clostridium*, *C. botulinum* is a gram-positive, anaerobic, spore-forming rod. *C. botulinum* spores are often very heat-resistant (e.g., they can often withstand boiling), a characteristic that plays a role in the development of many foodborne botulism outbreaks.

Isolates of *C. botulinum* are classified into seven types (designated A–G), depending upon the botulinum neurotoxin they produce; that is, serologic variation exists between botulinum neurotoxins made by different *C. botulinum* isolates. For unexplained reasons, virtually all cases of human botulism, whether foodborne, infant, or wound (see below), are caused by *C. botulinum* isolates belonging to types A, B, E, and (rarely) F. Types C and D isolates frequently cause botulism in animals. It has recently been recognized that occasional isolates of two other clostridial species, *C. barati* and *C. butyricum*, also produce botulinum neurotoxin; however, *C. botulinum* isolates appear to be responsible for most cases of human botulism.

Reservoir and Transmission

C. botulinum spores are found in soils throughout the world. This ubiquitous presence of *C. botulinum* spores in soil represents the reservoir for botulism and facilitates the contamination of food, the intestines, or wounds with *C. botulinum* spores. This contamination can occur either by direct contact with spore-containing soil or by inhalation or deposition of airborne spores picked up from this soil.

Human botulism develops in two ways. Foodborne botulism usually results from consumption of a food containing botulinum progenitor toxin (see below); that is, this illness is usually an intoxication that does not involve toxin production inside the host. In the United States, the widespread use of preservatives such as nitrites by the commercial food industry has reduced the occurrence of foodborne botulism to only 10 to 20 cases a year. Furthermore, this widespread use of preservatives in commercial foods has shifted the food vehicle responsible for most cases of foodborne botulism in the United States to home-preserved or home-prepared foods. Home-prepared fish and other seafoods have been a particularly common food vehicle in recent foodborne botulism outbreaks occurring in the United States, Canada, and Japan.

In contrast to foodborne botulism, wound botulism and infant botulism result from the in vivo production of progenitor toxin, that is, these forms of botulism are true infections requiring the presence of viable *C. botulinum* cells in the body. A major difference between these two *C. botulinum* infections is the mechanism of entry of *C. botulinum* into the body: wound botulism results from the entrance of *C. botulinum* spores or cells into open wounds, while infant botulism usually results from the ingestion of viable *C. botulinum* cells or spores into the gastrointestinal (GI) tract. Infant botulism now ranks as the most common form of botulism in the United States, where about 100 cases occur yearly. While infant botulism usually develops following ingestion of airborne spores, it has also been associated with the ingestion of honey contaminated with *C. botulinum* spores or cells. Wound botulism is the rarest form of human botulism, with only about 200 cases reported worldwide, and is increasingly associated with dirty needles and syringes used by drug users.

Virulence Factors

The flaccid paralysis symptoms of human botulism are caused by the botulinum neuro-toxins, whose action has already been described in this chapter. In foodborne botulism and infant botulism, botulinum neurotoxins are initially present in the lumen of the GI tract as part of a "progenitor toxin." Progenitor toxin is a large complex composed of one molecule of a botulinum neurotoxin and one or more nonneurotoxic proteins of *C. botulinum*. The nonneurotoxic components of progenitor toxin are important for pathogenesis, since they stabilize and protect the complexed botulinum neurotoxin from the acidity of the stomach and from degradation by intestinal proteases.

Some strains of *C. botulinum* produce additional toxins besides a botulinum neuro-toxin. For example, some *C. botulinum* strains produce C2 toxin, which causes an ADP-ribosylation of host actin. This effect, which can lead to a collapse of the cytoskeleton, induces fluid and electrolyte loss from the GI tract. Whether C2 or other "nonneurotoxic" toxins of *C. botulinum* play any role during the early course of botulism remains unclear; however, it is well established that they are not responsible for the hallmark symptoms of botulism: flaccid paralysis.

The resistance of *C. botulinum* spores to heat and other stresses should also be considered a virulence factor, since this trait allows *C. botulinum* to survive the incomplete cooking or preservation of foods. Surviving spores in improperly prepared foods can germinate into new bacterial cells, which will then produce botulinum toxin in these foods.

Pathogenesis

In foodborne botulism, illness usually follows ingestion of the progenitor toxin present in foods. Following its absorption from the intestines into the circulation, progenitor toxin dissociates to free botulinum neurotoxin. This free botulinum neurotoxin then binds to susceptible neurons at cholinergic synapses. Once the light chain of botulinum neuro-toxin has been internalized into the cytoplasm of these neurons, it exerts its proteolytic action, blocking the exocytosis of acetylcholine. Consequently, autonomic and neuro-muscular transmission are impaired, resulting in flaccid paralysis.

Symptoms of foodborne botulism usually develop within a day or so of the ingestion of progenitor toxin. However, this incubation period is dependent on the dose of ingested toxin and can range from as little as several hours to as much as 8 days. In approximately 33% of cases, the first symptoms of botulism are nonspecific GI symptoms such as nausea, vomiting, and diarrhea. More typically, the initial symptoms of foodborne botulism involve the head, face, mouth, and throat; they include diplopia, dry mouth, pupillary abnormalities, ptosis, dysphagia, and dysarthria. During the development of these initial symptoms of flaccid paralysis, constipation often occurs. As the paralysis develops further, the patient may suffer from potentially fatal respiratory paralysis or cardiac arrest. Although improved therapeutic efforts are helpful, the mortality rate for botulism remains high (see Resolution of Clinical Case). One particularly unfortunate aspect of botulism is that the patient typically remains fully conscious until shortly before death.

Except for their initial steps, the pathogeneses of infant botulism and of wound botulism generally resemble that of foodborne botulism. Infant botulism develops because of the relative instability of the normal microbial GI flora in neonates, which sometimes allows *C. botulinum* cells to colonize an infant's GI tract. Once *C. botulinum* cells become established in an infant's GI tract, they begin to produce progenitor toxin. Progenitor toxin can then be absorbed by the intestines, with subsequent events occurring as described for foodborne botulism. The initial symptoms of infant botulism include

*Ptosis is the inability to raise the eyelid, **dysphagia** is the inability to swallow, and **dysarthria** is the inability to speak properly. All three result from paralysis of the muscles involved in these processes. Usually this results from the lack of proper innervation (as occurs during botulism, where botulinum toxin disrupts stimulatory neurotransmitter release at the neuromuscular junction).*

The importance of normal GI flora in preventing the colonization of the human GI tract by C. botulinum *is also illustrated by the fact that adults receiving antibiotic therapy (which can disrupt the normal GI flora) have occasionally become colonized by* C. botulinum; *that is, these antibiotic-treated adults essentially develop "infant botulism."*

constipation (which is often overlooked), followed by lethargy, diminished movement, weak cry, and poor appetite. Wound botulism occurs when *C. botulinum* cells contaminate a wound and begin producing botulinum neurotoxin in the wound, which then results in flaccid paralysis similar to other forms of botulism.

Diagnosis

The initial diagnosis of any form of botulism should be made on clinical grounds. Unless a large outbreak of foodborne botulism occurs in which many people simultaneously become sickened with similar symptoms, the clinical diagnosis of botulism is often difficult, because the early nonspecific symptoms of this illness are easily confused with other neurologic disorders and most physicians have had little experience with this illness. Nevertheless, a prompt clinical diagnosis of botulism is imperative because delays can postpone the administration of effective therapy and increase the probability of death for the patient.

Laboratory tests (e.g., serologic assays or mouse lethality bioassays) for detection of botulinum neurotoxins are available to confirm clinical diagnoses. These tests can be used to detect botulinum neurotoxins in the serum of a patient or in remaining aliquots of foods that have recently been ingested by the patient. These same tests can also be used to detect botulinum toxins in the bowel contents of an infant with infant botulism. However, since it takes time to perform these assays—samples usually must be shipped to the relatively specialized laboratories with the ability to perform these tests—a physician should not wait for laboratory results to confirm the diagnosis before starting therapy for botulism.

With respect to culturing food or feces for *C. botulinum*, viable *C. botulinum* is often absent from contaminated foods (remember: foodborne botulism is often an intoxication), and, therefore, culturing foods for *C. botulinum* is not commonly performed. The intestinal contents of infants suspected of suffering from infant botulism can be cultured for *C. botulinum*; the detection of *C. botulinum* is meaningful, since this bacterium is not normally present in the GI flora of humans.

Treatment and Prevention

The currently used botulinum antitoxin contains antibodies against types A, B, and E botulinum neurotoxins, that is, against the botulinum neurotoxins involved in most cases of human botulism.

Antimicrobial agents are not routinely administered for cases of foodborne or infant botulism.

Antitoxin is usually administered for therapy against all forms of botulism. In cases of wound botulism, antimicrobial therapy should also be administered into the wound to kill the *C. botulinum* cells and prohibit further in vivo production of botulinum neurotoxin. Supportive care, particularly respiratory support, is also very important in managing botulism and in preventing secondary infections, which can lead to pneumonia or other illnesses.

Foodborne botulism is best prevented by rigid adherence to proper food preparation procedures, particularly during home preparation of foods. It is notable that while the spores of *C. botulinum* are often resistant to boiling, the neurotoxin itself is quite heat-labile: 10–20 min at 100°C will inactivate botulinum neurotoxin. Most cases of infant botulism are difficult to prevent, since they apparently involve inhalation and swallowing of *C. botulinum* spores from the air. However, one step that can be taken to reduce the occurrence of infant botulism is not to give honey, which may contain *C. botulinum* spores, to infants under 1 year of age.

RESOLUTION OF CLINICAL CASE

Despite the clinic's best efforts, the man died the next day.

This case illustrates a typical scenario for foodborne botulism, which is often caused by improperly prepared home-processed vegetables, fruits, meats, and seafood. This illness is particularly prevalent in Alaska, where home-processed foods are often a dietary staple. A good candidate for the outbreak depicted in this case is the smoked fish, which is often preserved in airtight plastic that can produce an anaerobic environment favorable for the growth of *C. botulinum*.

Failure to adhere to proper food preparation conditions can allow *C. botulinum* spores to survive the home preparation of foods; after these spores germinate, the resultant *C. botulinum* cells will produce botulinum progenitor toxin in foods. Unless the food is thoroughly cooked (e.g., at 100°C for 10–20 min) before ingestion, foodborne botulism may then result.

Because of the extreme potency of the botulinum neurotoxins, some victims have died after merely sampling a small amount of neurotoxin-contaminated food. In general, the more botulinum neurotoxin a person ingests, the faster he or she will develop symptoms of botulism, and the more serious the symptoms will be (the symptoms of this man are typical of foodborne botulism). When high doses of a botulinum neurotoxin are ingested, death can occur quickly. This apparently was the situation with the oil company executive.

Improved respiratory support has helped reduce the mortality rate for botulism from about 60% to about 20%. If given promptly after the onset of symptoms, antitoxin may prevent the progression of paralysis. As mentioned earlier, treatment must be given on the basis of clinical diagnosis and should not be delayed for laboratory confirmation. Federal or state public health laboratories usually must perform this testing, using approaches described previously in the chapter. In the case of this executive, the correct diagnosis was not made and botulinum antitoxin was not administered, a lapse that possibly contributed to the fatal outcome. Botulism should certainly have been diagnosed when other persons sharing the same meal developed similar symptoms. Unfortunately, many or most foodborne botulism outbreaks involve a single case, which can be difficult to diagnose early enough for optimal therapy to be given.

REVIEW QUESTIONS

Directions: For each of the following questions, choose the **one best** answer.

1. Which one of the following statements about fragment A of diphtheria toxin is correct?

    (A) It binds directly to the diphtheria toxin receptor

    (B) It acts by inactivating ribosomes

    (C) It is eventually internalized into the host cell cytoplasm

    (D) It has monoglucosyltransferase activity

    (E) It catalyzes an increase in intracellular cyclic adenosine monophosphate (cAMP) levels

2. Which one of the following toxins would cause a massive proliferation of T cells and subsequent high levels of systemic tumor necrosis factor-α (TNF-α)?

    (A) Tetanus toxin

    (B) *Escherichia coli* heat-stable enterotoxin

    (C) *Streptococcus pyogenes* pyrogenic exotoxins A and C

    (D) Shiga toxin

    (E) *Pseudomonas* exotoxin A

3. Botulinum neurotoxins have which of the following characteristics?

    (A) They induce spastic paralysis

    (B) They are heat-labile

    (C) They act by adenosine diphosphate (ADP)-ribosylating neuronal docking proteins

    (D) They must be produced in vivo to cause illness

    (E) They block the release of inhibitory neurotransmitters in the CNS

4. Which one of the following toxin:action pairings is correct?

    (A) Tetanus toxin:highly specific protease that cleaves a neuronal docking protein

    (B) Shiga toxin:increases cyclic guanosine monophosphate (cGMP) levels

    (C) Diphtheria toxin:adenosine diphosphate (ADP)-ribosylates ribosomes

    (D) Streptolysin O:has phospholipase C activity

    (E) Cholera toxin:ADP-ribosylates the Gi protein of the adenylate cyclase system

5. Which one of the following statements about botulism is correct?

    (A) This illness is always acquired by ingestion of contaminated food

    (B) This illness is rarely fatal

    (C) Initiation of treatment is usually delayed until the return of laboratory results

    (D) Treatment of this illness always involves administration of antibiotics

    (E) This illness involves a flaccid paralysis resulting from an inhibition of acetylcholine release

ANSWERS AND EXPLANATIONS

1. **The answer is C.** Option A is incorrect because it is the B (not A) fragment of diphtheria toxin that binds to the diphtheria toxin receptor. Option B is incorrect because fragment A inhibits protein synthesis by inactivating elongation factor-2, not by inactivating ribosomes (remember: shiga toxin inactivates ribosomes). Option D is incorrect because fragment A has ADP-ribosyltransferase activity (remember: *C. difficile* toxins A and B have monoglucosyltransferase activity). Option E is incorrect because fragment A does not cause an increase in intracellular cAMP levels (remember: cholera toxin, *E. coli* heat-labile enterotoxin, and pertussis toxin increase cAMP levels).

2. **The answer is C.** Superantigens induce a massive T-cell proliferation and TNF-α release; of the listed toxins, the *S. pyogenes* pyrogenic toxins A and C are the only superantigens. Tetanus toxin is a proteolytic neurotoxin. *E. coli* heat-stable enterotoxin acts by inducing an increase in intestinal cGMP levels. Shiga toxin shuts down host protein synthesis by inactivating ribosomes. Pseudomonas exotoxin A shuts down host protein synthesis by ADP-ribosylating elongation factor-2.

3. **The answer is B.** Botulinum neurotoxins are heat-labile, which means that thorough cooking of foods will reduce the occurrence of foodborne botulism. Option A is incorrect because botulinum neurotoxins induce a flaccid, not spastic, paralysis. Option C is incorrect because botulinum neurotoxins cleave, not ADP-ribosylate, neuronal docking proteins. Option D is incorrect because foodborne botulism is often an intoxication involving botulinum neurotoxin that had been produced in foods (not in vivo). Option E is incorrect because botulinum toxins act by interfering with the release of acetylcholine (a stimulatory neurotransmitter), primarily at neuromuscular junctions.

4. **The answer is A.** Option B is incorrect because shiga toxin inactivates ribosomes, that is, it does not increase cGMP levels. Option C is incorrect because diphtheria toxin ADP-ribosylates elongation factor-2, not ribosomes. Option D is incorrect because streptolysin O forms pores but does not have enzymatic activity. Option E is incorrect because cholera toxin ADP-ribosylates the Gs protein (not Gi protein) of the adenylate cyclase system.

5. **The answer is E.** Option A is incorrect because there are nonfoodborne forms of botulism, including wound and infant botulism. Option B is incorrect because there is still a significant (approximately 20%) mortality rate associated with botulism. Option C is incorrect because treatment should be initiated on the basis of clinical diagnosis and should not be delayed for the return of laboratory results. Option D is incorrect because antibiotics are rarely given to patients suffering from foodborne or infant botulism.

21 SEPSIS

Karen A. Norris, Ph.D.

CHAPTER OUTLINE

Introduction of Clinical Case
Sepsis
- Pathogenesis of Sepsis
- Host Factors Related to Sepsis
- Management of Sepsis
Resolution of Clinical Case
Review Questions

INTRODUCTION OF CLINICAL CASE

A 10-month-old boy with a history of sickle cell disease was brought to the pediatrician's office at 11:30 A.M. with a history of several days of upper respiratory infection symptoms and a high fever (104°F) the previous night. In the office, he was febrile (105°F) with tachypnea (rapid respiratory rate) and, after receiving ibuprofen for fever, was sent directly to the hospital for admission to rule out sepsis. The patient arrived at the pediatric unit about 1:00 P.M. Additional information obtained at that time revealed that he recently had not received a couple of doses of his daily penicillin prophylaxis. On examination, he was noted to be lethargic but able to drink his bottle. Blood and cerebrospinal fluid (CSF) cultures were obtained, and broad-spectrum antibiotics were ordered. At 2:00 P.M. the patient underwent a generalized seizure.

SEPSIS

The induction of the host inflammatory response, as a component of both the innate and the acquired immune responses, is of prime importance in early control of the infectious process. The orchestration of recognition, attack, and elimination of an invading pathogen is tightly regulated and is quite efficient under most circumstances. In some situations, however, innate defenses are overwhelmed by the infectious agent, and an extremely vigorous and potentially harmful inflammatory response ensues. This may occur at a localized site (see Chapter 22) or on a systemic level.

Several terms have been used over the years to describe this systemic inflammatory response to infection: sepsis, septic shock, septicemia, and endotoxic shock. As the understanding of the pathogenesis and physiology of this syndrome has progressed, a consensus definition of sepsis and its related disorders has been adopted by the American College of Chest Physicians and the Society of Critical Care Medicine. Systemic inflammatory response syndrome (SIRS) has been adopted as the broad term to describe the physiologic changes and symptoms that occur as a result of a systemic inflammatory response. SIRS can be initiated by either an infectious or a noninfectious stimulus (Figure 21-1). The term sepsis refers to a subset of SIRS that is caused by an infectious agent.

> SIRS may result from an infectious or noninfectious process.

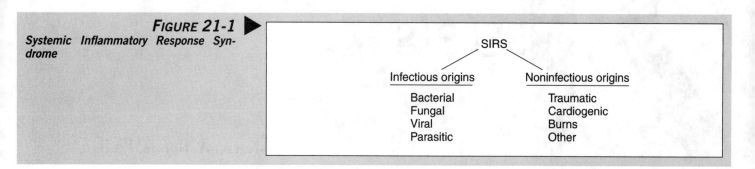

FIGURE 21-1 ▶
Systemic Inflammatory Response Syndrome

SIRS is a dynamic process that is identified in patients with two or more of the following: fever or hypothermia, tachycardia, tachypnea, and white blood cell count abnormalities. A patient may progress from sepsis to severe sepsis, as defined by decreased blood pressure, diminished perfusion of tissues (leading to hypoxia), and organ dysfunction. Septic shock hemodynamics are defined as increased cardiac output and greatly decreased peripheral vascular resistance despite attempts to restore the fluid balance. As a result of hemodynamic derangements, multiple organs may sustain damage and may fail to maintain function. This situation is referred to as multiple organ dysfunction and, in severe situations, may eventually lead to multiple organ failure and death.

Sepsis is a subset of SIRS that is initiated by an infection.

Sepsis is often initiated by the proliferation of microorganisms at a localized site, and through tissue invasion or damage, microbes or microbial products reach the bloodstream, thus initiating a systemic inflammatory response. It should be noted, however, that microorganisms may be present in the bloodstream in some infections without resulting in sepsis. The terms bacteremia, viremia, fungemia, and parasitemia refer to the presence of viable microorganisms (bacteria, viruses, fungi, and parasites, respectively) in the bloodstream, which may or may not lead to a septic state. Sepsis also may result from an overwhelming infection of a localized site (e.g., peritonitis) without direct inoculation of the bloodstream with viable microorganisms. For these reasons, as well as for better management of patients with sepsis, it is necessary to use consistent terminology to define sepsis and its sequelae based on the physiologic picture, as described above, rather than in microbiologic terms.

Pathogenesis of Sepsis

INITIATION OF THE INFLAMMATORY RESPONSE

The initial recognition of foreign microorganisms by the host immune system leads to an inflammatory response at the site of infection. This response generally efficiently contains the infection and promotes the antigen-dependent immune responses necessary to clear the infectious agent. In situations where the infection is not contained, whether because of the severity of the infection, the virulence of the microorganism, or an immunocompromised state of the host, microorganisms and their products can be disseminated via the lymphatics or bloodstream, leading to a systemic inflammatory response (Figure 21-2).

The inflammatory response is initiated by bacterial, fungal, parasitic, and helminthic pathogens and, in some cases, their secreted products. The best-characterized bacterial product capable of inducing septic shock in experimental animal models is bacterial endotoxin (lipopolysaccharide [LPS]). Until recently, gram-negative organisms accounted for most cases of sepsis, and endotoxin was found to be the principal mediator of the response (hence the term *endotoxic shock*).

The range of biologic effects of endotoxin is extraordinary. Endotoxin activates the alternate complement pathway, leading to the production of anaphylatoxins, and directly activates the coagulation cascades through interaction with factor XII. Endotoxin shed by the microorganisms also interacts with various cell types, including macrophages and endothelial cells, leading to the production of tumor necrosis factor–α (TNF-α), IL-1, prostaglandins, and other proinflammatory molecules. Many of these biologic effects of

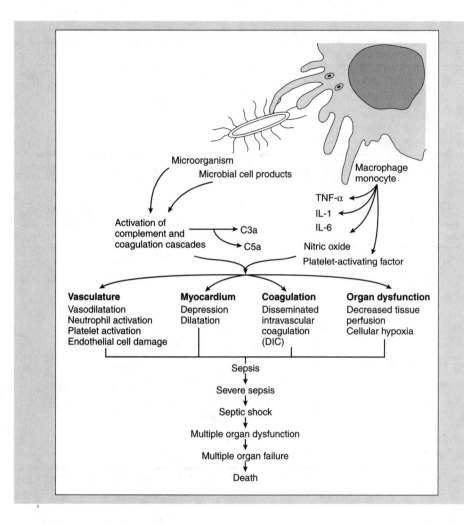

◀ **FIGURE 21-2**
Sequence of Events in Systemic Inflammatory Response. *TNF-α = tumor necrosis factor–α; IL = interleukin; DIC = disseminated intravascular coagulation; C3a, C5a = complement proteins.*

endotoxin are mediated through the lipid A moiety, which is generally conserved among gram-negative bacteria.

Other microbial products, including teichoic acid and peptidoglycan of gram-positive organisms, some bacterial exotoxins, and fungal cell wall components, are also capable of inducing a systemic inflammatory response when present in sufficient amounts in the vascular system. For example, superantigenic toxins (e.g., *Staphylococcus aureus* toxic shock syndrome toxin, pyrogenic toxins of group A streptococci; see Chapter 20) induce massive T-cell proliferation that leads to a large release of cytokines.

Cytokines. As illustrated in Figure 21-2, the interplay of the microorganism (or microbial products) with complement components and macrophages, monocytes, endothelial cells, and other cells typically leads to cellular activation and the production of several proinflammatory cytokines. Most importantly, the production of TNF-α and interleukin-1 (IL-1) has far-reaching effects on numerous cell types that contribute to the inflammatory response (Table 21-1). TNF-α and IL-1 are produced by several cell types, including monocytes, macrophages, endothelial cells, microglia, and astrocytes. In addition to its activating effects on reticuloendothelial cells, TNF-α inhibits myocyte contractility, which may contribute to cardiac dysfunction in patients with sepsis.

In addition to TNF-α and IL-1 (and in response to their production), many other factors are released that participate in the amplification of the inflammatory response, including IL-6, IL-8, platelet-activating factor (PAF), interferon-γ (IFN-γ), and metabolites of arachidonic acid (Table 21-2). These proinflammatory mediators affect the activation of immune cells and endothelial cells (by influencing vascular permeability), the mobility and adherence properties of leukocytes, the metabolic activity of a variety of cells, and cardiac function. Their amplifying effects can be extraordinarily far-reaching, causing metabolic and physiologic changes in almost every organ system.

The interaction of LPS with macrophages has been well characterized and involves binding of LPS by the serum LPS-binding protein and the cell surface receptor CD14. Subsequent cell-signaling events lead to "activation" of these cells, which is characterized by the release of cytokines as well as a heightened responsiveness to cytokines and other proinflammatory factors.

TNF-α and IL-1 are the principal host mediators of sepsis. Experimental injections of these cytokines in animals lead to a systemic inflammatory response with physiologic alterations, including fever, hypotension, and damage to endothelial cells, that resemble septic shock. The physiologic effects are dose dependent in that very high levels of circulating TNF-α and IL-1 correlate with increased mortality rates. In patients with sepsis, a very high level of TNF-α in the plasma often indicates a poor prognosis.

TABLE 21-1 ▶
Cell Targets of Tumor Necrosis Factor–α

Cell/Tissue Target	Primary Effect
Neutrophils	Activation
Endothelial cells	Activation
Liver	Production of acute-phase proteins
Muscle and fat	Catabolism
T and B lymphocytes	Costimulation
Hypothalamus	Fever

TABLE 21-2 ▶
Mediators of Sepsis

Mediator	Effect
TNF-α	Induces IL-1, IL-6, IL-8, PAF release; fever
IL-1	Fever; IL-6, IL-8 release; leukocyte migration
IL-6, IL-8	Neutrophil chemotaxis and activation, increased capillary permeability
PAF	Leukocyte activation, vascular permeability, platelet aggregation, decreased myocardial contractility
Hageman factor and clotting factors	Coagulation, fibrinolysis, complement activation
Complement	Neutrophil chemotaxis, vascular permeability
Leukotrienes	Increased vascular permeability, platelet aggregation, and neutrophil adhesion
Prostaglandins	Increased vascular permeability, fever
Nitric oxide	Vasodilator

Note. TNF-α = tumor necrosis factor–α; IL-1 = interleukin-1; PAF = platelet-activating factor.

Complement. The complement system plays a critical role in the early recognition of the presence of microorganisms and their products. Activation and amplification of the complement cascade has three beneficial effects for the host: (1) direct killing of the microbe by cell lysis, (2) coating the microorganism with opsonic proteins for increased efficiency of phagocytosis, and (3) the release of proinflammatory mediators, C3a, C4a, and C5a (anaphylatoxins). Activation of the complement cascade may occur by two different pathways, the classic and the alternate pathways. The alternate pathway represents an early, first line of defense against infection in that it may be activated by a variety of infectious agents or their cell products independent of antibody recognition and binding. Classic pathway activation generally requires recognition of microorganisms by specific antibodies. Both pathways contribute to the clearance of microorganisms and to the generation of a beneficial inflammatory response.

The anaphylatoxins have a variety of proinflammatory effects, including activation of mast cells and basophils leading to the release of histamine, and activation and increased chemotaxis of polymorphonuclear neutrophil leukocytes (PMNs; see Table 21-2). In a severe, overwhelming infection, the complement cascade is amplified to such an extent as to have deleterious effects. The effects of the anaphylatoxins and the events they stimulate lead to smooth muscle contraction, increased vascular permeability, and local endothelial cell damage. All of these events contribute to the maldistribution of fluids in the periphery, decreased venous return, and thus the hypotension that is characteristic of septic shock.

Coagulation System. The coagulation cascade may be initiated by microorganisms through direct interaction with coagulation factor XII (Hageman factor; see Table 21-2). This interaction results in a series of enzymatic reactions, ultimately leading to the production of fibrinopeptides, which increase the vascular permeability and chemotactic activity of leukocytes, thus contributing to the septic hemodynamic picture. The kinin system is also initiated by activated Hageman factor, ultimately leading to the production of bradykinin, a potent vasoactive agent. Bradykinin causes increased vascular permeability, contraction of smooth muscle cells, and vasodilatation. The clotting cascade can also contribute to the amplification of the complement cascade through the production of plasmin, a multifunctional protease that is involved in lysing fibrin clots but also can cleave the complement component C3 to its activated form. This interaction between plasmin of the coagulation cascade and C3 of the complement cascade leads to further amplification of complement activation and therefore increases proinflammatory events.

Other Mediators. Various other mediators are involved in initiating and sustaining the systemic inflammatory response, thus contributing to the hemodynamic derangement of sepsis by promoting vasodilatation, increased vascular permeability, and the induction of chemotaxis of leukocytes. Metabolites of the fatty acid arachidonic acid, leukotrienes and prostaglandins, are important mediators of vasodilatation and chemotaxis. β-Endorphin, a natural opiate produced by the pituitary gland in response to stress, appears to contribute to the hypotension associated with septic shock through its ability to depress cardiovascular function and increase vascular permeability. Nitric oxide is a short-lived, highly reactive product with potent vasodilating properties and is highly cytotoxic. It is produced constitutively in endothelial cells and some neurons and is up-regulated in response to calcium influx. Nitric oxide is also an inducible product of activated macrophages and contributes to the killing of microbial pathogens. High levels of nitric oxide produced by activated macrophages in sepsis can lead to massive vasodilatation and contribute to the progression to shock (see Table 21-2).

PROGRESSION OF SEPSIS

Although the progression from sepsis to shock and finally to multiple organ failure is a dynamic process, it primarily involves vascular disturbances. As discussed above, these events are increased vascular permeability, decreased peripheral vascular resistance, decreased venous return, decreased tissue perfusion, hypoxia, and cell death. In the initial stages, there may be an increase in cardiac output, an effort by the cardiovascular system to compensate for decreased peripheral blood pressure and diminished venous return. An effort is also made to preserve vital organs; thus, blood flow in the heart and brain are favored over other organs. Both of these responses contribute to diminished perfusion of peripheral tissues, leading to hypoxia and cellular damage. Initiation of the coagulation cascade on a systemic level (in response to widespread tissue damage and complement activation) leads to disseminated intravascular coagulation (DIC) and further tissue damage. Although the interplay of the various host responses is complex, the ultimate consequence is widespread tissue damage, leading to organ failure. Once these various host responses have been set in motion, it is likely that the proximal cause of multiple organ failure and death is the lack of down-regulation of the host inflammatory response rather than the progression of the initiating infection. Thus, prompt recognition and management of sepsis at the earliest stages is crucial. The stages in the progression of sepsis are summarized in Table 21-3.

DIC is a coagulation disorder characterized by widespread activation of the coagulation pathways, leading to the formation of microthrombi and deposition of fibrin in the microcirculation. Both events may lead to ischemia and tissue damage. A second consequence of DIC is consumption of platelets and clotting factors, resulting in a failure to control bleeding.

Host Factors Related to Sepsis

Although the medical and surgical advances in the last several decades, particularly the introduction of antibiotics, have allowed more critically ill patients to survive their underlying illness, many still succumb to multiple organ failure associated with shock. When septic shock became widely recognized as a cause of organ failure in these patients, it was primarily associated with gram-negative organisms that could be cultured from patients' blood. For this reason, the term sepsis was used interchangeably with gram-negative bacteremia. More recently, however, gram-positive organisms and nonbacterial pathogens (particularly fungi) account for more than half of the sepsis cases in the United States. Several factors may account for this shift, including the increased use of indwelling catheters and prosthetic devices, immunosuppression related to chemotherapy and acquired immunodeficiency syndrome (AIDS), and other underlying illnesses such as diabetes and cirrhosis.

There are approximately 400,000 cases of sepsis in the United States annually, many of which lead to death.

Certain host factors may predispose patients to sepsis caused by particular types of pathogens. As in the clinical case presented here, sickle cell anemia patients become

TABLE 21-3 ▶
Stages in the Progression of Sepsis

Initiation of inflammatory response
Increased arteriolar dilatation
Increased vascular permeability
Movement of fluids, cells, and solutes into peripheral tissues
Increased venous pooling
Decreased venous return

Compensatory response to altered hemodynamic state
Decreased effective cardiac volume
Increased cardiac output
Preservation of perfusion of vital organs (further decreasing blood flow to peripheral tissues)

Continued hypoperfusion of tissues
Anoxic injury leading to DIC and further tissue injury
Shock
Multiple organ failure
Death

Individuals with sickle cell disease are at increased risk for bacterial sepsis and meningitis, particularly that caused by the pneumococcus. The risk of acquiring pneumococcal meningitis is 300–500 times greater than that in children without sickle cell disease.

functionally asplenic because of multiple infarcts in the spleen, resulting in defective antibody production, and are therefore particularly susceptible to infections with encapsulated organisms such as *Streptococcus pneumoniae, Haemophilus influenzae,* and *Neisseria meningitidis* (see Chapter 18). Because of the danger of overwhelming infections with these organisms in the pediatric population, young patients with sickle cell disease are treated prophylactically with penicillin. Neutropenic patients are often highly susceptible to infections with gram-negative bacteria and fungal pathogens such as *Aspergillus* spp. and *Candida* spp. Patients with defects in T-cell immunity (e.g., AIDS patients) are particularly susceptible to pathogens that require cell-mediated immune response for control or clearance. For this reason, intracellular pathogens such as *Mycobacterium* spp. and viruses are particularly problematic in these patients.

Management of Sepsis

Patients with sepsis are treated in intensive care units, where continual monitoring is of prime importance. The components of treatment of septic shock are (1) antibiotics, (2) fluid replacement, (3) oxygen, and (4) drugs to promote vasoconstriction (vasopressors). Treatment with broad-spectrum antibiotics is recommended until culture information has been obtained, so that both gram-positive and gram-negative organisms will be covered. Prompt treatment with antibiotics is necessary, but it may not be sufficient to prevent the progression from sepsis to shock, which can occur rapidly, as in the clinical case presented here. Continued progression of the inflammatory response, even after the initiating infection is under control, suggests that down-regulation of cytokine-mediated responses may be dysfunctional in some situations or that the inflammatory response has progressed beyond the ability of the host's natural regulatory mechanisms. New methods of treating sepsis aim at promoting down-regulation of the inflammatory response to prevent end-stage organ damage of septic shock. Several clinical trials have attempted to dampen the effects of TNF-α or IL-1 using neutralizing monoclonal antibodies or receptor antagonists. These experimental treatments have met with limited success, most likely because of the complex interactions of mediators of sepsis, as discussed above.

RESOLUTION OF CLINICAL CASE

The patient was transferred to the pediatric intensive care unit and received antibiotics (ceftriaxone and vancomycin). Gram staining of the CSF showed gram-positive cocci. At 4:00 P.M., the patient experienced cardiac arrest and underwent cardiopulmonary resuscitation (CPR) for 5 minutes before recovering a stable heart rate. At 5:30 P.M., the patient underwent a second, prolonged cardiac arrest, and extensive attempts at resuscitation were unsuccessful. His blood and CSF cultures were subsequently found to be positive for penicillin-sensitive *S. pneumoniae.*

REVIEW QUESTIONS

Directions: For each of the following questions, choose the **one best** answer.

1. Which of the following predisposes an individual to sepsis?

    (A) Breach of anatomic barriers

    (B) Neutropenia

    (C) Genetic defects in complement components

    (D) Chemotherapy with bone marrow cytotoxic agents

    (E) All of the above

2. Which one of the following statements is true?

    (A) Sepsis refers to the presence of viable microorganisms in the bloodstream

    (B) Sepsis refers to the presence of viable microorganisms in localized sites in the body

    (C) The role of tumor necrosis factor–α (TNF-α) in sepsis is the down-regulation of proinflammatory cytokine synthesis

    (D) TNF-α and interleukin 1 (IL-1) are primary mediators of systemic inflammatory response syndrome

    (E) Septic shock is characterized by profound hypertension

3. The initiation of the complement cascade

    (A) requires antigen-specific immunoglobulin

    (B) occurs exclusively in the spleen

    (C) occurs exclusively in the liver

    (D) results from binding complement components to bacteria and bacterial cell products

    (E) is inhibited by the protease plasmin of the coagulation cascade

4. A major consequence of the elicitation of host inflammatory response to infectious agents is

    (A) increased vascular permeability

    (B) induction of septic shock

    (C) induction of systemic inflammatory response syndrome (SIRS)

    (D) detriment to the host, which must be immediately controlled with anti-inflammatory drugs

    (E) polyclonal T-cell activation

ANSWERS AND EXPLANATIONS

1. **The answer is E.** Options A, B, C, and D describe situations of immunologic defects that result in decreased function of innate host defense effector mechanisms and are all predisposing factors to sepsis.

2. **The answer is D.** TNF-α and IL-1 are the primary mediators of the systemic inflammatory response. In experimental systems, TNF-α and IL-1 alone can induce a shock-like syndrome. Options A and B are incorrect because sepsis is defined as the systemic inflammatory response induced by microorganisms, not by the anatomic site of infection. Option C is incorrect because one of the primary influences of TNF-α is the up-regulation of pro-inflammatory mediators such as IL-1, IL-6, and IL-8. Option E is incorrect because septic shock is characterized by profound hypotension, resulting in part from maldistribution of blood.

3. **The answer is D.** The complement cascade may be initiated when complement components bind to microorganisms or their cell products. Option A is incorrect because initiation of the alternate pathway occurs in the absence of specific immunoglobulins and so represents an early host defense mechanism. Options B and C are incorrect because complement proteins are present in the plasma, and therefore activation is not specific to the liver or spleen. Option E is incorrect because the complement cascade may be initiated by cleavage of C3 by plasmin, thus linking the complement and coagulation cascades.

4. **The answer is A.** Several factors (such as the anaphylatoxins and the kinins) produced during an inflammatory response promote vascular permeability. It is important to note that the inflammatory response to an infection is a protective, beneficial host response, and in the context of a localized infection, the inflammatory response promotes clearance of the infectious agent. Options B and C are incorrect because the progression to SIRS and septic shock is the result of systemic inflammation when the infection is overwhelming and when there is a defect in the host's immune system, not as a general consequence of an inflammatory response. A polyclonal T-cell response does not generally follow the induction of an inflammatory response.

22 IMMUNOPATHOLOGIC CONSEQUENCES OF INFLAMMATION

JoAnne L. Flynn, Ph.D.

CHAPTER OUTLINE

Introduction of Clinical Case
Immunopathology in Response to Infection: Pathology vs. Protection
Mechanisms of Pathogen-Elicited Immunopathology
- Immune Complex Formation
- Cross-Reactive Antibodies
- Cell-Mediated Reactions: Granuloma Formation

Illustrative Pathogen: *Mycobacterium tuberculosis*
- Biologic Characteristics
- Reservoir and Transmission
- Virulence Factors
- Pathogenesis
- Diagnosis
- Prevention and Treatment

Illustrative Pathogen: *Schistosoma* spp.
- Biologic Characteristics
- Reservoir and Transmission
- Virulence Factors
- Pathogenesis
- Diagnosis
- Prevention and Treatment

Resolution of Clinical Case
Review Questions

INTRODUCTION OF CLINICAL CASE

A 60-year-old man visited the clinic complaining of a persistent cough, night sweats, and some difficulty breathing during the past 3 months. His temperature at this visit was 100°F, and blood tests showed a normal leukocyte count. A purified protein derivative (PPD; tuberculin) skin test was placed and sputum was obtained for staining and culturing. The patient volunteered that previous PPD skin test results had been positive for 30 years. Acid-fast bacilli were observed in the sputum following staining, and the patient was put in respiratory isolation. A chest x-ray showed a dense infiltrate within the right upper lobe, within which could be discerned a "highlight" consistent with a cavity. Two days later, the PPD test gave an induration of 15 mm.

- What infectious agent is responsible for this patient's symptoms?
- What does cavity formation signify?

- What special precautions must be taken with this patient?
- What is the significance of a 15-mm induration resulting from a PPD skin test?
- What is the treatment for this disease?

IMMUNOPATHOLOGY IN RESPONSE TO INFECTION: PATHOLOGY VS. PROTECTION

Following an encounter with a pathogen, the host mounts various immune responses, both innate and acquired, in an effort to eliminate the pathogen. For the most part, these responses are ultimately effective and clear the infection. However, in some cases, the immune response that is designed to eliminate the pathogen also results in damage to the host. A classic example is sepsis, as described in the preceding chapter. An immuno-pathologic response can occur in a variety of other ways and may be an unavoidable consequence of the effective response to an infection. In some infections, for example tuberculosis, the price paid for protection against disease can be tissue pathology. In other cases, the disease is the direct result of tissue damage caused by the host response to the infection, for example, schistosomiasis and hepatitis B virus (HBV). Additionally, damage to the host may result when the immune response against a pathogen also targets host tissues, as in the case of cross-reactive antibodies in such diseases as rheumatic fever, which can be a complication of untreated group A streptococcal infection (see Chapter 16). The development of vaccines against infections that can trigger harmful immune responses is challenging, as the vaccine strategy must avoid elicitation of antihost tissue responses. Thus, a thorough understanding of the interaction of pathogen and host is often required before a safe and effective vaccine can be developed.

MECHANISMS OF PATHOGEN-ELICITED IMMUNOPATHOLOGY

Immune Complex Formation

Immune complexes can result when antibody binds soluble antigen and forms a matrix. The large antibody–antigen complexes that form in the presence of sufficient antibody are cleared by cells bearing a receptor for antibody (the Fc receptor). When antigen is in excess, it is not adequately coated by antibody, and these small immune complexes are not removed by reticuloendothelial cells. Immune complexes continue to circulate in the blood and can deposit in tissues and small blood vessels, leading to inflammation and tissue damage. Inflammation is initiated by complement activation at the site of immune complex deposition. Complement activation results in polymorphonuclear neutrophil (PMN) cell and monocyte infiltration. The production and release of proinflammatory molecules by phagocytes and the discharge of degradative enzymes from the PMNs contribute to tissue damage.

One common form of immune complex–mediated disease is glomerulonephritis, occurring when immune complexes are deposited in the glomeruli of the kidneys. This is an important complication of group A streptococcal infection. Immune complexes form during the acute infection, and deposition continues after the infection is resolved, with glomerulonephritis occurring 1 or 2 weeks later. This is thought to be due to the continuous release of microbial antigens, perhaps during a subpatent or chronic infection. Immune complex deposition and glomerulonephritis can also occur during other infections, such as with *Plasmodium* spp. (malaria) and *Treponema pallidum* (during secondary syphilis).

Cross-Reactive Antibodies

Microbial antigens that mimic host antigens can give rise to cross-reactive antibodies. These antibodies can cause host tissue damage, and it is thought that some autoimmune diseases are actually caused by antibodies against microbial antigens that can also bind to host tissue. The most widely recognized disease considered to be due to antigenic cross-reactivity between host and pathogen is rheumatic fever, which can follow group A streptococcal infection of the throat. Antibodies against streptococcal antigens cross-react with heart tissue and can result in myocarditis. Repeated streptococcal infections can cause recurrent rheumatic fever attacks. The advent of antibiotic treatment for group A streptococcal infections has drastically reduced the incidence in industrialized countries, but rheumatic fever continues to be a major cause of heart disease in developing countries (see Chapter 16).

Cell-Mediated Reactions: Granuloma Formation

Cell-mediated immune responses (i.e., those involving T cells) are necessary for the successful elimination of most pathogens. When a cell-mediated immune response is mounted, inflammation, lymphocyte and macrophage recruitment, and macrophage activation result. These responses, while required to control and eliminate an infection, can be responsible for pathology also. In particular, chronic infections with intracellular pathogens can lead to an ongoing cell-mediated immune response, with a resulting pathology. A classic example of the response to a chronic infection is granuloma formation. A granuloma is a collection of macrophages, often fused to form a giant multinucleated cell surrounded by lymphocytes, which acts to contain and localize an infection within a tissue (Figure 22-1). The granuloma is a pathologic reaction, which is often a necessary component of the successful immune response to a pathogen (e.g., tuberculosis). In some cases, granulomas formed in response to microbial antigens form the pathologic basis for disease caused by that microbe (e.g., schistosomiasis). Granuloma formation can result from infection with various bacteria, parasites, and fungi.

Microorganisms That Cause Granulomatous Disease	
Organism	**Disease**
Mycobacterium tuberculosis	Tuberculosis
Mycobacterium leprae	Leprosy
Bartonella henselae	Cat scratch disease
Coccidioides immitis	Coccidioidomycosis
Histoplasma capsulatum	Histoplasmosis
Schistosoma species	Schistosomiasis

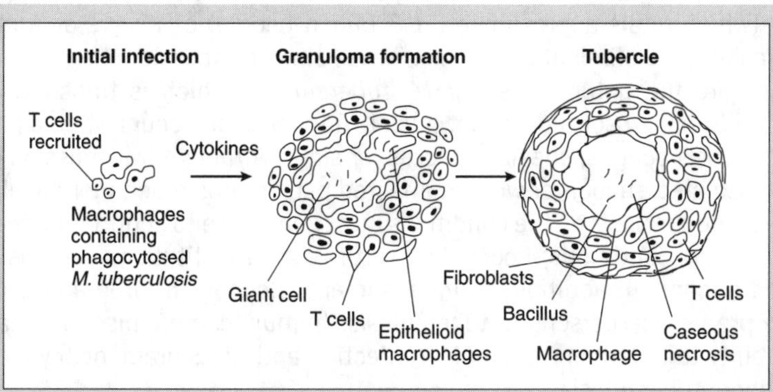

◀ **FIGURE 22-1**
Granuloma Formation in Tuberculosis

Granulomas form in response to a microbial antigen, often to intracellular pathogens. Mononuclear cells are recruited to the site of infection, as are specific T lymphocytes. The T cells produce cytokines, which act on the macrophages containing the pathogen at the center of the granuloma. In addition, cytolytic T cells can lyse the infected macrophages, releasing bacteria to be taken up by activated macrophages within the granuloma. Thus, the granuloma acts locally to control the infection and to prevent the spread of the pathogen to the rest of the tissue. An unfortunate side effect of this is localized pathology and some loss of host tissue.

Two fungal infections, caused by the dimorphic fungi *Histoplasma capsulatum* and *Coccidioides immitis*, resemble tuberculosis both in symptoms and in pathology. *H. capsulatum* is found in river valleys in the central United States, while *C. immitis* is prevalent in the southwestern United States. *H. capsulatum* causes pulmonary infections and is asymptomatic in approximately 60% of those infected. Granuloma formation occurs in response to a chronic infection, as occurs with *Mycobacterium tuberculosis* (see below), and immunocompromised persons can "reactivate" the chronic infection, with serious consequences.

ILLUSTRATIVE PATHOGEN: *Mycobacterium tuberculosis*

Biologic Characteristics

Tuberculosis is caused by a bacterium, *M. tuberculosis*, which is an aerobic, non–spore-forming, nonmotile bacillus. It is rod-shaped and tends to clump in culture and histologic specimens, giving the appearance of groups of rods. As described in Chapter 1, Figure 1-9, mycobacteria are neither gram-positive nor gram-negative but are instead termed acid-fast bacilli (AFB). When stained with a phenolic red dye, mycobacteria retain the red color even upon acid-alcohol decolorization. This characteristic is likely due to the high lipid content of their cell wall, which forms a waxy outer covering for the bacteria. This unique cell wall makes mycobacteria resistant to environmental factors and many antibacterial agents. Although *M. tuberculosis* can be propagated in laboratory media, pathogenic mycobacteria are very slow-growing, with a doubling time of 16–18 hours in liquid media (compared with less than 1 hour for most human pathogens) and an estimated doubling time in the host of 16–24 hours. These factors have made the genetic study of *M. tuberculosis* very difficult, and genetic systems for studying the pathogenesis of this organism have been described only recently. In addition, the slow growth rate of *M. tuberculosis* prevents rapid definitive diagnosis of infection.

> The slow rate of mycobacterial growth prevents rapid diagnosis of infection. The **Bactec method** of assessing mycobacterial growth allows diagnosis within 2 weeks. A sputum (or other) specimen is treated with NaOH to kill most bacteria; mycobacteria survive this treatment. The Bactec bottle containing liquid medium with radioactive carbon source is inoculated with the treated specimen. As the mycobacteria grow, radioactive CO_2 is given off and measured. The amount of radioactive CO_2 corresponds to the growth rate. This method cannot distinguish among the various mycobacteria, but it is used to test for susceptibility to antibiotics.

Reservoir and Transmission

Tuberculosis kills approximately 3 million people worldwide each year, and one-third of the world's population is infected with *M. tuberculosis*. Infection with *M. tuberculosis* can result in active or latent tuberculosis. Active tuberculosis within 2 years of infection occurs in a small percentage of infected people. Only those with active tuberculosis are infectious to others. Most *M. tuberculosis*–infected people are latently infected and are not infectious. However, reactivation of infection occurs in approximately 10% of latently infected persons, resulting in active, contagious tuberculosis. Thus, the latently infected population (which totals approximately 1.7 billion people) can serve as a reservoir of infection, making the elimination of this disease almost impossible to imagine.

Humans are the natural host for *M. tuberculosis*, which is transmitted via the respiratory route in aerosolized droplet nuclei. Transmission occurs when a person with active tuberculosis coughs, speaks, sneezes, or sings. Although transmission can occur following an isolated encounter with an infected person, it is much more likely to occur following repeated exposure. The conditions most conducive to contracting tuberculosis are crowded living conditions, poor urban settings, and institutions such as homeless shelters and prisons. In addition, malnourishment, alcoholism, drug abuse, and other factors can predispose persons to tuberculosis. Immunocompromise is a major factor in susceptibility to tuberculosis, and HIV infection and AIDS dramatically increase the susceptibility to tuberculosis.

> Although this form is rarely seen these days, tuberculosis can also be caused by Mycobacterium bovis, *which is a bovine pathogen. In* fact, *transmission from the ingestion of contaminated milk was common until the advent of pasteurization.*

Virulence Factors

Very few, if any, proven virulence factors have been identified in *M. tuberculosis*. In part, this is due to the difficulty in performing genetic experiments with mycobacteria. *M. tuberculosis* does not seem to possess obvious or classic virulence factors, such as toxins. In order to cause disease, the bacillus needs to be able to survive in the macrophage; the factors that dictate macrophage survival could be considered virulence factors. The bacterium is taken up by phagocytosis into the macrophage, and it resides in a phagosome. Experimentally, it has been shown that uptake is partially mediated by both complement and mannose receptors on macrophages. The complex, lipid-rich cell wall probably protects the organism in the hostile environment of the macrophage. Fusion of the phagosome with the lysosome appears to be inhibited by *M. tuberculosis*, which would prevent the bacteria from coming into contact with the contents of the lysosome. The mechanism by which this occurs is unknown. Acidification of the phagosome has been reported to be inhibited by *M. tuberculosis*, providing a more hospitable environment for the bacillus. The respiratory burst and reactive oxygen intermediates (oxygen radicals, H_2O_2, etc.) are not particularly effective against *M. tuberculosis*. Instead, reactive nitrogen intermediates, such as nitric oxide, are capable of killing *M. tuberculosis* bacilli. Nitric oxide is produced by activated murine macrophages, although the importance of this antimycobacterial mechanism in human macrophages remains to be proved. As discussed below, the host immune response to *M. tuberculosis* participates in the disease by causing a pathologic state and destruction of host tissue. The persistent nature of the infection contributes to disease by resulting in a chronic inflammatory response. Various components of the mycobacterial cell wall cause the production of inflammatory cytokines, such as tumor necrosis factor-α (TNF-α) and interleukin-1 (IL-1). These molecules and other cytokines participate in the pathogenesis of tuberculosis and also result in the low-grade fever that characterizes this disease.

Pathogenesis

Most persons infected with *M. tuberculosis* develop a cell-mediated immune response against the pathogen. This can be detected by a skin test for a delayed-type hypersensitivity response against mycobacterial PPD, which is a standard diagnostic test for exposure to *M. tuberculosis*. A positive PPD test result (induration at the site of PPD injection) does not mean that the person has active tuberculosis, just that he or she was exposed to and infected with the bacillus. Only those with active tuberculosis are infectious to others. A small percentage of people, particularly those with weakened immune systems, may develop active tuberculosis a short time after exposure. Most PPD-positive people do not develop active disease, but harbor the organism for their lifetime. In about 10% of those PPD-positive persons, the infection will be reactivated at some later time and become active tuberculosis. The host factors responsible for maintaining latent *M. tuberculosis* infection and those that allow reactivation are unknown at this time. Cell-mediated immune responses involving T cells and macrophage activation are certain to be important in preventing reactivation. In support of this hypothesis, immunosuppression due to age, drugs, or another infection contributes to the reactivation of latent tuberculosis. Persons infected with HIV have a greatly increased risk of reactivation, even before CD4 T cell levels become significantly diminished.

> *A PPD skin test result is generally read as positive if induration (not merely redness) at the site of placement is 10 mm or greater. In AIDS patients, the induration may be smaller because of waning T-cell responses.*

M. tuberculosis is primarily a respiratory pathogen, although infection can occur in any tissue in the human body. The disease can be pulmonary, extrapulmonary, or miliary (disseminated). In the normal course of infection, *M. tuberculosis* bacilli are inhaled into an alveolus and ingested by alveolar macrophages. The bacterium may be destroyed by the macrophage, or it may establish an infection and multiply. The infection is spread hematogenously, and many tissues can be seeded with the organism. Bloodborne bacilli are usually deposited in the apical sections of the lungs. The multiplying bacteria are taken up by other macrophages and monocytes that may be attracted to the site of infection by factors released by infected macrophages. Resting (nonactivated) macrophages are not capable of killing intracellular *M. tuberculosis* bacilli. Activation of macrophages requires a cell-mediated immune response to be mounted against the infection. This occurs 1 to 3 weeks following infection; T cells specific for mycobacterial antigens migrate to the site of infection, and a granuloma forms around the infected macrophages. The macrophages in the center of the granuloma can be destroyed by the bacteria or by the immune response against the bacteria and form a necrotic center in the granuloma. This necrotic center causes pathology and loss of viable tissue in the lungs. The initiation of a T-cell response and formation of the granuloma in most cases prevent the further rapid replication and spread of the infection. It is not clear whether replication of the mycobacteria is completely halted within the granuloma, or whether it continues at a very low rate. With containment of the infection, healing and fibrosis occur, with eventual scar formation around the granuloma; this is also referred to as a tubercle. Although such a lesion is less than desirable, granuloma formation is essential to the successful control of *M. tuberculosis* infection. When the immune system is compromised in some manner, reactivation of the bacilli contained within the granuloma occurs, and bacteria replicate and spread to other parts of the organ. In active pulmonary tuberculosis, significant pulmonary pathologic changes are seen, with cavity formation, necrosis, and actual liquefaction of lung tissue. Bacteria grow well in damaged lung tissue. When liquefaction of a lesion occurs, the contents, including large numbers of

M. tuberculosis bacteria, can spill into the bronchus and then are spread to other people when the patient breathes or coughs.

Extrapulmonary tuberculosis occurs less frequently than pulmonary tuberculosis. Tuberculosis can occur in almost any organ or site in the body. Lymphatic and pleural tuberculosis are the most common extrapulmonary forms of infection, but genitourinary, skeletal, and meningeal tuberculosis are also seen. Miliary tuberculosis is progressive disseminated hematogenous tuberculosis and can be acute or chronic. Both miliary and extrapulmonary tuberculosis are more common in AIDS patients than in the general population of PPD-positive persons. Children are also more susceptible to extrapulmonary and miliary tuberculosis.

Since *M. tuberculosis* is an intracellular pathogen, the immune response to *M. tuberculosis* requires T cells, while an antibody response plays a minor, if any, role. CD4 T cells, and possibly CD8 T cells, participate in control of the infection through the production of macrophage-activating cytokines and by killing infected cells. The cytokine interferon-γ (IFN-γ), produced by T cells, activates macrophages in conjunction with other cytokines or bacterial products. Macrophage activation is essential for control of the infection. TNF-α and other cytokines also play important roles in the response to this infection.

Immunocompromised persons, such as those infected with HIV, are more susceptible to initial infection with *M. tuberculosis*, to active tuberculosis shortly after infection, and to the reactivation of latent tuberculosis infection. The AIDS epidemic has collided with the large number of tuberculosis cases worldwide to create a public health problem of great magnitude. Pulmonary tuberculosis in HIV-positive individuals can be very similar to that in HIV-negative patients, if the CD4 T cell levels are still high in the HIV-positive patient. However, in more immunocompromised HIV-positive patients, pulmonary tuberculosis is often notable for the lack of cavitation and infiltrates in the lower or middle lobes of the lungs. Extrapulmonary and miliary tuberculosis are also common in AIDS patients. Tuberculosis can occur throughout the body, including the lymphatics, liver, bone, genitourinary system, and gastrointestinal system.

Diagnosis

The symptoms of active tuberculosis include coughing, dyspnea, fever (often night sweats), fatigue, anorexia, and weight loss. In contrast to acute pneumonia, the symptoms can linger for many months before a patient seeks medical help. A skin test with mycobacterial proteins (PPD) is usually placed; a positive reaction indicates exposure to or infection with *M. tuberculosis*, although it does not indicate active infection. A chest x-ray is performed in cases of suspected tuberculosis. An infiltrate in the upper lobe is characteristic of tuberculosis, although infiltrate can also be observed in the lower lobes. In some cases, a lesion or cavity can be distinguished. If the patient is producing sputum, it is stained for AFB. The bacteria will stain as slightly bent red rods on a blue background. Fluorochrome stains for AFB are often used for sputum samples. Sputum specimens are also cultured for mycobacteria. In cases where sputum cannot be obtained, bronchial washings obtained by bronchoscopy are stained and cultured. The slow-growing nature of this organism can delay definitive diagnosis, and screening for antibiotic susceptibility of the organism can take many weeks.

Prevention and Treatment

Before the advent of antibiotic therapy for tuberculosis, only half of tuberculosis patients survived. Tuberculosis is generally amenable to antibiotic treatment, although drug-resistant strains have become a problem in recent years. Successful treatment requires a course of two to four antibiotics for 6 months to a year. Drug resistance is often the result of noncompliance with the antibiotic regimen. The front-line antituberculosis drugs are isoniazid, rifampin, pyrazinamide, and ethambutol. Although a few other drugs are available, the cell wall of mycobacteria makes them very resistant to most antibiotics. Strains of *M. tuberculosis* that are resistant to multiple antituberculosis drugs have been isolated in the United States and other countries; patients infected with such strains have a 50% mortality risk. Clearly, more chemotherapeutic options for tuberculosis are necessary.

---

*HIV-positive patients who present with symptoms of tuberculosis may be more difficult to diagnose, since pulmonary tuberculosis may have a different appearance on chest x-rays. Confounding the diagnosis further, HIV-positive patients may be PPD-negative on skin test, owing to anergy (nonreactivity to T-cell antigens). For this reason, an **anergy panel** may be placed on HIV-positive patients when a PPD test is placed. The anergy panel consists of antigens to which most people are commonly exposed: mumps, Candida (yeast), trichophyton. If a patient does not respond to these antigens, a negative result from the PPD test is meaningless.*

Acid-fast staining is performed by fixing a sample (sputum, culture, CSF) on slide and flooding the slide with phenol-based red stain (carbolfuschin). The slide is then treated with acid-alcohol and counterstained with blue dye. Bacteria, except acid-fast bacteria, do not retain the dye in the presence of acid. Mycobacteria retain the red dye, even when washed with acid, probably because of their lipid-rich cell walls, and stain red on a blue background. This method is not very sensitive, since at least 5000 bacilli/mL sputum must be present to be detected by direct microscopy.

Although an attenuated mycobacterial strain, BCG (bacille Calmette-Guérin) is used worldwide (although not currently in the United States) as a vaccine against tuberculosis, the effectiveness of BCG has been questioned. Its efficacy in various studies ranges from 70% protection to no protection at all. A better vaccine is needed to prevent the spread of tuberculosis in developing and developed countries. Given the large numbers of cases and deaths due to tuberculosis, such a vaccine would have a major impact on health worldwide.

Fluorochrome stains are also used to identify acid-fast organisms in patient samples. The concept is similar to that of acid-fast staining, except that the stain used is auramine-O or auramine-rhodamine. The bacteria appear yellow or orange when viewed with a fluorescent microscope. This type of staining makes detection of the bacteria in the sample faster than standard acid-fast staining since screening of the sample can be performed at a lower magnification.

ILLUSTRATIVE PATHOGEN: *Schistosoma* spp.

Biologic Characteristics

The primary blood flukes responsible for schistosomiasis include *Schistosoma mansoni*, *S. japonicum*, and *S. haematobium*. These flatworms are a major cause of disease, infecting more than 200 million people worldwide. The life cycle of this parasitic worm (helminth) is shown in Figure 22-2 and involves an adult worm stage in humans, which reproduces sexually to produce eggs. These eggs are excreted by the human host, and hatch in fresh water to form motile miracidia. The miracidia penetrate the body of the intermediate host, a snail. Inside the snail, asexual reproduction results in the production of large numbers of motile cercariae, infectious to humans. During invasion of the skin, the cercariae transform into schistosomulae, which migrate to the liver and lungs, where they mature into adult worms. The *S. mansoni* and *S. japonicum* worms spread through the venous system to take up residence in the portal or mesenteric vessels; *S. haematobium* resides in the vesical plexus of the urinary tract.

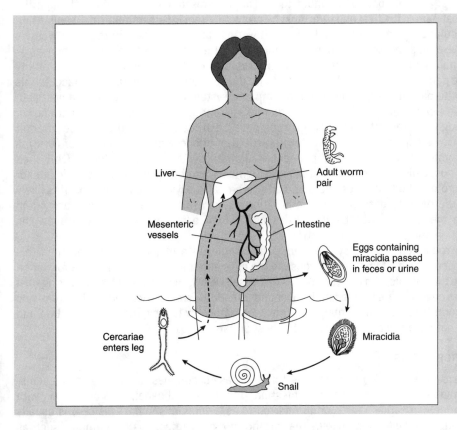

◄ **FIGURE 22-2**
Schistosoma *Life Cycle*

Reservoir and Transmission

There are endemic regions in Africa, Asia, and South America; different species are prevalent in different areas (Table 22-1). Each species of schistosome has its own specific intermediate host snail, and the distribution of *Schistosoma* species is depen-

Schistosomiasis

TABLE 22-1 ▶

Schistosoma species	Geographic Distribution	Final Habitat in Host	Site of Pathology
S. mansoni	Arabia Africa South America Caribbean	Mesenteric blood vessels	Intestines Liver
S. Japonicum	Japan China Philippines	Mesenteric blood vessels	Intestines Liver
S. haematobium	Africa Middle East	Vesical plexus	Ureter Bladder

dent on the snail prevalence in each area. Although it is estimated that many people (primarily immigrants) in the United States are infected with schistosomes, the absence of the snail intermediate host prevents spread of the disease in this country.

As discussed above, the *Schistosoma* eggs are excreted in the feces or urine of infected humans and hatch in fresh water to release a form infectious to snails. The infectious cercariae form, which emerges from snails, can penetrate human skin and usually infects humans who have frequent contact with contaminated water. Thus, the method of disposal of human waste and the amount of contact a society has with contaminated water play large roles in transmission of the infection.

Virulence Factors

The mechanisms that provide the *Schistosoma* parasite with the ability to survive within the host are not completely understood. The schistosomula must migrate through the bloodstream to the liver and thus must be protected from innate immune mechanisms, in particular the complement system. Adult worms can live for years in the blood vessels and also must possess mechanisms that protect them from host immune responses. A fascinating mechanism possessed by both schistosomula and adult worms is the ability of the parasite to "kidnap" host proteins and display them on the parasite surface. In this way, the parasite can "hide" from the immune system by masquerading as a host cell. The full extent of host antigens that can be appropriated by the parasite is not known, although several different host antigens have been identified on the surface of adult worms. Perhaps the best-studied example is that of decay accelerating factor (DAF), a host protein that prevents complement-mediated lysis of host cells. Human DAF, shed from host cells, is inserted into the parasite membrane by means of a glycolipid anchor and protects both schistosomula and adult worms from lysis by complement. It is likely that the parasite has evolved several other mechanisms to evade host immunity, and these mechanisms can be thought of as "virulence factors" in that they allow the infection and the disease to continue.

Production of eggs by the adult schistosomes is a major virulence factor in this infection. The host immune response to the eggs and the resulting granuloma formation cause the pathology in this disease, as discussed below. However, the response is against excess eggs that are trapped in the liver and intestines, are not excreted, and therefore do not contribute to further infection. Thus, the pathology is a byproduct of infection and does not have obvious benefits for the host or parasite.

Pathogenesis

Schistosoma infection can result in three disease syndromes: dermatitis, acute schistosomiasis, and chronic liver and intestinal disease. Initial penetration of the skin with cercariae can cause a rash, often referred to as "swimmer's itch." This rash is usually caused by *Schistosoma* species that are not normally infectious for humans, such as those from birds, although it can also occur following infection with human schistosomes. The rash occurs in previously sensitized individuals and results from cercariae that die in the dermis. This is an additional example of pathology resulting from the immune response against a microbe. An acute infection, also known as Katayama fever, can occur 2–3 weeks following infection, with fever, lymphadenopathy, and hepato-splenomegaly. This syndrome is more commonly seen with *S. japonicum* infections. Usually recovery is spontaneous, although in cases of heavy infection, Katayama fever can lead to death. The major consequence of schistosomiasis is the chronic liver, intestinal, and bladder disease caused by the immune response to the schistosome eggs.

Adult worm pairs living in vessels produce eggs, which are excreted. Eggs that are not excreted are carried away by the bloodstream and lodge in the liver and intestines, where a strong granulomatous response against the egg antigens is evoked. The granulomas are T cell–mediated and form in response to soluble egg antigens secreted by the miracidia within the eggs. The inflammatory cells recruited to the site of egg deposition cannot ingest the eggs, and a chronic inflammatory response ensues. The granulomatous inflammation is very strong in acute infection, but it becomes down-modulated to some extent during chronic infection. These granulomas contain eosinophils, a hallmark of worm infections. The granulomas eventually become fibrotic and can cause extensive pathology in the liver and intestines. The chronic inflammation and fibrosis in some heavily infected individuals can result in portal hypertension, hepatosplenomegaly, and gastrointestinal rupture and bleeding. *S. hematobium* causes a similar inflammation of the bladder. Thus, the response of the host to a byproduct of infection (eggs) is the key player in the pathologic changes of schistosomiasis.

Diagnosis

In diagnosing patients outside endemic areas, it is most relevant to take a travel history to determine potential sources of contact with reservoir snails. A definitive schistosomiasis diagnosis is made by microscopic identification of eggs in the stool or urine. However, the number of eggs excreted can be fairly small. Rectal biopsy with subsequent microscopic examination for eggs may also be performed. Immunologic tests do not provide information on the intensity of infection, nor do they differentiate between active and past infections. They are therefore of less use in the diagnosis of schistosomiasis.

Prevention and Treatment

Studies suggest that effective resistance to infection or reinfection may develop after 5–15 years of exposure. Vaccines against *Schistosoma* infections are the subject of research, but none are currently available. Prevention of infection and reinfection are next to impossible in endemic areas, where sanitation may be a problem, and people have constant contact with contaminated water. Attempts to eradicate the snail reservoir have been ineffective.

Effective drug management of schistosomiasis has become a reality in the past few years. Praziquantal, a broad-spectrum antihelminthic drug, is safe and effective against the major human schistosome infections. It can be administered orally as a 1-day treatment, which allows for effective treatment of people in areas that are difficult to serve with medical care. Praziquantal results in parasitologic cure and reduction of the egg burden, and it has only few and minor side effects.

RESOLUTION OF CLINICAL CASE

On the basis of the sputum containing AFB, the positive PPD skin test result, and the chest x-ray results, the presumptive diagnosis is pulmonary tuberculosis caused by reactivation of a prior infection. The patient was given a four-antibiotic regimen consisting of isoniazid, rifampicin, pyrazinamide, and ethambutol. Two weeks later, the culture of the sputum samples revealed *M. tuberculosis* bacilli. Two subsequent sputum specimens were negative for AFB, and the patient was removed from isolation. Drug susceptibility test results came back 2 more weeks later, indicating a drug-susceptible *M. tuberculosis* strain. The patient's antibiotic regimen was reduced to isoniazid and rifampin for 9 months.

REVIEW QUESTIONS

Directions: For each of the following questions, choose the **one best** answer.

1. The most common cells for replication of *Mycobacterium tuberculosis* in the host are
   - **(A)** hepatocytes
   - **(B)** endothelial cells
   - **(C)** CD4 T cells
   - **(D)** macrophages
   - **(E)** CD8 T cells

2. Correct treatment for active tuberculosis entails
   - **(A)** 6–12 months with antimycobacterial-specific antibiotics
   - **(B)** 2–6 weeks with antimycobacterial-specific antibiotics
   - **(C)** corticosteroid treatment
   - **(D)** chest x-ray and purified protein derivative (PPD) skin test
   - **(E)** vaccination with bacille Calmette-Guérin (BCG)

3. Most people infected with *Mycobacterium tuberculosis* have which of the following characteristics?
   - **(A)** They are *not* purified protein derivative (PPD) skin test-positive
   - **(B)** They experience symptoms of active disease within 2 years
   - **(C)** They do not experience symptoms of active disease throughout their lifetime
   - **(D)** They reactivate a latent infection some time after infection
   - **(E)** They are infectious to others

4. The emergence of drug-resistant strains of *Mycobacterium tuberculosis* is probably due to
   - **(A)** HIV infection
   - **(B)** Noncompliance with drug regimen
   - **(C)** bacille Calmette-Guérin (BCG) vaccination
   - **(D)** Poor or crowded living conditions

5. *Mycobacterium tuberculosis* is very resistant to chemical agents, drying, and acid removal of dyes due to
   - **(A)** endospore formation
   - **(B)** high lipid content of its cell wall
   - **(C)** lack of cell wall
   - **(D)** a polysaccharide capsule
   - **(E)** its inability to grow outside host cells

6. Which one of the following statements is true regarding schistosomiasis?
   - **(A)** *Schistosoma* infections are less prevalent in the United States because the insect vector for the parasite does not thrive here
   - **(B)** Granulomas occur primarily in response to the adult worm form
   - **(C)** Egg antigen causes granuloma formation in the liver and intestines
   - **(D)** Excreted eggs are infectious to humans
   - **(E)** Adult worms live within macrophages in the human host

ANSWERS AND EXPLANATIONS

1. **The answer is D.** Macrophages are the most common cell for mycobacterial infection and replication in vivo. Option A is incorrect because *M. tuberculosis* infection of hepatocytes is not observed in vivo. Option B is incorrect because although infection of endothelial cells can be observed in vitro, macrophages are much more easily infected. Infection of endothelial cells is not generally observed in vivo. Options C and E are incorrect because T cells are not infected by *M. tuberculosis* bacilli.

2. **The answer is A.** Successful treatment of tuberculosis requires long-term administration of 2–4 antimycobacterial drugs. Option B is incorrect because a short course of 2–6 weeks of antibiotic treatment is ineffective against this slow-growing organism. Option C is incorrect because corticosteroid treatment can exacerbate, not eliminate, *M. tuberculosis* infection. Option D is incorrect because the chest x-ray and PPD skin test are diagnostic methods, not treatments. Option E is incorrect because BCG vaccination does not act against established disease.

3. **The answer is C.** Ninety percent of people infected with *M. tuberculosis* never experience active disease, but instead have latent infection. Option A is incorrect because infected people are generally PPD-positive, which simply indicates exposure to infection. Option B is incorrect because only a small percentage (approximately 5%) of infected people have active tuberculosis within 2 years of infection. Option D is incorrect because only approximately 10% of infected people reactivate the latent infection during their lifetime. Option E is incorrect because only those with active tuberculosis (but not latent tuberculosis) are infectious to others.

4. **The answer is B.** Noncompliance with the long-term drug regimen allows drug-resistant strains to emerge. Option A is incorrect because HIV infection has no effect on drug resistance, although people with HIV are more susceptible to tuberculosis. However, drug treatment of tuberculosis in the AIDS population is remarkably effective. Option C is incorrect because BCG vaccination plays no role in drug resistance. Option D is incorrect because although poor or crowded living conditions contribute to the spread of tuberculosis and could contribute to the *spread* of drug-resistant organisms, they do not contribute to the emergence of such organisms.

5. **The answer is B.** The unique and lipid-rich cell wall of mycobacteria contributes to the resistance of these organisms to many environmental elements. Option A is incorrect because mycobacteria do not form endospores. Option C is incorrect because mycobacteria do have a cell wall. Option D is incorrect because mycobacteria do not have a polysaccharide capsule, although there is some evidence that polysaccharides are attached to the cell wall. In any case, these polysaccharides do not contribute to the environmental resistance of the mycobacteria. Option E is incorrect because mycobacteria can grow outside host cells.

6. **The answer is C.** Granulomas form in response to egg antigen, and these eggs are lodged in the liver and intestines. Option A is incorrect because the vector for *Schistosoma* is a snail, not an insect. These snails are not found in the United States. Option B is incorrect because adult worms do not promote granuloma formation and are not found in tissues, but in blood vessels. Option D is incorrect because the form of the parasite infectious to humans is the cercariae, excreted from snails, not the eggs, which are harbored and excreted by humans. Option E is incorrect because adult worms live within blood vessels and are not intracellular.

PART V: GENETICS OF MICROBIAL VIRULENCE

OVERVIEW

The contribution of virulence factors to microbial pathogenesis has been extensively discussed in previous chapters. It now should be obvious that (1) the virulence genes a pathogen carries and expresses strongly influence the kind of disease that pathogen causes and that (2) different pathogens (or even different isolates of the same pathogen) often have considerably different repertoires of virulence genes.

Why is there so much variation in the virulence genes present in different pathogens or even in different isolates of the same pathogen? At least for pathogenic bacteria, this diversity can largely be explained by the fact that many virulence genes are present on mobile genetic elements, such as plasmids, phages, and transposons (see Chapter 5). The association of many virulence genes with mobile genetic elements helps to limit the presence of individual virulence genes to certain bacteria, because mobile genetic elements are often specific for one particular bacterial species or closely related species.

While mobile genetic elements typically cannot spread virulence genes to distantly related bacteria, they are helpful for transferring virulence genes within a bacterial species (and sometimes to related species). However, reliance on mobile genetic elements for intraspecies transfer of virulence genes has some potential limitations. First, some extrachromosomal mobile genetic elements (particularly some low-copy-number plasmids) are unstable, that is, these DNA elements can be lost at relatively high frequency during growth of the bacterial cell. A second potential limitation of associating virulence genes with mobile genetic elements is that some mobile genetic elements (notably lytic phages) can kill their bacterial host. Virulence genes present on a strictly lytic phage would typically be of little pathogenic value to the bacterial cell, since that bacterium would probably undergo phage-induced death before it could establish an infection.

To overcome the drawbacks of associating virulence genes with mobile genetic elements, many important virulence genes have become located on phages or transposons that can stably integrate into the bacterial chromosome without causing death of their bacterial host. This is termed lysogeny. Chapter 23 examines several examples (e.g., *Corynebacterium diphtheriae*), illustrating how lysogeny contributes to bacterial pathogenesis.

Earlier chapters of this book have emphasized that virulence is often multifactorial, that is, many pathogens need to express several different virulence factors to cause disease. If each virulence gene required by a bacterial pathogen with multifactorial virulence were carried on a separate mobile genetic element, that bacterium would need to acquire and maintain a large number of different mobile genetic elements in order to be fully virulent. This potential problem has been overcome, in many cases, by the emergence of mobile genetic elements that carry multiple virulence genes. If one of these mobile genetic elements carrying several virulence genes integrates into the bacterial chromosome (lysogeny), this integration results in the formation of a "pathogenicity island," a region of chromosomal DNA rich in virulence genes (Chapter 23).

Once virulence genes have been acquired and are being stably maintained in a pathogenic bacterium, their expression often becomes highly regulated. Tight regulation of virulence gene expression makes good "pathogenic sense" for the bacterial pathogen, since virulence factors are typically needed only at certain times, for instance, after the bacterial pathogen has encountered the human host. Several important signaling mechanisms that bacteria use to sense their environment, including their presence in the human host, is discussed in Chapter 24. That chapter particularly focuses on two-component regulatory systems, which allow the bacterium to respond to environmental signals, and quorum-sensing regulatory systems, which allow the bacterium to respond to bacterial population density. Chapter 24 also discusses how different regulatory systems sometimes "cross-talk" to achieve even more precise regulation of virulence genes.

Finally, Chapter 24 discusses the process of coordinate regulation, which allows a pathogenic bacterium to simultaneously turn on and turn off expression of a number of different virulence genes. Coregulating virulence gene expression is an excellent strategy for the pathogenesis of those bacteria that need to express multiple virulence factors to cause disease, that is, coordinate regulation helps to ensure that all necessary virulence factors are produced when needed during infection.

23 ROLE OF MOBILE GENETIC ELEMENTS IN BACTERIAL VIRULENCE

CHAPTER OUTLINE

Introduction of Clinical Case
Role of Mobile Genetic Elements in Virulence
• β-Phage, Lysogeny, and Diphtheria
Illustrative Pathogen: *Corynebacterium diphtheriae*
• Biologic Characteristics
• Reservoir and Transmission
• Virulence Factors
• Pathogenesis
• Diagnosis
• Prevention and Treatment
Pathogenicity Islands
• Mobile Genetic Elements Transfer Pathogenicity Islands Between Bacterial Cells
Illustrative Pathogen: *Vibrio cholerae*
• Biologic Characteristics
• Reservoir and Transmission
• Virulence Factors
• Pathogenesis
• Diagnosis
• Prevention and Treatment
Resolution of Clinical Case
Review Questions

INTRODUCTION OF CLINICAL CASE

In 1994, a 67-year-old American man visited Russia on a month-long business trip. At the midpoint of his trip, he experienced a 99.2°F fever and a sore throat. Upon examination at the local physician's office, the tonsils and lateral pharynx were erythematous, and there was a patchy, white exudate on both tonsils. This exudate could be dislodged or picked up with a tongue depressor. A few shotty (less than 1 cm) nodes were palpated in each anterior cervical chain. A culture of the exudate was taken, and the man was reassured that if the culture were positive for group A streptococci, an antibiotic would be prescribed.

The culture turned out negative for group A streptococci. The man, whose condition had not improved, was told not to worry because he had a viral pharyngitis that would soon resolve. Instructions for symptomatic relief (e.g., saline gargles) were given.

The man returned to the Russian clinic several days later because his symptoms still had not resolved. He was admitted to the local hospital with a fever of 100.5°F and multiple enlarged lymph nodes in both anterior cervical chains. Examination of his throat showed a confluent light gray membrane, which covered the tonsils and the lateral and posterior pharynx. This membrane was tough and not easily dislodged—when attempts were made to remove it with a tongue depressor, bleeding occurred. The membrane was cultured, and the man was given a β-lactam antibiotic. The man was monitored by an electrocardiogram (ECG), which initially showed nonspecific ST-segment and T-wave changes.

- From what disease did this man suffer?
- What pathogen causes this illness?
- How does this pathogen cause this illness?
- Why did this treatment fail?
- What role do mobile genetic factors play in this illness?

ROLE OF MOBILE GENETIC ELEMENTS IN BACTERIAL VIRULENCE

Mobile genetic elements, including plasmids, phages, and transposons, were introduced in Chapter 5. In addition to their role in spreading antimicrobial resistance (see Chapter 5), mobile genetic elements also contribute to bacterial pathogenesis. As illustrated in Table 23-1, many bacterial virulence genes are located on mobile genetic elements, which contribute to phenotypic diversity by facilitating the rapid spread of these virulence factor genes through a bacterial species (and sometimes even to related species). Furthermore, the presence of multiple mobile genetic elements, each carrying its own virulence genes in a given bacterial species, often provides sufficient phenotypic diversity to enable individual isolates of that species to become specialized for causing different diseases. For example, *Escherichia coli* isolates associated with urinary tract infections usually carry the PAI I or PAI II pathogenicity islands, which are believed to be chromosomally integrated mobile genetic elements. PAI I and PAI II each carry the genes encoding P pili, which are important for the adherence of *E. coli* to the urinary tract epithelium, and hemolysin, which contributes to the damage and inflammation associated with urinary tract infections (UTIs) [see Chapter 12]. In contrast, ETEC strains of *E. coli*, which cause the watery diarrhea of traveler's diarrhea, carry a plasmid encoding the CFA I/II adhesins and the heat-labile and heat-stable enterotoxins. This ETEC plasmid illustrates that some plasmids often encode bacterial virulence factor genes; phages can also be important for distributing virulence genes, as discussed below.

TABLE 23-1 ▶

Examples of Virulence Factors Whose Genes Are Known to be Carried on Mobile Genetic Elements

Virulence Factor	Mobile Genetic Factor Carrying the Gene Encoding This Virulence Factor
Tetanus toxin	Plasmid
Yops of *Yersinia* spp.	Plasmid
Heat-labile and heat-stable enterotoxin in ETEC strains	Plasmid
CFA I/II adhesins	Plasmid
Shiga toxin in EHEC strains	Phage
Diphtheria toxin	Phage
Staphylococcal enterotoxin A	Phage
Streptococcal erythrogenic toxins	Phage
Cholera toxin	Phage

β-Phage, Lysogeny, and Diphtheria

Like mammalian cells, bacterial cells are susceptible to viral infections. There are two potential outcomes, lytic or lysogenic, when a bacterial virus (also known as a bacteriophage) infects a bacterial cell (Figure 23-1). In a lytic infection, large numbers of progeny phages accumulate in the bacterial cytoplasm, eventually causing the infected bacterial cell to lyse and release these progeny phages, which are then free to infect other susceptible bacterial cells. Alternatively, an infecting phage sometimes can integrate its DNA into the bacterial chromosome, a situation referred to as lysogeny. Typically, a lysogenized bacterial cell does not lyse but survives, in part, because there is no production of progeny virus. Therefore, lysogeny provides a genetic mechanism that allows the lysogenized bacterial cell, and most of its progeny, to stably carry and express phage-encoded virulence genes indefinitely into the future. However, under certain specific environmental conditions, the integrated phage DNA (referred to as a prophage) can be induced to leave the chromosome and replicate into new infectious phage particles, which can infect other bacterial cells.

Typically, each bacterial virus is only able to infect certain bacteria (e.g., corynephages infect only the gram-positive bacterium Corynebacterium*).*

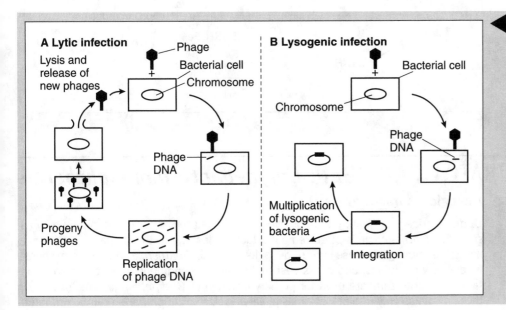

◀ **FIGURE 23-1**
Outcomes of Phage Infections of Bacterial Cells. *(A) Typical lytic infection; note that the host bacterial cell dies. (B) Typical lysogenic infection; note that these infected bacteria survive and that the phage DNA is then stably passed on to progeny bacterial cells. Each progeny bacterium carries a copy of the phage DNA. Occasionally the integrated phage DNA in an individual lysogenized cell will mobilize and give rise to new infectious phage particles, which can then infect other bacterial cells.*

One excellent example illustrating the contribution of lysogeny to virulence is provided by the disease diphtheria. The symptoms of this illness, caused by the bacterium *Corynebacterium diphtheriae*, result from the expression of diphtheria toxin. The gene encoding diphtheria toxin is carried by a corynephage, named β-phage, that can lysogenically infect *C. diphtheriae* cells. Lysogenic infection with β-phage leads to a population of *C. diphtheriae* cells that stably produces diphtheria toxin.

C. diphtheriae cells lysogenized with β-phage DNA express significant amounts of diphtheria toxin only when growing in a low-iron environment, such as exists in the human body. This iron-mediated regulation of diphtheria toxin expression is controlled by a repressor protein (Figure 23-2) that is encoded by a gene located on the *C. diphtheriae* chromosome (i.e., expression of the phage-encoded diphtheria toxin gene is regulated by a bacterial gene product). What is the mechanism by which iron regulates diphtheria toxin expression? As shown in Figure 23-2, *C. diphtheriae* cells growing in a high-iron environment accumulate significant amounts of iron in their cytoplasm. These high intracellular iron levels facilitate the binding of iron to the diphtheria toxin repressor; with this bound Fe^{2+}, the repressor then recognizes and binds as a dimer to the promoter region of the diphtheria toxin gene, inhibiting transcription. However, when *C. diphtheriae* cells are growing in an iron-poor environment and the concentration of cytoplasmic iron drops, the bound iron dissociates from the repressor, causing the repressor protein to "fall off" the promoter region of the diphtheria toxin gene. This allows RNA polymerase unimpeded access to the promoter region of the diphtheria toxin gene so that transcription of the diphtheria toxin gene significantly increases.

FIGURE 23-2

Regulation of Expression of C. diphtheriae Toxin by Iron. *(A) When intracellular iron levels rise as* Corynebacterium diphtheriae *grows in iron-rich conditions, some of this cytoplasmic* Fe^{2+} *binds to one or more molecules of the diphtheria toxin repressor protein (DTXR). A DTXR:Fe^{2+} complex, consisting of* Fe^{2+} *and a DTXR dimer, then binds to the promoter region (P) of the diphtheria toxin gene (tox), blocking the interaction of RNA polymerase with P and thus inhibiting transcription of tox. (B) When intracellular iron levels fall as* C. diphtheriae *grows in limiting iron conditions, the bound* Fe^{2+} *dissociates from the DTXR dimer, causing this repressor to fall off P. This allows RNA polymerase access to P, which leads to increased transcription of the tox gene.*

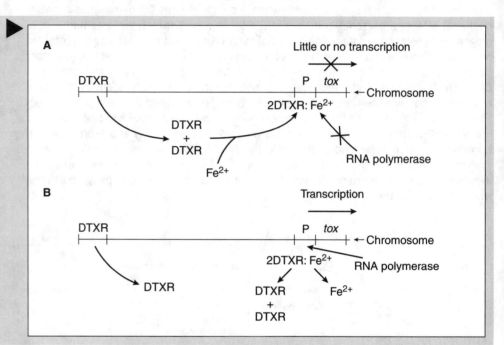

ILLUSTRATIVE PATHOGEN: *Corynebacterium diphtheriae*

Arrangements of C. diphtheriae cells
(1000 × magnification)

A "Chinese letters"

B Palisades

Three biotypes (mitis, gravis, and intermedius) of C. diphtheriae *can also be differentiated on the basis of biochemical reactions and hemolysis.*

Biologic Characteristics

C. diphtheriae is a small, gram-positive, club-shaped rod. After undergoing binary fission, *C. diphtheriae* cells often remain attached, leading to the formation of arrangements resembling "Chinese letters" or "palisades." *C. diphtheriae* does not form spores, is relatively fastidious, and grows best under aerobic conditions. Selective media containing tellurite salts are used for primary isolation of *C. diphtheriae*, which grows on these media as gray to black colonies of varying sizes. *C. diphtheriae* can be differentiated from other species of *Corynebacteriae* on the basis of biochemical reactions.

Reservoir and Transmission

C. diphtheriae causes two forms of infection: nasopharyngeal diphtheria and cutaneous diphtheria. Both forms of diphtheria result from the transmission of aerosolized droplets containing viable, toxigenic *C. diphtheriae* cells. When a contaminated droplet contacts broken skin (e.g., at the site of a cut or an ulcer), cutaneous diphtheria develops. This cutaneous infection is rare in the United States but sometimes occurs in homeless alcoholic men living on the street. When a contaminated droplet is inhaled, nasopharyngeal diphtheria develops. This form of diphtheria is also now rare in the United States.

Humans are the only natural host for *C. diphtheriae* and also represent the only known reservoir of this pathogen. Nontoxigenic *C. diphtheriae* can be found in the throats of healthy humans. It is possible that some people immunized with diphtheria toxoid, who are themselves protected from diphtheria, might harbor toxigenic *C. diphtheriae* isolates in their throats or on their skin. If so, these carriers would represent a reservoir for toxigenic isolates that could cause diphtheria in susceptible (nonimmune) hosts.

Virulence Factors

In order to cause disease, *C. diphtheriae* needs only to colonize the nasopharynx or skin and to produce diphtheria toxin.

Colonization Factors. Surprisingly little is known about the colonization factors of *C. diphtheriae.*

Diphtheria Toxin. The structure and action of diphtheria toxin were discussed in detail in Chapter 20. As a quick review, diphtheria toxin is an A-B fragment toxin that binds to host cells and then internalizes via receptor-mediated endocytosis. Following normal acidification of the endocytic vesicle containing diphtheria toxin, the A fragment of diphtheria toxin escapes into the cytoplasm, where it shuts down host cell protein synthesis by catalyzing an NAD-dependent, ADP-ribosylation of elongation Factor 2 (an important component of eukaryotic protein synthesis). The crucial role that diphtheria toxin plays in causing the symptoms of diphtheria is evident from two observations: (1) nontoxigenic *C. diphtheriae* are not a significant cause of human infections, and (2) successful immunization with purified diphtheria toxoid (see below) provides complete protection against diphtheria.

Pathogenesis

Following colonization of a person's nasopharynx or skin, *C. diphtheriae* starts producing diphtheria toxin. Approximately 1–7 days after infection, sufficient diphtheria toxin is present to cause localized necrosis at the site of infection. In nasopharyngeal diphtheria, this necrosis results in initial malaise and sore throat and triggers an inflammatory reaction that causes fever and enlargement of the cervical lymph nodes. At the site of infection (the throat or skin), this toxin-induced necrosis and inflammation leads to the formation of an adherent pseudomembrane composed of *C. diphtheriae* cells, fibrin, necrotic epithelial cells, lymphocytes, polymorphonuclear leukocytes, and erythrocytes. This pseudomembrane starts as a soft exudate that can easily be wiped off the host tissue, but with time it becomes thicker and more adherent so that any attempt to dislodge the pseudomembrane now causes bleeding. When it extends to the larynx and trachea during nasopharyngeal diphtheria, the pseudomembrane can block a patient's airway, causing death by suffocation. This more commonly occurs in children because of their smaller air passages.

C. diphtheriae cells remain localized on the mucosal epithelium; as an extracellular pathogen, it rarely or never invades deeper tissues. However, during diphtheria, the internal organs can become seriously damaged from diphtheria toxin that has been absorbed from the throat or skin into the circulation. The heart is particularly sensitive to diphtheria toxin; diphtheritic myocarditis often leads to death from complete atrio-ventricular heart block, congestive heart failure, or cardiogenic shock. Diphtheria toxin can also damage the nervous system, particularly during later stages of diphtheria. These cardiac and neural problems are somewhat more common in nasopharyngeal diphtheria than in cutaneous diphtheria.

Diagnosis

The initial diagnosis of diphtheria needs to be made quickly on clinical grounds so that antitoxin therapy can be effective in limiting toxin-induced damage and increase the patient's chance for survival. Clinical diagnosis of this disease is complicated by the rarity of diphtheria in most industrialized nations.

Definitive diagnosis of diphtheria involves a two-step laboratory confirmation process. First, *C. diphtheriae* cells are isolated from the throat or skin using a selective medium containing tellurite salts, which inhibit the growth of many normal flora in the nasopharynx. If *C. diphtheriae* is isolated, these bacteria must then be shown to produce diphtheria toxin; diphtheria toxin expression can be demonstrated by serologic tests or animal toxicity assays.

Prevention and Treatment

It is essential that treatment for diphtheria include both antitoxin therapy to neutralize diphtheria toxin already circulating in the body and antimicrobial therapy to eliminate the *C. diphtheriae* cells producing this toxin.

One hundred years ago, diphtheria ranked as a leading cause of death, particularly in

The enlargement of cervical lymph nodes during diphtheria often becomes highly noticeable, a condition referred to as bull-neck.

Diphtheria toxin has two effects on the heart: it depresses myocardial contractility (myocarditis), and it interrupts the conduction of electrical impulses from the atria to the ventricles, producing various abnormal rhythms. The total block of impulses from atria to ventricles is termed heart block. This condition is highly lethal because without stimulation from above the ventricles contract only 30–40 times per minute, which is usually insufficient to sustain life (cardiogenic shock). Lesser conduction defects and/or myocarditis may cause a backing up of blood into the lungs (pulmonary edema) or peripheral veins (congestive heart failure).

Peripheral neuritis occurs in about 10% of patients with diphtheria; most commonly the cranial nerves are involved. However, peripheral nerves, usually motor nerves, may also be involved, which can result in paralysis of respiratory muscles.

Because many adults develop hypersensitivity to diphtheria toxoid, the amount of diphtheria toxoid present in adult booster injections is usually much lower than the dose received in the childhood DPT vaccine. These adult booster injections also usually contain tetanus toxoid to boost immunity against tetanus simultaneously as well.

children. However, this illness has been virtually eliminated from most developed countries practicing widespread immunization with diphtheria toxoid. Protection against diphtheria is first induced during childhood using the diphtheria, pertussis and tetanus (DPT) vaccine (see Chapter 29); diphtheria immunity in adults is then boosted every 10 years. Earlier in this chapter it was mentioned that some reservoirs of toxigenic *C. diphtheriae* may still exist, even in developed countries practicing widespread immunization. Therefore, it is essential that universal immunization against diphtheria continue to be a public health goal in all areas of the world. The public health importance of continuing diphtheria immunization in industrialized countries is illustrated by the massive outbreak of diphtheria that occurred in Russia in 1994. This epidemic, which killed several thousand people and sickened tens of thousands more, followed a breakdown in vaccination programs upon the dissolution of the former Soviet Union.

PATHOGENICITY ISLANDS

Unlike β-phage, which apparently carries only a single virulence gene, some mobile genetic elements carry entire sets of virulence genes. Segregating a block of virulence genes onto a single mobile genetic element makes good "pathogenic sense," particularly for those bacterial pathogens that need to express multiple virulence factors in order to cause disease (i.e., localizing many or all of the virulence genes needed for pathogenicity onto one mobile genetic element means that the bacterial pathogen does not have to acquire several different mobile genetic elements independently to exhibit full virulence).

An individual "virulence" plasmid often encodes multiple virulence factors. For instance, as mentioned earlier in this chapter, some ETEC strains carry a plasmid encoding heat-labile enterotoxin, heat-stable enterotoxin, and a CFA adhesin (see Chapter 12). However, mobile genetic elements carrying virulence factor genes need not be maintained as extrachromosomal DNA; mobile genetic elements are also thought to be involved in the clustering of virulence genes that occurs on the chromosome of many bacterial pathogens. Such regions of the chromosome rich in virulence genes are referred to as pathogenicity islands and are thought to result from chromosomal integration of a mobile genetic element. Several examples of pathogenicity islands are shown in Table 23-2. This table illustrates several important points about pathogenicity islands: (1) pathogenicity islands have been identified in taxonomically diverse bacteria, ranging from the gram-negative Enterobacteriaceae (e.g., *Salmonella* spp.) to the gram-positive, spore-forming anaerobe *Clostridium difficile*; (2) a single bacterial cell can carry more than one pathogenicity island (e.g., some *Salmonella* spp. cells contain both the SPI-1 and SPI-2 pathogenicity islands); and (3) the genes encoding type III secretion systems of gram-negative bacteria are often located on pathogenicity islands (see Chapter 13).

It is believed that SPI-1 is important for the invasion of Salmonella *spp. into epithelial cells, while SPI-2 is involved in the survival of* Salmonella *spp. inside macrophages.*

TABLE 23-2 ▶
Examples of Pathogenicity Islands

Bacteria	Pathogenicity Island	Virulence Functions Encoded by This Pathogenicity Island
Uropathogenic strains of *Escherichia coli*	PAI-1 PAI-2	Hemolysin, P-fimbriae Hemolysin, P-fimbriae, other toxins
EPEC strains of *E. coli*	LEE	Type III secretion system, attachment and effacement
Salmonella spp.	SPI-1	Invasion of epithelial cells, type III secretion systems
Clostridium difficile	PaLoc	Toxins A and B
Vibrio cholerae	CTX	Cholera toxin, ZOT, ACE, and a colonization factor

Note. ZOT = zonula occludens toxin; ACE = accessory cholera enterotoxin.

Mobile Genetic Elements Transfer Pathogenicity Islands Between Bacterial Cells

As introduced above, most (if not all) pathogenicity islands are believed to be located on mobile genetic elements that can be horizontally transferred from bacterial cell to bacterial cell. In some cases, this transfer probably even occurs between bacteria belonging to different species, although this transfer may be less efficient. One important piece of evidence suggesting that mobile genetic elements are involved in the transfer of pathogenicity islands is the observation that the nucleotide base composition of DNA present in pathogenicity islands usually differs from the DNA base composition found in the remainder of that pathogen's chromosomal DNA.

The exact genetic mechanisms by which most pathogenicity islands are horizontally transferred between bacteria remain unclear. However, one genetic mechanism for transfering pathogenicity islands has now been identified in *Vibrio cholerae*, the bacteria causing cholera. Recent studies have shown that the *V. cholerae* CTX pathogenicity island, which contains virulence genes encoding cholera toxin (see Table 23-2), two other accessory enterotoxins named ZOT and ACE, and a colonization factor, is encoded by a filamentous phage named CTXφ. When a nontoxigenic *V. cholerae* isolate is lysogenically infected by CTXφ, the CTX pathogenicity island becomes stably integrated into the bacterial isolate's chromosome so that the lysogenized *V. cholerae* isolate now stably expresses the CTX virulence factors. Through mechanisms that are not yet completely understood, this CTX genetic element sometimes is tandemly duplicated (present in two adjacent copies) and may even undergo amplification (i.e., many copies of CTX may be present in each cell), possibly allowing for increased expression of CTX genes.

The CTXφ phage uses toxin-coregulated pilus (TCP) as its receptor for infecting *V. cholerae* cells. Although not encoded by CTXφ, TCP is itself an important virulence factor that helps mediate the adherence of *V. cholerae* to intestinal epithelial cells. Since *V. cholerae* cells synthesize large amounts of TCP in the intestines, CTXφ infection of *V. cholerae* cells may occur at significant frequency in vivo (i.e., a pathogenic isolate of *V. cholerae* may be able to convert nonpathogenic isolates to full virulence inside the human intestines). It is also interesting that the expression of both TCP and the CTXφ-encoded virulence factors is controlled by the ToxR regulatory system (see below) [i.e., the ToxR regulatory system, which is not itself encoded by CTXφ, regulates the expression of most *V. cholerae* virulence genes, including the phage-borne CTX genes].

> *Horizontal transfer of bacterial DNA refers to the transfer of DNA between two independent (perhaps nonrelated) bacterial cells; this contrasts to vertical transfer, where DNA is transferred from a parent cell to its progeny during binary fission.*

> *Although all DNA is composed of four nucleotide bases, the base composition (i.e., the percentage of DNA composed of G+C residues vs. A+T residues) varies between different bacterial species. For example, the G+C content of* Pseudomonas aeruginosa *is about 67%, while the G+C content of the pathogenic* Clostridia *is only about 25%. Whatever G+C ratio is present in a particular bacteria's chromosome, the same base composition tends to be maintained relatively uniformly throughout all regions of that chromosome. Thus, the fact that pathogenicity islands (which are often sizeable—more than several thousand bases) have a significantly different base composition from the rest of an isolate's chromosome suggests that these "islands" represent integrated mobile genetic elements.*

ILLUSTRATIVE PATHOGEN: *Vibrio cholerae*

Biologic Characteristics

The genus *Vibrio* includes highly motile, gram-negative, slightly curved ("comma-shaped") rods. These facultative anaerobes are usually halotolerant or even halophilic. *Vibrio* spp. are oxidase-positive, so they do not belong to the Enterobacteriaceae (see Chapters 5, 12, 13, and 24).

The genus *Vibrio* includes several pathogenic species (see Appendix 3), of which *V. cholerae*, the cause of cholera, is the most medically important. *V. cholerae* can be distinguished from other *Vibrio* species by biochemical reactions.

V. cholerae isolates are serotyped on the basis of differences in their O antigen (see Chapter 1). It was once believed that only those cholera toxin–positive *V. cholerae* isolates possessing an O1 antigen could cause epidemic cholera. However, in the past 10 years, cholera toxin–positive isolates expressing the O139 antigen have also emerged as an important cause of epidemic cholera. *V. cholerae* isolates belonging to other serogroups are typically cholera toxin–negative and therefore do not cause full-blown cholera; however, these "non-O1/non-O139" isolates often produce other types of enterotoxins and thus may still cause a mild-to-moderate gastrointestinal illness.

> *Halotolerant means that an organism is salt-tolerant. This is an important trait of* Vibrio *spp. because these bacteria often have a marine reservoir (i.e., they commonly exist in salt or brackish waters).*

> *V. cholerae O1 isolates can be subdivided into two biotypes, classical and el tor, on the basis of their biochemical and biologic properties. Both O1 biotypes can cause cholera, although el tor strains are considered responsible for most current cases of cholera.*

Reservoir and Transmission

A distinctive epidemiologic feature of cholera is its tendency to occur in massive outbreaks, called pandemics, which spread throughout much of the world. We are currently in the seventh or eighth pandemic since the first cholera pandemic was recognized in 1817. Transmission of *V. cholerae* during a pandemic usually occurs by the ingestion of water or food contaminated with human feces. Infected humans play an important role in this transmission, since patients with acute cholera often secrete enormous numbers (10^8 bacterial cells per gram of feces) of *V. cholerae* cells in their stools; this facilitates the entrance of these bacteria into a water supply, which in turn further perpetuates the epidemic.

Like other *Vibrio* species, the major natural reservoir for *V. cholerae* is believed to be estuary waters; however, most estuarine isolates are cholera toxin–negative. Furthermore, long-term carriage of *V. cholerae* by people or animals is unusual. It is fairly common for people living in areas with endemic cholera to become transiently colonized (without disease symptoms) by cholera toxin–positive isolates. These asymptomatically colonized individuals likely represent an important reservoir of pathogenic *V. cholerae* isolates.

> *The fact that people in endemic cholera areas can be colonized by fully virulent strains of* V. cholerae *without experiencing illness is probably due to naturally induced immunity from prior exposure to this bacterium.*

Virulence Factors

The following virulence factors contribute to the ability of *V. cholerae* cells to cause full-blown cholera.

Cholera Toxin. Cholera toxin–negative *V. cholerae* isolates are rarely or never involved in severe diarrhea, which illustrates that cholera toxin is responsible for causing the major diarrheic symptoms of epidemic cholera. The molecular action by which this ADP-ribosyltransferase induces massive fluid and electrolyte losses from the small intestine has already been described in Chapter 20. (Briefly, recall that cholera toxin adenosine diphosphate [ADP]–ribosylates the Gs regulatory protein of the intestinal adenylate cyclase system, which causes this stimulatory protein to activate continuously adenylate cyclase. The resultant rise in intestinal cyclic adenosine monophosphate [cAMP] levels then leads to a massive loss of fluid and electrolytes from the intestines.)

Accessory Enterotoxins. Although *V. cholerae* needs to produce cholera toxin to cause the massive diarrhea of epidemic cholera, this bacteria also produces several other enterotoxins that can contribute to gastrointestinal symptoms. The existence of these "accessory" enterotoxins first became apparent in vaccine trials involving pathogenic *V. cholerae* strains that had been genetically engineered so that their cholera toxin genes were deleted. When these attenuated vaccine strains were administered to human volunteers, the subjects still experienced mild-to-moderate diarrhea, which was later shown to be caused by accessory enterotoxins.

The accessory enterotoxins produced by *V. cholerae* include zonula occludens toxin (ZOT) and accessory cholera enterotoxin (ACE). ZOT increases leakage of water and electrolytes into the intestinal lumen by affecting the tight junctions (also known as the zonula occludens) between intestinal enterocytes. ACE may act by inserting into intestinal membranes and forming an ion channel.

As mentioned, the genes encoding both ACE and ZOT are present on the same CTXφ phage that carries the cholera toxin genes (i.e., upon lysogeny, a *V. cholerae* cell simultaneously acquires the genes for all three of those enterotoxins).

Colonization Factors. There are several virulence factors implicated in the intestinal colonization of *V. cholerae*: (1) Toxin-coregulated pili (TCP) are adhesins that appear to be essential for intestinal colonization by *V. cholerae*. (2) *V. cholerae* cells produce several other adhesin proteins, including both fimbrial (e.g., hemagglutinins) and afimbrial (e.g., outer membrane proteins) adhesins. (3) The O1 strains of *V. cholerae* are nonencapsulated. However, the O139 strains produce a polysaccharide capsule that contributes to the binding of these isolates to the intestines. (4) Lipopolysaccharide (LPS) contributes to the adherence of O1 strains to the intestines. (5) Flagella allow *V. cholerae* cells to move through the intestinal mucus to reach the intestinal epithelium. Nonmotile mutants of *V. cholerae* have greatly diminished virulence.

Regulators of Virulence Factor Expression. Many of the *V. cholerae* virulence factors described above are coordinately expressed (see Chapter 24) under certain environmental conditions. A model for the coordinate expression of *V. cholerae* virulence genes is shown in Figure 23-3. When ToxR, a transmembrane protein, senses certain environmental stimuli, a portion of ToxR extending into the bacterial cytoplasm binds to the promoter region of certain *V. cholerae* genes, increasing the transcription of those genes. In particular, the activation of ToxR increases the transcription of ToxT, which is itself a transcriptional activator. Once expressed, ToxT binds to the promoter region of many *V. cholerae* virulence genes, leading to increased expression of cholera toxin, TCP, and several other virulence factors.

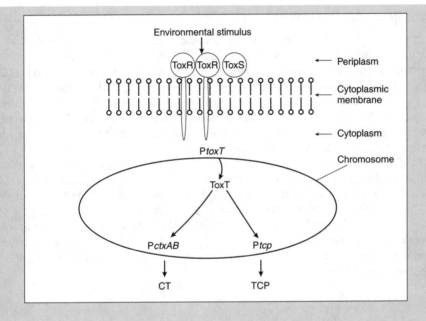

◀ **FIGURE 23-3**
ToxR-Regulated Expression of Virulence Factors in Vibrio cholerae. *An environmental stimulus (e.g., temperature, osmolarity, pH) activates ToxR, which is a transmembrane protein. This activation apparently involves the formation of a dimer between two ToxR molecules; this dimerization process is assisted by another V. cholerae protein called ToxS. Once activated, the cytoplasmic portion of the ToxR dimer then interacts with sequences in the promoter region (P) of the ToxT gene to increase transcription of the ToxT protein. This protein then interacts with sequences near the promoter region of several virulence factor genes (e.g., ctxAB), which encode the subunits of cholera toxin (CT) and tcp, which encodes the adhesin TCP (toxin-coregulated pilus). Although not shown in this figure, ToxR may also directly bind to sequences in the ctxA/B promoter region and cause some transcription of the ctxA/B gene. However, ToxT seems to be much more efficient than ToxR in stimulating CT expression.*

Pathogenesis

When ingested in contaminated food or water, *V. cholerae* immediately encounters the acid barrier of the stomach. If the ingested dose of bacteria is sufficiently large, some *V. cholerae* cells survive this exposure to the stomach and their passage into the small intestines, where they move through the intestinal mucus layer (via their flagella) and attach to intestinal epithelial cells (via TCP and other adhesins). Once this initial colonization has been established, the attached *V. cholerae* cells multiply and produce cholera toxin, which then binds to and affects the small intestinal enterocytes. As described in Chapter 20 and briefly reviewed above, cholera toxin primarily acts by increasing cAMP levels in enterocytes, which leads to a severe loss of fluids and electrolytes into the intestinal lumen. This effect is clinically manifested as the profuse watery diarrhea that is the hallmark of severe cholera.

The diarrheic symptoms of cholera typically develop suddenly following an incubation period of several hours to several days, depending (at least in part) on the number of bacteria ingested. The severity of diarrhea during cholera also varies from mild or moderate to severe. In part, the severity of cholera symptoms probably depends on the virulence of the *V. cholerae* isolate involved, as well as the dose of *V. cholerae* cells ingested. In severe cases of cholera (referred to as cholera gravis), which can represent up to 15% of cases in an outbreak, the rate of diarrheal fluid loss approaches 1 L/hr! In such severe cases, the stool is pale gray, with flecks of fecal material and a slightly fishy odor. The patient may also vomit and have poor skin turgor and sunken eyes. A person with cholera becomes extremely thirsty but remains mentally alert. Because *V. cholerae*

*This stool is referred to as **rice-water stool** because of its color and the small flecks of material it contains.*

During severe cholera, the skin on the hands and feet becomes wrinkled as if immersed in water for a long period; on the hands this is sometimes referred to as washerwoman's hands.

does not invade the intestinal epithelium, patients suffering from cholera have little or no fever, and their stools do not contain elevated levels of blood or leukocytes.

The massive loss of fluids and electrolytes that occurs during severe cases of epidemic cholera often leads to tachycardia, hypotension, and vascular collapse. These effects are often rapidly fatal unless proper therapy is given.

Diagnosis

The initial diagnosis of cholera must be made quickly on clinical grounds so treatment can be started promptly. The laboratory can culture the stool and perform biochemical tests on stool isolates to confirm the clinical diagnosis.

Prevention and Treatment

The primary treatment of cholera involves rapid restoration of the normal fluid and electrolyte balance. In severe cases of cholera, this involves intravenous administration of an electrolyte solution; the World Health Organization (WHO) recommends lactated Ringer's solution (Table 23-3), which should be supplemented with additional potassium chloride. Patients with mild-to-moderate cases of cholera are treated with oral rehydration solution. Antimicrobials (e.g., tetracyclines) are helpful for lessening the severity of symptoms, shortening the duration of disease, and reducing the length of time that a patient excretes V. cholerae cells in the stools.

Epidemic cholera is strongly associated with poor sanitation. Proper water treatment is particularly important in controlling this illness. Parenteral cholera vaccines have been licensed for many years, but these vaccines have several side effects (fever, localized pain, headache) and provide only moderate (approximately 50%) protection for short periods (about 3–6 months). In consideration of these facts, use of these parenteral cholera vaccines is not advocated by the WHO. Oral vaccines containing live attenuated V. cholerae strains produced by genetic engineering appear promising and are now undergoing field trials.

Oral rehydration effectively treats many cases of cholera because this illness does not produce histopathologic damage to the small intestine; therefore, the small intestine retains its absorptive function. Since intestinal electrolytes and glucose transport are coupled, orally administering a solution rich in glucose and electrolytes results in considerable glucose uptake, which stimulates electrolyte uptake. This then osmotically drives the uptake of fluid into the body (i.e., given time, the solution can restore the fluid and electrolyte balance of cholera patients). Intravenous fluids must be given to seriously dehydrated cholera victims; this approach restores fluid and electrolyte balances much more quickly than oral rehydration. Individuals with severe cholera may die before orally administered fluids and electrolytes are absorbed.

TABLE 23-3 ▶

Electrolyte Concentrations of Solutions Used to Treat Cholera

Solution	Electrolyte Concentration (mmol/L)				
	Sodium	Potassium	Chlorine	Base	Glucose
Lactated Ringer's solution	130	4[a]	109	28	—
Oral rehydration solution	90	20	80	30	111

[a] Usually supplemented with additional potassium for use in cholera therapy.

RESOLUTION OF CLINICAL CASE

On the day following his admission to the hospital, the businessman developed atrial fibrillation and died the next day in complete heart block and cardiogenic shock. The laboratory reported that C. diphtheriae was present in the pharyngeal specimen.

All indications were that this man was suffering from nasopharyngeal diphtheria, which is caused by toxigenic strains of C. diphtheriae. However, absolute confirmation of this diagnosis requires demonstrating that these pharyngeal isolates can express diphtheria toxin, which is important because only toxin-positive C. diphtheriae isolates are pathogenic.

From the information provided, it is unclear whether or not the attending physician ever recognized that this man was suffering from diphtheria. Early pharyngeal diphtheria is not distinctive. It is characterized by a mild pharyngitis, which may demonstrate a soft exudate that can be easily wiped off. There is nothing that distinguishes this presentation from that of group A streptococcal infection or viral pharyngitis, both of which are much more common than diphtheria. However, given the epidemic of diphtheria occurring in Russia in 1994, this diagnosis should have been considered.

Whether or not the physician recognized this illness as diphtheria, the treatment was obviously ineffective. Treating diphtheria with antimicrobials alone is incorrect therapy; by the time the symptoms of diphtheria become apparent, significant amounts of diphtheria toxin have probably entered the circulation. Since antimicrobial agents do not protect against circulating diphtheria toxin, an essential component of diphtheria treatment involves the administration of equine antitoxin to neutralize the circulating diphtheria toxin. Antimicrobial agents are also administered in order to clear *C. diphtheriae* from the throat and stop the further production of diphtheria toxin.

The patient must first be tested for allergy to horse serum before administering equine antitoxin.

Since this man was from the United States, it is almost certain that he had received immunization against diphtheria sometime in the past. However, the immunity afforded by the initial DPT vaccination series administered during childhood (see Chapter 28) wanes with time and must be periodically boosted, particularly in elderly patients, whose immune system function may be deteriorating. Therefore, it seems probable that this businessman either had not received a booster vaccine against diphtheria/tetanus recently or, if he had recently received a booster, he had not responded because of some underlying immunocompromising condition.

REVIEW QUESTIONS

Directions: For each of the following questions, choose the **one best** answer.

1. A 47-year-old American woman experienced vomiting and severe diarrhea immediately following her return from a business trip to Peru. When she was rushed to the emergency room, the physician determined that this woman had no fever; microscopic evaluation of her watery gray stool showed a few erythrocytes and no polymorphonuclear leukocytes. Culture of this stool revealed gram-negative, oxidase-positive, comma-shaped rods. These bacteria were facultative anaerobes. Which one of the following statements about this situation is correct?

   (A) A highly effective vaccine is currently licensed to prevent this woman's illness

   (B) The pathogen responsible for this woman's illness is a member of the Enterobacteriaceae

   (C) The pathogen responsible for this woman's illness invades the intestinal epithelium

   (D) This woman's symptoms are primarily induced by endotoxin

   (E) Antibiotic therapy alone is not sufficient treatment for this illness

2. Which one of the following statements about cholera and diphtheria is true?

   (A) Both cholera and diphtheria are caused by bacterial pathogens that stain blue with the Gram stain

   (B) The bacterial pathogens responsible for both cholera and diphtheria primarily have zoonotic reservoirs

   (C) The initial step in the pathogenesis of both cholera and diphtheria involves the adherence of the responsible pathogens to an epithelial surface

   (D) The symptoms of both cholera and diphtheria are primarily induced by adenosine diphosphate (ADP)-ribosyltransferases that inhibit host protein synthesis

   (E) The symptoms of both cholera and diphtheria result from pathogens that invade the epithelium

3. Which one of the following statements about pathogenicity islands is correct?

   (A) Pathogenicity islands rarely carry genes encoding virulence factors

   (B) A single bacterial cell can carry only one pathogenicity island

   (C) Pathogenicity islands can be transferred only between cells of the same species

   (D) The G+C ratio of DNA in pathogenicity islands typically differs from the G+C ratio of the remaining DNA on the bacterial chromosome

   (E) Pathogenicity islands are present only in gram-negative pathogens

4. Which one of the following statements best characterizes diphtheria toxin?

   (A) It is encoded by a bacterial gene present in all *Corynebacterium diphtheriae* isolates

   (B) Its expression is regulated by a gene that is encoded by a lysogenic phage

   (C) It is expressed best when *C. diphtheriae* is present in a low-iron environment

   (D) It is one of several *C. diphtheriae* toxins, all of which are essential for causing the disease diphtheria

5. Which one of the following statements is correct?

   (A) The only virulence-associated genes transferred on mobile genetic elements are toxin genes

   (B) ToxR regulates only the expression of virulence factor genes encoded by the CTXφ phage

   (C) β-Phage can infect almost all gram-positive bacteria

   (D) Expression of diphtheria toxin is regulated by an iron-binding repressor protein that is encoded by a chromosomal gene found in all *Corynebacterium diphtheriae* cells

ANSWERS AND EXPLANATIONS

1. **The answer is E.** On the basis of her symptoms and the microbiologic results, this patient apparently has cholera. While antimicrobial therapy is considered useful for fighting cholera, it is essential that therapy for cholera include the quick restoration of proper fluid and electrolyte balances. Option A is incorrect because currently licensed cholera vaccines are *not* highly effective. Option B is incorrect because *Vibrio cholerae*, the cause of cholera, is oxidase-positive. To belong to the Enterobacteriaceae, a bacterium must be oxidase-negative. Option C is incorrect because *V. cholerae* is not an invasive pathogen—it is an extracellular pathogen that remains localized on the surface of the intestinal epithelium during pathogenesis. Option D is incorrect because the symptoms of cholera are primarily caused by an exotoxin (cholera toxin).

2. **The answer is C.** Option A is incorrect because while *C. diphtheriae* (the cause of diphtheria) is gram-positive, *V. cholerae* (the cause of cholera) is gram-negative. Option B is incorrect because *C. diphtheriae* is not known to have a significant zoonotic reservoir. In periods between epidemics, the reservoir for *V. cholerae* is less clear. However, one reservoir during these periods may be marine crustaceans. Option D is incorrect because while both cholera toxin and diphtheria toxin (the toxins primarily responsible for inducing the symptoms of cholera and diphtheria, respectively) are ADP-ribosyltransferases, only diphtheria toxin inhibits protein synthesis (cholera toxin activates the adenylate cyclase system). Option E is incorrect because neither *V. cholerae* nor *C. diphtheriae* invades an epithelial surface.

3. **The answer is D.** Option A is incorrect because pathogenicity islands do carry virulence genes (in fact, they often carry blocks of virulence genes). Option B is incorrect because some *Salmonella* spp. cells, for example, carry two different pathogenicity islands. Option C is incorrect because the similarity between genes of pathogenicity islands in different species strongly suggests that these genetic elements have been transferred between species. Option E is incorrect because pathogenicity islands have also been found in *Clostridium difficile*, a gram-positive bacterium.

4. **The answer is C.** Option A is incorrect because the diphtheria toxin gene is present only in *C. diphtheriae* isolates that have been lysogenized with β-phage. Option B is incorrect because the expression of diphtheria toxin is regulated by a bacterial gene, not by a β-phage gene. Option D is incorrect because diphtheria toxin appears to be the only *C. diphtheriae* toxin required for the pathogenesis of diphtheria.

5. **The answer is D.** Option A is incorrect because nontoxin genes (e.g., genes encoding type III secretion systems) are also present on pathogenicity islands. Option B is incorrect because ToxR also regulates other genes not encoded by the CTXφ phage (e.g., the gene encoding toxin coregulated pili [TCP], which is not encoded by CTXφ, is regulated by ToxR). Option C is incorrect because β-phage is a corynephage that specifically infects *Corynebacterium*.

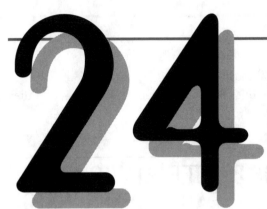

24 REGULATION OF BACTERIAL VIRULENCE FACTOR EXPRESSION

CHAPTER OUTLINE

Introduction of Clinical Case
Regulation of Bacterial Virulence Factor Expression
- Two-Component Regulatory Systems
- Quorum-Sensing Regulatory Systems
- Interactions between Quorum-Sensing Systems and Two-Component Regulatory Systems
Illustrative Pathogen: *Salmonella* **spp.**
- Biologic Characteristics
- Reservoirs and Transmission
- Virulence Factors
- Pathogenesis
- Diagnosis
- Prevention and Treatment
Resolution of Clinical Case
Review Questions

INTRODUCTION OF CLINICAL CASE

A 32-year-old American tourist who worked as a restaurant chef in New York City visited Nepal for a hiking trek through the Himalayas. Near the end of his vacation he became ill with a low-grade fever and constipation. After a few days he felt better and was able to return to the United States.

A week after his return he developed a fever, which increased each day. Within a few days he experienced headache, malaise, myalgia, anorexia, nausea, sore throat, and cough; his constipation continued. At the emergency room, his temperature was 102.3°F. His pulse rate was 72 beats/min. Examination revealed rose spots on the anterior part of his chest. The abdomen was slightly tender on palpation; there was no rebound tenderness. The edge of the liver was felt 2 cm below the right costal margin in the midclavicular line. The tip of the spleen could be palpated below the left costal margin on deep inspi-

> **Rose spots** are slightly raised, discrete, irregular pink macules, 2–4 mm in diameter, that blanch on pressure. They occur in crops of 5–15, usually on the anterior chest wall, last for 3–4 days, then fade, leaving no scars.

ration. The stool was negative for occult blood. A complete blood count revealed anemia and leukopenia (white blood cell [WBC] count, 2880/mm^3) with a normal differential count. A blood culture was performed and showed gram-negative, lactose-negative rods that were later identified as *Salmonella typhi*.

- From what disease was this man suffering?
- How is this disease acquired?

- Is this disease common in industrialized countries?
- Are the virulence factors involved in this disease produced constitutively, or is their expression regulated?

REGULATION OF BACTERIAL VIRULENCE FACTOR EXPRESSION

Many bacterial pathogens express some, or all, of their virulence factors only after receiving an environmental signal associated with the presence of the human host. Once this environmental signal is received, these bacterial pathogens often simultaneously "turn on" the expression of several different virulence factors. Such coregulation of virulence factor expression is referred to as coordinate regulation. Coordinate regulation makes good "pathogenic sense," particularly for those bacteria that spend time outside the host (e.g., in soil, water, sewage, food), because (1) it helps ensure that all necessary virulence factors are available when needed (i.e., during infection in the host), and (2) it prevents the wasteful production of virulence factors when these bacteria are growing outside the host. Some bacterial pathogens coordinately regulate the expression of their virulence factors using a single regulatory element, which is referred to as a global regulator. In other bacteria, coordinate regulation of virulence factor expression is achieved by means of several different regulatory systems that act in concert.

The regulation of virulence factor expression by bacterial pathogens may be very finely tuned, with different sets of virulence factors being produced as the pathogen encounters new host microenvironments. For example, when a salmonella cell becomes localized within a professional phagocyte, this bacterium starts expressing genes that, while unnecessary for extracellular growth or growth in epithelial cells, are required for survival and growth inside the inhospitable phagocyte. At the same time, this salmonella cell stops expressing other genes that had been needed during the early steps of salmonella infection (e.g., for invasion of the intestinal epithelium) but do not contribute to growth or survival inside phagocytes.

Bacteria sense their presence in the host (or in particular host microenvironments) through several types of environmental stimuli, including temperature, pH, nutrient concentrations (e.g., iron), and osmolarity. While laboratory studies usually assess the responsiveness of a bacterial pathogen to a single type of environmental signal, it is likely that most pathogens sense and respond to several stimulatory signals in vivo.

Once an appropriate environmental signal has been received, a pathogenic bacterium can use several different regulatory mechanisms to "turn on" virulence factor expression. One example of an important sensory regulatory system that can control virulence factor expression has already been introduced in Chapter 23: the fur/fur-like repressor system. Fur/fur-like repressor systems involve an iron-binding repressor that, in response to changes in environmental iron concentrations, either binds to (under high iron conditions) or dissociates from (under low iron conditions) gene promoters, thus leading to decreased or increased transcription, respectively, of these fur-regulated genes. The regulation of diphtheria toxin expression by an iron-binding repressor, as described in Chapter 23, represents an example of a fur-like repressor that plays an important role in pathogenesis.

Two other sensing systems, two-component regulatory systems and the quorum-sensing systems, also play an important role in controlling bacterial virulence factor expression.

Fur stands for *ferric uptake repressor.*

Studies have shown that not all genes regulated by two-component regulatory systems, fur/fur-like systems, or quorum-sensing systems encode classic virulence factors (e.g., toxins). It is possible that these regulated products play a subtle, still unknown role in infectious disease.

TWO-COMPONENT REGULATORY SYSTEMS

Two-component regulatory systems have been found in both gram-positive and gram-negative pathogens (Table 24-1). These signal transduction systems have been shown to regulate many bacterial functions, including the expression of important virulence

Pathogen	Two-Component Regulatory System	Regulated Virulence Factors
Bordetella pertussis	BvgA/BvgS	Filamentous hemagglutinin, other fimbriae, pertussis toxin, adenylate cyclase
Vibrio cholerae	ToxR/ToxS[a]	Cholera toxin and, through ToxT[a], many other virulence factors such as TCP pili
Clostridium perfringens	VirR/VirS	α toxin, θ toxin (perfringolysin O), proteases, sialidase
Salmonella spp.	PhoP/PhoQ	Factors needed for survival inside phagocytes
Staphylococcus aureus	AgrC/AgrA	Increases expression of toxins (e.g., α toxin)

[a] Recall from Chapter 23 that the ToxR/ToxS system is an atypical two-component regulatory system because ToxR and ToxS together sense environmental stimuli. Furthermore, the transcriptional activator for this system (ToxR) is not a cytoplasmic protein but instead is anchored in the plasma membrane with a cytoplasmic tail that can bind to promoters of ToxR-regulated genes. Another unusual feature of this system is that environmental stimulation of ToxR does not appear to involve phosphorylation. Finally, stimulation of ToxR leads to the expression of another transcriptional activator, ToxT, which then turns on many virulence genes.

factors such as toxins. The first component of these regulatory systems is the sensor protein, which is a transmembrane protein (a protein that spans the plasma membrane); when stimulated by the proper environmental signal, this sensor protein usually undergoes a conformational change that activates its cytoplasmic histidine kinase domain. This activation causes phosphorylation of the second component of the two-component regulatory system, which is typically a cytoplasmic protein that functions as a transcriptional regulator. Once phosphorylated, this transcriptional regulator activates the expression of some genes (Figure 24-1) but represses the transcription of other genes.

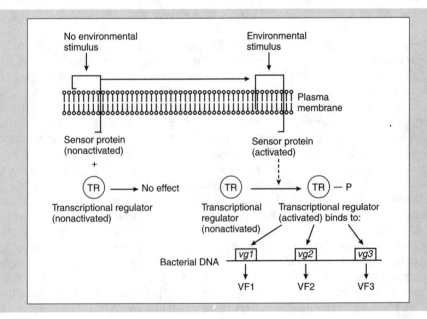

FIGURE 24-1
Activation of Virulence Genes by Two-Component Regulatory Systems. *When a proper environmental stimulus activates the membrane sensor protein, a transcriptional regulator (TR) is phosphorylated, producing an activated transcriptional regulator (TR-P). TR-P then binds to the promoters of virulence genes, increasing the expression of virulence genes (VG). Consequently, the pathogen now produces large amounts of virulence factors (VF).*

The involvement of two-component regulatory systems in regulating virulence gene expression can be fairly complicated. For example, it is now clear that a single bacterial cell can carry more than one type of two-component regulatory system (e.g., cells of *Salmonella* spp. often carry both the PhoP/PhoQ two-component regulatory system [described below] and the PmrA/PmrB two-component regulatory system). Since different two-component regulatory systems can sometimes cross-talk, the expression of a single virulence gene may be controlled by more than one type of two-component regulatory system. Additionally, it has also become clear that some two-component regulatory systems can regulate the activity of other two-component regulatory systems, or even regulate the activity of different types of regulatory systems. For example, the activation of ToxR (the transcriptional activator of a two-component regulator in *Vibrio cholerae*; see Chapter 23) increases the transcription of ToxT, a member of the AraC class of transcriptional regulators, which leads to increased expression of many *V. cholerae* virulence factors.

Transcriptional regulators of the AraC class are named for the first recognized regulator of this class, the Escherichia coli *araC product, which controls the arabinose operon.*

PhoP/PhoQ System of Salmonella spp. One of the best studied two-component regulatory systems is the PhoP/PhoQ system of *Salmonella* spp., wherein PhoP functions as the transcriptional regulator and PhoQ functions as the membrane sensor. PhoP/PhoQ appears to be essential for the pathogenesis of a salmonella infection, since PhoP/PhoQ mutants are avirulent for both humans and mice. Activation of PhoP/PhoQ leads to increased expression of some genes (at least 21 *pag* [PhoP-activated genes] have been identified) but the repression of other genes (referred to as *prg* genes [PhoP-repressed genes]).

PhoP/PhoQ mutants do not survive inside phagocytic cells in vitro, strongly suggesting that one major function of this two-component regulatory system is to facilitate survival of salmonella cells inside phagocytes. Consistent with this, laboratory studies have shown that the PhoP/PhoQ system responds to the environmental conditions (e.g., low magnesium ion and low calcium ion conditions) found inside acidified phagosomes. Thus, PhoP/PhoQ is probably silent when salmonella cells are outside the host and during the early stages of infection, but it becomes activated upon the entrance of these bacteria into phagocytes. Activation of PhoP/PhoQ increases the expression of *pag* genes, which are needed for survival inside acidified phagosomes (the intracellular location where salmonellae primarily survive and proliferate in phagocytes), but it also decreases the expression of *prg* genes, whose products contribute to survival in the environment and/or during early stages of infection but become unnecessary once salmonellae are localized inside phagosomes. For example, activation of PhoP/PhoQ has been shown to decrease the expression of a *prg* gene involved in invasion; because continued expression of an invasion gene by salmonella already internalized in phagocytes would be wasteful, repression of this invasion gene by activated PhoP/PhoQ makes good "pathogenic sense."

Not all PhoP/PhoQ-regulated genes are classic virulence factors; for example, some are involved in metabolic activities. The pathogenic role, if any, of such genes remains unclear.

How does activation of the PhoP/PhoQ system contribute to the increased survival and growth of salmonella inside phagocytes? Although the answer to this question is not yet totally clear, it appears that PhoP/PhoQ activation promotes the survival of salmonella inside phagocytes, at least in part by increasing the ability of these bacteria to resist antimicrobial peptides found in the phagosomes of phagocytic cells. The results of recent studies suggest that there are at least two PhoP/PhoQ-regulated pathways by which salmonella resist the antimicrobial peptides of phagosomes. Resistance to antimicrobial peptides such as CAP37 and CAP57 involves, at least in part, activation of the PmrA/PmrB two-component regulatory system of salmonella by PhoP/PhoQ. In turn, this activated PmrA/PmrB regulatory system increases the expression of enzymes that can modify salmonella lipopolysaccharide (LPS). The resultant modified LPS possesses decreased electrostatic affinity for antimicrobial peptides, which contributes to the survival of salmonella inside phagocytes because it results in decreased amounts of antimicrobial peptides binding to the outer membrane of these bacteria. However, LPS modifications do not explain all PhoP/PhoQ-mediated resistance of salmonella to antimicrobial peptides. The ability of salmonella to resist the defensin family of antimicrobial peptides appears to result from increased expression of PhoP/PhoQ-regulated outer membrane proteins, such as PagC. The molecular mechanisms by which these outer membrane proteins offer protection against defensins are not yet clear.

Antimicrobial peptides include peptides such as the defensins, azurocidin (CAP37), and bactericidal/permeability-increasing protein (CAP57). These are cationic, amphipathic peptides that kill microorganisms by forming pores or solubilizing membranes. In gram-negative bacteria, they bind to the outer membrane by electrostatic interactions with LPS and can then traverse to the cytoplasmic membrane. Thus, antimicrobial peptides act by affecting both the outer and the cytoplasmic membranes of gram-negative bacteria.

Quorum-Sensing Systems

Many bacterial pathogens must reach a critical density inside the host before causing disease. Until this required population level is reached, it is wasteful for the pathogen to produce certain virulence factors (particularly those needed later in infection). In response, some pathogens sense their population density and adjust their gene expression accordingly, using a process called quorum sensing.

Quorum sensing typically involves the production and secretion of one or more autoinducers, which are small organic molecules (e.g., peptides or members of the homoserine lactone family). When the population density reaches threshold levels, sufficiently high concentrations of the autoinducers become present in the microenvironment of the pathogenic bacteria to enable one or more transcriptional regulators to be activated, leading to the expression of virulence factors.

An excellent example of a bacterium that utilizes quorum sensing during its pathogenesis is the opportunistic pathogen *Pseudomonas aeruginosa* (see Chapter 5). As shown in Figure 24-2, when sufficient numbers of *P. aeruginosa* become present at a site in the body, threshold levels of an autoinducer (designated PAI-1) diffuse into the *P. aeruginosa* cell. This results in the activation of a transcriptional regulator (designated LasR) that directs the increased expression of some virulence factors, including exotoxin A (see Chapters 5 and 20). This activated LasR also directs the synthesis of another autoinducer (designated PAI-2), as well as a second transcriptional regulator (Rh1R). When the autoinducer PAI-2 binds to Rh1R, this transcriptional regulator becomes activated and increases the expression of additional virulence factors (e.g., elastase).

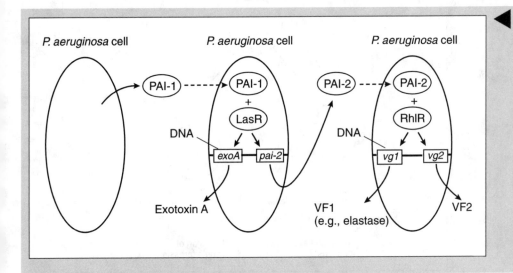

◀ **FIGURE 24-2**
Quorum-Sensing System of Pseudomonas aeruginosa. *P. aeruginosa constitutively produces and secretes an autoinducer (PAI-1). At high densities of* P. aeruginosa *cells, sufficient amounts of PAI-1 enter these bacteria to activate a transcriptional regulator named LasR. The activated LasR:PAI-1 complex then binds to the promoters of some virulence genes (e.g., the gene for exotoxin A, exoA), as well as genes (pai2) involved in the production of a second autoinducer, PAI-2. PAI-2 can then bind to a second transcriptional regulator, Rh1R; the activated Rh1R:PAI-2 complex then recognizes the promoters of additional virulence genes (vg), leading to increased expression of virulence factors (VF), including elastase.*

Interactions between Quorum-Sensing Systems and Two-Component Regulatory Systems

As mentioned earlier in this chapter, virulence gene expression is often subject to control by multiple regulatory systems. Such an overlap in regulatory mechanisms probably provides the bacterium with very tight control over the timing and levels of virulence gene expression. In this regard, recent studies have established *Staphylococcus aureus* as a model for understanding interactions that occur between quorum-sensing regulatory systems and two-component regulatory systems. *S. aureus* produces a small autoinducing peptide during its growth (Figure 24-3). As large numbers of *S. aureus* cells become present in the host, the concentration of this autoinducing peptide eventually reaches threshold concentrations, so that there is significant binding of this peptide to AgrC, which is the sensor component of the AgrC/AgrA two-component regulatory system of *S. aureus*. Binding of autoinducing peptide to AgrC causes activation of the AgrC/AgrA system, which results in increased expression of toxins but decreased expression of certain cell surface proteins. Interestingly, recent studies have shown that different *S. aureus* strains may produce slightly different autoinducing peptides as well as slightly different AgrC molecules. Consequently, the AgrC/AgrA system of an individual *S. aureus* cell becomes activated only by the binding of autoinducing peptide produced by itself or

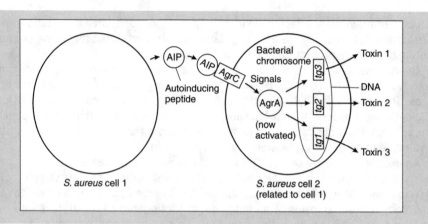

FIGURE 24-3 ▶
Quorum-Sensing System of Staphylococcus **aureus.** S. aureus *produces an autoinducing peptide (AIP) that can bind to, and activate, the AgrC membrane sensor protein of similar* S. aureus *isolates. This binding induces AgrC to phosphorylate the AgrA transcriptional regulator, which leads to increased expression of several toxins. (Although it is not shown in this figure, AIP can also induce the repression of other genes, including genes encoding some surface proteins that served as virulence factors earlier in infection but apparently are unimportant by the time* S. aureus *reaches high densities in vivo.)*

by a closely related *S. aureus* isolate. If the isolate's AgrC binds the autoinducing peptide produced by an unrelated *S. aureus* isolate, no activation of AgrC occurs, and toxin expression by the isolate will be inhibited (Figure 24-4).

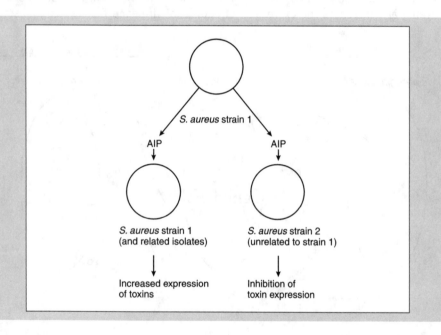

FIGURE 24-4 ▶
Differential Effects of Autoinducing Peptide on Similar and Dissimilar Staphylococcus **aureus Isolates.** *Production of autoinducing peptide (AIP) by* S. aureus *strain 1 activates expression of virulence factors (e.g., toxins) by* S. aureus *strain 1 and related strains, but inhibits virulence factor expression by dissimilar* S. aureus *strains (e.g., strain 2).*

ILLUSTRATIVE PATHOGEN: *Salmonella* spp.

Biologic Characteristics

Salmonella spp. are gram-negative bacteria that belong to the Enterobacteriaceae. These bacteria are motile, rod-shaped, facultative anaerobes that do not utilize lactose but usually produce H_2S. *Salmonella* spp. are facultative intracellular pathogens that can survive (at least transiently) inside nonactivated phagocytes as well as epithelial cells.

Although many different schemes have been used to classify the *Salmonella* spp., it is most straightforward to consider them as two groups: the typhoid salmonella (particularly *S. typhi*) and the nontyphoid salmonella (e.g., *S. enteritidis, S. typhimurium*).

Reservoirs and Transmission

Nontyphoid Salmonella. The nontyphoid salmonella (particularly *S. enteritidis* and *S. typhimurium*) are responsible for salmonella gastroenteritis (also known as salmonella food poisoning), which is one of the most common infectious diseases in industrialized

Salmonella typhi generally produces only trace amounts of H_2S. This trait can be useful for distinguishing this bacterium from other Salmonella *spp., which generally produce substantial amounts of H_2S.*

countries. At least 50,000 cases of foodborne salmonella gastroenteritis are documented each year in the United States, but estimates suggest that the true incidence of this illness is probably in the range of millions of cases per year. Most cases of salmonella gastroenteritis involve transmission by foods, but this illness can also be acquired by ingestion of fecally contaminated water. Salmonella food poisoning typically results from improper food handling, particularly from incomplete cooking of foods. People with low or no stomach acid (hypochlorhydria) are at particular risk for developing disease from nontyphoid salmonella.

The prevalence of food poisoning caused by nontyphoid salmonella can be explained in large part by these bacteria having a zoonotic reservoir that includes nearly all common food animals. Therefore, it is not surprising that poultry, poultry products (e.g., eggs), and improperly pasteurized milk rank among the most common food vehicles for salmonella gastroenteritis. However, these bacteria can also be acquired from household pets, particularly turtles but also dogs and cats.

Although the infectious dose of nontyphoid salmonella is relatively high (i.e., $\sim 10^6$ vs. 10–1000 for *Shigella* spp.), these bacteria can also be spread from person to person by the fecal–oral route, which contributes to the common occurrence of salmonella gastroenteritis among several members of a family and among patients in a hospital ward or nursing home. Such person-to-person transmission of nontyphoid salmonella is significantly aided by the ability of these bacteria to achieve a carrier state in some people, particularly because carriers may be asymptomatic even while they are continuously shedding viable (and infectious) nontyphoid salmonella in their feces.

Typhoid Salmonella. While typhoid fever is no longer common in most industrialized countries because of hygienic improvements, it remains an important cause of disease in less developed countries. In developed countries, people with this illness are often travelers who have recently returned from foreign countries where typhoid fever is endemic.

The typhoid salmonella (primarily *S. typhi* and *S. paratyphi*) have only a human reservoir and are commonly transmitted by the fecal–oral route, usually by contaminated food or water. As with the nontyphoid salmonella, it is fairly common for a carrier state to develop, particularly in individuals with gallstones. These human carriers represent a significant reservoir for typhoid fever.

Virulence Factors

There are several important virulence factors implicated in the pathogenesis of a salmonella infection.

Lipopolysaccharide (LPS). This important molecule contributes in several ways. First, LPS helps extracellular *Salmonella* spp. resist bile and complement. Second, as mentioned previously, recent studies suggest that modified LPS plays an important role in the intracellular survival of salmonella by providing resistance against certain antimicrobial peptides. Finally, the endotoxic activity of LPS is a major contributor to inflammation, which is considered responsible for most of the gastrointestinal (GI) symptoms and fever associated with salmonella infections.

Type III Secretion Systems and Effector Molecules. *Salmonella* spp., like many gram-negative bacteria (see Chapter 13), encode type III secretion systems, which can directly introduce effector molecules into the host cell. In *Salmonella* spp., these type III secretion systems are present on pathogenicity islands (see Chapter 23). Two different type III secretion systems have been identified in *Salmonella* spp. (note that it is possible for a single salmonella cell to carry both of these type III expression systems):

1. The Inv/Spa system (see Chapter 13) introduces effector proteins into the host cell, thereby stimulating a host signal transduction cascade that promotes the entry of salmonella into intestinal epithelial cells.
2. The Spi/Ssa system is thought to contribute to the survival of salmonella inside macrophages (although other virulence factors also appear to contribute to the survival of salmonella in macrophages).

One taxonomic system that has been used for classifying *Salmonella* species is the Ewing system, which recognizes only three *Salmonella* spp.: S. typhi, S. choleraesuis, and S. enteritidis. Another classification system is the Kauffman-White scheme, which (on the basis of differences in O, H, and Vi antigens) recognizes approximately 1500 different *Salmonella* spp.! The most recent taxonomic scheme recognizes two *Salmonella* spp.: S. enterica (which includes most of the major human pathogens) and S. bongori. S. enterica contains several subspecies and serovars (e.g., S. enterica subsp. enterica serovar typhimurium).

The molecular details of how the effector proteins associated with salmonella type III secretion systems exert their effects on host cells are not yet clear.

PhoP/PhoQ. This two-component regulatory system was described earlier in this chapter. In addition to being essential for the survival of salmonella inside phagocytes, PhoP/PhoQ also regulates the genes involved in the entry of salmonella into epithelial cells and phagocytes.

PagC and Other Outer Membrane Proteins. The PhoP/PhoQ-regulated synthesis of PagC and other outer membrane proteins appears to be important for salmonella resistance against defensins and thus for the survival of these bacteria inside macrophages.

Adhesins. *Salmonella* spp. produce both fimbrial and afimbrial surface adhesins (see Chapter 12) that probably assist in the attachment of these bacteria to the intestinal epithelium.

Enterotoxins. Although several reports have indicated that at least some salmonella isolates produce an enterotoxin, the importance of such toxins to pathogenesis remains unclear and controversial. It is generally believed that inflammation, not an enterotoxin, accounts for most (if not all) gastrointestinal symptoms associated with salmonella infections.

Virulence Antigen. The Vi antigen is a capsular polysaccharide produced by most strains of *S. typhi* and by some strains of *S. paratyphi*. The contribution of the Vi capsular antigen to the pathogenesis of typhoid salmonella infection remains unclear, but the Vi capsule does exhibit antiopsonic properties.

Flagella. The ability to produce flagella (composed of flagellin protein; see Chapter 1) is thought to allow *Salmonella* spp. to move through the intestinal mucus and gain access to the intestinal epithelium. Interestingly, while most salmonella isolates are able to produce two antigenically different types of flagella, termed phase variation, they only express one of these two flagella types at a time (Figure 24-5).

FIGURE 24-5 ▶

Salmonella spp. Phase Variation. *The ability of* Salmonella *spp. cell to repeatedly switch back and forth between the expressions of two antigenically different types of flagella is referred to as phase variation. Phase variation results from the "flip-flopping" of the promoter region for one of the two flagellin genes in the salmonella isolate. In one orientation, this promoter is functional, leading to the transcription and expression of one type of flagellin as well as the expression of a repressor that binds to the distant promoter of a gene encoding a second type of flagellin (expression of the repressor halts expression of this second flagellin gene). However, when this promoter region "flip-flops," the promoter becomes oriented in such a way that transcription of the first type of flagellin gene and repressor cannot occur. Consequently, transcription of the second flagellin gene now proceeds, because this gene carries its own promoter and is no longer subjected to repression.*

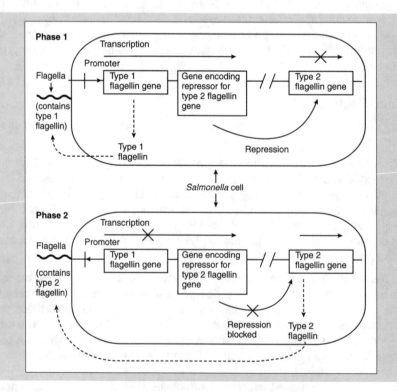

Pathogenesis

Nontyphoid Salmonella. The ingestion of large numbers of nontyphoid salmonella (usually in contaminated food or water) permits some of these bacteria to survive their transit through the stomach. After viable organisms enter the small intestines, they move through the intestinal mucus and adhere to the intestinal epithelium, where they invade both enterocytes and M cells. This intestinal invasion is mediated by the Inv/Spa type III secretion system (see Chapter 13); the effector proteins of this type III secretion system alter, through incompletely understood mechanisms, host cell signal transduction pathways that result in membrane ruffling, which stimulates macropinocytosis and facilitates the entry of nontyphoid salmonella into epithelial and M cells.

Once they are present inside intestinal epithelial cells, nontyphoid salmonella remain localized in an endosome (unlike the *Shigella* spp., which escape from an endosome into the cytoplasm; see Chapter 13). This endosome gradually translocates from the apical to the basal side of the intestinal epithelial cell; during this translocation process, the nontyphoid salmonella acclimate to their new intracellular environment and even replicate. Contact of the endosome with the basolateral membrane of the enterocyte or M cell results in the release of nontyphoid salmonella into the lamina propria.

In the lamina propria, nontyphoid salmonella are often phagocytosed by macrophages and other professional phagocytes. Their entry into the phagosomes of professional phagocytes is sensed by their PhoP/PhoQ two-component regulatory system (and possibly other sensor-regulator systems), which triggers changes in gene expression that facilitate survival in the harsh intracellular environment of the phagocyte. For example, these intracellular salmonella become more resistant to stresses present in the phagolysosome (e.g., low pH and the presence of cationic antimicrobial peptides such as defensins). PhoP/PhoQ contributes to the survival of nontyphoid salmonella inside phagocytes by means of several mechanisms, which (as previously described) include (1) inducing LPS modifications that inhibit the binding of antimicrobial peptides such as CAP37 and CAP57 and (2) inducing the synthesis of outer membrane proteins (such as PagC) that somehow inhibit defensin-mediated killing.

In immunocompetent individuals, the presence of nontyphoid salmonella in the lamina propria induces a strong inflammatory response that is considered responsible for most, or all, of the symptoms that characterize salmonella food poisoning. These symptoms, which include mild-to-moderate fever and GI symptoms (diarrhea and abdominal cramps), typically persist for about a week before resolving. Ultimately this inflammatory response benefits the host by preventing the spread of nontyphoid salmonella beyond the GI tract and eventually by helping to clear the infection.

By contrast, when immunocompromised individuals unable to mount a strong cell-mediated immune response become infected with nontyphoid salmonella (particularly *S. choleraesuis*), these bacteria often disseminate throughout the body, producing septicemia and possibly death. Nontyphoid salmonella are a particularly notable cause of septicemia and death in AIDS patients.

Typhoid Salmonella. The pathogenesis of infection with typhoid salmonella is generally similar to that of infection with nontyphoid salmonella up to the point where these bacteria become present in the lamina propria. In contrast to nontyphoid salmonella cells, which are usually restricted to the intestines of immunocompetent individuals (where they are killed after a few days), typhoid salmonella cells typically disseminate beyond the intestines (even in immunocompetent individuals) and then survive in the human body for several weeks. Because this dissemination involves the transport of typhoid salmonella from the intestines before these bacteria can multiply to high levels or before the intestinal immune system can become fully activated, the initial symptoms of typhoid fever are relatively mild (low-grade fever, constipation). This dissemination involves the transport of typhoid salmonella via the lymph or the blood to the reticulo-endothelial system (particularly the liver), where these bacteria multiply for 1–2 weeks, a period corresponding to the incubation time for typhoid fever. During this incubation period, symptoms remain relatively mild.

When a threshold burden of typhoid salmonella becomes present in reticulo-endothelial tissue, these bacteria suddenly emerge into the blood and bile, triggering the onset of full-blown typhoid fever. Large numbers of typhoid salmonella in the blood may lead to septic shock (see Chapter 21), abscesses in distant organs, or organ failure. This bacteremia also contributes to the prolonged high (i.e., ~104°F) temperature that is typical of typhoid fever. At this time, large numbers of typhoid salmonella are re-introduced into the intestines through contaminated bile. Because the intestinal im-

The molecular basis for the greater ability of typhoid vs. nontyphoid salmonella to survive inside macrophages and to disseminate (in immunocompetent people) remains unclear.

Many students are familiar with the infamous Typhoid Mary, a cook in a New York City restaurant early in the 20th century. Epidemiologists eventually established that, as a chronic carrier of Salmonella typhi, Typhoid Mary was responsible for several outbreaks of typhoid fever. Faced with a major public health threat, authorities gave Typhoid Mary a choice between removal of her gallbladder or prison—and she chose prison! After 3 years in jail, Typhoid Mary was released after promising not to work as a cook in the future. However, she assumed a new name and resumed work as a cook in restaurants and hotels. Several years later, Typhoid Mary was arrested after epidemiologic investigations identified her as the source of several new outbreaks of typhoid fever. She was sent back to prison, where she died 23 years later.

Typhoid salmonella are excreted in the urine of approximately 25% of patients, which means that the urine of typhoid fever patients should be considered potentially infectious.

mune system was exposed to typhoid salmonella only 1–2 weeks earlier, this second exposure often induces a vigorous inflammatory response in the intestines that can result in diarrhea and, more importantly, in intestinal granuloma or abscess formation and hemorrhage. If perforation of the intestines results from this inflammation, normal GI flora may enter the patient's abdomen, resulting in life-threatening peritonitis. Because of the tendency for typhoid fever to result in effects such as intestinal hemorrhage, septic shock, or organ failure, this illness has a mortality rate of 10%–20% without antimicrobial therapy. In the absence of antimicrobial therapy, activated macrophages (along with the development of an appropriate humoral immune response) are critical for recovery from typhoid fever.

As mentioned previously, some people (particularly those with gallstones) become carriers of typhoid salmonella. Although these individuals may not experience disease symptoms, they still represent a significant public health threat because they are persistently shedding infectious typhoid salmonella in their feces.

Diagnosis

The laboratory plays an important role in diagnosing all salmonella infections. The presence of gram-negative, lactose-negative rods on a selective medium such as MacConkey agar (see Appendix 1) suggests the presence of *Salmonella* or *Shigella* spp., which can then be easily differentiated on the basis of motility (*Shigella* spp. are nonmotile, while *Salmonella* spp. are motile), H_2S production, and other biochemical properties. If it is warranted for epidemiologic reasons, salmonella isolates can be further characterized by serologic testing (e.g., different strains of salmonella can be distinguished on the basis of their O, H, and, if present, Vi antigens).

Nontyphoid Salmonella. Stool cultures are highly informative because they typically test positive for *Salmonella* spp. throughout the course of salmonella food poisoning. In addition to fecal cultures, the identification of a salmonella food poisoning outbreak can be assisted by the determination of epidemiologic parameters (such as incubation times and symptoms) of the outbreak or by isolating *Salmonella* spp. from suspected food vehicles. For diagnosing cases of septicemia from nontyphoid salmonella, blood cultures are extremely important.

Typhoid Salmonella. Because blood cultures usually test positive for typhoid *Salmonella* spp. earlier than either stool or urine cultures, most cases of typhoid fever are also initially identified on the basis of positive blood cultures. The diagnosis of typhoid fever may also be assisted by clinical observations, such as the characteristic rash ("rose spots") on the patient's abdomen.

Prevention and Treatment

Nontyphoid Salmonella. Views differ as to whether antimicrobial therapy should be used to treat cases of salmonella food poisoning in immunocompetent individuals. Many physicians believe that antimicrobial therapy may actually contribute to the development of the carrier state in persons with gastroenteritis. Otherwise, treatment for salmonella gastroenteritis is symptomatic (e.g., rehydration). In contrast, antimicrobial therapy is always essential for treating septicemia involving nontyphoid salmonella.

Because no effective vaccine is currently available to protect against salmonella food poisoning, this illness is best controlled by adhering to good sanitary practices (e.g., proper food storage and processing) and by cooking foods completely.

Typhoid Salmonella. Because of the life-threatening nature of typhoid fever, prompt and effective antimicrobial therapy is essential for treating this disease. When administered early in the course of typhoid fever, antimicrobial therapy can significantly decrease the severity and duration of symptoms, can dramatically reduce fatalities, and may decrease the likelihood that the carrier state will develop. Unfortunately, the antimicrobial therapy of typhoid fever (or septicemia caused by nontyphoid salmonella) is becoming more difficult because of increasing problems with antibiotic resistance.

Antimicrobial therapy does not always resolve the carrier state (particularly in individuals with gallstones); when antimicrobial therapy cannot clear carriers of *S. typhi*, it may be necessary to remove the carrier's gallstones or even surgically remove the gallbladder.

For many years a parenterally administered, killed whole-cell *S. typhi* vaccine has been available for "preventing" typhoid fever. However, this parenteral vaccine frequently causes side effects, and its efficacy is unclear. In response, a live, attenuated, oral typhoid fever vaccine (see Part VII) has recently been licensed. While the efficacy of this new vaccine is not yet completely clear, it is available for use in Third World countries where typhoid fever remains a major public health problem. In industrialized countries where typhoid fever is no longer common, sanitary measures (e.g., good hygienic practices by food preparers) provide the front-line defense against this illness.

> *Because salmonella are facultative intracellular pathogens, an effective salmonella vaccine needs to develop both cellular and humoral immune responses. Killed bacterial vaccines, such as the traditional typhoid fever vaccine, do not usually result in the development of potent cellular immune responses (see Part VII).*

RESOLUTION OF CLINICAL CASE

This individual was suffering from typhoid fever (also known as enteric fever), which is usually caused by *S. typhi*. As described in the chapter, *S. typhi* (which only has a human reservoir) is transmitted by the fecal–oral route, usually by contaminated food or water. In contrast to most cases of nontyphoid salmonella infection, which are limited to moderate fever and GI symptoms, *S. typhi* eventually causes bacteremia that may result in the localization of typhoid salmonella in various organs, especially the gallbladder, bone, and soft tissue, producing cholecystitis, osteomyelitis, and abscesses, respectively. The intestines also become involved in this disease as typhoid salmonella are reintroduced by contaminated bile from the gallbladder.

In typhoid fever, an elevated temperature first appears about 1–2 weeks after infection and increases slowly, in a stepwise fashion, over several days. Fever is soon accompanied by flu-like symptoms, including malaise, anorexia, myalgia, arthralgia, cough, sore throat, and headache. By the end of the first week of symptoms (2–3 weeks after initial exposure to *S. typhi*), there is sustained fever, confusion, cough, sore throat, chest pain, anorexia, and vomiting. The symptoms of bronchitis may be prominent because of the dissemination of *S. typhi* to the lungs. Constipation is common, but diarrhea may develop later in this disease. Physical examination may reveal relative bradycardia for the height of the temperature, rose spots, abdominal tenderness, hepatomegaly, and splenomegaly. Later in the course of typhoid fever, metastatic or focal infection may occur. Anemia is common. Leukopenia or a normal white blood cell count (which would be unusual in other forms of bacteremia) is typically seen.

As described in the chapter, the diagnosis of typhoid fever rests on the isolation of *S. typhi*, usually from the blood, but the bacterium may also be recovered from rose spots, stool, urine, and bone marrow. Examination of the serum for antibodies against salmonella O and H antigens (Widal's test) is not very reliable. Because of the ubiquitousness of salmonella and cross-reactions between the various species and serotypes, antisalmonella antibodies are fairly common in the general population. Furthermore, the titers of these antibodies can rise in other, non-salmonella infections.

Since antibiotic resistance is fairly common among salmonella, the choice of antibiotic for treating typhoid fever should be guided by susceptibility testing. Nonresistant typhoid fever is usually managed with a 2- to 4-week course of chloramphenicol. Ampicillin, trimethoprim-sulfamethoxazole, third-generation cephalosporins, and fluoroquinolones are all reasonable alternatives but may be slightly less effective than chloramphenicol. The relapse rate, even in appropriately treated disease, may approach 10%.

As also mentioned in the chapter, a carrier state may follow symptomatic disease or asymptomatic infection with any salmonella, including *S. typhi*. The usual site of persistence is the gallbladder, and the organism is excreted in the stool, serving as a source of new infections. The incidence of positive stool cultures following infection with *S. typhi* is about 50% at 1 month, 20% after 2 months, and 10% after 3 months; chronic carriage for more than 1 year occurs in about 3%. Food handlers, such as the chef in this clinical case, should not be allowed to return to that line of work until two weekly stool cultures are negative. In some cases, it may be necessary to resort to several courses of antibiotics, and even cholecystectomy, in an attempt to terminate the carrier state.

REVIEW QUESTIONS

Directions: For each of the following questions, choose the **one best** answer.

1. Thirty-six hours after ingesting some contaminated food, a 17-year-old woman in Illinois developed a moderate fever, abdominal cramps, and diarrhea. These symptoms persisted for about a week and then subsided without any further illness. Fecal culture identified the responsible pathogen as an H_2S-positive, lactose-negative, oxidase-negative, motile, gram-negative rod. Considering this clinical scenario, which one of the following statements is correct?

   (A) This woman's illness was probably typhoid fever

   (B) This woman may have continued shedding viable pathogens in her stools for the next several weeks after her illness subsided

   (C) The pathogen responsible for this woman's illness has only a human reservoir

   (D) This woman's illness is not currently common in the United States

   (E) The pathogen responsible for this woman's illness does not invade the intestinal epithelium

2. Which one of the following statements about two-component regulatory systems is correct?

   (A) Two-component regulatory systems can activate, but can never repress, bacterial gene expression

   (B) Two-component regulatory systems always act independently of quorum-sensing regulatory systems

   (C) A single bacterial cell can carry only one type of two-component regulatory system

   (D) Two-component regulatory systems can sometimes sense the difference between intracellular and extracellular environments

   (E) Only gram-negative bacteria use two-component regulatory systems

3. Which one of the following statements about quorum-sensing systems is correct?

   (A) They involve production of an autoinducer, which is usually a large protein

   (B) They become activated at low bacterial population densities

   (C) They always induce decreased expression of virulence genes

   (D) They are found only in gram-negative bacteria

   (E) They can sometimes regulate virulence gene expression without the autoinducer entering the bacterial cytoplasm

4. Which one of the following statements about PhoP/PhoQ is correct?

   (A) It refers to a quorum-sensing system present in most *Salmonella* spp.

   (B) It cannot increase the expression of salmonella genes involved in modifying the structure of lipopolysaccharides (LPS)

   (C) It cannot increase the expression of salmonella genes encoding outer membrane proteins

   (D) It is not required for the survival of *Salmonella* spp. inside phagocytes

   (E) It is important for the resistance of *Salmonella* spp. to defensin-mediated killing

5. Which one of the following statements about typhoid fever is correct?

    (A) This disease has a zoonotic reservoir

    (B) This disease is typically diagnosed by the use of fecal culture

    (C) This disease is never transmitted by asymptomatic human carriers

    (D) This disease remains quite common in industrialized countries

    (E) This disease involves dissemination of bacteria beyond the gastrointestinal tract

ANSWERS AND EXPLANATIONS

1. The answer is B. Option A is incorrect because the woman's symptoms and the geographic location (i.e., typhoid fever is not common in the United States) strongly suggest that she was ill with salmonella gastroenteritis, not typhoid fever (if she had been sick with typhoid fever, her illness would have recurred after 1–2 weeks, with much more severe symptoms). Option C is incorrect because nontyphoid salmonella have a zoonotic reservoir. Option D is incorrect because salmonella gastroenteritis is extremely common in the United States, where there are probably millions of cases of this illness each year. Option E is incorrect because all salmonella (typhoid and nontyphoid) invade the intestines.

2. The answer is D. Option A is incorrect because the PhoP/PhoQ two-component regulatory system, for example, activates the expression of *pag* genes but represses the expression of *prg* genes. Option B is incorrect because, for example, the AgrC/AgrA two-component regulatory system of *Staphylococcus aureus* can be activated by an autoinducer that is part of a quorum-sensing system. Option C is incorrect because salmonella carry both the PhoP/PhoQ and PmrA/PmrB two-component regulatory systems. Option E is incorrect because two-component regulatory systems have been identified in several gram-positive pathogens (e.g., *S. aureus*, *Clostridium perfringens*).

3. The answer is E. The autoinducer of *S. aureus* apparently regulates gene expression changes in this bacterium by binding to, and activating, the membrane sensor protein AgrC. Option A is incorrect because recognized autoinducers are all small molecules (either peptides or modified lactones). Option B is incorrect because quorum-sensing systems can increase the expression of many virulence genes (e.g., *S. aureus* toxin synthesis increases when the proper autoinducer is present). Option D is incorrect because quorum-sensing systems are found in both gram-positive (e.g., *S. aureus*) and gram-negative (e.g., *Pseudomonas aeruginosa*) pathogens.

4. The answer is E. Option A is incorrect because PhoP/PhoQ is a two-component regulatory system, not a quorum-sensing system. Option B is incorrect because PhoP/PhoQ does increase the expression of genes that can modify the structure of LPS (making the salmonella less susceptible to certain antimicrobial peptides). Option C is incorrect because PhoP/PhoQ can increase the expression of genes encoding outer membrane proteins (this effect is also important for resistance to certain anti-microbial peptides). Option D is incorrect because PhoP/PhoQ is important for the survival of salmonella in phagocytes (in large part because it promotes resistance to antimicrobial peptides).

5. The answer is E. Option A is incorrect because typhoid fever has only a human reservoir. Option B is incorrect because the diagnosis of typhoid fever usually depends primarily on blood cultures. Option C is incorrect because this illness can be transmitted by human carriers, some of whom may be asymptomatic. Option D is incorrect because typhoid fever is now uncommon in industrialized countries, although some cases still occur.

PART VI: HOST FACTORS AND THE OUTCOME OF INFECTION

OVERVIEW

INABILITY OF THE HOST TO CLEAR AN INFECTION

The vast majority of microbes that come into contact with healthy human beings every day are cleared by innate or specific host defenses. However, some microbial pathogens are able to persist within the host for extended periods of time and cause overt (symptomatic) disease by progressively degrading the immune status of the host. In other cases, these microbial pathogens cause escalating episodes of disease symptoms that eventually culminate in the debilitation of the host. In either case, the common theme is the ability of the microbial pathogen to persist within the host, culminating in serious disease. The persistence of a microbial pathogen within the human host can be viewed as the host's inability to clear the microbial pathogen. Part VI describes this ability to clear a microbial pathogen in four chapters.

In Chapter 25, *Mycobacterium leprae* (the causative agent of leprosy) and *Treponema pallidum* (the causative agent of syphilis) are discussed to underscore the consequences of failing to clear these pathogens in immunologically healthy individuals. Both of these organisms cause persistent disease that progresses to more serious disease as a function of the time in which an individual is infected. While leprosy and syphilis presently occur within the United States at relatively low morbidity rates, the contemporary medical community cannot ignore the prevalence of these infections worldwide, nor can it ignore the historical importance of these diseases.

Chapter 26 describes the association between persistent infectious diseases and cancer. A simplistic view of cancer is that it derives from one of two broad etiologies: (1) they are genetically preprogrammed or (2) they are induced upon exposure to carcinogens in the environment. Because we are constantly exposed to microbial pathogens as part of our environment, it follows that exposure to microbial pathogens may contribute to the transformation of eukaryotic cells—the first step in the development of cancer. The focus of Chapter 26 is the role that human papilloma virus (HPV) plays in transforming the host cell, which in turn can lead to the development of cervical cancer. A practical outcome of understanding the pathogenesis of HPV infection and its link to cervical cancer is the Pap smear, a test that looks for early signs of cervical cell transformation in sexually active women. It is estimated that the common use of the Pap smear has reduced the number of deaths from cervical cancer by 70%. In addition to viral paradigms, bacterial infections such as stomach ulcers caused by *Helicobacter pylori* (see Chapter 14) are also associated with cancer.

Chapter 27 discusses what is arguably the most socially and medically significant infectious disease of the past two decades, AIDS. The social and medical significance of this disease derives from the fact that AIDS was at one time closely associated with sexual transmission among the homosexual community and/or among intravenous drug abusers. The rapid spread of AIDS into the heterosexual community by sexual transmission and the fact that the disease is terminal in nearly all infected individuals have contributed to the significance of human immunodeficiency virus type 1 (HIV-1) infection. The immunopathology of HIV-1 infection is somewhat unique among microbial pathogens. This virus causes devastating disease by an indirect route, slowly impairing the function of the cellular immune system as the virus persists within the human host over the course of many years. During this period, the virus is infectious via the exchange of body fluids such as semen, vaginal secretions, and blood. This infectious condition does not kill the human host per se; rather the progressive impairment of the cellular arm of the immune response renders an HIV-1 infected individual increasingly susceptible to opportunistic microbial pathogens. As a result, diseases that were rarely seen in the past, such as encephalitis due to *Toxoplasma gondii* (Chapter 28), and diseases that were under reasonable control, such as mycobacterial infections (see Chapter 22), are now commonplace among people with AIDS and are the actual causes of death among HIV-1 infected individuals. It is safe to say that the prevention and management of HIV-1 infection will affect all of us, in some way, in the decade to come.

Chapter 28 describes an important concept in medical microbiology—opportunistic infections. We humans coexist with viruses, bacteria, and parasites. We are able to do so because of a highly evolved immune system that prevents the overgrowth of these microbial pathogens. However, when the opportunity arises (e.g., as a result of HIV-1 infection, see Chapter 27) these ubiquitous organisms can cause disease. In Chapter 28 fungal and parasitic disease are focused on as specific examples of opportunistic infections; however, it is emphasized in this chapter that all microbial pathogens—viral, bacterial, fungal, and parasitic—can be opportunistic. Furthermore, opportunistic infections are becoming increasingly important as medicine is required to micromanage important conditions such as old age, cancer, and a variety of illnesses. These clinical scenarios put patients in the position of confronting ubiquitous microbial pathogens while in a state of lowered immune defense, creating the possibility of opportunistic infection. As we find more ways to prolong life, opportunistic infection will surely become a problem of increasing importance.

25

CONSEQUENCES OF FAILURE TO CLEAR PATHOGENS: PERSISTENCE, LATENCY, AND THE CARRIER STATE

William F. Goins, Ph.D.

CHAPTER OUTLINE

Introduction of Clinical Case
Pathogens That Fail to be Effectively Cleared by the Host
Illustrative Pathogen: *Treponema pallidum*
- Biologic Characteristics
- Reservoir and Transmission
- Virulence Factors
- Pathogenesis
- Diagnosis
- Prevention and Treatment
Illustrative Pathogen: *Mycobacterium leprae*
- Biologic Characteristics
- Reservoir and Transmission
- Virulence Factors
- Pathogenesis
- Diagnosis
- Prevention and Treatment
Resolution of Clinical Case
Review Questions

INTRODUCTION OF CLINICAL CASE

A 47-year-old man went to see a dermatologist because of a rash that had been present on his palms for a week. The patient indicated that he had felt feverish and had experienced a loss of appetite around the time when the rash appeared. Physical examination revealed about a dozen, flat (macular), pinkish brown, 3–4 mm round lesions on both palms and similar lesions occurring less frequently on the soles of both feet. Upon questioning, the patient revealed that he noted a painless, shallow ulcer on his penis, just proximal to the glans, about 8 weeks prior to the development of the skin lesions. The ulcer healed on its own, thus the patient did not seek treatment at that time. The patient admitted that 3 weeks prior to the appearance of the penile lesion, he had traveled to a distant city on business and had availed himself of the services of a female sex worker without using a condom.

- What is the cause of this patient's symptoms?
- Are the temporal sequences of having unprotected sex, the occurrence of a penile lesion, and the development of a characteristic rash relevant for identification of the infectious agent associated with this patient's symptoms?
- Should this patient be administered an antibiotic at this time?

PATHOGENS THAT FAIL TO BE EFFECTIVELY CLEARED BY THE HOST

In **persistent infection**, the microorganism persists in the body by escaping host immune surveillance, often for extended periods or throughout life.

In most cases host immunity is effective in clearing bacterial, viral, fungal, and protozoan pathogens in response to acute infection. Sometimes, however, host defenses fail to eliminate the microorganisms properly, resulting in persistence of the pathogen. This persistence may ultimately lead to severe disease later in life (Table 25-1). In such cases, either the host defense is not sufficient to clear the infection or the invading pathogen somehow overcomes the gauntlet of host defense mechanisms in a manner that favors chronic disease. These types of infections are appropriately referred to as *persistent infections*.

TABLE 25-1 ▶

Persistent Pathogens

Microorganism	Sites of Persistence	Reactivation Disease
Bacteria		
Chlamydia trachomatis	Conjunctiva	Chronic eye disease and blindness
Rickettsia prowazekii	Lymph node	Reactivation tuberculosis
Salmonella typhi	Gall bladder	Cystitis
Mycobacterium tuberculosis	Macrophages in lung	Reactivation typhus and vasculitis
Mycobacterium leprae	Macrophages in lung and skin	Skin lesions and nerve damage
Treponema pallidum	Lymph nodes and disseminated	Neurologic disease
Protozoa		
Plasmodium vivax	Liver	Clinical malaria
Toxoplasma gondii	Lymphoid tissue, muscle, and brain	Neurologic disease
Trypanosoma cruzi	Blood and macrophages	Chronic disease
Viruses		
Epstein-Barr virus	B-cells	B-cell lymphomas
Herpes simplex virus	PNS neurons	Facial and genital lesions
Varicella zoster virus	PNS neurons and glia	Shingles and nerve damage
Human cytomegalovirus	T-cells and macrophages in lung and liver	Pneumonitis and retinitis
Human immunodeficiency virus	T-cells and dendritic cells in lymph nodes	AIDS
Hepatitis B virus	Liver	Chronic hepatitis
Human papillomavirus	Keratinocytes	Warts and malignant tumors[a]

Note. PNS = peripheral nervous system; AIDS = acquired immunodeficiency syndrome.
[a]Warts and tumors result from integration and persistence not reactivation.

Persistent infections are particularly important because they enable an infectious agent to exist within a specific human host over an extended time period without severely disabling the infected individual, which in turn allows these agents to remain present within the population. For example, persistently infected individuals, or *carriers*, may display little or no manifestations of clinical disease, yet act as reservoirs for the shedding of pathogens to other individuals. In some instances, low-level production of the pathogen occurs; however, the microorganism may be produced in a form that is not fully infectious and typically does minimal damage to the host until induced.

Pathogens employ a variety of techniques to evade clearance. Some pathogens (e.g., human immunodeficiency virus type 1 [HIV-1], mycobacteria, Epstein-Barr virus [EBV], human cytomegalovirus [HCMV], *Trypanosoma cruzi*) infect and persist in host cells involved in the immune response to pathogens (see Table 25-1). These persistent pathogens may exist in the absence of any clinical manifestation (latency), which makes diagnosis difficult, particularly when patient history of the distant past has been forgotten. Upon entering the latent state, no (or very low levels of) pathogen-specific antigens are generally synthesized. This allows pathogens like herpes simplex virus (HSV) to escape the host immune response. A variety of stimuli can cause these latent pathogens to reactivate and replicate, leading to severe and even fatal disease. Factors such as ultraviolet light, stress, hormones, drugs, trauma, and immune suppression may lead to reactivation of the virus as reported for HSV. Reactivation of latent pathogens is frequently observed in immunocompromised hosts such as transplant patients, patients receiving immunosuppressive drugs, and acquired immunodeficiency syndrome (AIDS) patients. Reactivation of latent pathogens often leads to the elimination of the inhabited cells (as with HIV), thereby further reducing the ability of the host to clear the microorganism.

Other mechanisms of pathogen persistence include strategies that induce autoimmune disease (e.g., streptococcal M-protein; see Chapter 16). Although rare, persistent pathogens are also associated with neoplasia, as seen with *Helicobacter pylori*, human papillomavirus (HPV), hepatitis B virus (HBV), and other infectious agents (see Chapter 26). The ability of a persistent pathogen to overcome the innate aspects of the host, such as disruption of the host's complement cascade observed with HSV and various streptococci (see Chapters 9 and 16, respectively), can affect efficient complement-mediated clearance. Other pathogens like influenzavirus, HIV, and *T. cruzi* evade the host response by undergoing antigenic variation in their crucial surface proteins, which are not only the major antigens seen by the host but are also molecules involved in the interaction of the pathogen with the host (see Chapter 16).

In this chapter, two pathogens that demonstrate the advantage of persistence are described. *Treponema pallidum* employs molecular mimicry to evade the host immune response and cause syphilis. *Mycobacterium leprae* avoids clearance by invading and altering the ability of infected cells to be properly phagocytized, culminating in the disease named leprosy. In the end, the ability of a pathogen to persist long-term within a human host provides time for the pathogen to select another susceptible host in which it can spread.

> A **carrier** is an infected individual who is either asymptomatic or displays minimal overt symptomatology. Casual carriers temporarily harbor (days to weeks) the pathogen, whereas chronic carriers harbor the pathogen for extended periods, sometimes for life.

> **Shedding** is the liberation of the microorganism from a persistently infected host, who may be asymptomatic.

> **Latency** is a type or stage of persistent infection in which a microorganism remains quiescent and causes no disease but retains the ability to reactivate and cause overt disease.

> **Reactivation** of a persistent or latent microorganism occurs when a latent pathogen is stimulated to actively replicate, usually resulting in overt disease. However, in some circumstances the recurrent disease can be asymptomatic.

ILLUSTRATIVE PATHOGEN: *Treponema pallidum*

T. pallidum is the causative agent of syphilis, a multifaceted disease of humans that progresses through a series of stages first described by Philippe Ricord in 1927. Syphilis is a disease of historical significance, with original reports of this disease dating back to sometime around the 16th century. When the disease first arose within the human population, it was an extremely virulent and rapid killer. Syphilis spread rapidly throughout the Old World and had a major influence on the outcomes of military endeavors because of its incidence, severity, and ability to decimate an army. Syphilis is thought to have been brought from Europe to the Americas by Christopher Columbus and his men. Eventually, the interaction between this microbial pathogen and its human host evolved into a disease of reduced severity during the early stages. This pathogen acquired the ability to persist in tissues of the host for extended periods in the absence of clinical disease, while retaining high rates of mortality in advanced disease. In effect, evolution has created a persistent pathogen that, rather than rapidly killing its host, quietly expands its reservoir in a manner that facilitates its spread.

Biologic Characteristics

T. pallidum is a spiral-shaped, motile microorganism that is a member of the heterogeneous group of spirochetes. Like another spirochete, *Borrelia burgdorferi* (see Chapter 8), *T. pallidum* does not stain using the conventional Gram stain because it is too thin to be observed by light microscopy. Instead, *T. pallidum* is observed using darkfield, immunofluorescent, or electron microscopy. This poses problems for the diagnosis of *T. pallidum* infection because these techniques are not routinely performed by most diagnostic laboratories.

T. pallidum *cannot be observed by Gram stain and cannot be isolated by standard bacterial culture techniques. This makes definitive diagnosis of syphilis difficult.*

T. pallidum is microaerophilic and replicates very slowly in vivo, possessing a doubling time of more than 30 hours. Like the other spirochetes, *T. pallidum* is not amenable for culture on standard bacteriologic media, which further complicates its diagnosis (see Diagnosis).

Electron microscopic evaluation of *T. pallidum* demonstrates the two-membrane organization typical of gram-negative bacteria. Similar to *B. burgdorferi*, these spiral- or corkscrew-shaped bioforms possess endoflagella within their periplasm, which accounts for their corkscrew-like appearance and movement (see Figure 1-10). In contrast, the *T. pallidum* outer membrane lacks the classic lipopolysaccharide (LPS) found in other well-characterized gram-negative bacteria. The outer sheath that encases *T. pallidum* contains a series of complex glycosaminoglycans (gags) similar to those found on various host cells. This molecular "face" facilitates the evasion of *T. pallidum* from host immunity by the strategy of molecular mimicry (see Chapter 16).

Reservoir and Transmission

Humans are the sole reservoir for *T. pallidum*. This pathogen is transmitted most frequently by direct sexual contact between sexual partners. At least one-third of all new cases of syphilis in the United States occur in homosexual males. Transmission during sexual contact occurs when the microorganism penetrates intact mucous membranes or enters through abrasions in the skin. Under the appropriate circumstances, *T. pallidum* can also be transmitted transplacentally from an infected mother to her fetus. In the case of congenital syphilis, transmission of the microorganism in the blood of the mother to the fetus occurs as early as 10 weeks after gestation. Transmission in utero can result in severe disease leading to miscarriage, stillborn birth, or death of the fetus. Infected infants who survive birth frequently display multiorgan dysfunction with considerable CNS complications. Even in asymptomatic infants, sequelae such as keratitis, arthritis, deafness, and CNS problems become prominent later in life. Interestingly, these sequelae are similar to those observed among asymptomatic infants who are infected in utero by HCMV (see Chapter 10).

T. pallidum *is typically transmitted between sex partners. This organism is also efficiently transmitted from mother to fetus. Syphilis transmitted between adult sex partners demonstrates symptoms that are distinct from those observed during in utero infection.*

Virulence Factors

An important feature of *T. pallidum* persistence involves the ability of the microorganism to avoid host immune surveillance, which *T. pallidum* accomplishes using molecular mimicry. The outer sheath of *T. pallidum* contains complex glycosylaminoglycans modified with sialic acid residues; the presence of these treponemal-encoded antigens, which resemble common molecules found on the surface of human cells, results in the blockage of both antibody-dependent cell-mediated cytotoxicity (ADCC) and complement-mediated lysis of *T. pallidum* infected cells. Additionally, *T. pallidum* encodes a hyaluronidase that allows for the breakdown of hyaluronic acid in host tissues, thereby enhancing the ability of the pathogen to invade the multitude of organs and tissues involved in tertiary disease.

Virulence factors of T. pallidum:
- *Molecular mimicry*
- *Glycosylaminoglycans*
- *Hyaluronidase*

Pathogenesis

Following its deposition onto the genital mucosa, *T. pallidum* gains access to subepithelial tissues through tiny cracks in the epithelial cell spaces. From this site, *T. pallidum* spreads to local lymph nodes and eventually to the blood over a period of about 3 weeks. After an incubation period of 2–10 weeks, a painless syphilitic chancre characteristic of primary syphilis develops at the site of infection due to inflammation and necrosis resulting from a response by neutrophils, T-cells, and macrophages against *T. pallidum* (Table 25-2). The chancre heals spontaneously over a period of 2–6 weeks, even in the absence of antibiotic treatment.

◀ **TABLE 25-2**
Clinical Stages of Syphilis

Stage	Time Course	Manifestations	VDRL/ RPR +[a]	FTA +[a]
Primary	2–10 weeks	Syphilitic chancre on genitals, asymptomatic	76%	85%
Secondary	3–6 weeks	Maculopapular rash, CNS involvement, mucous membrane lesions	99%	100%
Latent				
Early	< 1 year	None	Similar to secondary	
Late	> 1 year	None	Similar to tertiary	
Tertiary	3–30 years	Neurosyphilis: asymptomatic, meningovascular, dementia, tremors, dysarthria, unsteady gait, locomotor ataxia, urinary incontinence, impotence, optic atrophy	70%	98%
		Cardiovascular: thoracic aorta aneurysm, aortic valve insufficiency		
		Syphilitic granulomas: gumma formation of skin, bone, testes, liver, brain, and heart		

Note. VDRL = Venereal Disease Research Laboratory; RPR = rapid plasma reagin; FTA = fluorescent treponemal antibody.
[a] Percentage of patients that test positive.

The microorganism then disseminates in the blood, localizing to blood vessels and spreading to the skin, liver, joints, lymph nodes, muscles, and brain over a period of 3–6 weeks. Approximately 25%–50% of these patients develop some observable clinical symptoms associated with secondary syphilis (Table 25-3); however, a significant number of patients remain asymptomatic at this stage of the disease. Secondary syphilis frequently manifests itself as a maculopapular rash over the palms and feet, but lesions can appear on any part of the body. This skin rash heals spontaneously (i.e., without treatment) over the course of 2–6 weeks.

Following symptomatic or asymptomatic secondary syphilis, the disease progresses into a state of latency in which there are no clinical manifestations of disease, and the microorganism resides within local lymph nodes and the spleen. During the latent period, which can last from 3–30 years, infected individuals can only be accurately diagnosed using a treponemal-specific test, since the nontreponemal tests are less sensitive in patients with latent syphilis or even in those that have progressed into tertiary disease. Individuals in early latency (less than 1 year post–secondary disease) can be effectively treated with antibiotic therapy, however, treatment of patients in late latency (more than 1 year post–secondary syphilis) is exceedingly difficult.

The microorganism continues to persist in a latent state in about 30% of all patients with tertiary syphilis, even in those not treated with antibiotics. However, in 30%–40% of all latently infected patients, the pathogen reactivates and begins to replicate actively, spread, and penetrate various tissues of the body. Tertiary syphilis manifests itself as either (1) the development of granulomatous lesions or gumma of the skin, bone, liver, testes, and other tissues, (2) degenerative CNS disease or neurosyphilis, (3) cardiovascular lesions and heart failure (see Table 25-2), or (4) a combination of these manifestations. Gumma formation appears to be the result of a cell-mediated hypersensitive response to treponemal antigens involving chronic inflammation, since these lesions contain very few spirochetes compared to the skin lesions characteristic of primary and secondary disease. Tertiary syphilis displays an extremely high incidence of mortality mainly resulting from the vast complications associated with CNS invasion, which markedly alters the success of antibiotic therapy. Even with intensive antibiotic regimens, individuals afflicted with tertiary syphilis suffer increased morbidity.

TABLE 25-3 ▶

Clinical Manifestations of Secondary Syphilis

Manifestation	Frequency
Skin	90%
Rash	
Macular	
Maculopapular	
Papular	
Pustular	
Condyloma latum	
Generalized lymphadenopathy	
Pruritus	
Constitutional symptoms	70%
Fever of unknown origin	
Malaise	
Pharyngitis	
Anorexia	
Arthralgias	
CNS involvement	40%
Asymptomatic	
Symptomatic	
Headache	
Meningitis	
Ocular disease	
Diplopia	
Decreased vision	
Otitis	
Tinnitis	
Vertigo	
II–VIII cranial nerve damage	
Mouth and throat	35%
Mucous patches	
Erosions	
Ulcers	
Kidney	Rare
Glomerulonephritis	
Nephrotic syndrome	
Gastrointestinal tract	Rare
Hepatitis	
Intestinal wall invasion	
Joints and bone	Rare
Arthritis, osteitis, and periostitis	

Diagnosis

Physical examination can aid in the diagnosis of syphilis. A syphilitic chancre appears on the genitals of patients with primary syphilis; however, in many women this painless lesion may not be noticed. Because many patients with secondary syphilis are asymptomatic and patients with latent syphilis display no clinical manifestations of disease, this method is not definitive for the diagnosis of syphilis.

Standard in vitro culturing techniques are ineffective for growth of this microorganism, precluding its use to amplify and purify *T. pallidum*. Silver staining or darkfield examination of material from either the ulcerated chancre in patients with primary syphilis or skin lesions in patients with secondary syphilis is an effective measure in the diagnosis of *T. pallidum*. However, this approach is ineffective for examining oral lesions in patients with secondary syphilis because of the presence of commensal spirochetes in the mouth.

The most reliable tests for the differential diagnosis of *T. pallidum* include serologic tests for the presence of nontreponemal antibodies or for the presence of treponemal-specific antibodies. *T. pallidum* infection stimulates the synthesis of a distinct non-

Nontreponemal antibodies against cardiolipin are used in the RPR and VDRL tests. These serologic assays have the advantage of being inexpensive and the disadvantage of being only 76% positive in syphilis patients. The FTA test uses a fluorescently labeled antibody to T. pallidum and has the advantage of being very sensitive, but it is expensive.

treponemal antibody that is referred to as *reagin* (why syphilis induces this antibody is not known). This antibody is directed at a cellular lipid antigen (cardiolipin) associated with mitochondria. The Venereal Disease Research Laboratory (VDRL) and rapid plasma reagin (RPR) tests assay for the presence of nontreponemal antibodies, which are present in about 76% of patients with primary syphilis and in almost all patients with secondary syphilis (see Table 25-2). However, the sensitivity of these nontreponemal assays in identifying patients with latent syphilis reduces dramatically as the period of latency increases. This loss in sensitivity is probably due to the fact that active replication of the microorganism leads to synthesis of the nontreponemal antibodies. Since active replication of *T. pallidum* does not occur during latency, the host response dissipates over time. The most accurate serologic tests for syphilis use immunofluorescent procedures to test for the presence of treponemal-specific antibodies in the host. The fluorescent treponemal antibody (FTA) test can be used as a reliable diagnostic tool throughout all of the sequential stages characteristic of the progression of syphilis (see Table 25-2). A combination of nontreponemal (VDRL or RPR) and treponemal-specific (FTA) tests are routinely employed for *T. pallidum* differential diagnosis.

Prevention and Treatment

As with any sexually transmitted disease, increased awareness and prevention through the use of condoms during sexual intercourse can limit the spread of syphilis. This is especially important because of asymptomatic shedding of the pathogen during the primary stage of the disease. Follow-up of sexual contacts of an infected individual represents an important method of controlling further spread of the microorganism.

Although the lesions associated with primary and secondary syphilis are usually self-resolving, antibiotic treatment is necessary for blocking progression to the tertiary stage of the disease. Penicillin is an extremely effective antibiotic for treating individuals with primary, secondary, and early latent syphilis. For patients allergic to penicillin, tetracycline or doxycycline can be employed. Penicillin can also be used to treat patients with tertiary disease; however, these individuals frequently suffer irreversible damage to the brain, heart, or liver before antibiotic clearance of the pathogen occurs. In addition, reactivated *T. pallidum* located in some privileged sites, such as the CNS, remains difficult to treat even with high doses of penicillin administered intravenously. Until the onset of AIDS, the number of individuals with syphilis had decreased. The increased incidence of syphilis in AIDS patients has complicated the treatment of this group of infected individuals, as the combination of drugs they are taking to combat HIV infection are not always well tolerated and sometimes leave the individual feeling worse than if they were not on any medication.

ILLUSTRATIVE PATHOGEN: *Mycobacterium leprae*

M. leprae is the causative agent of leprosy. This is a multifaceted disease originally described by G. A. Hansen in 1873, although lepers have been documented throughout human history. These individuals were shunned and isolated by society, even though in reality patients afflicted with *M. leprae* are poorly infectious, that is, not readily capable of spreading the disease. The incidence of leprosy is extremely low in the United States; however, the disease is of substantial significance in the Third World, where it displays high morbidity and mortality. It is estimated that 12–15 million people are afflicted with leprosy worldwide.

Biologic Characteristics

M. leprae, like *M. tuberculosis*, is a member of the *Mycobacterium* genus (see Chapter 22), which includes bacteria that are neither true gram-negative nor gram-positive organisms. However, the single membrane of these bacteria makes them more similar to gram-positive bacteria. All *Mycobacterium* species possess a high lipid content that is localized at the cell surface in the form of "waxes" that enable these microorganisms to resist germicides and drying, but this distinct feature does not confer resistance to heat. The waxy nature of their cell walls prohibits the microorganism from taking up most stains and dyes, making identification by simple Gram-staining procedures difficult. The predominant component of the waxy layer is mycolic acid, a β-hydroxy fatty acid linked covalently to the cell wall. Because of this unique cell coat, special staining procedures employing heat, detergent, and acid treatment are required. The Ziehl-Neelsen acid-fast staining technique allows for a strong dye to be retained after these microorganisms are decolorized with acid.

M. leprae is a strict aerobe that grows slowly, possessing a doubling time of more than 24 hours. M. leprae grows best at low temperatures, which may explain some of the microorganism's growth characteristics in the human host, where, as an obligate intracellular pathogen, it preferentially grows in the skin and the extremities.

Reservoir and Transmission

Humans represent the sole reservoir for M. leprae. The exact route of transmission of M. leprae remains to be determined, yet this bacterium seems to require close contact and unusually high inoculums to achieve colonization. It is thought that M. leprae can be spread by aerosol, similar to M. tuberculosis, since lepromatous patients can shed the bacilli from their nasal septa. AIDS patients display an increased susceptibility to infection with M. leprae; these individuals also show an increased incidence of reactivation.

Virulence Factors

M. leprae is able to avoid immune surveillance by persisting in macrophages; this ability to establish persistence is probably aided by the bacterium's slow-growth characteristics. In addition, the microorganism possesses phenolic glycolipid in the "waxy" cell wall that aids blocking of oxidative killing of infected cells by macrophages. M. leprae can also activate T-suppressor cells, thereby altering the T-cell response, which ultimately determines how the disease manifests itself in the host. Alternatively, M. leprae inactivates the C5a chemotoxin component of the complement cascade. As during infection with M. tuberculosis, two clear clinical spectra exist for leprosy, and individuals may demonstrate varying degrees of both.

Pathogenesis

Following entry, M. leprae disseminates in the blood, invades endothelial cells of blood vessels and mononuclear cells, and persists in macrophages to evade host defenses. The pathogen then spreads to the skin, nasal septa, Schwann cells, and other tissues throughout the body.

Lepromatous Leprosy. Lepromatous leprosy is similar to primary tuberculosis in that both disorders are manifested by the lack of cell-mediated immunity (afflicted individuals lack delayed type hypersensitivity [DTH] responses to mycobacterial antigens). Also like primary tuberculosis, many microorganisms are present within the infected tissues during lepromatous leprosy. The lepromatous form is characterized clinically by the loss of eyebrows, with thickening and enlargement of nares, ears, and cheeks. Nerve involvement results in a loss of sensation which eventually leads to the development of lesions of the face and extremities, where the lower temperatures allow for more vigorous replication of the pathogen. These inadvertent lesions can lead to secondary infections that result in bone resorption, mutilating lesions, and even disfigurement.

Tuberculoid Leprosy. Tuberculoid leprosy resembles secondary tuberculosis in that cell-mediated immunity to disease is effective with the activation of macrophages and the presence of a Mycobacterium-specific DTH response. In addition, the macular skin lesions present on the face and extremities associated with tuberculoid leprosy display very few bacilli in the lesions, similar to that seen with secondary tuberculosis. Peripheral nerve cell damage occurs as a result of a T-cell response to the pathogen, which can be extremely severe.

Diagnosis

Diagnosis of leprosy caused by *M. leprae* is largely based on physical examination and patient history. Since the organism cannot be cultured, isolation and purification by standard in vitro techniques used for other *Mycobacterium* species such as *M. tuberculosis* are not effective. Although Gram stain cannot be employed, material from lesions can be examined using the Ziehl-Neelsen acid-fast staining method. Sensitive polymerase chain reaction (PCR) and antigen detection kits are in development for the accurate identification of this pathogen.

Prevention and Treatment

Identification and early treatment is the key for controlling the spread of *M. leprae*. Multidrug therapies employing dapsone, a specialized sulfone, and rifampin, which is effective against intracellular pathogens, are given for many months because sulfone resistance represents a significant problem in the treatment of *M. leprae*. Clofazimine can be used in the treatment of sulfone-resistant leprosy. As with *M. tuberculosis*, multidrug approaches are designed to avoid the selection of antibiotic-resistant mutants. Patients with tuberculoid disease are easier to treat than those with the lepromatous form; however, even with treatment many residual side effects including permanent nerve damage are prevalent. The bacille Calmette-Guérin (BCG) vaccine has met with limited success in treating leprosy patients.

RESOLUTION OF CLINICAL CASE

The patient's blood was drawn for a RPR test, which turned up positive at a titer of 1:64, and a FTA test, which was also positive. A serologic test for antibodies to HIV was negative. The diagnosis of secondary syphilis based on the physical examination and patient history was confirmed by the nontreponemal RPR and treponemal-specific FTA tests. The patient was treated with a single dose of benzathine penicillin G and was instructed to take probenicid, which retards penicillin excretion, orally for 14 days. The rash on the patient's palms and soles disappeared over the next week.

REVIEW QUESTIONS

Directions: For each of the following questions, choose the **one best** answer.

1. Which of the following statements about persistent infection is true?
    (A) Persistently infected individuals serve as a reservoir for the infectious agent
    (B) Persistent infection results in death of the host
    (C) Persistence cannot occur in the presence of a host immune response
    (D) Reactivation cannot occur in immune suppressed hosts
    (E) Drug or vaccine therapies are always able to treat persistent pathogens

2. The best treatment for a patient with primary syphilis is
    (A) no treatment, as the chancre will heal spontaneously
    (B) oral dosing with acyclovir
    (C) intramuscular injection of penicillin G
    (D) oral dosing with tetracycline
    (E) oral dosing with lincomycin

3. Which of the following statements concerning tertiary syphilis is true?
    (A) It can be readily cured with simple antibiotic therapy
    (B) It can be definitively diagnosed with the RPR or VDRL tests
    (C) It is usually asymptomatic or less severe than secondary syphilis
    (D) It is characterized by multiorgan disease
    (E) It does not require antibiotic therapy because it is self-resolving

4. Secondary syphilis can be definitively diagnosed by
    (A) culturing of *Treponemal pallidum* on blood agar plates
    (B) culturing of *T. pallidum* in human macrophages
    (C) Gram-staining material from palm lesions
    (D) darkfield examination of material from oral lesions
    (E) VDRL, RPR, and FTA assays

5. *Mycobacterium leprae* persists in the human host by
    (A) infecting hepatocytes of the liver
    (B) infecting mononuclear cells
    (C) infecting and establishing latency in neurons
    (D) inactivating the C3b component of the complement cascade
    (E) molecular mimicry of host proteins

Note. Abbreviations used in the questions: RPR = rapid plasma reagin; VDRL = Venereal Disease Research Laboratory; FTA = fluorescent treponemal antibody.

ANSWERS AND EXPLANATIONS

1. **The answer is A.** Persistence of the pathogen enables a reservoir for spread of the microorganism. Option B is incorrect because most persistent pathogens do little or no damage to the host during their persistence; however, they may cause severe disease and death following reactivation. Option C is incorrect because microorganisms have developed methods to persist by evading host immune surveillance, thereby avoiding clearance. Option D is incorrect because immune suppression such as that seen with human immunodeficiency virus (HIV) or *M. tuberculosis* frequently results in reactivation of the pathogen and disease progression. Although antibiotic or drug therapies can be effective treatments for some persistent pathogens such as *Mycobacterium leprae* or *Treponema pallidum*, they can only control the spread and severity of others such as HIV and herpes.

2. **The answer is C.** Penicillin G is the antibiotic of choice for treating syphilis. Option A is incorrect because even though the primary syphilitic chancre heals spontaneously, without antibiotic treatment the patient is 70% likely to progress through the secondary and tertiary stages of syphilis resulting from persistence of the microorganism. Option B is incorrect because the antiviral drug acyclovir is a DNA polymerase inhibitor that is effective against herpes simplex virus. Option D is incorrect because even though a broad-spectrum antibiotic like tetracycline can be employed against *Treponema pallidum*, the microorganism is far more sensitive to penicillin, making it the drug of choice in treating syphilis. Option E is incorrect because lincomycin is effective in treating gram-positive bacteria, and *T. pallidum* is gram-negative.

3. **The answer is D.** Tertiary syphilis usually involves multiorgan disease resulting from reactivation, renewed replication, and spread of the microorganism to the heart, brain, liver, skin, testes, and bone. Option A is incorrect because even radical antibiotic therapy is frequently ineffective in treating patients with tertiary syphilis because of the spread of the microorganism and invasion of privileged tissues such as the CNS. Option B is incorrect because the two nontreponemal antibody tests (VDRL and RPR) are not as sensitive with tertiary patients as they are in detecting individuals with primary or secondary syphilis, and they frequently give negative results. Option C is incorrect because disease associated with tertiary syphilis is extremely severe, involving multiple organs and resulting in the death of the patient. Option E is incorrect because untreated patients rarely fail to develop clinically apparent tertiary syphilis, and antibiotic regimens may not be successful in treating tertiary disease.

4. **The answer is E.** The VDRL and RPR assays are nontreponemal tests that detect host cell antibodies found in 99% of all patients with secondary syphilis. The FTA test detects the presence of treponemal-specific antibodies present in 100% of all individuals with secondary syphilis and is the best confirmatory test. Options A and B are incorrect because it has been impossible to culture *T. pallidum*. Option C is incorrect because even though palm lesions in secondary syphilis contain many spirochetes, *T. pallidum* stains poorly or not at all in Gram stain. Option D is incorrect because even though darkfield examination can readily detect *T. pallidum*, many commensal spirochetes exist within the oral mucosa and complicate the differential diagnosis of *T. pallidum*.

5. **The answer is B.** *M. leprae* evades the host defense system by infecting and persisting in host mononuclear cells in a manner similar to *M. tuberculosis*. Option A is incorrect because liver hepatocytes are not a target for *M. leprae* but are for *Plasmodium vivax*. Option C is incorrect because even though reactivated *M. leprae* causes severe nervous system damage, it does not initially infect neurons or persist in nervous system tissue like herpes simplex virus. Option D is incorrect because *M. leprae* affects the C5a component of the host's complement cascade, whereas herpes simplex virus alters the C3b component. Option E is incorrect because *M. leprae* does not employ molecular mimicry as *Treponema pallidum* does to evade host immune surveillance.

26 ROLE OF BACTERIA AND VIRUSES IN TUMORIGENESIS

CHAPTER OUTLINE

Introduction of Clinical Case
Tumorigenesis
• Mechanisms of Tumor Formation
• Bacteria in Human Tumorigenesis
• Viruses in Human Tumorigenesis
Illustrative Pathogen: Human papillomavirus
• Biologic Characteristics
• Reservoir and Transmission
• Virulence Factors
• Pathogenesis
• Diagnosis
• Prevention and Treatment
Resolution of Clinical Case
Review Questions

INTRODUCTION OF CLINICAL CASE

A 26-year-old woman visited her gynecologist for the first time in several years. She gave a history of dyspareunia (pain during sexual intercourse) over the past 6 months. She related that she was sexually active, using oral contraceptive pills as her primary method of contraception. She did not use barrier methods. She admitted to having a dozen sexual partners since her past gynecologic checkup. Up to this point, her examinations had been entirely unremarkable.

On physical examination, the physician noted several small papular lesions on her labia minor, which whitened with the application of 5% acetic acid. They were painful to the touch. As part of her routine care, the physician did a Papanicolaou (Pap) smear, took cultures for gonorrhea and *Chlamydia*, and counseled her to have a human immunodeficiency virus (HIV) test taken, which she consented to do.

> Although acetowhite staining is not specific for HPV infection, clinically normal tissue infected with HPVs often turn white after brief exposure to 5% acetic acid (vinegar).

A week later, her test results were returned. Scanning them, her physician saw that her gonorrhea and *Chlamydia* cultures were negative. However, her Pap smear result was read as low-grade squamous intraepithelial lesion (LSIL). The physician paused to consider what to tell the patient about her result.

- What is the likely cause of her genital lesions and her abnormal Pap smear?
- What is the prognostic significance of LSIL? What are the other elements of this Pap smear grading scale?
- What treatments are possible for the genital lesions? What efficacy do these treatments carry?

TUMORIGENESIS

The term neoplasm refers to a group of cells that have lost the normal controls of growth and proliferation. All cellular growth is finely tuned by a complex interplay of signals that regulate the ability of the cell to undergo the appropriate number of divisions and differentiation necessary for function. When appropriate, these same processes may also cause apoptosis, or programmed cell death. Some cell types reach a mature stage and simply maintain themselves for the life of the organism, such as neurons in the central nervous system. Other tissues, such as intestinal epithelia, constantly divide and slough off cells as they renew the absorptive and protective lining of the gut. When this regulated growth is disrupted within the cell, normal controls are lost (either suddenly or as part of a slow process), and unregulated, unstoppable growth begins. These cells are said to have been *transformed*. Growing masses of transformed cells are commonly referred to as neoplasia, or more generically as tumors. Terms commonly used in tumor biology are defined in Table 26-1.

TABLE 26-1 ▶
Terms and Definitions Used to Describe Tumors and Tumor Biology

Term	Definition
Tumorigenic	Giving rise to the formation of a tumor, either benign or malignant. The term is synonymous with oncogenic.
Benign tumor	A loss of growth controls of normal cells, giving rise to a tumor. Such tumors do not undergo metastasis (see next definition). While potentially dangerous by mechanically interfering with adjoining organs, frank invasion of adjacent tissue does not occur.
Malignant tumor	A tumor capable of sloughing cells from its primary growth site and promoting the spread to other sites (metastasis). Malignant tumors can invade and destroy neighboring tissues.
Neoplasm	New and abnormal growth. The term is used to describe any kind of tumor.
Oncogene	A gene whose product, an oncoprotein, transforms a normal cell. For oncogenic DNA viruses, the viral oncogene is a gene essential for virus replication. Among the avian oncogenic retroviruses (oncoviruses), the viral oncogene is a mutated cellular proto-oncogene that has been incorporated into the viral genome by recombination.
Proto-oncogene	A normal cell gene that, if *improperly* expressed or regulated (usually) because of a mutation, becomes a functioning oncogene. The regulated expression of unaltered proto-oncogenes facilitates important cellular reactions and does not cause cell transformation.
Tumor suppressor gene	A cellular gene whose protein product can suppress the action of one or more oncogenes.

All tumors—from solid masses such as osteosarcoma to dermoid ovarian tumors to hematogenously spread leukemia—are characterized by disordered growth, though each type of neoplasm has different characteristics with respect to growth rate, alteration of cellular markers, and elaboration of new products. There are many ways to classify tumors, but the primary division among neoplasia and tumors is *benign* versus *malignant*. Benign tumors generally grow slowly, without a significant alteration in normal surface markers, and tend to acquire a capsule of fibrous tissue as they homogeneously enlarge in a direct radial growth pattern. Malignant tumors, commonly called cancers, tend to have higher rates of growth, undergo a more severe loss of normal markers, and have heterogeneous growth patterns. They are rarely encapsulated, and their ability to spread to distant sites (metastasize) contributes to their often poor prognosis. Malignant tumors may also elaborate products not normally seen in that tissue, such as calcitonin elaborated by bronchogenic carcinoma. Though the dividing line between benign and malignant is frequently clear, certain tumors have characteristics that fall between the two definitions (e.g., borderline ovarian tumors, which have the slow-growth characteristics of benign tumors but may metastasize over time, as a malignant tumor does). Neoplasia occurs in every tissue in the body, with a predilection for those sites where frequent turnover of tissue may predispose those cells to neoplastic transformation. Bacteria and viruses identified with the formation of malignant tumors are presented in Table 26-2.

◀ **TABLE 26-2**
Bacteria and Viruses Associated with Tumorigenesis

Organism	Type of Cancer
Bacteria	
Helicobacter pylori	Adenocarcinoma and lymphoma of the stomach
Bartonella quintana	Microscopic bacillary angiomatosis lesions characterized by tumor-like capillary lobules
Viruses	
Hepatitis B virus	Hepatocellular carcinoma
Hepatitis C virus	Hepatocellular carcinoma
HTLV-1 virus	Leukemia
Epstein-Barr virus	Lymphoma
Human herpesvirus type 8	Kaposi's sarcoma
Human papillomavirus types 16 and 18	Cervical cancer

Note. HTLV-1 = human T-cell leukemia virus type 1.

Mechanisms of Tumor Formation

The formation of tumors relies on the loss of normal control of cell growth. Though a few tumors are known to result from single events that cause this loss of control, most occur after a multistep process that favors neoplastic transformation. Virtually all the steps in tumor formation involve regulation of cellular DNA transcription. These events can involve point mutations—activating a proto-oncogene—or larger events, such as the t9;22 chromosomal translocation known as the Philadelphia chromosome (implicated in chronic myelogenous leukemia). Generally, tumors arise from a combination of many cellular events in a lengthy temporal sequence, as has been well documented for colon cancers.

Currently, tumors are thought to occur by two general mechanisms: direct and indirect. Indirect tumorigenesis involves the intracellular process described above. However, direct methods, mediated by outside sources, may occur. The rare but recognized tumorigenic potential of microbes is classified under direct tumorigenic mechanisms. The manner in which a microbial agent can directly cause cell transformation is envisioned to occur in one of four ways (Figure 26-1):

1. By *direct expression* of the product of an oncogene (i.e., oncoprotein) carried by a microbe. Either the oncogene is a gene carrying out an essential microbial function (e.g., papillomavirus replication proteins) or it may be a transduced and altered proto-oncogene (e.g., avian oncoviruses).

2. By mutating a crucial cellular gene. For example, the insertion of a viral DNA sequence into a tumor suppressor gene inactivates it. This is an example of *insertional inactivation* of a functional gene sequence.

3. By activating the overexpression of a proto-oncogene. For example, if a retroviral genome's long terminal repeats (LTRs) contain promoter sequences which, upon

insertion immediately upstream of a (normally unexpressed) proto-oncogene, unregulate expression of that proto-oncogene, it may effectively turn its product into an oncoprotein. This phenomenon is called *cis*-activation.

4. By producing a product, presumably a protein, that can activate the promoter or by enhancing sequences of a cellular gene, thereby upregulating its expression. This *trans*-activation may result in the same outcome as described in *cis*-activation.

Certain microbial agents are associated with the induction of cancer without possessing oncogenes or the ability to activate or inactivate cellular genes directly. The correlation between these agents and cancer presumably involves the ability of these agents to trigger events indirectly that result in the transformation of normal cells. Such events may include chronic inflammation and damage to a tissue, which may cause increased cellular proliferation or even dysplasia of the normal tissue. This increased rate of mitotic activity, along with altered growth in dysplastic tissues and possible free radicals produced by accompanying inflammatory cells, may increase the probability of mutations occurring, which activate oncogenes and produce neoplasia.

FIGURE 26-1 ▶

Mechanisms of Viral Oncogenesis. *Four direct means by which a viral genome or a product of a viral genome can transform a normal cell into a cancer cell.*

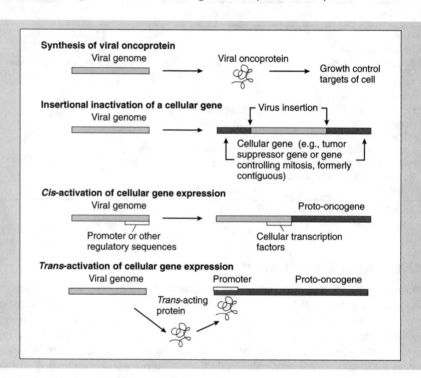

Bacteria in Human Tumorigenesis

Helicobacter pylori is a prime example of an infectious agent that can predispose the host toward neoplasia (see Table 26-2). While several explanations of the pathogenesis of gastric and duodenal ulcers were hypothesized before the 1980s, that decade saw the strong identification of *H. pylori* as the causative agent of stomach ulcers (see Chapter 14). Effective antibiotic treatment of infection was conclusively shown to cure many patients of their ulcers. In the following years, a convincing role has been found for *H. pylori* in several different gastrointestinal diseases, including gastric and duodenal ulcers, hypertrophic gastropathy, and nonulcer dyspepsia.

In 1994, the World Health Organization identified *H. pylori* as a definitive or class I carcinogen, based on the large body of collected clinical evidence linking the progression of ulcer disease to chronic gastritis to adenocarcinoma and lymphoma of the stomach. Since most gastric ulcers are thought to be caused by *H. pylori*, the importance of this bacterium in stomach cancer is clear. The association of *H. pylori* infection with a three- to eightfold higher risk of gastric carcinoma also buttressed this conclusion. Though other factors certainly contribute to the progression of stomach cancer, the role of *H. pylori* seems firm.

Helicobacter pylori is a slender, spirally curved, gram-negative rod that is motile and microaerophilic. This organism has been linked to ulcers and stomach cancers.

The mechanism by which *H. pylori* induces tumorigenesis is believed to involve chronic inflammation. This inflammation results in three tumorigenic events: recruitment of inflammatory cells and their toxic free radicals to the site; increased cellular proliferation in response to the chronic inflammation; and changes in the local environment that may potentiate the ability of certain carcinogens, such as *N*-nitroso compounds, to cause mutations. The end result of these inflammatory processes is a predisposition to cancer. Strikingly, one particular type of cancer, the mucosa-associated lymphoid tissue tumor (MALToma), can actually regress with effective antibiotic treatment—a convincing argument for the role of *H. pylori* in the production of gastric carcinoma.

Viruses in Human Tumorigenesis

Several different families of viruses have been linked to the development of neoplasia in humans: Adenoviridae, Herpesviridae, Papovaviridae, Retroviridae, and others (see Table 26-2). These viral agents may cause persistent infections and may progress to malignancy. Some of them are indirectly tumorigenic because they induce an inflammatory reaction (e.g., hepatitis B and C viruses), and others are directly tumorigenic through the activation of oncogenes (e.g., human papillomavirus [HPV], human T-cell leukemia virus type 1 [HTLV-1]). Certain viruses are tumorigenic only in the background of host immune suppression, while others cause tumors in immunocompetent individuals.

Like *H. pylori*, hepatitis B and C viruses (HBV and HCV) are considered carcinogens by virtue of the increased risk of hepatocellular carcinoma among persistently infected patients with chronic active hepatitis. While genes in HBV and HCV express a protein that *trans*-activates other viral (and potentially other cellular) genes, there is no solid evidence that either virus directly transforms cells. The current thinking is that HBV and HCV cause an immune-mediated, chronic inflammation in the liver, with the resulting cell damage eventually giving rise to transformation and hepatocellular carcinoma. Whereas successful antibiotic treatment of *H. pylori* decreases the risk of gastric adenocarcinoma and may actually regress MALTomas and other lymphoid cancers, HBV and HCV infection cannot be treated as effectively. However, effective vaccination for the prevention of HBV infection is feasible (see Chapter 29) and represents a significant public health effort toward protection from this virus. Though no effective HCV vaccine exists, education of at-risk populations about the risks of acquiring HCV and strategies to avoid infection may help reduce the incidence of this virus as well.

HTLV-1, a human retrovirus, and Epstein-Barr virus (EBV), a human herpesvirus, are two additional examples of viruses closely associated with human cancers. Both viruses illustrate the typical association of viral infection with neoplasia; that is, neoplasia occurs in some but not all people infected with these viruses. HTLV-1 is clearly associated with a form of adult T-cell leukemia, but it is not the sole cause, nor does it progress to malignancy in every person infected. Likewise, EBV has been strongly linked to the development of several hematologic malignancies, including Burkitt's lymphoma (a B-cell tumor), Hodgkin's disease, and anaplastic nasopharyngeal carcinoma. DNA and oncogenes of EBV can be identified in the tumor cells of these patients. Again, though EBV is prominent in these tumors, infection with EBV does not commonly progress to neoplasia. Many have theorized that certain cofactors, infectious or genetic, may predispose certain individuals to cancer.

A growing area of study in the tumorigenic potential of viruses is their effect on the immune-suppressed patient. EBV can cause tumors in immunocompromised hosts. These tumors are invariably associated with EBV DNA sequences, and these viral sequences are most likely the driving tumorigenic force in these cells. Disturbingly, these tumors tend to be refractory to current chemotherapy and treatment. Another example of this phenomenon comes from HIV, where it has recently been found that gene sequences from human herpesvirus type 8 (HHV-8) can be identified by polymerase chain reaction (PCR) from Kaposi's sarcoma lesions, as well as body cavity lymphomas found in acquired immunodeficiency syndrome (AIDS). In this situation, HHV-8 is most likely not directly tumorigenic, as it lacks transforming potential in laboratory studies; rather, it may be another example of a relatively nonpathogenic virus that, in the immunosuppressed patient, becomes a cofactor in cellular transformation.

ILLUSTRATIVE PATHOGEN: Human papillomavirus

One of the best examples of an infectious agent that potentiates the development of cancer is HPV. These viruses produce a variety of lesions and have been implicated in the development of a common gynecologic neoplasm.

Biologic Characteristics

Papillomaviruses, a subfamily of the Papovaviridae family (papovaviruses) of DNA viruses, contain more than 70 distinct viral types that infect humans. All papovaviruses possess unique plasmid-like dsDNA genomes, which are enclosed in a nonenveloped icosahedral protein capsid. The HPV genome contains eight open reading frames in the early (E) region and two in the late (L) region, coding for proteins that govern replication (E1), transformation (E6 and E7), and capsid proteins (L1 and L2). E6 and E7, which are expressed early in viral replication, are examples of viral oncogenes that interact with host sequences to produce alteration of growth.

> *The HPV family is divided into genotypes (types). All members of this virus family have a similarly organized viral genome; however, the sequences that make up this genome may be quite different.*

The more than 70 types of HPV may be generally divided in several ways. One convenient way to categorize them is into the *cutaneous* types (generally not oncogenic) and the *mucosal* types (may be oncogenic). Among the cutaneous HPV isolates, types 1, 2, and 4 cause most common warts and plantar warts, while HPV types 3, 10, 28, and 41 can cause flat warts. Some mucosal HPV types may cause nononcogenic lesions in sites other than the genitalia; types 6 and 11 can be found on the genitalia, the conjunctiva, and even the respiratory tract. However, they have no strong association with cancer. Conversely, types 16 and 18 have been found to have a strong association with not only cervical cancer but vulvar cancer as well.

> *HPV types 16 and 18 are strongly associated with cervical and vulvar cancer. For example, HPV genomic DNA sequences are found in approximately 80% of cervical carcinomas in the United States.*

Reservoir and Transmission

HPV infects only human beings, and transmission is through intimate contact. This may be through minor skin abrasions for cutaneous HPV types, through vertical transmission from mother to infant for respiratory papillomas, and finally through sexual contact for mucosal HPV types. Cutaneous lesions exhibit several different clinical presentations, all of which are nontumorigenic and which often regress spontaneously. Mucosal HPV types also cause a range of clinical disease—from flat or exophytic lesions on the vulva or penis to plaque-like lesions of the cervix. They generally do not regress, however, and often progress to more serious disease. The mucosal strains are highly transmissible, and as such represent a significant sexually transmitted disease in the United States and throughout the world (see Chapter 9). The only effective prevention of transmission occurs with barrier methods of protection, which deny the virus access to host skin or mucosa.

Virulence Factors

HPV has evolved a mechanism similar to that in the herpesviruses: its genome may remain latent within infected cells for long periods of time. Thus, even in the absence of clinically apparent disease, the viral genomes may persist in epithelial cells. In carcinoma secondary to HPV infection, all or part of the viral genome has usually been integrated into the host DNA. Within these transformed cells, active transcription of the E6 and E7 oncogenes is found. These oncoproteins have been demonstrated to sequester, respectively, the tumor suppressor proteins p53 and Rb. Inactivation of these proteins further predisposes cells to genetic instability and mutation, which leads to unregulated cellular proliferation and neoplastic transformation. Thus, the E6 and E7 proteins represent definitive virulence factors with respect to HPV tumorigenesis.

> *The retinoblastoma (Rb) and p53 genes are termed* tumor suppressor genes *because they encode proteins that play a role in regulating mitosis; if they are inactivated by oncoproteins, cell transformation is possible.*

Pathogenesis

HPV has a strict tropism for epithelial cells. They infect the cells of the basal epithelium through damaged skin, and as epithelial cells are pushed to the surface through continued proliferation of deeper cell layers, HPV virions are assembled and exit the sloughing apical cell layer of the epithelium (Figure 26-2). In cutaneous infections, the basal keratinocytes typically mature until their death in the stratum corneum, the topmost layer of cells in skin. In these infections, there is hypertrophy of all layers except the basal layer, with HPV found as episomal elements distinct from cellular DNA. The epithelial cells often demonstrate a small shrunken nucleus inside a vacuolized cell (koilocytosis). The hypertrophy of cell layers and the specific type of virus often determine the clinical nature of the lesion in the skin.

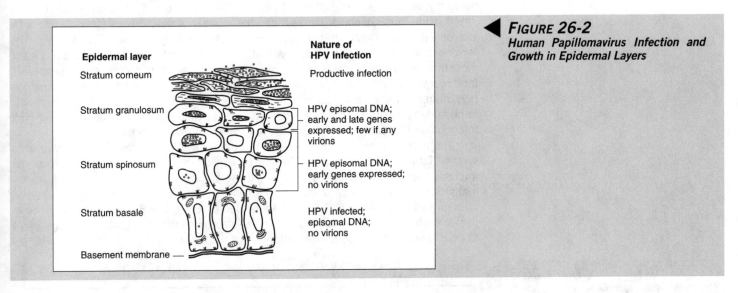

FIGURE 26-2
Human Papillomavirus Infection and Growth in Epidermal Layers

The process of infection and cellular proliferation in mucosal infection often produces lesions similar in appearance to those of cutaneous types, with exophytic lesions being common. Oncogenic HPV types can integrate their genomes into chromosomal DNA. These lesions, when they progress to more serious disease, show increasing degrees of cellular dysplasia, with the basal layer being affected first. As the disease progresses an increasing amount of the total epithelium is occupied by dysplastic cells. This progression from normal epithelium to increasing amounts of dysplasia to carcinoma in situ to invasive cancer is the basis for the screening tests that are used for early detection and treatment of cervical lesions. However, it is important to note that until invasive cervical cancer is present, the progression is not entirely predictable. Many lesions remain at one stage, some progress, and some even regress. The chances of progression increase with the level of dysplasia, and once invasive cervical cancer is established, it never regresses.

The pathogenesis of HPV infection is influenced by the type of virus. It is also influenced by host factors, such as immune competency. Evidence from immunosuppressed patients shows that HPV tends to be more aggressive and progresses more quickly and uniformly to cancer. Indeed, invasive cervical cancer has become one of the defining diagnoses for clinical AIDS, demonstrating an important role for the immune system in the control of infection.

Diagnosis

HPV infection is identified by clinical examination with or without histologic examination of material obtained at biopsy. The typical presentation of warts, whether they be flat, plantar, or larger exophytic lesions, is a common identifier for HPV. It is important to realize, however, that HPV infection may be subclinical or may result in other forms of cellular dysplasia. While surveillance for cutaneous forms is important, the identification and diagnosis of mucosal lesions is vital in at-risk populations. Examination of the genital areas for manifestations of HPV infection is an important screening tool. The typical appearance of external genital warts (condyloma acuminatum) is of flesh-colored to gray, hyperkeratotic, exophytic papules on the skin, either sessile (flat) or attached to a broad peduncle (base). They may range in size from a millimeter to several centimeters. They may involve the anus, the exterior genitalia in men and women, and the vaginal or cervical mucosa in women. In women, exterior lesions are an important clue to the possibility of internal genital lesions. Though most external warts are painless, itching and burning may be experienced. In women, external or internal infection is often accompanied by dyspareunia.

One of the most important aids to diagnosis of female genital lesions of HPV is the Pap smear. This simple test involves the scraping of cervical and endocervical cells and the examination of these cells' morphologic features by a qualified pathologist. Since its introduction, the Pap smear has reduced the number of deaths from cervical cancer by almost 70%. It is estimated that if all women regularly received Pap smears, the incidence of cervical cancer could virtually be eliminated. The Pap smear can detect more than 90% of early cervical neoplasia, and combined with colposcopy (a procedure for direct visualization of the cervix with chemical treatment applied to enable visualization of areas of abnormal epithelium), it is a powerful screening tool. It is particularly important for sexually active women, who are at the highest risk for acquiring HPV infection and its subsequent sequelae, to get regular Pap smears.

The most common system for the reporting of Pap smear results is the Bethesda system (Table 26-3). This system classifies the result in six general categories. The most important for HPV infection is group 4, those smears showing squamous cell abnormalities. Older systems often classified smears by level of dysplasia or by the cervical intraepithelial neoplasia (CIN) 1-2-3 scale (Table 26-4). The Bethesda system encompasses both scales and allows the physician to correlate the result with the likely degree of dysplasia present and its likely outcome for the patient.

TABLE 26-3 ▶

Bethesda System for Papanicolaou Smear Grading

Category	Description	CIN Equivalent	Dysplasia Equivalent
Group 1	Findings within normal limits	None	None
Group 2	Infections	None	None
Group 3	Reactive or reparative atypia	None	None
Group 4	Squamous cell abnormalities		
	Squamous atypia	None	None
	Low-grade SIL	HPV or CIN 1	Mild
	High-grade SIL	CIN 2 or 3	Moderate or severe
	Squamous cell carcinoma	Not applicable	Not applicable
Group 5	Glandular cell abnormalities	Not applicable	Not applicable
	Atypia of undetermined significance		
	Adenocarcinoma		
Group 6	Nonepithelial malignancy	Not applicable	Not applicable

Note. CIN = cervical intraepithelial neoplasia; SIL = squamous intraepithelial lesions.

TABLE 26-4 ▶

Natural History of Cervical Intraepithelial Neoplasia (CIN)

	Regression[a]	Persistence[b]	Progress to CIS[c]	Progress to Invasion[d]
CIN 1	57%	32%	11%	1%
CIN 2	43%	35%	22%	5%
CIN 3	32%	<56%		>12%

[a] Regression refers to the dysplasia pathologic state decreasing or disappearing over time.
[b] Persistence refers to the dysplasia pathologic state staying the same over time.
[c] Progress to CIS refers to the dysplasia progressing to carcinoma in situ.
[d] Progress to invasion refers to the dysplasia progressing to cervical or metastatic cancer.

Prevention and Treatment

Only limited antiviral therapy is available for HPV infection. Cutaneous warts, though unsightly, are relatively harmless and regress of their own accord. The treatments available for cutaneous warts—over-the-counter remedies, cryotherapy, and laser surgery—

are generally not warranted unless significant disability and pain are present. None of them destroy HPV specifically; they simply destroy the tissue in which the virus resides.

The treatment of mucosal HPV is somewhat more aggressive, given the higher potential for tumorigenesis. Podophyllin or trichloroacetic acid applied topically may be somewhat effective but can be painful. Electrosurgery and cryotherapy are also used. Injection of interferon-α into the lesion is now available but is also quite painful. The primary prevention of mucosal lesions remains barrier methods of contraception and a reduced number of sexual partners.

Cervical lesions suspected on Pap smear should routinely be confirmed with colposcopy. Once a lesion is identified, it may be removed with cryotherapy if small, and excision if large. Cervical punch biopsy for staging and cone excision are available for further treatment. A mainstay of treatment remains frequent follow-up Pap smears, typically every 3 months for 1 year, to check for further atypia.

RESOLUTION OF CLINICAL CASE

The patient's abnormal Pap smear was most likely related to her external genital warts. These lesions were almost certainly due to HPV exposure from one of her sexual partners, and the physician's first recommendation was strict use of barrier contraception. The physician offered to treat her external lesions with a combination of podophyllin and cryotherapy, which though uncomfortable has a good chance of reducing them. For treatment of her LSIL (which could have corresponded to simple HPV infection or CIN 1), the physician counseled her that nearly 60% of these lesions regress, but that as a precaution she should undergo colposcopy for examination of her cervix. The colposcopist would perform a punch biopsy of any suspicious areas, and she could then be monitored with frequent Pap smears as follow-up. If histopathologic examination of the biopsy specimen gave much worse results than her Pap smear, she may need further follow-up. The physician also strongly warned her that there might be other inapparent lesions present and that she needed to be sure to examine her vulva for new lesions and to get regular Pap smears from that time on.

REVIEW QUESTIONS

Directions: For each of the following questions, choose the **one best** answer.

1. Which one of the following statements about human papillomavirus (HPV) is correct?
    (A) HPV cannot be transmitted from one human to another
    (B) HPVs contain single-stranded DNA genomes
    (C) Warts rarely evolve into carcinomas
    (D) HPV infection can be successfully treated with antiviral agents
    (E) HPV types 1, 2, and 4 are highly associated with cervical cancer

2. A man complaining of stomach ulcers was successfully cured by antimicrobial therapy. Which one of the following is *most accurate* about his condition?
    (A) His ulcers are most likely caused by a double-stranded DNA virus and can progress to cancer
    (B) His ulcers are most likely caused by a single-stranded RNA virus, which will resolve in the absence of antimicrobial therapy
    (C) His ulcers can be associated with gram-negative, motile bacteria and can progress to adenocarcinoma and lymphoma of the stomach
    (D) His ulcers can be associated with gram-positive, toxin-producing bacteria and can progress to adenocarcinoma and lymphoma of the stomach
    (E) His ulcers can be associated with gram-positive, motile bacteria and will resolve independent of antimicrobial therapy

3. The phenotype of a neoplastic cell is most accurately described by which of the following statements?
    (A) Neoplastic cells typically divide faster than normal cells
    (B) Neoplastic cells typically exhibit unregulated growth
    (C) Neoplastic cells always arise from cellular hypertrophy
    (D) Neoplastic cells always contain portions of viral DNA
    (E) Neoplastic cells are never associated with bacterial or viral infections

4. A Pap smear performed on a sexually active woman with a history of genital warts was submitted to the pathology laboratory. The laboratory report indicated that she had a low-grade squamous intraepithelial lesion (LSIL). Which of the following statements is most accurate about this woman's condition?
    (A) Her Pap smear result could be associated with an infection by human papillomavirus type 16 or 18
    (B) This woman has incurable cervical cancer
    (C) Her genital warts can be treated with antibiotic therapy, which should also improve her Pap smear result
    (D) LSIL, as shown by Pap smear, generally progresses to cancer
    (E) Her LSIL is probably unrelated to her sexual activity

5. Which of the following viral or bacterial pathogens is associated with tumorigenesis?
    (A) *Neisseria gonorrhoeae*
    (B) *Vibrio cholera*
    (C) Hepatitis B virus
    (D) *Haemophilus influenzae*
    (E) Respiratory syncytial virus

ANSWERS AND EXPLANATIONS

1. **The answer is C.** It is true that warts rarely evolve into carcinomas. Option A is incorrect because HPV is highly transmissible as a sexually transmitted disease and is transmissible from warts as well. Option B is incorrect because the genome is double-stranded. Option D is incorrect because there is no specific antiviral treatment for HPV. Option E is incorrect because HPV types 16 and 18 are highly associated with cervical cancer; types 1, 2, and 4 are generally associated with common and plantar warts.

2. **The answer is C.** *Helicobacter pylori* is a gram-negative, motile bacteria that causes ulcers that can progress to cancer. The resolution of the patient's ulcers following antimicrobial treatment is consistent with *H. pylori* as the etiologic agent. Option A is incorrect because no DNA virus has been linked to ulcers and subsequently to cancer. Option B is incorrect because no RNA virus has been linked to ulcers, and these viruses would not be treatable with antimicrobial therapy. Option D is incorrect because there are no gram-positive, toxin-producing bacteria that are known to cause ulcers and that are associated with cancer. Option E is incorrect because there are no gram-positive bacteria linked to ulcers.

3. **The answer is B.** All neoplastic cell growth results from the loss of normal cellular control. Options A, C, and D are sometimes true of neoplasia, but not always. Option E is incorrect because, as this chapter describes, there are several instances in which bacteria or viruses are associated with neoplasia.

4. **The answer is A.** HPV types 16 and 18 are associated with LSIL. Option B is incorrect because an LSIL result does not mean that the woman had cancer. Option C is incorrect because genital warts are caused by a virus and are not susceptible to antimicrobial therapy. Option D is incorrect because LSIL, as shown by a Pap smear result, progresses to invasive cancer in only 1% of all cases. Option E is incorrect because LSIL is linked to HPV, which is a common sexually transmitted disease.

5. **The answer is C.** Hepatitis B virus is linked to hepatocellular carcinoma (see Table 26-2). Options A, B, D, and E all concern bacterial or viral pathogens that are associated with significant disease, but in each case the diseases that they cause are not linked to cancer.

27 ACQUIRED IMMUNODEFICIENCY SYNDROME

CHAPTER OUTLINE

Introduction of Clinical Case
Acquired Immunodeficiency Syndrome
• Discovery of an Emerging Virus Disease
• Magnitude of the Epidemic
Lentiviruses
• General Characteristics
• Nature of Infection
Illustrative Pathogen: HIV-1
• Biologic Characteristics
• Reservoir and Transmission
• Virulence Factors
• Pathogenesis
• Diagnosis
• Treatment and Prevention
Resolution of Clinical Case
Review Questions

INTRODUCTION OF CLINICAL CASE

A 37-year-old man came to the emergency room complaining of fever and cough. The patient was in good health until two weeks previous, when he began to feel warm at various intervals during the day. One week previous, he developed a frequent (every few minutes), dry cough. On three occasions during that week, he experienced fevers of 99.8°, 102.5°, and 101.4°F. In

> **Crackles** indicate the presence of fluid in the aveoli; an absence of dullness to percussion suggests a lack of serious inflammation in the lung.

the emergency room, his temperature was 101.1°F. Chest examination revealed crackles at the bases of both lungs posteriorly but no dullness to percussion. The rest of the physical examination was unremarkable. Total and differential blood counts were normal. A chest x-ray showed a diffuse, bilateral, hazy infiltrate in all lung fields except the apices bilaterally. An arterial blood gas determination revealed partial pressure of oxygen (PaO_2) of 59 mm Hg (normal = 75–100 mm Hg).

Upon persistent questioning, the patient acknowledged that he was gay and tested positive for human immunodeficiency virus (HIV) infection 8 years ago. At that time, he was informed that (1) he did not have acquired immunodeficiency syndrome (AIDS),

(2) his immune system was functioning well, and (3) no treatment was necessary, but that he should have periodic follow-up medical examinations. After moving to another city, he abandoned medical checkups.

- How did this man contract HIV?
- Would it have been appropriate to administer antiviral chemotherapy immediately after determining the patient was HIV-positive?
- What is the long-term prognosis for this patient?
- What measures, if any, should this patient take to prevent transmitting HIV to others?

ACQUIRED IMMUNODEFICIENCY SYNDROME

Discovery of an Emerging Virus Disease

In the late 1970s a peculiar pattern of disease symptoms was observed in New York City and San Francisco. Young adults were afflicted with generalized lymphadenopathy and unusual opportunistic infections, including mycobacterial infections (see Chapter 22), fungal infections (see Chapter 28), toxoplasmosis (see Chapter 28), and pneumocystis pneumonia. Some of these patients also suffered from a form of cancer, Kaposi's sarcoma, formerly occurring only in elderly men of Mediterranean or equatorial African ancestry. At first the disease seemed confined primarily to homosexual men, but it soon became clear that other populations, including intravenous drug users, hemophiliacs, and Haitian immigrants, also constituted high-risk groups. By 1981, two important facts became evident: (1) virtually all victims exhibited a severe deficiency in their cellular immunity, and (2) the number of cases was increasing rapidly. By 1983, a novel retrovirus called lymphadenopathy-associated virus (LAV) was isolated in France. Shortly thereafter, researchers in the United States reported their discovery of human T-cell lymphotropic virus III (HTLV-III). Subsequent investigations suggested that these viruses were one and the same and that HTLV-III was likely recovered from cell cultures contaminated with the French virus isolate. This virus is currently called human immunodeficiency virus type 1 (HIV-1) and is recognized as the etiologic agent of acquired immunodeficiency syndrome (AIDS). Later, a second virus, HIV-2, closely related to simian immunodeficiency virus (SIV), was also found to cause AIDS in certain parts of the world.

Magnitude of the Epidemic

The following statistics apply to HIV infection and clinical AIDS: (1) There are over 22 million cases worldwide, and over half have occurred in sub-Saharan Africa; (2) it is estimated that there are over 16,000 new HIV infections worldwide every day; (3) it is estimated that in 1999 there will be 40,000 new HIV infections in the United States; (4) in 1994–1995, AIDS was the leading killer of 25- to 44-year-old men and the third leading cause of death in women of the same age in the United States; (5) the rate of new infections is increasing fastest among heterosexual men and women (in Africa, most cases occur in heterosexual people); (6) in developed countries, high-risk groups continue to be men practicing promiscuous, unprotected sex with other men, and intravenous drug users (IDU); (7) since the introduction of tests for anti-HIV antibodies, the threat of spreading HIV by the parenteral introduction of blood or blood products has been dramatically reduced; and (8) the introduction of multidrug therapy in developed countries, particularly the use of viral protease inhibitors, has dramatically contributed to an improved quality of life for HIV-infected individuals.

LENTIVIRUSES

General Characteristics

The Retroviridae family of retroviruses is composed of three subfamilies: the oncoviruses, the lentiviruses, and the spumaviruses (Table 27-1). Only members of the onco- and lentiviruses cause human disease.

◀ **TABLE 27-1**
Human Retroviruses

Subfamily	Groups	Viruses	Diseases
Oncoviruses	Human T-cell lymphotropic viruses (C-type particles)	HTLV-1 HTLV-2	Adult T-cell lymphoma Hairy cell leukemia?
Lentiviruses	Human immunodeficiency viruses	HIV-1 HIV-2	AIDS
Spumaviruses	Human spumaviruses (foamy viruses)	HSV[a]	None

[a] Human spumaviruses, sometimes referred to as human foamy viruses (HFV) are commonly isolated from human beings, but their association with a given disease has never been established. They are not cytotoxic, although infected cells exhibit abnormal vacuolization.

Lentiviruses possess several unique characteristics. First, their wedge-shaped nucleocapsid (Figure 27-1), although similar to that of spumaviruses, is distinct from the spherical nucleocapsid of oncoviruses. Second, whereas most oncoviruses possess only *Gag, Pol,* and *Env* genes, human lentivirus genomes contain *Gag, Pol,* and *Env* plus at least 6 other genes. Of these other genes, *tat* and *rev* encode regulatory proteins that are essential for virus growth (Table 27-2). The other four accessory genes, *nef, vpr, vpu,* and *vif,* are not required for virus growth in tissue culture but play important, albeit not fully understood, roles in pathogenesis. Third, lentiviruses can kill infected cells unlike other retroviruses that either cause cell transformation (some oncoviruses) or grow without causing cytotoxicity (certain oncoviruses and spumaviruses).

In addition to the Gag, Pol, *and* Env *genes, the human oncoviruses HTLV-1 and HTLV-2 possess two regulatory genes,* tat *and* rev.

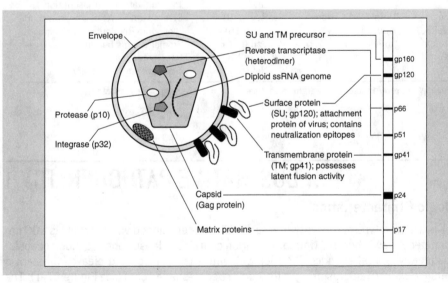

◀ **FIGURE 27-1**
Schematic Representation of Human Immunodeficiency Virus. *This figure depicts HIV (left) and most of its structural proteins after electrophoretic separation in a polyacrylamide gel (right). Viral glycoproteins are designated with a gp prefix. gp160 is the precursor to SU (gp120) and TM (gp41). Some minor core proteins are not shown. Detection of p24 and gp160 or gp120 or gp41, using patient sera, constitutes a positive Western blot test result.*

Nature of Infection

Lentiviruses attach to cells possessing suitable receptor (e.g., CD4) and coreceptor molecules. After fusion of the viral envelope and plasma membrane and consequent entry of the nucleocapsid into the cytoplasm, the lentivirus RNA genome is reverse transcribed into a dsDNA molecule. This plasmid-like molecule enters the nucleus and becomes integrated into a cellular chromosome as a provirus (see Chapter 3). The provirus may remain quiescent for long periods of time and is passed to daughter cells during mitosis. However, the exact role viral latency plays in the pathogenesis of AIDS remains controversial (see Pathogenesis below). During productive infection, the provirus is transcribed to form full-length RNA transcripts that are multiply spliced (by default) to form mRNAs encoding Tat, Rev, and other accessory proteins. Tat proteins move to the nucleus where they interact with the U3 region of the 5′ proviral long terminal repeat (LTR), thereby stimulating transcription by 50- to 100-fold. As Rev protein concentration increases, it blocks the multiple splicing of the full-length transcripts, increasing the generation of unspliced mRNA, which synthesizes Gag and Pol proteins, and singly spliced mRNA, which encodes the Env proteins (SU and TM). With the formation of the Gag and Pol proteins in the cytoplasm, nucleocapsids begin to form at the inside surface of regions of the plasma membrane in which the Env proteins are embedded. Virus particle assembly involves the budding of these nucleocapsids through the plasma membrane. Inside these premature particles, the protease (PR) cleaves the nucleocapsid precursor proteins, resulting in the distinctive wedge-shaped nucleocapsid characteristic of the mature, infectious lentivirus particle.

TABLE 27-2 ▶
Summary of Genes and Proteins of HIV

Gene	Formation of mRNA	Precursor Protein	Viral Protein (MW)	Viral Function
gag	Unspliced genomic RNA	Gag (p55)	CA (p24) NC (p8) MA (p17)	Capsid virus budding Nucleocapsid packaging of RNA Matrix
pol	Unspliced genomic RNA	Gag-Pol (p160	RT (p66; p51) IN (p32) PR (p11)	Reverse transcriptase Integrase Protease
env	Singly spliced mRNA	Env (gp160)	SU (gp120)	Virus attachment, tropism, neutralization epitopes
			TM (gp41)	Membrane fusion
Same as viral protein	Multiply spliced mRNA	None	Tat (p14) Rev (p19) Vpr (p15) Vpu (p16) Vif (p23) Nef (p27)	Transactivation of transcription Blocks viral RNA splicing, transport of some RNA out of nucleus Promotes virus budding Infectivity T-cell activity; infectivity

Note. MW = protein molecular weight in thousands; p = protein; gp = glycoprotein.

ILLUSTRATIVE PATHOGEN: HIV-1

Biologic Characteristics

HIV-1 is the prototype of the lentivirus subfamily. The enveloped virus particle is 100 nm in diameter. A newly budded (immature) virion contains a dense spherical nucleocapsid. Subsequently, a viral-encoded PR packaged with the nucleocapsid cleaves the capsid precursor protein (Gag), resulting in its unique wedge-shaped core (see Figure 27-1). The HIV-1 genome, like that of all retroviruses, is composed of two identical copies of a positive-sense ssRNA molecule. One or more short stretches of complementary sequences allow the two molecules to anneal to each other. Approximately 5–10 copies of the reverse transcriptase (RT) and integrase (IN) proteins are contained within the nucleocapsid. Unlike oncovirus genomes, the HIV-1 genetic map is complex (Figure 27-2). Retroviral gene expression involves virtually all the mechanisms discussed in Chapter 3, including splicing, proteolytic processing to form different functional proteins from a

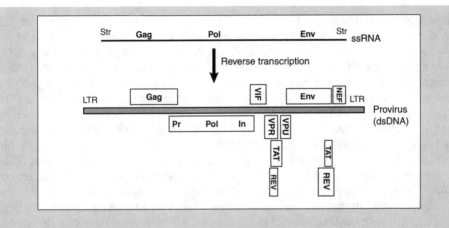

FIGURE 27-2
Reverse Transcription of Human Immunodeficiency Virus Genome. Reverse transcription of the HIV genome results in a provirus with the same genetic map but a long terminal repeat (LTR) in lieu of the short terminal repeat (Str) on the viral ssRNA genome. The prototypic retroviral structural genes are printed horizontally. The Gag and Pol proteins are translated directly from the full-length RNA transcript made from the provirus. The exons of the regulatory and accessory genes are printed vertically and, like that of the ENV gene, their mRNA molecules are formed by splicing of the full-length RNA transcript. Only the Gag, Pol, and Env genes are shown on one of the two copies of the viral ssRNA genome (top line).

common precursor, and ribosomal read-through and/or frameshifting to escape stop codons so that different precursor proteins in different amounts can be made. Unspliced genomic ssRNA molecules direct the synthesis of only the Gag precursor protein (p55) or the Gag-Pol precursor (p160) protein (see Table 27-2). The mRNA encoding the envelope precursor protein (gp160) is created after a single splicing event of the genomic ssRNA transcript before it leaves the nucleus. The mRNAs for the regulatory and accessory proteins are formed only when a genomic-length ssRNA transcript is multiply spliced in any one of several ways (see Figure 27-2). In this manner, HIV utilizes all three open reading frames of its genome to produce virus-specific proteins.

Reservoir and Transmission

The only reservoir for HIV-1 is human beings. Transmission is by parenteral introduction of contaminated fluids into the body by injection or by unprotected sexual activities. Although infectious mucosal fluids may contain virions, infected mononuclear cells, particularly macrophages, may be of greater importance. There is evidence that during the early stages of HIV-1 infection, the virus population is largely macrophage tropic, whereas later virus isolates exhibit lymphotropism. HIV-1 can be transmitted from mother to child in utero, by breast feeding, or in the process of birthing. Antiviral therapy, by reducing the virus burden in the mother, can significantly decrease the likelihood of transmission of the virus to her newborn.

Virulence Factors

Despite extensive knowledge of the structure and replication of HIV, the identity of viral products responsible for pathogenicity remains elusive. The virion membrane protein, SU, clearly determines the tropism of HIV for lymphocytes or macrophages. It also possesses most of the antigenic sites that elicit neutralizing antibodies, although at least one neutralization epitope resides on the TM envelope protein (see Table 27-2). Viral regulatory proteins, particularly Tat and Rev, play crucial roles in activating and regulating virus gene expression and the production of virions. It remains to be determined how the accessory HIV genes, such as *nef* and *vif,* influence the ability of HIV to infect and kill specific immune cells.

Pathogenesis

The dogma describing how HIV elicits clinical disease (AIDS) begins with the factors that determine the tropism of HIV for helper lymphocytes and macrophages. For HIV-1, the viral surface envelope protein (SU) binds to the CD4 receptor. However, for fusion and nucleocapsid penetration to occur, a second interaction between the viral SU protein (see Figure 27-1) and a second plasma membrane chemokine coreceptor must ensue. The coreceptor on lymphocytes is called CXCR4; on macrophages it is called CCR5. SU

The absence of a coreceptor (homozygous condition) can result in an HIV infection in which there is a prolonged or indefinite period of clinically inapparent disease (i.e., long-term nonprogressive infection).

Neutralizing antibodies are those molecules that can block the ability of a virus to infect cells. *Cytotoxic T-cells* attack and destroy virus-infected cells displaying viral antigens on their surface.

protein-coreceptor interaction permits the TM protein to mediate the fusion of the viral envelope with the cell's plasma membrane, translocating the nucleocapsid into the cell. HIV-2, which is confined primarily to West Africa, also requires the CD4 receptor but may utilize coreceptors different than those used by HIV-1. These findings indicate that to successfully infect CD4 positive (CD4+) cells, HIV-1 requires both CD4 and one of a family of chemokine receptors that normally play a role in inflammatory reactions. Unlike oncoviruses, which only successfully infect dividing cells, HIV-1 can infect nondividing CD4+ macrophages and kill dividing CD4+ T-lymphocytes. However, when infected T-cells are activated to divide, virus production results. As the level of virus increases in lymph nodes, liver, spleen, and peripheral blood, cytotoxic (CD8+) T-lymphocytes (CTL) and specific neutralizing antibodies are produced. These immune responses control but do not eliminate virus production. During this phase, usually 1–2 months after initial infection, the patient may experience an acute, influenza-like disease for several weeks (Figure 27-3). With the resolution of the acute phase illness, a period of clinical latency ensues. This period can last 1–10 years, during which there is inapparent disease. Although infectious virus may be undetected in the blood, billions of T-cells are being destroyed daily, particularly in the lymph nodes, with the concurrent production of an estimated 10^9–10^{10} virions per day. This virus is rapidly cleared by the reticulo-endothelial system. The absence of frank disease suggests that an equilibrium exists between virus production, the turnover of the lymphocyte population, and other elements of the immune system such as antibody production. Viral latency may play a limited but important role whereby infected cells escape immune attack.

FIGURE 27-3 ▶

Pathogenesis of Human Immunodeficiency Infection. Changes in CD4+ counts and onset of clinical syndromes are depicted on the left. The average time course of disease progression, according to 1998 statistics, is shown on the right.

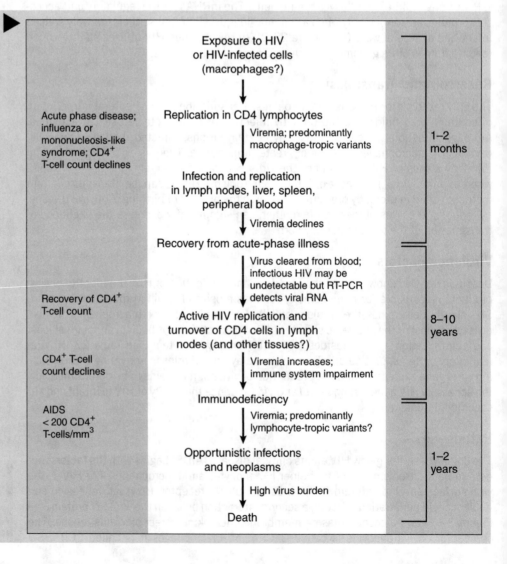

Because of the error-prone retroviral RT and the functional plasticity of its attachment protein (SU or gp120), virus variants with altered CTL and antibody epitopes are constantly produced. In response, the immune system mounts successive antibody and cellular immune responses against these variants, a process that may continue for many years. Eventually, mutant viruses emerge with increased virulence, possibly as a consequence of their ability to escape recognition by CTL and antibody responses. Likewise, under the selective pressure of chemotherapy, drug-resistant viruses evolve. As the virus burden becomes excessive, the rate of CD4+-lymphocyte killing exceeds their replacement, causing the helper T-cell population to drop below a threshold consistent with normal immune function. The subsequent immune impairment permits (1) a variety of opportunistic pathogens to gain a foothold, and (2) cancers such as Kaposi's sarcoma and lymphomas to develop. In addition, approximately half of HIV-infected patients develop an HIV encephalitis or encephalopathy (e.g., AIDS dementia complex) with neuropsychiatric signs. Although the nature of this syndrome remains obscure, it is probably the consequence of infected T-cells or macrophages entering the brain and permitting HIV to directly or indirectly infect and kill brain cells.

The capacity of HIV to continually generate mutants or variants in a single infected patient results in a virus population so diverse (no two virions contain identical genetic codes) that it is considered a quasispecies.

Diagnosis

The diagnosis of HIV infection, but not AIDS, is generally made by the detection of anti-HIV antibodies in serum by enzyme-linked immunosorbant assay (ELISA) and confirmed by the more tedious but more reliable Western blot assay. Other available tests include virus isolation in cultures of activated macrophages or T-lymphocytes, detection of specific viral antigens by ELISA, and the identification of HIV-specific sequences in blood or tissue fractions using a reverse transcriptase–polymerase chain reaction (RT-PCR) technique. Recent advances indicate that RT-PCR can be used to measure the amount of virus in the blood (i.e., virus burden). Because there is a direct correlation between the amount of virus and the rate of disease progression, direct measurements of the virus burden are useful in assessing the extent of disease as well as the effectiveness of antiviral chemotherapeutic regimens.

RT-PCR is a methodology that uses a purified reverse transcriptase (RT) to synthesize a dsDNA copy of one or more ssRNA molecules. For subsequent analysis, millions of copies of the dsDNA molecules are generated by a heat-resistant DNA polymerase and suitable oligonucleotide primers (polymerase chain reaction).

Currently, a diagnosis of AIDS requires a combination of evidence of HIV infection and (1) a CD4+ T-cell count of less than 200/mm^3 or (2) a diagnosis of one or more opportunistic infections or diseases. The criteria used to make an AIDS diagnosis are summarized in Table 27-3.

Treatment and Prevention

Current treatment protocols call for the early use of a combination of antiviral drugs to inhibit virus production and minimize the selection for resistant virus mutants. In approximately 80% or more of HIV-infected patients, a triple-drug combination using two different RT inhibitors and a protease inhibitor dramatically reduces the virus burden for several years. Just how long this therapeutic regimen will suppress virus production remains to be determined. Current antiviral drugs block two different stages of the virus growth cycle: (1) reverse transcription of the RNA genome into a dsDNA provirus using drugs such as zidovudine (AZT), lamivudine (3TC), and didanosine (ddI); and (2) viral-specific proteolytic processing using viral protease inhibitors such as indinavir, nelfinavir, retronavir, or saquinavir.

It is now recognized that anti-HIV chemotherapy with a single drug, while transiently reducing the virus burden, promotes the rapid emergence of drug-resistant HIV mutants.

Unfortunately, many HIV-infected patients do not benefit from this potentially effective combination therapy because of (1) direct toxic effects to blood cells, (2) unpleasant side effects such as nausea and headache, (3) expense of the drugs, and (4) failure of patients to adhere to a strict regimen of self-medication multiple times each day for years.

*The use of drug cocktails containing both viral reverse transcriptase and protease inhibitors is termed **highly active antiretroviral therapy (HAART)**.*

RT-PCR can be used periodically to monitor therapeutic effectiveness by quantitating the virus burden in the blood. For example, an increase in the amount of bloodborne virus during chemotherapy usually signals the emergence of drug-resistant viruses. Early treatment of women with zidovudine (AZT) during pregnancy and birth reduces the transmission of HIV from mother to neonate by 70%.

Recently, the potency of protease inhibitors has increased to the point where the "pill burden" has been reduced to one or two daily.

Prevention of HIV infection relies primarily on education. Users of injectable drugs must understand the high risks associated with the use of contaminated syringes and

TABLE 27-3 ▶

Criteria for the Diagnosis of Acquired Immunodeficiency Syndrome (AIDS) among Adolescents and Adults

Confirmed HIV infection, as indicated by repeatedly reactive screening tests for HIV antibody (e.g., enzyme immunoassay) with specific antibody identified by the use of supplemental tests (e.g., Western blot); or the direct identification of virus in host tissues by isolation of HIV or detection of its specific antigens, and

either

CD4+ (helper) T-cell count less than 200 cells/mm³

or any one of the following:

HIV-associated clinical syndrome:
- HIV wasting syndrome: profound involuntary weight loss plus either chronic diarrhea or chronic weakness and documented fever
- Encephalopathy (dementia), HIV related

Superimposed opportunistic infection:
- Candidiasis of bronchi, trachea, or lungs
- Candidiasis, esophageal
- Coccidioidomycosis, disseminated or extrapulmonary
- Cryptococcosis, extrapulmonary
- Cryptosporidiosis, chronic intestinal (greater than 1-month duration)
- Cytomegalovirus disease (other than liver, spleen, or lymph nodes)
- Cytomegalovirus retinitis (with loss of vision)
- Herpes simplex: chronic ulcers (greater than 1-month duration); or bronchitis, pneumonitis, or esophagitis
- Histoplasmosis, disseminated or extrapulmonary
- Isosporosis, chronic intestinal (greater than 1-month duration)
- *Mycobacterium avium* complex (MAC) or *M. kansasii*, disseminated or extrapulmonary
- *M. tuberculosis*, pulmonary or extrapulmonary
- *Pneumocystis carinii* pneumonia
- Pneumonia, recurrent
- Progressive multifocal leukoencephalopathy (PML)
- *Salmonella* septicemia, recurrent
- *Toxoplasma* encephalitis

Neoplasm:
- Cervical cancer, invasive
- Kaposi's sarcoma
- Lymphoma, Burkitt's or immunoblastic
- Lymphoma, primary, of brain

needles. Likewise, all persons, particularly those practicing promiscuous sex, must recognize that HIV is a sexually transmitted disease and that its transmission can be thwarted (but not entirely eliminated) by using condoms.

RESOLUTION OF CLINICAL CASE

Virtually all PCP occurs in highly immunocompromised individuals, including transplant recipients and cancer patients on cytotoxic chemotherapy.

The patient was admitted to the hospital for further tests. A T-lymphocyte subset count showed his CD4+ T-cell concentration was 185/mm³ (normal = 500–1900/mm³). Cultures of bronchial lavage fluid were negative for bacteria and fungi. The virus laboratory also failed to identify any pathogens. A diagnosis of *Pneumocystis carinii* pneumonia (PCP) was made based on a diffuse, bilateral, symmetric pneumonia in a relatively young individual with only minimal signs; the negative results of the bacterial, fungal, and viral cultures supported this diagnosis. The patient was treated with sulfamethoxazole and trimethoprim (Bactrim) for presumptive PCP. Given his CD4+ cell count of less than 200/mm³ and his opportunistic PCP infection, he was diagnosed as having AIDS. Highly active antiretroviral therapy (HAART) was initiated using three drugs: zidovudine (AZT), lamivudine (3TC), and saquinavir. Fortunately, the drugs did not elicit intolerable toxic reactions. Over the next two weeks, his pneumonia resolved, his CD4+ cell count rose to 250/mm³, and he was released from the hospital.

REVIEW QUESTIONS

Directions: For each of the following questions, choose the **one best** answer.

1. Vaccine development against HIV infection and the prevention of AIDS remains a significant challenge because
   - **(A)** HIV uses a protease to cleave its precursor proteins
   - **(B)** HIV replicates in lymphoid cells
   - **(C)** the envelope proteins of HIV fail to elicit neutralizing antibodies in infected humans
   - **(D)** the virion membrane protein (SU) of HIV can exist in many variant forms, thus thwarting the immune system's capacity to eradicate the virus
   - **(E)** virulence factors for HIV have not been clearly delineated

2. Which one of the following justifies a clinical diagnosis of AIDS?
   - **(A)** CD4$^+$ count of 190/mm^3 and a positive Western blot assay for anti-HIV antibodies
   - **(B)** Serologic evidence of HIV infection and an upper respiratory infection
   - **(C)** Kaposi's sarcoma and herpesvirus retinitis
   - **(D)** Systemic fungal infection and a CD4$^+$ count of 133/mm^3
   - **(E)** CD4$^+$ count of 190/mm^3 and tuberculosis

3. Lentiviruses are unique among retroviruses because they
   - **(A)** possess a reverse transcriptase
   - **(B)** synthesize a provirus
   - **(C)** cause Kaposi's sarcoma
   - **(D)** have a nucleocapsid morphologically unlike any other retrovirus
   - **(E)** can kill the cells they infect

4. The importance of the CD4 molecule in HIV pathogenesis is that
   - **(A)** HIV infection results in the proteolytic hydrolysis of the CD4 molecules in infected lymphocytes
   - **(B)** HIV induces an autoimmune reaction in which uninfected cells possessing this molecule are destroyed
   - **(C)** HIV infection causes lymphocytes to be produced in which there are no CD4 molecules
   - **(D)** HIV commonly attaches to the CD4 molecule, permitting infection
   - **(E)** the immune response to HIV infection is to produce soluble CD4 molecules to thwart the progression of the virus

5. The most sensitive indicator of the extent of virus infection in an AIDS patient is the
   - **(A)** number of CD4$^+$ lymphocytes in the blood
   - **(B)** amount of virus in the blood
   - **(C)** ratio of CD4$^+$ to CD4$^-$ cells in the blood
   - **(D)** presence or absence of neutralizing antibodies to HIV
   - **(E)** number of CD4$^+$ macrophages in the blood

Note. HIV = human immunodeficiency virus; AIDS = acquired immunodeficiency syndrome.

ANSWERS AND EXPLANATIONS

1. **The answer is D.** During HIV infection, random mutations introduced by the error-prone reverse transcriptase result in the synthesis of altered forms of SU, allowing these virus mutants to escape previous immune responses. Options A and B, although true statements, are immaterial to vaccine development. Option C is incorrect because neutralizing antibodies do form in infected persons and probably account in part for the reduction in circulating virus during clinical latency. Option E is incorrect because it is pure speculation that the identification of viral virulence factors will materially affect vaccine development.

2. **The answer is A.** There must be evidence of HIV infection and a CD4+ T-cell count of less than 200/mm³. In the absence of direct evidence of HIV infection, an AIDS diagnosis cannot be made. Options C, D, and E are incorrect because opportunistic diseases with or without an accompanying reduced CD4+ count do not constitute an AIDS diagnosis; they may or may not indicate an immunodeficiency, the etiology of which remains to be determined. Option B is incorrect because an upper respiratory disease (e.g., the common cold) is not considered an opportunistic infection; in the absence of a reduced CD4+ cell count and other disease manifestations, AIDS would not be the diagnosis.

3. **The answer is E.** Other retroviruses either transform cells (certain oncoviruses) or are not cytotoxic (some oncoviruses and spumaviruses). Options A and B are incorrect because all retroviruses possess a reverse transcriptase and synthesize a proviral DNA. Option C is incorrect because Kaposi's sarcoma occurs in the absence of HIV infection and not all HIV-infected persons suffer from this cancer. Its association with AIDS is a consequence of a compromised immune system and not directly caused by HIV. Option D is incorrect because lentiviruses and spumaviruses share the same nucleocapsid morphology.

4. **The answer is D.** The principal receptor for HIV is the CD4 molecule on the surface of helper T-lymphocytes, macrophages, and other cells. Option A is incorrect because the protease of HIV acts to specifically process viral and not cellular proteins. Option B is incorrect because autoimmune responses to CD4 are not a pathogenetic feature of HIV infection. Option C is incorrect because HIV does not prevent the proper maturation of lymphocytes but eventually kills more helper lymphocytes than the body can manufacture. Option E is incorrect because CD4 molecules are integral membrane proteins and are not secreted from cells even after HIV infection.

5. **The answer is B.** The best single indicator of how the HIV infection is progressing is the amount of virus in the peripheral blood. Option A is incorrect because the number of CD4+ T-cells becomes important when it drops below 200/mm³, but it is not as sensitive an indicator of the progression of disease as the virus burden. Option C is incorrect because the ratio of CD4+ to CD4− cells is less useful than the absolute number of CD4+ cells. Option D is incorrect because AIDS patients typically have neutralizing antibodies to HIV, so this parameter has not proven useful in assessing the disease's progress. The number of CD4+ macrophages does not correlate with disease progression (option E).

28 OPPORTUNISTIC INFECTIONS

CHAPTER OUTLINE

Introduction of Clinical Case
Opportunistic Infections
- Immunosuppression and Opportunistic Infection
- Types of Immunosuppression

Illustrative Pathogen: The Fungi
- Biologic Characteristics
- Cutaneous and Subcutaneous Mycoses
- Systemic Mycoses
- Opportunistic Mycoses

Illustrative Pathogen: *Toxoplasma gondii*
- Biologic Characteristics
- Reservoir and Transmission
- Virulence Factors
- Pathogenesis
- Diagnosis
- Prevention and Treatment

Resolution of Clinical Case
Review Questions

INTRODUCTION OF CLINICAL CASE

A 24-year-old pregnant woman was referred to an infectious disease specialist by her obstetrician because of infectious mononucleosis occurring in the third month of pregnancy. The patient had had a low-grade fever and a mild sore throat for about 1 week. A complete blood count showed a leukocyte count of 10,500/μL (normal: 5000–10,000) with 55% lymphocytes (normal: 16%–45%) and 12% atypical lymphocytes (normal: none). The result of a monospot test for heterophile antibodies was negative.

The patient was a housewife and had

> **Mononucleosis** *is a general description of an infection caused by Epstein-Barr virus (EBV), cytomegalovirus (CMV), acute toxoplasmosis, streptococcal pharyngitis, hepatitis B virus (HBV), or human immunodeficiency virus (HIV). Signs of mononucleosis include fever, sore throat, headache, white patches on the back of the throat, swollen "glands" in the neck, general exhaustion, and lack of appetite.*

had no contact with anyone known to have infectious mononucleosis. She had obtained a kitten from the animal shelter about 3 weeks earlier and had trained the kitten to use a litter box, which the patient changed.

Physical examination revealed a temperature of 99.8°F. There were numerous shotty (< 1 cm) nodes in the anterior and posterior cervical chains bilaterally. Neither the liver nor the spleen was palpable, and the rest of the examination was noncontributory. Liver function tests were mildly elevated. Specific Epstein-Barr virus (EBV) serology revealed the presence of antibody to EBV nuclear antigen (EBNA) and immunoglobulin G (IgG) antibody to EBV capsid antigen (VCA), but these antibody titers indicate infection with EBV in the remote past. IgG antibody to cytomegalovirus (CMV) was present at a titer of 1:64, also indicating infection with CMV in the remote past. IgM antibody against *Toxoplasma gondii* was present at a titer of 1:1024 in the absence of any IgG antibody.

- Why was this patient referred by her obstetrician to an infectious disease specialist?
- What is the most probable etiologic agent responsible for this patient's symptoms?

Monospot Test. The *monospot test* is a rapid blood test that detects the presence of heterophile antibodies—antibodies that nonspecifically react against proteins or cells from another species. For reasons that are poorly understood, such antibodies increase in the blood after infections by various microorganisms, especially viruses. Since viruses are usually difficult to detect and quantitate, heterophile tests are useful screening methods for viral infections. Heterophile antibodies are so named because they can react with antigens from unrelated species. EBV-associated infectious mononucleosis heterophile antibodies belong to the IgM class. They are present in 60%–70% of patients in the first week of clinical illness and in 80%–90% by 3 months after onset of symptoms in most patients, but persist in some patients for up to 12 months. In 15%–20% of patients with EBV-associated infectious mononucleosis, heterophile antibody test results are negative. This rate is even higher in children younger than 4 years, approaching 50% in some studies. Although a variety of infections can produce heterophile antibodies (e.g., mumps, malaria, rubella) the concentrations of heterophile antibodies achieved during these disease processes are much lower than in patients with EBV-associated infectious mononucleosis.

OPPORTUNISTIC INFECTIONS IN MEDICAL MICROBIOLOGY

Opportunistic infections are those caused by the normal flora of the human host, or by transient microbes, when the host is immunocompromised. The two most important factors in these types of infections are exposure and opportunity (hence, *opportunistic infection*).

The human body, which is made up of $\sim 10^{13}$ human cells, routinely harbors $\sim 10^{14}$ microorganisms. These microbes constitute a relatively stable normal microbial flora, with specific microbes inhabiting specific sites of the body during extended periods in an individual's life (see Chapter 11). In addition, individuals are transiently exposed to microbes every day through contact with pets, dust, aerosols, and other substances. In point of fact, we coexist with microbes, most of which are *not* pathogens. However, the opportunity for these normally nonpathogenic microorganisms to cause infection arises when exposure occurs at a time when the host defense mechanisms are compromised. This is particularly true in today's medical era, when mechanical (e.g., catheterization) and pharmacologic (e.g., immunosuppressive drugs) interventions, which compromise the host immune system, are in common use. While these methods of intervention alleviate the immediate symptoms of noninfectious diseases, they can subvert the host's normal resistance to infection.

Immunosuppression and Opportunistic Infection

Any time host defenses are compromised, a person becomes susceptible to opportunistic infection. The immune defenses consist of a series of coordinately organized strategies that can be classified as two components: (1) innate defense mechanisms that are constitutively produced and (2) a highly specific and inducible response, referred to as specific immunity. The molecular participants in innate immunity are present before exposure to microbial pathogens and are not enhanced by prior exposure to the microbial pathogen; in addition, innate immunity is unable to discriminate one microbial pathogen from another. In contrast, specific immunity is capable of discriminating microbial pathogens from host molecules and is enhanced at each encounter with the microbial pathogen. These two systems act synergistically to eliminate microbial pathogens; thus a breach in any aspect of these immune defenses renders an individual susceptible to opportunistic infection. Table 28-1 provides examples of the relationship between disruptions in host defenses and opportunistic pathogens.

The risk of opportunistic infection in immunocompromised persons is largely determined by the interaction of two factors: (1) the nature of the immunosuppression and (2) exposure to opportunistic pathogens. If the "net state" of immunosuppression is severe enough, even minor exposure to the most innocuous opportunistic microbe can result in a life-threatening infection. The "net state" of immunosuppression is a complex function comprising several conditions, including the degree and duration of the immunosuppressed condition. Consequently, different patterns of opportunistic infection emerge. For example, during the first few weeks after the onset of the immunosuppressed state the major risk of infectious disease is posed by rapidly growing viral and bacterial pathogens. The more rare fungal and protozoan infections generally occur only after a prolonged immunosuppressed state.

◀ **TABLE 28-1**
Examples of Opportunistic Pathogens Associated with a Disrupted Host Defense

Deficits in immunity at the host/environment barrier
- Burns breach the epidermal layers, allowing deeper tissues of the host to become infected with *Pseudomonas aeruginosa* (associated with soil, plants, and water), which creates significant infectious complications for burn victims.
- Catheterization gives microbial organisms access to deeper tissues of the host. As a result, *P. aeruginosa*, *Escherichia coli*, *Staphylococcus aureus*, and other pathogens that are part of the hospital environment, commonly cause urinary tract infection and sepsis in hospital patients.
- Disruption of the normal microbial flora (e.g., by administration of antimicrobial therapy) allows normal flora such as *S. aureus*, *Clostridium difficile*, and *Candida albicans* to cause localized (e.g., epidermal, intestinal, vaginal) disease.

Deficits in innate immune defenses
- Complement deficiencies are associated with susceptibility to bacterial infections. Individuals with C3 deficiencies are susceptible to pyogenic infections, whereas those deficient in the C5b–C9 components are susceptible to infection by pathogenic *Neisseria* spp.
- Granulocyte abnormalities are associated with *S. aureus* infection of the skin, lymph nodes, or other visceral organs.
- Neutropenia predisposes individuals to bacteremia (caused by a variety of bacteria), bacterial pneumonia (e.g., *P. aeruginosa* pneumonia), and systemic mycosis (caused by a variety of fungi).

Deficits in specific immune defenses
- T-cell malfunction or depletion results in tuberculosis caused by *Mycobacterium* spp., candidiasis caused by *Candida albicans*, cryptococcosis caused by *Cryptococcus immitus*, histoplasmosis caused by *Histoplasma capsulatum*, cryptosporidiosis caused by *Cryptosporidum parvum*, pneumocystis pneumonia caused by *Pneumoncystis carinii*, toxoplasmosis caused by *Toxoplasma gondii*, and others.

Types of Immunosuppression

DEFICITS IN HOST DEFENSES AT THE HOST/ENVIRONMENT BARRIER

The largest and, arguably, most important barrier separating the sterile spaces of the human host from opportunistic microbial pathogens is the skin. Compromise of this barrier may occur as a consequence of cuts, burns, or mechanical manipulation (e.g., needles or surgery). A breach in this layer presents the opportunity for local flora to access the sterile spaces. For example, intravenous catheters can introduce *Staphylococcus epidermidis*, a member of the local flora, into the bloodstream, resulting in septicemia. Patients who experience cutaneous burns are very susceptible to bacterial infection because the necrotizing skin tissue that results from a burn is an excellent bacterial growth medium. *Staphylococcus aureus* and *Pseudomonas aeruginosa* are ubiquitous within the environment and therefore have access to this necrotizing tissue. Consequently, complications of burn infections are often the result of *S. aureus* and *P. aeruginosa*.

The disruption of local commensal flora on mucosal surfaces can facilitate the establishment of an opportunistic pathogen on mucosal surfaces because instead of coexisting with the host, the normal flora now cause disease. This is a common occurrence in the intestine, sometimes as the result of antibiotic therapy. Pseudomembranous colitis caused by the opportunistic pathogen *Clostridium difficile* is an example of a disease caused by antibiotic therapy (see Chapter 11). Another example of the medical consequences resulting from disruption of the commensal flora has been described for bacterial vaginosis. Lactobacilli are bacteria associated with a healthy vagina. Displacement of these bacteria by antibiotic suppression or douching can result in the overgrowth of anaerobic bacteria, resulting in bacterial vaginosis.

Some mucosal tissues are highly differentiated and function to remove microbial pathogens mechanically. For example, the lung uses a combination of mucus production by goblet cells and ciliary activity of the respiratory epithelial cells to trap and transport microbial pathogens out of the pulmonary compartment. Disrupting this innate defense mechanism predisposes individuals to *P. aeruginosa* lung infections such as those described for cystic fibrosis patients (see Chapter 5). In addition, individuals with a deficiency in their ability to secrete IgA are more prone to contract sinus infections, pneumonia, or gastrointestinal illnesses.

DEFICITS IN INNATE IMMUNE DEFENSES

Complement Deficiencies. Individuals lacking a fully functional complement system are often susceptible to infection. For example, those with homozygous deficiency of factor C3 or the C3b inactivator (factor I) commonly suffer repeated pyogenic infections with gram-negative and gram-positive organisms. The association between these recurrent pyogenic infections (e.g., streptococcal disease) and C3 deficiency demonstrates the central role of C3 in maintaining normal host defenses. C3 is required for the opsonization of foreign organisms because the C3b fragment acts as a bridge between these organisms and surface receptors on neutrophils and macrophages.

Interruption of complement activation at the C3 step also prevents progression to the late stages of the complement cascade in which the C5b–C9 complex is formed. This complex, termed the membrane attack complex (MAC), is responsible for complement-mediated bacterial lysis. As part of this cascade, the chemotactic factor C5a, which functions to localize leukocytes to the site of infection is also generated. Persons with deficiencies of late-stage MAC complement components are unusually susceptible to systemic *Neisseria* spp. infections involving gonococci or meningococci, suggesting that complement-mediated opsonization and bacteriolysis are important factors in the host's resistance to *Neisseria* spp.

Granulocyte Abnormalities. Defects in granulocyte structure and function are associated with an increased frequency of bacterial infection, particularly recurrent abscesses of the skin, lymph nodes, and visceral organs caused by *S. aureus* or various gram-negative bacilli. However, the most common granulocyte defect is a decrease in the absolute number of neutrophils (neutropenia). This commonly occurs in patients with leukemia or aplastic anemia or in patients treated with radiation or various forms of chemotherapy. Neutropenic individuals frequently have bacteremia and bacterial pneumonias. If the neutropenia occurs over an extended period, there is an increased risk of fungal infection caused by *Candida* spp. and *Aspergillus* spp. The absolute level of circulating neutrophils required to maintain a sterile intracellular environment is unclear, but the risk of infection is significantly increased when neutrophil levels fall to $<1000/mm^3$, is further increased when they fall to levels of $<500/mm^3$, and becomes maximal at levels $<100/mm^3$. The relationship between opportunistic infectious diseases and leukocyte count is shown in Figure 28-1.

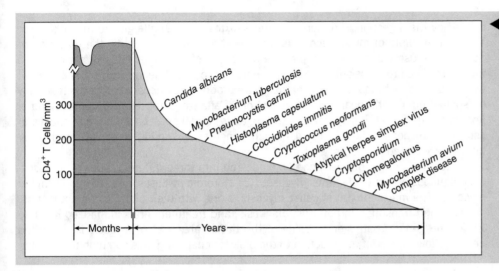

FIGURE 28-1
Opportunistic Infections as a Function of CD4+ Count. *Graphical representation demonstrating the occurrence of opportunistic infections as a function of CD4+ count (Y-axis). Because the CD4+ count typically decreases slowly over time in immunosuppressed individuals (e.g., individuals with HIV-1 infection), this relationship is also shown as a function of time (X-axis).*

DEFICITS IN SPECIFIC IMMUNE DEFENSES

Hypogammaglobulinemia. Patients with hypogammaglobulinemia fail to produce adequate amounts of opsonizing and bactericidal antibody after either immunization or natural exposure to an antigen. This deficiency is associated with a particular susceptibility to serious bacteremia, pneumonia, and sinusitis caused by the encapsulated bacteria *Streptococcus pneumoniae, Haemophilus influenzae,* and *Neisseria meningitidis.* In addition, patients with this deficiency have an increased susceptibility to infection with the parasite *Giardia lamblia,* the fungus *Pneumocystis carinii,* and enteroviruses (including poliovirus and rotavirus). Patients with multiple myeloma and chronic lymphocytic leukemia are most likely to present with hypogammaglobulinemia.

Abnormalities in Cell-Mediated Immunity. Depressed cell-mediated immunity causes an increased incidence and severity of infection by pathogenic microbes capable of establishing chronic intracellular infection, including *Mycobacterium* spp., *Salmonella* spp., *Listeria* spp., fungi (most commonly *Candida* spp. but also *P. carinii* and *Cryptococcus neoformans*), various viruses (particularly herpes, vaccinia, and measles virus), and parasites such as *T. gondii* and *Cryptosporidium parvum.* Depressed cellular immunity is common in adult patients with lymphoma (especially those with Hodgkin's disease), patients who have received an organ transplant, and those with acquired immunodeficiency syndrome (AIDS).

Opportunistic infection that results from nonpathogenic bacteria is not dealt with at length in this chapter. Many of them have been discussed elsewhere in this text (e.g., see Chapters 5, 10, 11, 15, 22, and 27) and their opportunistic strategies for causing infection have been described. Humans are exposed to these microbial agents on a daily basis, typically without experiencing pathologic symptoms. However, when given the opportunity, fungi and the parasites represent significant contributors to infectious disease. Because of this association, the fungi and *T. gondii* (a parasitic pathogen) serve as the illustrative pathogens for this chapter.

ILLUSTRATIVE PATHOGEN: The Fungi

The fungi are important etiologic agents of infectious diseases, particularly opportunistic disease. They represent a large and complex group of eukaryotic pathogens with a diverse and complicated biology. Therefore, this chapter focuses only on the general characteristics of fungal disease and the student is referred to more detailed texts that focus specifically on the science of mycology.

We encounter fungi everyday. They are ubiquitous and are used in the production of many food sources, including bread, cheese, and wine. In addition to infections (referred to as mycosis), fungi cause two noninfectious diseases: (1) mycotoxicosis, intoxications caused by the ingestion of preformed fungal toxins, and (2) allergies to fungal spores. The best example of mycotoxicosis is the condition brought about by the ingestion of poisonous mushrooms. For example, the mycelium of the fungus *Amanita* grows as a mushroom and produces amanitin and phalloidin, two potent hepatotoxins that are lethal when ingested by humans. Also, aflatoxins are produced by *Aspergillus flavus* that grow on spoiled grains and peanuts. The ingestion of aflatoxins causes liver damage and is implicated in human hepatic cancer. Allergies to fungal spores are common causes of asthmatic responses (i.e., a rapid bronchoconstriction mediated by IgE) and other immune-mediated reactions.

Infectious fungal diseases can be organized into three different types of diseases: (1) cutaneous and subcutaneous mycoses, (2) systemic mycoses, and (3) opportunistic mycoses. The major fungi that cause mycosis, along with their biologic characteristics, reservoir and transmission patterns, diagnosis, and treatment are summarized in Table 28-2. The general pathogenic profile of the three categories of mycosis is described below, following a brief introduction to the biologic characteristics common to all fungi.

Biologic Characteristics

Chitin composes the cell wall of fungi and is a homopolymer of N-acetylglucosamine.

In addition to being eukaryotic pathogens, fungi differ from prokaryotic pathogens in the production of two different, and unique, structural components. Chitin, not peptidoglycan, constitutes the fungal cell wall and thus is not a target of bacterial cell wall synthesis inhibitors. Further, the fungal cell membrane contains ergosterol and zymosterol, unlike bacterial pathogens, which do not contain sterols (with the exception of the *Mycoplasma* spp.) and unlike the human cell membrane, which contains predominantly cholesterol. The selectivity of antifungal agents such as amphotericin B, ketoconazole, fluconazole, itraconazole, and myconazole exploits this difference in membrane composition by selectively binding to, or inhibiting the synthesis of, ergosterol and zymosterol. Most (but not all) fungi that cause human disease exist as two distinct morphotypes—yeasts and molds (see Chapter 1). Recall that yeasts are unicellular organisms that reproduce by asexual budding. Molds grow as long hyphae that intertwine to form a mycelium. Medically important fungi are often (but not always) dimorphic, that is, they exist as molds at ambient temperatures but as yeasts at room temperature. Most fungi are obligate aerobes, and their natural habitat is the environment, the human host being the exceptional environment.

*Many fungi are **dimorphic**: they can exist as either yeast or molds, depending on the conditions in which they are grown.*

Cutaneous and Subcutaneous Mycoses

Cutaneous mycoses are fungal infections of the dead layer of the skin, the epidermis, the hair, or the nails. Subcutaneous mycoses are fungal infections of the subcutaneous tissue.

Cutaneous Mycoses. Dermatophytoses are chronic diseases caused by fungal infections of only superficial keratinized structures and include dandruff, athlete's foot, jock itch, and ringworm. The most important dermatophytes (i.e., fungi that cause dermatophytoses) are *Epidermophyton* spp., *Microsporum* spp., and *Trichophyton* spp. They are spread from individual to individual by direct contact. *Microsporum* spp., the causative agents of ringworm, can also be spread from infected pets such as dogs and cats. Heat and humidity favor these infections, which generally result in the formation of papules and vesicles, causing skin scales and thickened broken nails.

Dermatophytes grow only in the superficial keratin layer of the skin, using keratin as a nutritional source. They are not dimorphic and exist only as molds. Furthermore, they do not invade the underlying tissue. The growth of these organisms at the site of infection is normally inhibited by fatty acids produced by the sebaceous glands. However, when a disruption of this microenvironment occurs, fungi are allowed to colonize these sites. For most dermatophytes, the lesions (e.g., skin scales) that ensue are the result of an inflammatory response to the fungal growth. Alternatively, hyper- and hypopigmentation of the skin may also occur as the result of some fungal diseases (e.g., tinea versicolor and tinea nigra).

Sabouraud's agar is a solid medium that selects for the growth of fungi and selects against the growth of bacteria.

To diagnose the cutaneous mycoses, skin scales can be examined microscopically in a 10% solution of potassium hydroxide (KOH). The demonstration of hyphae suggests a cutaneous fungal infection. Growth of fungal organisms on Sabouraud's agar (a media that

TABLE 28-2 ▶
Summary of Major Fungal Pathogens

Major Fungal Pathogen	Distinguishing Biologic Characteristics	Reservoir and Transmission	Diagnosis	Treatment
Cutaneous and subcutaneous mycoses				
Dermatophytoses (*Depidermophyton*, *Trichophyton*, and *Microsporum* spp.)	Infect only superficial keratinized structures, not deeper tissue; cause ringworm, jock itch, athlete's foot	Spread by direct contact from human to human; *Microsporum* spp. can be transmitted by animals (e.g., dogs and cats)	Scrapings of skin or nail placed in 10% KOH show microscopic hyphae	Antifungal creams including myconazole
Sporothrix schenckii	Subcutaneous dimorphic fungi causing rose gardener's disease (a.k.a. sporotrichosis)	Spread by the subcutaneous introduction of these organisms into the skin, such as by the prick of a rose thorn; causes a local papule or ulcer	Round or cigar-shaped budding yeast observed microscopically in tissue specimens	Oral potassium iodide or itraconazole
Systemic mycoses				
Coccidioides immitis	Dimorphic fungus that exists as a mold in soil, but as a yeast in tissue; causes coccidioimycosis, (a.k.a., valley fever, or desert rheumatism)	Endemic to the soils of the arid regions of the Southwest (U.S.) and Latin America; inhalation is the major mode of transmission	"Spherules" filled with yeast endospores are seen in tissues examined microbiologically; skin tests with fungal extract result in a delayed type hypersensitivity response	Amphotericin B is used for existing lung infection
Histoplasma capsulatum	Dimorphic fungus that exists as a mold in soil, but as a yeast in tissue; causes histoplasmosis; produces a characteristic capsule	Endemic to the soils of the Ohio and Mississippi River valleys, particularly if these soils contain large concentrations of bird droppings; found within macrophages	Oval yeasts within macrophages derived from tissue biopsy specimens or bone marrow aspirates; serologic and skin tests also available	Oral ketoconazole is beneficial for progressive lung lesions; amphotericin B is the drug of choice for disseminated disease
Blastomyces dermatitidis	Dimorphic fungus that exists as a mold in soil, but as a yeast in tissue; causes blastomycosis	Endemic in North and Central American soils; spread by inhalation	On tissue biopsy, thick-walled yeast cells with broad-based buds are seen microscopically	Itraconazole and amphotericin B are potential treatments
Opportunistic mycoses				
Candida spp.	Not dimorphic, oval yeast with a single bud; part of the normal mucosal flora; the causative agent of thrush, vaginitis, and chronic mucocutaneous candidiasis	Only fungi of medical importance that are part of the local human flora, which explains why it is not dimorphic	In mucosal exudates or inflamed tissues, budding yeast with pseudohyphae are seen microscopically	Fluconazole for flush, nystatin for skin infections, and ketoconazole for mucocutaneous candidiasis
Aspergillus spp.	Not dimorphic, exist only as molds; causes aspergillosis	Widely distributed in nature and spread to humans by aerosols	Microscopic examination of infected tissue demonstrates molds with septate, branching hyphae	Amphotericin B is the treatment of choice, but not very effective

Note. KOH = potassium hydroxide.

is selective for the growth of fungi) can also be used to identify this organism. Prevention of the cutaneous mycoses can be accomplished by keeping the skin cool and dry. Topical application of antifungal agents (see Chapter 4) is effective in treating these types of infections.

Subcutaneous Mycoses. Fungi that cause subcutaneous mycotic infection grow in soil and on vegetation and find their way into the subcutaneous tissue after trauma to the skin. *Sporothrix schenckii* causes a disease that is typical of the subcutaneous mycoses. This dimorphic fungus exists on thorny plants such as roses and gains access to the subepithelial spaces through the prick of a thorn. The immune response to the growing fungi results in the formation of a localized ulcer. It is susceptible to antifungal treatment and can be prevented by wearing gloves while gardening.

Systemic Mycoses

In the United States, blastomycosis, coccidioidomycosis, and histoplasmosis are the major causes of systemic mycotic infection in the normal human host. These infections share several characteristics: (1) Infections occur in specific geographic areas where the infecting agents are found in the soil and can be aerosolized; (2) the usual portal of entry of these infections is the respiratory tract; (3) the fungal agent in each case is dimorphic, existing in nature as a mold with infectious spores and differentiating into yeast or other specialized forms in the lungs; (4) clinical manifestations and pathogenic events closely resemble those of tuberculosis, and asymptomatic pulmonary infection is common; and (5) an intact cell-mediated immune response is critical for control, and the absence thereof is correlated with a high risk for disseminated disease.

Blastomycosis. This disease is a systemic mycosis of humans and dogs that is caused by the dimorphic fungus *Blastomyces dermatitidis*. Blastomycosis is endemic in the southeastern and south-central regions of the United States, and several pockets of infection extend northward along the Mississippi and Ohio Rivers. Blastomycosis occurs in patients of all ages but is most often found in young and middle-aged adults. The incidence of this disease is more frequent in persons who spend extended periods of time outdoors. The natural habitat of *B. dermatitidis* appears to be the moist soil associated with waterways enriched with animal excreta. Primary infection results from the inhalation of fungal conidia (an asexual reproductive form of *B. dermatitidis*) that become airborne when soil is disturbed. The median incubation period between inhalation and primary symptoms is 45 days.

Coccidioidomycosis. This disease is caused by the dimorphic fungus *Coccidioides immitis*. This organism is a natural inhabitant of the soil and is endemic in arid regions of the southwestern United States. In this environment, *C. immitis* grows as a mold composed of a mesh of septate hyphae with alternating arthrospores and empty (i.e., containing no nuclei) cells. These arthrospores are readily aerosolized and can be infectious when inhaled.

Within the mammalian host, the highly infectious arthrospores mature into spherules, the definitive tissue pathogen. The spherules grow to 20–100 mm³; a mature spherule contains hundreds of endospores. On rupture of a mature spherule, endospores are discharged into the tissue and differentiate to form new spherules. In individuals with an intact cellular immune system, granuloma formation (see Chapter 22) effectively limits the spread of these organisms within the host. Infection of the lungs is often asymptomatic and is evident only by a positive skin test result (i.e., injecting a small amount of *C. immitis* antigen into the skin results in a local reaction) and the presence of antibodies specific for *C. immitis*. Some infected individuals have influenza-like symptoms, with fever and cough. About 50% of infected individuals have lung lesions that are visible on radiographs, and ~10% demonstrate erythema nodosum (EN) and arthralgia (muscle ache). However, in persons with deficits in cell-mediated immunity, dissemination throughout the body can occur, resulting in infection of almost any organ. These individuals generally have a negative skin test result and lack antibody to *C. immitis* antigens.

Diagnostically, the skin and antigen tests are the most useful means of detecting exposure of a healthy individual to *C. immitis*. Tissue specimens observed microscopically demonstrate spherules. Culture of these tissues on Sabouraud's agar incubated at 25°C

Sporothrix schenckii causes sporotrichosis, a subcutaneous mycotic infection that is an occupational hazard for rose gardeners.

Coccidioidomycosis is known as valley fever in the San Joaquin Valley of California and as desert rheumatism in Arizona. These two regions have a particularly high burden of Coccidioides immitis associated with the soil.

Erythema nodosum (EN) manifests as red, tender nodules on the arms and legs. It is the result of a delayed type hypersensitivity response to fungal antigens such as those expressed by Coccidioides immitis. EN is not specific for coccidioidomycosis; it occurs in other granulomatous diseases such as histoplasmosis, tuberculosis, and leprosy.

shows hyphae with arthrospores. No treatment is needed in asymptomatic or mild lung infection. Amphotericin B is used for persistent lung infection or for disseminated disease.

Histoplasmosis. This disease is caused by the dimorphic fungus *Histoplasma capsulatum*, which grows as a mold in soil in many areas of the world, particularly in soil enriched with the fecal material of chickens, starlings, and bats. In the United States, the endemic area is mainly the Ohio and Mississippi River valleys but also extends eastward into Virginia and Maryland. Disease occurs when fungus-laden soil is disturbed, thus creating an aerosol which contains infectious spores. Although histoplasmosis has long been associated with farming and rural activities, epidemic histoplasmosis is now being reported with increasing frequency among urban and suburban populations. For example, when the soil in and around a starling roost or accumulations of bat droppings is disturbed, large numbers of susceptible individuals are exposed through the inhalation of infectious *H. capsulatum* spores.

As a mold *H. capsulatum* forms two types of asexual spores: (1) tuberculate macroconidia, with typical thick walls and finger-like projections (this characteristic is important in the laboratory identification of this fungus), and (2) microconidia, which are smaller, thin, smooth-walled spores that, if inhaled, can establish an infection. Inhaled microconidia are engulfed by macrophages and develop into yeast forms. In tissues, *H. capsulatum* develops into an oval budding yeast found within a macrophage. Growing within macrophages, these organisms can disseminate throughout the body, especially to the liver and spleen. In most healthy individuals, the infection is localized by granuloma formation and most infections are asymptomatic. With intense exposure of healthy individuals (e.g., those working in a chicken house or a bat-infested cave), flu-like symptoms or a pneumonia may result. In individuals with severe deficits in their cell-mediated immune response (e.g., AIDS patients), disseminated histoplasmosis can develop. Among AIDS patients, early disseminated histoplasmosis is commonly manifested as ulcerated lesions on the tongue.

Diagnosis of *H. capsulatum* is made by the microscopic examination of tissue biopsies or bone aspirates for the presence of oval yeast within macrophages. Cultures propagated at room temperature on Sabouraud's agar will demonstrate hyphae with tuberculate microconidia. Serologic tests can detect exposure, and a positive skin test result against histoplasmin (a mycelial extract) is indicative of exposure but not necessarily of infection. As with coccidioidomycosis, no therapy is needed for asymptomatic or mild lung infections. However, if these infections progress to disseminated disease, amphotericin B is used.

Opportunistic Mycoses

The systemic mycoses described above can all cause at least mild infections in apparently healthy individuals. However, in many ways they can also be considered opportunistic infections because when the opportunity presents itself, as in a depressed immune system, these microbial pathogens usually give rise to more serious and disseminated fungal disease. The opportunistic fungi described below differ from the systemic mycoses in that they have worldwide distribution (recall that most systemic mycoses are endemic to a given area) and, under normal circumstances, do not normally cause disease. However, in individuals whose natural defense mechanisms have been disrupted, both local and disseminated infections may occur.

Candidiasis. This disease is the most common opportunistic fungal infection and is most commonly caused by *Candida albicans*. This fungus is the causative agent of thrush, vaginitis, and mucocutaneous candidiasis, among other diseases. *C. albicans* is part of the normal mucosal flora of the upper respiratory, gastrointestinal, and female genital tracts. When the host defenses are impaired, disease caused by *C. albicans* may ensue. For example, overgrowth of *C. albicans* in the mouth produces white patches and is commonly referred to as thrush. Disruption of the normal flora of the vagina may result from the use of antibiotics or by an impaired immune system associated with diabetes, resulting in vulvovaginitis. Mucocutaneous candidiasis occurs when fingers and nails are repeatedly immersed in water. This can result in thickening or loss of the nail. In immunosuppressed individuals, *C. albicans* can disseminate to many organs or cause chronic mucocutaneous candidiasis and endocarditis.

The diagnosis of candidiasis can be accomplished by the microscopic demonstration of budding yeasts and pseudohyphae (elongated yeasts that closely resemble short hyphae) in tissues or exudates. Cultures grow on Sabouraud's agar at body temperature or room temperature only as yeasts. Because *C. albicans* is part of our normal flora, healthy individuals uniformly have a positive skin test result for this organism, and a person who does not respond to this skin test is suspected of having an impaired cellular immune response. Treatment of thrush typically involves fluconazole, treatment of skin lesions utilizes topical application of antifungal drugs such as nystatin or clotrimazole, while the treatment of disseminated candidiasis consists of either amphotericin B or fluconazole.

Aspergillosis. This disease is caused by *Aspergillus* spp., particularly *Aspergillus fumigatus*. These organisms exist only as molds, that is, they are not dimorphic, and are widely distributed in nature. They grow on decaying vegetation, forming airborne spores. They cause infections of the skin, eyes, ears, and other organs. Because of their propensity to grow as molds, even at body temperature, within the lungs these fungi commonly cause fungus balls apparent on radiologic examination.

Invasive aspergillosis most frequently gains access to the lungs by inhalation; however, injuries to the skin may also introduce this fungus into susceptible hosts. On gaining access, *Aspergillus* spp. may disseminate to other organs. Quantitative and functional defects in circulating neutrophils are two important risk factors for the development of invasive aspergillosis. For example, neutropenia resulting from cytotoxic chemotherapy and systemic corticosteroids is a common predisposing factor for invasive aspergillosis.

Tissue biopsy specimens taken from suspected sites of infection show septate, branching hyphae when examined microscopically. Positive culture of these organisms on selective agar is not confirmatory for disease because colonization of the host is so common. A fungus ball present in the sinus or in the pulmonary cavity can be surgically removed, and antifungal treatment is then given. Invasive aspergillosis is treated with amphotericin B. However, because of the impaired immune status of the host, antifungal treatment for these diseases is often not successful.

Cryptococcosis. *Cryptococcus neoformans* is the causative agent of cryptococcosis, which commonly manifests as cryptococcal pneumonia and meningitis in immunocompromised individuals, particularly patients suffering from AIDS. This organism is an oval, budding yeast that is surrounded by a thick polysaccharide capsule. *C. neoformans* is not dimorphic, existing only as a yeast. This organism occurs widely in nature and thrives in soil containing bird (particularly pigeon) droppings. Human infection results from inhalation of the organism.

Cryptococcus neoformans breaks the dimorphic rule of fungal pathogens because it exists only as a yeast.

C. neoformans can be detected in infected cerebral spinal fluid (CSF) by mixing the specimen with India ink. Because the capsule repels the India ink, the yeast cell is seen microscopically surrounded by a round unstained area. Cryptococcal meningitis is treated with a combination of amphotericin B and fluconazole.

ILLUSTRATIVE PATHOGEN: *Toxoplasma gondii*

T. gondii is the etiologic agent responsible for toxoplasmosis. This is an obligate intracellular protozoal parasite of worldwide distribution that can infect nearly all animals, making it one of the most widely distributed eukaryotic pathogens, which explains why *T. gondii* is such an important opportunistic infection.

Biologic Characteristics

Although all animals can harbor *T. gondii*, cats are the definitive host. The sexual life cycle occurs in the feline intestine, leading to oocysts (the infectious form of this organism), which are shed in the feces. The oocysts are ingested by intermediate hosts (including animals and humans), where they develop into trophozoites. Trophozoites enter the circulation and gain access to body tissues, where they form a cyst. Acquisition by humans is by the ingestion of either material contaminated with cat feces or the cysts present in undercooked meat (pork, mutton, beef) of other intermediate hosts. The vast majority of *T. gondii* infections are inapparent; ~40% of the normal adult population has IgG antibody to *T. gondii* with no history of previous illness.

Reservoir and Transmission

As described above, humans typically acquire *T. gondii* infections by ingestion. These infections may also be spread transplacentally or via blood transfusion or organ transplantation. Ingestion of contaminated water has also been implicated as a means of infection.

Virulence Factors

Specific virulence factors expressed by *T. gondii* have not been well described because of the complexity of this parasitic pathogen. Clearly, the opportunistic nature of this organism implicates the importance of an intact immune response for preventing disease.

Pathogenesis

Digestive enzymes in the human intestinal tract liberate *T. gondii* trophozoites. Parasitemia results when trophozoites penetrate the intestinal mucosa and invade the bloodstream. Subsequently, trophozoites infect other organs and tissues, where they can invade and replicate in any nucleated cell. Eventually, the trophozoites may form cysts (encyst). Although encysted parasites remain viable for many decades, they are clinically silent, or latent. If the initial infection occurs during pregnancy, parasitemia can cause transplacental infection of the fetus. Although toxoplasmosis is extremely common, most acquired and congenital infections are subclinical and are revealed only by the presence of antibodies.

In the normal adult host, clinically apparent disease presents most commonly as lymphadenopathy. In some patients, fever, pharyngitis, hepatosplenomegaly, abnormal liver function, and atypical lymphocytosis may occur. Therefore, toxoplasmosis is considered in the diagnosis of heterophile-negative infectious mononucleosis, along with cytomegalovirus, various hepatitis viruses, and human immunodeficiency virus. Uncommonly, toxoplasmosis may cause meningoencephalitis, pneumonitis, or myocarditis in the normal host.

In the immunocompromised host, reactivation of either remote infection or primary infection usually manifests as a necrotizing encephalitis with either focal or diffuse involvement clinically. In AIDS patients, in particular, toxoplasmosis usually manifests as multiple brain abscesses. When primary toxoplasmosis occurs in the pregnant woman, the risk to the fetus depends on fetal age: ~10% in the first trimester to 60% in the third trimester. However, fetal infection acquired early in gestation is most likely to result in severe damage. Since the vast majority of cases in adults are asymptomatic, there is usually no indication of maternal infection until an infant is born with congenital toxoplasmosis. Even when acute maternal infection is diagnosed, treatment of the fetus is problematic because antiparasitic therapy is teratogenic.

Diagnosis

Because of the difficulty in culturing *T. gondii*, serologic testing is used for the diagnosis of toxoplasmosis. These tests measure IgG antibodies and are positive 1–3 weeks postinfection. Because positive titers persist for many years after exposure, a definitive diagnosis of *T. gondii* requires seroconversion, which is defined as a fourfold rise in antibody titer when compared with titers determined before the appearance of disease symptoms. In cases in which only post-symptom serum is available, a high titer (>1:1000) is compatible with acute toxoplasmosis. The complement fixation (CF) test usually reverts to negative 2–4 years after infection; CF titers of 1:16 are compatible with acute toxoplasmosis. The IgM fluorescent antibody (IgM-FA) test has proved very useful in the diagnosis of acute toxoplasmosis. IgM-FA titers become positive within 1–2 weeks of infection, however because these elevated antibody titers usually persist only for weeks to months, a single significant titer (>1:80) establishes the diagnosis of recent toxoplasmosis. The demonstration of trophozoites in tissues is diagnostic of active infection but this can rarely be accomplished except in a brain biopsy specimen examined by electron microscopy.

Prevention and Treatment

The prevalence of infection varies greatly in different population groups and geographic regions; most surveys suggest an increasing incidence of infection with age. In the United

States, serologic evidence of *Toxoplasma gondii* infection may be seen in ~50% of the population. Standard therapy for toxoplasmosis consists of a combination of the folate synthesis pathway inhibitors, sulfadiazine, and pyrimethamine (see Chapter 4). However, pyrimethamine is teratogenic, and there is no evidence that sulfadiazine alone is efficacious.

RESOLUTION OF CLINICAL CASE

Based upon the laboratory results the obstetrician concluded that the diagnosis was acute toxoplasmosis. This was consistent with the high titers (>1:1000) specific for *Toxoplasma gondii*, the lack of high titers to CMV and EBV antigens, the immunocompromised condition associated with pregnancy, and the mother's history of exposure to cat feces. The patient was advised that during the first trimester, there was a ~10% chance that the fetus had been infected and that if fetal infection had occurred, the outcomes might include fetal death, neurologic damage, and chorioretinitis. Since effective antibiotic therapy is itself teratogenic, the only sure preventive measure is therapeutic abortion. The patient elected to undergo ultrasound examination of the fetus immediately, and monthly thereafter, in a search for hydrocephalus, intracranial calcifications, and other signs of damage. No signs of fetal damage were detected by ultrasound examinations, and the patient delivered a full-term, normal infant.

REVIEW QUESTIONS

Directions: For each of the following questions, choose the **one best** answer.

1. A patient with hypogammaglobulinemia is predisposed to infection by which one of the following microbial pathogens?

    (A) Hepatitis B virus

    (B) *Clostridium difficile*

    (C) *Neisseria meningitidis*

    (D) *Treponema pallidum*

    (E) *Chlamydia trachomatis*

2. A 23-year-old medical student presents to the physician's office in Florida with a 2-week history of malaise, low-grade fever (99°F–101°F), and an intermittent cough producing some blood. He is a social smoker (2 packs per week) who spends his summers in free clinics treating migrant farm workers in the San Joaquin Valley. His human immunodeficiency virus (HIV) status is negative, and a recent tuberculin tine test result is also negative. Which one of the following infectious agents is the likely cause of this student's symptoms?

    (A) Atypical *Mycobacterium* spp.

    (B) *Histoplasma capsulatum*

    (C) *Toxoplasma gondii*

    (D) *Coccidioides immitis*

    (E) *Candida albicans*

3. A 12-year-old boy undergoes bone marrow transplantation for acute lymphocytic leukemia and is receiving extended treatment with corticosteroids. Two months after transplant, he develops a high spiking fever (104°F) and a productive cough. Radiographic evaluation reveals a well-demarcated cavity in the right middle lobe. Microscopic examination of the sputum reveals septate, branching hyphae. Which one of the following microbial pathogens is most likely responsible for this child's symptoms?

    (A) *Aspergillus fumigatus*

    (B) *Pneumocystis carinii*

    (C) *Candida albicans*

    (D) *Coccidioides immitis*

    (E) *Mycobacterium tuberculosis*

4. Toxoplasma encephalitis is most likely to occur in which one of the following patients and clinical scenarios?

    (A) A healthy adult who has a history of smoking

    (B) A sexually active high school student

    (C) A fetus that contracted the disease in the third trimester of gestation

    (D) A farmer from the Ohio River Valley

    (E) Migrant farm workers

5. Complications from burn infections are most likely to arise from which one of the following organisms?

    (A) *Pseudomonas aeruginosa*

    (B) *Haemophilus influenzae*

    (C) *Clostridium perfringens*

    (D) *Clostridium tetani*

    (E) *Neisseria meningitidis*

ANSWERS AND EXPLANATIONS

1. **The answer is C.** A high proportion of antibodies specific for the meningococcal capsule is correlated with protection from infection. Option A is incorrect because hepatitis B virus is not linked to the circulating levels of antibodies in serum. Option B is incorrect because *Clostridium difficile* is a gastrointestinal illness that occurs independently of antibody levels. Option D is incorrect because protection from disease caused by *Treponema pallidum*, the causative agent of syphilis, is not known to be dependent on antibody levels. Likewise, option E is incorrect because *Chlamydia trachomatis*, the causative agent of chlamydial infection, is not known to be dependent on antibody levels.

2. **The answer is D.** *Coccidioides immitis* is associated with the cough, fever, and exposure in the San Joaquin Valley. Option A is incorrect because the patient reported a negative tine test result. Option B is incorrect because *Histoplasma capsulatum* is a systemic mycosis associated with the Ohio River Valley. Option C is incorrect because *Toxoplasma gondii* does not cause the cough and associated fever described in the question. Option E is incorrect because *Candida albicans* infections are not manifested by the symptoms described.

3. **The answer is A.** The symptoms (high fever and cough) and the laboratory findings (radiologic evidence of a fungal mass in the lung, and the presence of septate branching fungi) are consistent with an *Aspergillus fumigatus* infection of an immunocompromised host. Option B is incorrect because *Pneumocystis carinii* causes a systemic mycosis and would not show hyphae in a sputum sample. Option C is incorrect because *Candida albicans* typically causes a cutaneous infection rather than a fungal mass, as was seen on the radiograph. The hyphae in the sputum and the radiologic findings also are not consistent with *Coccidioides immitis*, making D incorrect, or *Mycobacterium tuberculosis*, making E incorrect.

4. **The answer is C.** It is quite common for a fetus to contract toxoplasma encephalitis in the third trimester from a benign infection of the mother. Option A is incorrect because no relationship exists between smoking and toxoplasma encephalitis. Option B is incorrect because there is no relationship between sexual activity and toxoplasma encephalitis. Option D is incorrect because there is no known association between an Ohio River Valley farmer and toxoplasma encephalitis. Option E is incorrect because there is no association between migrant farm workers and toxoplasma encephalitis.

5. **The answer is A.** *Pseudomonas aeruginosa* is ubiquitous in the environment and commonly causes infections of burn wounds. Option B is incorrect because *Haemophilus influenzae* is generally a respiratory pathogen. Option C is incorrect because *Clostridium perfringens* is generally associated with foodborne illnesses or histotoxic infections. Option D is incorrect because *Clostridium tetani* causes deep wound infections. Option E is incorrect because *Neisseria meningitidis* affects the spinal meninges, not skin or flesh.

PART VII: VACCINE PRINCIPLES

OVERVIEW

PASSIVE & ACTIVE IMMUNIZATION

Immunization represents one of the most successful and important approaches to preventing infectious diseases. The two basic types of immunization used by public health officials are passive immunization and active immunization.

Passive immunization involves the administration of immune serum globulin (gamma globulin) containing protective antibodies. This approach is now successfully used to prevent or treat several illnesses (e.g., rabies). One potential drawback of passive immunization is that it may lead to serious hypersensitivity reactions, such as serum sickness or anaphylactic shock.

The likelihood of a serious hypersensitivity reaction increases significantly when the immune serum used for passive immunization is of animal (e.g., equine) origin. Therefore, it is preferable to use an immune serum (or purified antibodies) of human origin for passive immunization.

Active immunization involves the administration of a vaccine, a biological material that stimulates the vaccine recipient's own immune system to mount a protective immune response. The efficacy of active immunization is obvious: several devastating infectious diseases (e.g., diphtheria, tetanus, polio) have been virtually eliminated (at least in the United States) by universal vaccination. Besides protecting the vaccine recipient, vaccination sometimes indirectly protects unvaccinated individuals through the herd immunity phenomenon. Herd immunity develops when a large percentage of a population becomes immune to a pathogen, whether through vaccination or natural disease-acquired immunity. The presence of a large number of immune individuals in a population makes it more difficult for the pathogen to find a susceptible host, causing the presence of the pathogen to drop significantly, which in turn makes it less likely that any remaining susceptible hosts will encounter the pathogen.

PROPERTIES OF A USEFUL VACCINE

Despite the well-documented public health effectiveness of vaccination, the development of new vaccines lagged, for many years, behind the development of new or improved antimicrobial agents. However, a renaissance in vaccine research has occurred over the past 15 years. This revived activity in vaccine research was spurred on, in large part, by the increasing problems of treating infectious diseases resulting from, for example, antimicrobial resistance, and the high costs of some antimicrobial therapies (e.g., HIV chemotherapy). Already, a number of highly effective, new, infectious disease vaccines have resulted (see Chapter 28) from this resurgence of vaccine research, and a number of additional vaccines now making their way through the licensing pipeline are likely to be available in the near future.

What are the desirable properties of a useful vaccine? What are the general principles of vaccination? What types of vaccines are used in medicine? A useful vaccine should induce substantial, long-lasting protection against an important or common disease, without inducing significant side effects. Further, if the vaccine is to be used for universal immunization, it should be stable, relatively inexpensive to produce, and administerable in one or a few doses.

Unfortunately, vaccines do not always meet such high standards. For example, Chapter 29 discusses how the traditional diphtheria-pertussis-tetanus (DPT) vaccine has been used for many years, despite the fact that the pertussis component induces adverse reactions in many vaccine recipients. Public health officials have justified the continued use of this vaccine on the basis of epidemiologic studies showing that adverse reactions from the traditional DPT vaccine were less common and usually less severe than pertussis itself. Fortunately, a better pertussis vaccine is now available (see Chapter 29).

VACCINATION PRINCIPLES

A useful vaccine needs to elicit the proper type of immune response against the proper microbial antigens in the proper location in the body. For example, to protect against cholera (a disease involving a noninvasive pathogen that attaches to the intestinal epithelium and there produces an enterotoxin; see Chapter 23), a vaccine would have to generate a strong intestinal immunoglobulin A (IgA) response directed against both cholera toxin and adhesins.

Typically, humoral immunity plays a particularly important role in protecting against those bacterial illnesses that are primarily mediated by toxins (e.g., tetanus). In contrast, a vaccine often needs to induce cell-mediated immunity (perhaps together with humoral immunity) to protect against many other infections, particularly those involving intracellular pathogens (e.g., *Salmonella* spp.).

The age of the vaccine recipient is an important consideration for vaccination. Several pathogens show a predilection for causing illness in children and the elderly; these epidemiologic associations result, in large part, from the suboptimal functioning of the immune system in the very young and very old. In particular, young children have a difficult time responding to T-cell independent antigens. This limited ability is clinically significant because bacterial capsules, which are important virulence factors (see Chapter 18), are usually composed of polysaccharides. The fact that polysaccharides are typically T-cell independent antigens helps explain why many of the important bacterial pathogens in young children (e.g., *Haemophilus influenzae* type b, *Streptococcus pneumoniae, Neisseria meningitidis,* K1 strains of *Escherichia coli*) are encapsulated. This has an important practical consequence for vaccination; that is, while purified capsules can often induce protective immunity in older children or adults, such T-cell–independent vaccines do not work well in the young children who are at greatest risk for contracting the diseases caused by many encapsulated bacteria.

Fortunately, recent studies have revealed that covalently coupling a polysaccharide capsule to a T-cell–dependent antigen (such as a protein) converts that capsule to a T-cell–dependent antigen. Since even infants respond reasonably well to T-cell–dependent antigens, these capsular conjugate vaccines can be used in children as young as several months of age to induce a protective immune response against encapsulated bacteria. Besides lowering the age of vaccination, converting capsules to a T-cell–dependent immune response through conjugation also yields more desirable immune responses than can be obtained using capsules alone. Chapter 29 describes how the benefits of conjugating capsules to T-cell dependent antigens are now being exploited to produce new, highly effective vaccines that protect against encapsulated bacteria.

T-cell–dependent antigens generally result in better memory for the immune system and trigger a stronger secondary immune response on re-exposure to the antigen.

VACCINE COMPOSITION

Currently, licensed vaccines consist of several types of biologic materials: subunit vaccines, killed whole pathogen vaccines, and live vaccines.

Subunit Vaccines

Some vaccines consist of a limited number of purified microbial components. Bacterial subunit vaccines can be toxoids, adhesins, or capsules. Viral subunit vaccines typically contain protein subunits, which are often viral structural proteins.

Subunit vaccines are generally the safest type of vaccine, since no infectious pathogen is administered, and only a defined number of highly purified materials that are known to be nontoxic are included as components of these vaccines. Some subunit vaccines (e.g., the tetanus and diphtheria components of the DPT vaccine) consist wholly or partially of bacterial toxoids, which are purified bacterial toxins that have been altered (e.g., by formalin treatment) to lose toxicity, while retaining antigenicity.

Killed Whole Pathogen Vaccines

Some licensed vaccines (e.g., Salk polio vaccine, the pertussis component of traditional DPT vaccine) contain intact killed pathogens, either bacteria or viruses. Such killed pathogen vaccines are inherently less safe than subunit vaccines. Although these killed vaccines are noninfectious (if prepared properly), they often induce side effects resulting from their relatively "dirty" nature, that is, some toxic components may retain their activity in these vaccines even after the killing process, such as occurs in the pertussis component of the traditional DPT vaccine.

Live Vaccines

A number of licensed vaccines, particularly viral vaccines, consist of live microorganisms that have been attenuated for virulence, that is, the vaccine strain is less virulent than natural disease-causing strains of the same microorganism. Because live attenuated microorganisms usually persist longer in the body than either whole killed pathogens or purified microbial subunits, the immune system generally has a better opportunity to see and respond to live vaccines relative to other vaccines. This means that live vaccines can usually be given in fewer doses and with less microorganisms per dose. Further, live vaccines usually induce a stronger immune response, particularly a stronger cell-mediated immune response, than other vaccines. Finally, when live vaccines are used, there is potential for spread of attenuated microorganisms from a vaccine recipient to unvaccinated individuals, which improves herd immunity.

The most obvious disadvantage of live vaccines is safety. There is always the potential that a live vaccine attenuated for immunocompetent individuals may still be sufficiently virulent to cause disease in immunocompromised individuals. Depending on the genetic nature of the attenuation, there is also the possibility that an attenuated microorganism may revert to virulence, causing, rather than preventing, disease.

29 BACTERIAL AND VIRAL VACCINES

CHAPTER OUTLINE

Introduction of Clinical Case
Principles of Vaccinology
- Live Attenuated Vaccines
- Dead Vaccines
- Subunit Vaccines

Vaccine Administration
- Combined Vaccines
- Negative Aspects of Vaccination

Illustrative Pathogen: *Bordetella pertussis*
- Biologic Characteristics
- Reservoir and Transmission
- Virulence Factors
- Pathogenesis
- Diagnosis
- Prevention and Treatment

Illustrative Pathogen: Poliovirus
- Biologic Characteristics
- Reservoir and Transmission
- Virulence Factors
- Pathogenesis
- Diagnosis
- Prevention and Treatment

Illustrative Pathogen: Varicella-zoster virus
- Biologic Characteristics
- Reservoir and Transmission
- Virulence Factors
- Pathogenesis
- Diagnosis
- Prevention and Treatment

Resolution of Clinical Case
Review Questions

INTRODUCTION OF CLINICAL CASE

A 58-year-old American-born businessman was referred to an infectious diseases specialist because of an intractable cough. Five weeks previous he had developed a "cold," consisting of low-grade fever, a runny nose, and conjunctivitis, which had persisted for about 2 weeks. Just when these symptoms began to improve, the patient developed a dry, hacking cough. He experienced 4–6 episodes of coughing each hour, day and night, and was exhausted from lack of sleep. Each paroxysm (coughing spasm) lasted up to 5 minutes and was so continuous that it left him short of breath. Between episodes, he felt well except for a tingling sensation in the throat. Aside from the paroxysm, the physical examination was entirely normal. A chest x-ray was normal. A sputum culture was obtained for microbiologic characterization, blood was obtained for serologic studies, and the patient was started on erythromycin.

Arrangements were made with the microbiology laboratory to obtain a "cough plate" on Bordet-Gengou medium, which eventually proved to be negative. However, the patient's serum contained a high titer of antibody to both *Bordetella pertussis* filamentous hemagglutinin and pertussis toxin, as measured by enzyme-linked immunosorbent assay (ELISA). The patient slowly improved on erythromycin therapy.

- What etiologic agent is causing his symptoms?
- Should the patient be given an antiviral or an antibacterial drug at this time?
- What is the underlying cause of the patient's paroxysms?
- Could vaccination have prevented this patient's illness?

PRINCIPLES OF VACCINOLOGY

Table 29-1 summarizes the viral and bacterial vaccines that have been developed by traditional methods and that are currently approved for human use within the United States.

TABLE 29-1 ▶

Vaccines Approved for Human Use within the United States

Type	Vaccine
Live attenuated	
Viral	Vaccinia, yellow fever, polio (OPV), measles, mumps, rubella, adenovirus, varicella-zoster, rotavirus
Bacterial	Bacille Calmette-Guérin, *Salmonella typhi* Ty21a
Inactivated whole organism	
Viral	Influenza, rabies, Japanese encephalitis, polio (EIPV), hepatitis A
Bacterial	*Bordetella pertussis* (P), *Vibrio cholerae*, *S. typhi*, *Borrellia burgdorferi* (canine use)
Subunit	
Viral	Influenzavirus HA and NA, hepatitis B soluble antigen (HbsAg)
Bacterial	Capsular polysaccharide:
	Streptococcus pneumoniae
	Haemophilus influenzae
	Neisseria meningitidis serotypes A and C
	S. typhi Vi carbohydrate
	Polysaccharide-protein conjugate:
	H. influenzae type b (Hib)
	Acellular pertussis (aP)
	Toxoids:
	Clostridium tetani
	Corynebacterium diphtheriae
Combination	
Viral	Measles, mumps, rubella (MMR)
Bacterial	Diphtheria, tetanus, pertussis (DTP or DTaP)

Note. OPV = orally administered poliovirus vaccine; EIPV = enhanced inactivated poliovirus vaccine; HA = hemagglutinin; NA = neuraminidase.

Live Attenuated Vaccines

As mentioned in the overview, the immune response to live attenuated vaccines is long-lived and requires only a limited number of vaccinations. The disadvantage of this vaccine method is that live attenuated organisms can infect and cause disease, particularly in immunocompromised individuals. Also, they can spread to people who are not targeted for vaccination. This unintended spread may be a benefit if vaccination of other individuals by person-to-person spread can be achieved without illness, but it may be a problem if the vaccine causes disease in immunocompromised individuals.

Live attenuated vaccines can be obtained using several different approaches. One of these is prolonged passage of the microbial pathogen either in culture or in nonhuman hosts. For example, the oral polio vaccine (OPV, commonly referred to as the Sabin vaccine) was obtained after prolonged passage of polioviruses in nonhuman primates and in tissue culture. The bacille Calmette-Guérin (BCG) vaccine for the prevention of tuberculosis was created by passing a strain of *Mycobacterium bovis* on routine laboratory medium for several years. In spite of the marginal effectiveness of the BCG vaccine in protecting against tuberculosis, it is commonly used outside of the United States. It is not used within the United States because individuals receiving the vaccine test positive for the tuberculosis skin test (see Chapter 22). Public health officials within the United States concur that the benefits of this test for tuberculosis exposure outweigh the benefits afforded by the BCG vaccine and therefore do not recommend its use.

Another approach toward attenuation is exemplified by the recently licensed vaccine for the prevention of salmonellosis. *Salmonella typhi* vaccine strain (Ty21a) was generated from a wild-type strain grown in the presence of a specific mutagen. The resultant mutations incurred by this strain render it unable to establish a sustained infection but still allow it to evoke a vigorous and protective immune response.

Another means by which to accomplish attenuation is to deliver a pathogenic microorganism by a route that renders the microorganism nonpathogenic. For example, while natural adenoviral infections usually are acquired by inhalation, the adenovirus vaccine delivers the same pathogenic virus by ingestion. Given by this route, the virus does not cause disease but instead evokes a substantial immune response that protects the host from natural infection. Similar methods of attenuation have been used to create vaccines for the prevention of mumps, measles, and rubella that are now part of the standard childhood vaccine regimen. Most recently, this attenuation strategy has been applied to the current chickenpox (Var) vaccine.

Dead Vaccines

The alternative to a live vaccine is a dead vaccine. The primary method of creating a dead vaccine is through chemical inactivation and purification of subunits. The general properties of live versus dead vaccines are summarized in Table 29-2.

TABLE 29-2
Advantages and Disadvantages of Live Versus Dead Vaccines

Property	Live	Dead
Stimulation of an immune response	Effective upon a minimal number of administrations	Requires multiple administrations
Infectious nature of the vaccine	Infectious	Noninfectious
Incidence of adverse reaction to vaccine administration	Can cause infection in immunocompromised individuals	Common for certain vaccine formulations (e.g., pertussis component of DTP vaccine)

Chemically Inactivated Vaccines. A second traditional method for preparing a vaccine is inactivation of the virus or bacterium, which is generally accomplished by treating whole virus or bacterial preparations with a chemical cross-linker such as formaldehyde. Inactivated preparations of poliovirus (referred to as inactivated polio vaccine [IPV] or the Salk vaccine), influenzavirus, and rabies virus are in wide use. A drawback of many inactivated vaccines is that the viruses used were prepared from eukaryotic cells. For example, the early rabies vaccine was prepared from virus isolated from animal brain tissue. It was feared then that a cross-reactive immune response would be generated against host neurologic tissue because of small amounts of contaminating animal proteins found in the vaccine. These fears have now been mitigated by propagating the virus in tissue culture-adapted cell lines and by using highly purified viral preparations.

Whole-cell inactivation has been used in the preparation of vaccines for the prevention of several bacterial infections (see Table 29-1). Of these, only the pertussis vaccine (P) is in broad use, and this vaccine is associated with adverse side effects. Inactivated vaccines have several disadvantages: (1) the amount required to immunize a host is high relative to a live attenuated vaccine, (2) whole-cell inactivated vaccines have to be given repeatedly to achieve and maintain protection, (3) inactivation is a problem for gram-negative bacterial vaccines because a substantial amount of endotoxin is delivered as part of these vaccination protocols, and (4) chemical modification of the inactivated microbial pathogens can destroy antigenic epitopes that are critical for generating a protective immune response.

Subunit Vaccines

Td is a vaccine formulation that includes only the tetanus and diphtheria toxoids, as distinguished from the DTP or DTaP vaccines that also include a pertussis component. This vaccination is recommended to boost adults' immunity against tetanus and diphtheria as it wanes over time. It is recommended that Td boosters be administered at 10-year intervals to maintain protection against these diseases.

An approach known as toxoiding has been used for preparing vaccines against two important bacterial diseases, tetanus and diphtheria (see Chapters 20 and 23, respectively), that are mediated by secreted, enzymatically active exotoxins. Diphtheria and tetanus toxoids are prepared by formalin treatment of *Corynebacterium diphtheriae* and *Clostridium tetani* culture supernatants, which contain high concentrations of each exotoxin. This chemical modification inactivates the enzymatic activity of these exotoxins while preserving their antigenicity; thus, the term *toxoid*. The primary series of tetanus and diphtheria vaccination is administered in the form of a diphtheria, tetanus, and pertussis (DTP) combined vaccine as part of the childhood immunization regimen (see Table 29-3). After this primary series of DTP vaccinations is completed, it is recommended that the tetanus and diphtheria vaccine (Td) be given every 10 years. Toxoiding is an effective means of creating a vaccine and is largely responsible for the control of tetanus and diphtheria in the United States today. Unfortunately, this approach is confined to only a limited number of microbial diseases whose pathogenicity is mediated by a single toxin.

Fractionation of molecular determinants from a pathogen to produce subunits often achieves several important objectives: (1) it effectively disables the viability of the microbial pathogen, while preserving or, in the case of some capsular polysaccharide antigens, enhancing the antigenicity of these virulence determinants; (2) it allows the construction of vaccines containing only "safe" molecules that do not induce side effects; and (3) a protective immune response is engendered that uncouples the algorithm of transmission, colonization, and pathology that is characteristic of the infectious diseases.

Fractionation of viruses into molecular subunits is routinely used to generate a vaccine against influenzavirus (see Chapter 17). This vaccine contains neuraminidase (NA) and hemagglutinin (HA) components that are extracted from the viral envelope. This approach is also used for the vaccine against the hepatitis B virus (HBV), in which noninfective viral particles (HBsAg) are used as immunogens. As described in Chapter 10, hepatitis B is a viral disease transmitted through blood and body fluids. The risk for contracting HBV is greatest among health care workers, male homosexuals, sexually active individuals, intravenous drug users, and some ethnic groups and nationalities. Except for infants born to mothers with HBV infection, infants are not at great risk for developing this disease. So why is vaccination recommended for infants instead of adults for HBV? The answer is that attempts to vaccinate adults have been largely unsuccessful because it has proven difficult to persuade this at-risk group to take the vaccine. It is easier to reach children because vaccination can be tied to day care or elementary school enrollment. Therefore, for lifelong protection, the Centers for Disease Control and Prevention recommend that all infants be vaccinated before 15 months of age, in a vaccination series given at three different times in three different doses (see Table 29-3).

The ability to fractionate and purify capsular polysaccharides from those bacterial pathogens utilizing capsules as a component of their pathogenesis (see Chapter 18) has offered important contributions to vaccine development. Those bacteria for which a capsular vaccine is available are summarized in Table 29-1. As mentioned in the overview, the problem with capsular-polysaccharide-based vaccines is that, given alone, they are T-cell independent antigens. Children less than 2 years of age, who are in the process of developing a mature immune system, tend to respond poorly to these types of preparations. The relevance of this problem is perhaps best demonstrated by our experience with the *Haemophilus influenzae* type b (Hib) vaccine. Prior to administering the current version of the Hib vaccine in the United States in 1987, *H. influenzae* type b infection struck 1 child in every 200 before their fifth birthday. Of those afflicted, 12,000 children per year developed meningitis; 1 in 20 of these children died, and many other children suffered severe mental deficits, and infections of the joints, bones, soft tissues, throat, ears, membrane surrounding the heart (pericardium), and the lower respiratory tract. The polyribitolphosphate capsule was used as a subunit vaccine against this organism, but this vaccine did not protect infants from disease caused by *H. influenzae* type b because in this form it is a T-cell independent antigen. In 1990 the Food and Drug Administration (FDA) licensed the first *H. influenzae* vaccine effective in infants under a year old, the age group in which Hib infections are most damaging (see Chapter 7). The Hib vaccine is a conjugate vaccine that is made up of polyribitolphosphate capsular polysaccharide covalently linked to a protein carrier. In this formulation, the protein carrier directs T-cell help that allows an effective immunoglobulin G (IgG) antibody response to the capsular polysaccharide. The Hib conjugate vaccine is given in either three or four doses by the time a child is 12–18 months old. The implementation of the Hib conjugate vaccine has led to a substantial decrease in *H. influenzae* type b infections in the United States.

> *Hib vaccine is a **conjugate vaccine** made up of the polyribitolphosphate capsule associated with* H. influenzae *type b coupled to a carrier protein. Conjugation renders the carbohydrate, a T-independent antigen which is poorly immunogenic in young children, T-cell dependent, producing an effective vaccine that can be used in infants.*

Two other capsular polysaccharide vaccines in wide use effectively prevent disease caused by *Neisseria meningitidis* (see Chapter 16) and *Streptococcus pneumoniae* (see Chapter 18). These organisms are more prevalent in adults. Consequently, a capsular conjugate is not required to enhance the immunogenicity of these vaccines.

For many years, the whole-cell inactivated pertussis vaccine was included in the standard childhood DTP vaccination regimen. However, as described in this chapter, this vaccine was associated with adverse side effects. As a result, the acellular pertussis (aP) formulation, a protein subunit vaccine, was developed. This relatively new vaccine protects against whooping cough, a life-threatening disease, especially in children under 1 year of age. This new vaccine is made of protein subunits of the bacterium that are important for the pathogenesis of this organism. The general formulation of the aP vaccine varies depending on the manufacturer but includes purified pertussis toxin, filamentous hemagglutinin, pertactin, and other molecules referred to as agglutinins.

VACCINE ADMINISTRATION

While development of an effective vaccine is important, so is the ability to deliver these vaccines to the population at risk. In the United States, two significant populations most at risk for contracting serious infectious diseases are the very young and the very old.

One vaccine currently recommended for the elderly is for the prevention of disease caused by *Streptococcus pneumoniae*. This encapsulated organism is a common cause of pneumonia among the elderly. There are currently 83 different capsular types produced by this gram-positive pathogen. The current vaccine includes 23 of these capsular types, and it protects against 85%–90% of all *S. pneumoniae* infections. Pneumococcal infections among infants are also significant. However, the current pneumococcal vaccine is not recommended for infants because in its unconjugated form it elicits a T-cell independent immune response, which infants lack.

A second vaccine intended for the elderly and other high-risk populations is the influenzavirus vaccine. Because of the antigenic variation of this virus (see Chapter 17), annual immunization of groups at risk is recommended.

The near mandatory vaccination of children in the United States has virtually eradicated several diseases including polio, mumps, measles, tetanus, diphtheria, and Hib infections. The childhood vaccination schedule has changed in recent years and will continue to change as new vaccines are developed and as existing vaccines are reformulated. Table 29-3 represents the current schedule of vaccines that are recommended for children within the United States. One reason that childhood vaccination has been successful in the United States is the ensured compliance with these recommendations that is possible because almost all children are initially under the health care supervision of a pediatrician who administers vaccines. In addition, schools and day care facilities typically require up-to-date immunization records for attendance. A final element that contributes to vaccine compliance is affordability. It is estimated that the cost of vaccinating a child in the United States, as recommended in Table 29-3, is between $120 and $264. This cost is customarily covered by health insurance providers or any one of several social programs.

TABLE 29-3 ▶

Recommended Childhood Immunization Schedule[a] (United States, January–December 1999)

Vaccine	Age										
	Birth	1 mo	2 mos	4 mos	6 mos	12 mos	15 mos	18 mos	4–6 yrs	11-12 yrs	14–16 yrs
Hepatitis B[b]	Hep B										
			Hep B		Hep B					Hep B	
Diphtheria and tetanus toxoids and pertussis[c]			DTaP	DTaP	DTaP		DTaP		DTaP	Td	
***H. influenzae* type b[d]**			Hib	Hib	Hib	Hib					
Poliovirus[e]			IPV	IPV		Polio			Polio		
Rotavirus[f]			Rv	Rv	Rv						
Measles-mumps-rubella[g]						MMR			MMR	MMR	
Varicella[h]						Var				Var	

Note. ☐ = range of acceptable ages for vaccination; ⬭ = vaccines to be assessed and administered if necessary; ■ = incorporation of this new vaccine into clinical practice may require additional time and resources from health-care providers.

[a] This schedule indicates the recommended ages for routine administration of currently licensed childhood vaccines. Any dose not given at the recommended age should be given as a "catch-up" vaccination at any subsequent visit when indicated and feasible. Combination vaccines may be used whenever any components of the combination are indicated and its other components are not contraindicated. Providers should consult the manufacturers' package inserts for detailed recommendations.

[b] Infants born to hepatitis B surface antigen (HBsAg)-negative mothers should receive the second dose of hepatitis B (Hep B) vaccine at least 1 month after the first dose. The third dose should be administered at least 4 months after the first dose and at least 2 months after the second dose, but not before age 6 months. Infants born to HBsAg-positive mothers should receive Hep B vaccine and 0.5 mL hepatitis B immune globulin (HBIG) within 12 hours of birth at separate injection sites. The second dose is recommended at age 1–2 months and the third dose at age 6 months. Infants born to mothers whose HBsAg status is unknown should receive Hep B vaccine within 12 hours of birth. Maternal blood should be drawn at the time of delivery to determine the mother's HBsAg status; if the HBsAg test is positive, the infant should receive HBIG as soon as possible (no later than age 1 week). All children and adolescents (through age 18 years) who have not been vaccinated against hepatitis B may begin the series during any visit. Special efforts should be made to vaccinate children who were born in or whose parents were born in areas of the world where hepatitis B virus infection is moderately or highly endemic.

[c] Diphtheria and tetanus toxoids and acellular pertussis vaccine (DTaP) is the preferred vaccine for all doses in the vaccination series, including completion of the series in children who have received one or more doses of whole-cell diphtheria and tetanus toxoids and pertussis vaccine (DTP). Whole-cell DTP is an acceptable alternative to DTaP. The fourth dose (DTP or DTaP) may be administered as early as age 12 months, provided 6 months have elapsed since the third dose and if the child is unlikely to return at age 15–18 months. Tetanus and diphtheria toxoids (Td) is recommended at age 11–12 years if at least 5 years have elapsed since the last dose of DTP, DTaP, or DT. Subsequent routine Td boosters are recommended every 10 years.

[d] Three *Haemophilus influenzae* type b (Hib) conjugate vaccines are licensed for infant use. If Hib conjugate vaccine (PRP-OMP) (PedvaxHIB® or ComVax® [Merck]) is administered at ages 2 and 4 months, a dose at age 6 months is not required. Because clinical studies in infants have demonstrated that using some combination products may induce a lower immune response to the Hib vaccine component, DTaP/Hib combination products should not be used for primary vaccination in infants at ages 2, 4, or 6 months unless approved by the Food and Drug Administration for these ages.

[e] Two poliovirus vaccines are licensed in the United States: inactivated poliovirus vaccine (IPV) and oral poliovirus vaccine (OPV). The ACIP, AAFP and AAP recommend that the first two doses of poliovirus vaccine should be IPV. The ACIP continues to recommend a sequential schedule of two doses of IPV administered at ages 2 and 4 months followed by two doses of OPV at age 12–18 months and age 4–6 years. Use of IPV for all doses also is acceptable and is recommended for immunocompromised persons and their household contacts. OPV is no longer recommended for the first two doses of the schedule and is acceptable only for special circumstances (e.g., children of parents who do not accept the recommended number of injections, late initiation of vaccination that would require an unacceptable number of injections, and imminent travel to areas where poliomyelitis is endemic. OPV remains the vaccine of choice for mass vaccination campaigns to control outbreaks of wild poliovirus.

[f] The first dose of Rv vaccine should not be administered before age 6 weeks, and the minimum interval between doses is 3 weeks. The Rv vaccine series should not be initiated at age 7 months, and all doses should be completed by the first birthday. The AAFP opinion is that the decision to use rotavirus (Rv) vaccine should be made by the parent or guardian in consultation with the physician or other health-care provider.

[g] The second dose of measles, mumps, and rubella vaccine (MMR) is recommended routinely at age 4–6 years but may be administered during any visit provided at least 4 weeks have elapsed since receipt of the first dose and that both doses are administered beginning at or after age 12 months. Those who have not previously received the second dose should complete the schedule no later than the routine visit to a health-care provider at age 11–12 years.

[h] Varicella (Var) vaccine is recommended at any age on or after the first birthday for susceptible children (i.e., those who lack a reliable history of chickenpox [as judged by a health-care provider] and who have not been vaccinated). Susceptible persons aged ≥ 13 years should receive two doses given at least 4 weeks apart.

Unfortunately, infectious diseases remain a concern, especially among unimmunized infants. It is estimated that approximately 50% of all children in the United States are not fully immunized by the age of 2, and in some inner city areas only 10% of children have been properly immunized. Also, many infectious diseases of infants cannot be prevented by vaccination (e.g., pneumococcal disease, group B *N. meningitidis*).

Some vaccines are used in special, targeted populations other than children and the elderly. For example, the capsular meningococcal vaccine and the attenuated adenovirus vaccine are often administered to military personnel housed in crowded barracks where meningococcal and adenoviral diseases can flourish. Further, travelers going to areas in which cholera, typhoid fever, and hepatitis A are endemic often receive vaccinations against these diseases.

Combined Vaccines

Ideally, a vaccine should be potent enough to be given only once in an individual's life; this is unfortunately not the case for most current vaccines. Because patient compliance drops when repeated vaccinations are required, minimizing the number of these physician-patient interactions is an important factor in developing vaccine regimens. One way of confronting this problem is to administer vaccines in combinations. Two commonly used vaccine combinations are the measles, mumps, and rubella (MMR) vaccine and the diphtheria, tetanus, and cellular or acellular pertussis (DTP or DTaP) vaccines.

Negative Aspects of Vaccination

While vaccines afford tremendous benefits to our society, they are not without risks. Adverse consequences of vaccination associated with the pertussis, polio, and chickenpox vaccines have been known to occur in the past and are described in this chapter. So, how do we protect ourselves from vaccine-associated risks? The primary line of protection is government regulation. Like other drugs, any vaccine used within the United States has to be licensed by the FDA. This ensures that the vaccine has been tested and evaluated for safety and efficacy in the laboratory and in clinical trials. In 1986, Congress passed the National Childhood Vaccine Injury Act to help ensure vaccine safety and availability and to compensate people injured by vaccination. The act also requires that health care providers and vaccine manufacturers report certain serious adverse reactions they observe. The FDA and the Centers for Disease Control and Prevention keep track of these reports through the Vaccine Adverse Event Reporting System. The National Vaccine Injury Compensation Program also protects doctors and manufacturers from lawsuits. It is paid for by a tax levied on each vaccine sold for profit.

These strict safeguards allow for the development of the safest and most effective vaccines possible. However, even some licensed vaccines are controversial. In this chapter, three important infectious diseases—pertussis, polio, and chickenpox—are discussed. Both the argument for vaccination against the pathogen responsible for each of these diseases and the controversy regarding adverse consequences associated with these vaccines are presented.

> *MMR vaccine protects against three important childhood illnesses: measles, mumps, and rubella. These diseases are not described in this text because they are largely kept under control in the United States by the MMR vaccine. Mumps and measles are caused by closely related paramyxoviruses, ssRNA[−] viruses that contain an envelope. Rubella is caused by a togavirus. Togaviruses have a ssRNA[+] genome and an envelope. They replicate in the cytoplasm, not the nucleus.*

ILLUSTRATIVE PATHOGEN: *Bordetella pertussis*

Whooping cough, or pertussis, is a disease caused by the gram-negative bacillus *Bordetella pertussis*. Whooping cough derives its name from the characteristic "whoop" sound that occurs when the breathless patient rapidly draws in air following a paroxysm (spasm) of coughing.

Pertussis, once common in the United States, has been virtually eliminated in children by universal vaccination. While acute illness usually affects young children, there is a small but growing incidence of milder illness in adults. The illness of these older patients appears to result from the waning of vaccine-induced immunity.

Pertussis is often a severe illness in the very young. Periods of apnea (difficulty in breathing) occur in 40% of infants less than 1 year old. Pneumonia is found on chest x-ray in about 25% of infants less than 6 months of age but only in about 10% of children 1–4 years of age. In infected infants less than 6 months old, seizures that often lead to long-term neurologic problems are common. Among infants less than 6 months old, mortality resulting from a pertussis infection is approximately 0.5%. By contrast, aside from the prolonged period (up to a month or more) during which coughing spells continue to occur, serious complications in adults are not associated with *B. pertussis* infection. A striking feature of pertussis in young children is a marked lymphocytosis, which is absent in adults. In addition, as shown in Table 29-4, the characteristic "whooping" cough is more common in children. Although the number of reported cases of pertussis increased among all age groups during the 1980s, the most striking increases of this infection have occurred among adolescents and adults.

TABLE 29-4 ▶
Incidence of Signs and Symptoms of Pertussis in Adults and Children

Signs and Symptoms	Incidence (%)	
	Adults	Children
Protracted paroxysmal coughing episodes (worse at night)	100	100
Shortness of breath during coughing episodes	86	0
Tingling sensation in throat	86	0
Sleep disturbed by cough	57	100
"Whoop" sound with cough	7	40
Cyanosis with cough	0	40

Biologic Characteristics

B. pertussis and the closely related human pathogen *Bordetella parapertussis* belong to a small family of bacterial pathogens. Disease caused by *B. parapertussis* is rare relative to that caused by *B. pertussis*, so this section focuses only on the latter organism. *B. pertussis* is a strict aerobe with very specific growth requirements. Culture of this organism is typically accomplished by plating it on a rich agar medium such as Bordet-Gengou agar medium. *B. pertussis* is very sensitive to fatty acids and requires compounds such as starch to detoxify these fatty acids, so that it can grow. It also is very sensitive to chemical and physical agents in the environment and does not survive outside the body for an appreciable period.

Reservoir and Transmission

B. pertussis is thought to be exclusively a human pathogen. Unlike the closely related *H. influenzae*, which is routinely found as part of the normal mucosal flora (see Chapter 7), *B. pertussis* is rarely recovered from nasopharyngeal cultures of healthy persons. However, its definitive environmental niche has yet to be described. It has been speculated that the inability to recover *B. pertussis* from the nasopharynx may be a consequence of the ability of this organism to invade and survive within respiratory cells. This possibility requires further evaluation.

Virulence Factors

Virulence factors of B. pertussis:
- *Pertussis toxin*
- *Adenylate cyclase*
- *Filamentous hemagglutinin*
- *Tracheal cytotoxin*
- *Dermonecrotic toxin*
- *Lipooligosaccharide*
- *Pili*
- *Pertactin*
- *Phase variation and gene regulation*

Bacterial adhesins are associated with infection caused by *B. pertussis*. Like other gram-negative pathogens, pili are found on the cell surface of these organisms and are involved in bacterial attachment. In addition, pertactin, a protein associated with the *B. pertussis* outer membrane, is thought to participate as an afimbrial adhesin. The significance of pertactin for *B. pertussis* infection is demonstrated by the fact that purified preparations of this protein used as a vaccine in an animal model of *B. pertussis* infection offered protection from disease. In addition, filamentous hemagglutinin (FHA) is found on the cell surface of, and is secreted by, *B. pertussis*. FHA attaches to cilia by binding exposed lactose receptors on the host cell surface. However, the full role of FHA in the pathogenesis of *B. pertussis* is unclear. Like pertactin, FHA is significant for pathogenesis because the presence of antibodies against this molecule enhances the effectiveness of the acellular pertussis vaccine.

Many toxins have been described for *B. pertussis*. The most notable of these is pertussis toxin. Like several other exotoxins, pertussis toxin is organized as a characteristic 5B:1A subunit motif (see Chapter 20). However, the B pentamer of pertussis toxin is relatively unique since it consists of four nonidentical subunits termed S-2, S-3, S-4 (two copies), and S-5. As for the other 5B:1A subunit toxins, these B pentamers form the receptor-binding component of the pertussis toxin. The A subunit, designated S-1, traverses the plasma membrane after binding by the B subunit. Once intracellular, the A subunit adenosine diphosphate (ADP) ribosylates a critical cysteine residue on the G_i regulatory proteins involved in the control of host cell adenylate cyclase (and other host enzymes), resulting in increased intracellular cyclic adenosine monophosphate (cAMP) levels. These cAMP levels (and other effects) result in cellular dysfunction. *B. pertussis* expresses an adenylate cyclase that inserts into the host cell membrane. Interestingly, this toxin is activated by intracellular host calmodulin. Like pertussis toxin, activated adenylate cyclase increases the levels of cAMP within the cell. The increase of cAMP resulting from the effects of pertussis toxin and adenylate cyclase is associated with the inhibition of phagocytic cell oxidative responses (see Chapter 15) and the inhibition of natural killer cell activity. The dermonecrotic toxin is a high molecular weight protein that is not secreted by *B. pertussis* but is cell associated. Lysis of the bacterial cell releases this toxin, causing strong vasoconstrictive effects that may be important during the initial stages of pertussis infection. Tracheal cytotoxin is chemically related to a portion of the *B. pertussis* peptidoglycan, that is, the *N*-acetylmuramic acid–*N*-acetylglucosamine disaccharide and the tetrapeptide that is involved in the peptidoglycan cross-link (see Chapter 1). When this peptidoglycan breakdown product is incubated with ciliated tracheal cells in culture, the cells are destroyed in a matter of days. A lipid A-bearing lipooligosaccharide (LOS) is associated with the *B. pertussis* surface and has potent endotoxin activity.

Phase variation and gene regulation of many of these virulence factors are under the regulatory control of a single genetic locus that has been designated the bordetella virulence gene (*bvg*). This genetic locus uncodes a two-component regulatory system that allows for the expression of virulence genes in a coordinated fashion during the course of infection (see Chapter 24).

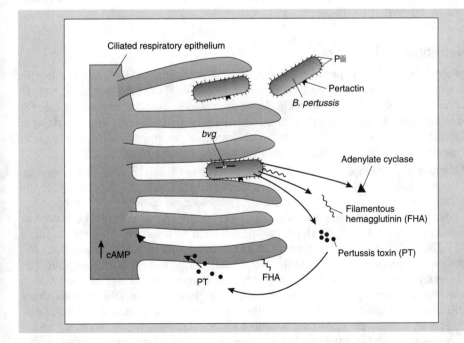

◀ **FIGURE *29-1***
***Pathogenesis* of Bordetella pertussis.** B. pertussis *attaches to a ciliated respiratory epithelium, using the adhesins pili and pertactin. Attached organisms secrete pertussis toxin (PT), filamentous hemagglutinin (FHA), and adenylate cyclase, which act on the host cell to cause pathology.* bvg = *bordetella virulence gene;* cAMP = *cyclic adenosine monophosphate.*

Pathogenesis

Upon gaining access to the respiratory tract through the inhalation of aerosol droplets from an infected individual, *B. pertussis* attaches to tufts of ciliated cells using pili and afimbrial adhesins (e.g., pertactin) [Figure 29-1]. This adherence may, in part, be effected by the synergistic action of FHA and surface-associated pertussis toxin, each acting as a bridge between a bacterium and a ciliary receptor. Once bound, these bacteria multiply on the surface of respiratory tract mucous membranes. After an incubation period of about 2 weeks, the *catarrhal stage* develops, with mild coughing and sneezing. During this stage, large numbers of organisms are spread by aerosolization, and the patient is highly infectious but not very ill. The *paroxysmal stage* follows, during which the cough develops its explosive character. Exhaustion, vomiting, cyanosis, and convulsions are associated with this stage. During the paroxysmal stage, *B. pertussis* is thought to deliver its repertoire of toxins, the activities of which produce many or all of the symptoms of pertussis. For example, lymphocytosis occurs when purified pertussis toxin is injected into animal models, and ciliary stasis (i.e., stopping the normal beating action of respiratory cilia) is consistent with the activities of adenylate cyclase toxin and tracheal cytotoxin. The necrotizing inflammation and leukocyte infiltration into the area of *B. pertussis* colonization is also characteristic of the congestion that is induced upon infection. The inflammatory response induced by LOS production also contributes to these symptoms. It is not clear which specific virulence factor causes the long-term paroxysmal coughing that occurs when *B. pertussis* can no longer be recovered.

Diagnosis

Pertussis should be suspected in any adult with a persistent cough lasting more than 2 weeks. The sensitivity of culture ranges from 15% to 80%, depending on when during the course of disease the culture is obtained (the likelihood of obtaining a positive culture is enhanced when using clinical specimens obtained within 4 weeks of the onset of symptoms). Appropriate clinical specimens for culturing *B. pertussis* include nasopharyngeal aspirates obtained using swabs containing dacron or calcium alginate (cotton swabs inhibit growth of *B. pertussis*). Direct fluorescent antibody staining to identify organisms directly in nasopharyngeal specimens has a sensitivity of about 60% and a specificity of 95% when performed by experienced personnel. Recent studies suggest that polymerase chain reaction (PCR) is 35%–70% sensitive and 87%–100% specific. However, as the disease progresses, the paucity of organisms makes detection by any method much more difficult.

Prevention and Treatment

Successful prevention of pertussis has been clearly demonstrated through effective vaccination of children using the DTP vaccine formulation. For cases diagnosed early in infection, treatment with erythromycin (for at least 14 days) is the drug of choice. For those individuals recently exposed to an individual with pertussis, prophylaxis with erythromycin is used. For patients intolerant to erythromycin, trimethoprim-sulfamethoxazole is an acceptable alternative for treatment or prophylaxis.

DTP Vaccine Controversy. The quality and acceptance of the DTP vaccine formulation have been variable, leading to a high incidence of adverse reactions associated with the inactivated whole-cell pertussis component of this vaccine. Several adverse reactions have been associated with DTP vaccination. These include minor local reactions such as pain, redness, and swelling. Systemic symptoms such as fever and fussiness occur in 50%–75% of DTP vaccine recipients but generally are self-limiting. Drowsiness and anorexia are also common. Persistent, inconsolable crying lasting 3 or more hours has also been reported after pertussis vaccination. Convulsions and lethargy have each been reported to occur at a frequency of about 1:1750 injections of DTP vaccine. Most convulsions are of short duration, self-limited, and usually associated with fever. Complete recovery from these convulsions almost always occurs, without persistent neurologic or developmental defects. These adverse reactions have been linked to the chemically inactivated whole-cell pertussis component of the DTP vaccine.

There has also been concern about the possible association between inactivated whole-cell pertussis vaccine and severe neurologic illness (including encephalopathy) occurring within 72 hours of vaccination in previously healthy infants. However, the risk of an association between this vaccine and neurologic illness is so small compared to the background rate for these types of events that no cause-and-effect relationship can be established. In spite of this, controversy regarding the safety of pertussis vaccine during the 1970s and the 1980s led to a large number of parents refusing the vaccine for their children. This in turn led to an increase in the number of pertussis cases. Because of these concerns, a safer, but more expensive, acellular pertussis (aP) vaccine has been introduced. Several epidemiologic analyses clearly indicate that the benefits of pertussis vaccination by either the DTP or the DTaP far outweigh any risks.

When pertussis vaccination is discontinued in an area, the incidence of pertussis increases markedly. In this regard, the DTaP vaccine is a significant development because it discourages adverse reactions.

ILLUSTRATIVE PATHOGEN: Poliovirus

Poliomyelitis (polio) is remembered by many as a frightening disease that was epidemic in the United States during the 1950s. According to statistics from the Centers for Disease Control and Prevention, more than 20,000 people—mostly children—were afflicted with this disease in 1952. The first symptoms of polio are a sore throat, headache, and a stiff neck. These symptoms can quickly progress to paralysis of the lower limbs and chest, making walking and breathing difficult.

Biologic Characteristics

Poliomyelitis virus (poliovirus) is a member of the Enterovirus group, one of five genera of the Picornaviridae family (see Chapter 3). The other virus groups contained in the Enterovirus group include coxsackie A and B, the echoviruses, and other enteroviruses. In fact, the distinction among certain of these viruses, such as specific coxsackieviruses and echoviruses, is so ambiguous that all new enteroviruses are now designated enterovirus and given a specific number (e.g., enteroviruses 68–72). All picornaviruses are nonenveloped, icosahedral, nucleocapsid particles containing ssRNA[+]. Once delivered into the cytoplasm, the uncoated viral RNA acts as a messenger RNA (mRNA) molecule and directs the synthesis of viral proteins (Figure 29-2). These proteins include the viral RNA-dependent RNA polymerase needed for replicating the viral genome, as well as the four structural proteins that form the capsid. All enteroviruses are sensitive to heat inactivation (50°C for 30 min) but are acid stable, thus surviving transit through the stomach to the intestinal tract.

Polioviruses share certain common antigens. However, due to unique neutralizing epitopes, these viruses segregate into three distinct serotypes; immunization to a member of each serotype is required to protect against poliomyelitis.

The Centers for Disease Control and Prevention report that an estimated 30 million nonpolio Enterovirus infections cause aseptic meningitis, hand-mouth-and-foot disease, and nonspecific upper respiratory disease annually.

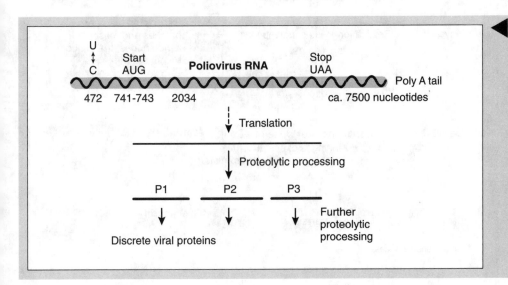

◄ **FIGURE 29-2**
Critical Sites on Poliovirus Genomic RNA Strongly Influence Neurovirulence. *A mutation at position 472 of the type 3 Sabin poliovirus, in which a cytidylic acid (C) replaces a uridylic acid (U), results in increased neurovirulence. To a significant but lesser extent, a base substitution at position 2034 resulting in a phenylalanine replacing a serine also increases neurovirulence. For types 1 and 2 polioviruses, amino acid changes in the proteins derived from P3 precursor proteins (not shown) also can influence neurovirulence.*

Because humans are the only reservoir for polioviruses, the World Health Organization (WHO) initiated a vaccination program in 1985 to eliminate wild-type polioviruses from the human population by the year 2000. WHO has made dramatic progress towards its goal; only 10 cases of polio are seen in the U.S. per year, all of which are vaccine related.

Reservoir and Transmission

Polioviruses naturally infect only human beings. Experimentally, other primates such as rhesus monkeys can be inoculated with resulting neurologic disease, which provides an animal model for studies of pathogenesis. Natural transmission is primarily by the fecal-oral route because, as the name implies, all enteroviruses grow in the gut and are excreted in the feces. Inside the home, fecal contamination of food and water provides an efficient mode of spread from infected individuals to others. Outside the home, prior to the introduction of vaccines, virus transmission was often traced to contaminated water in swimming pools or at public beaches. Shellfish (e.g., oysters), which filter and concentrate microbial agents present in water, may also play a role in the spread of enteroviruses.

Virulence Factors

Molecular biologic studies on the serotype 3 Sabin strain used in the live attenuated, oral vaccine revealed two sites on the viral genome that are major determinants of neurovirulence. A single nucleotide change can render a neurovirulent viral isolate attenuated (see Figure 29-2). For example, a mutation in the 5′ noncoding region of the virion RNA is thought to alter the three-dimensional conformation of the 5′ noncoding domain of the viral RNA. This conformational change affects the efficacy with which the viral RNA molecule can act as a mRNA. Another base change causes the substitution of one amino acid for another in one of the capsid proteins, influencing neurovirulence. The exact mechanism by which this mutation affects neurovirulence is unproven but may affect the efficiency with which the virus particle penetrates the cell or with which the viral genome is released from the capsid into the cytoplasm. Similar studies with poliovirus serotypes 1 and 2 have confirmed these findings. Other subtle alterations of the viral genome that influence neurovirulence of the serotype 1 and 2 viruses have also been identified.

Pathogenesis

After polioviruses are ingested, they initially infect the tonsils and other lymphoid cells in the oropharynx (Figure 29-3). Once swallowed, the virus survives the acid pH of the stomach and passes into the intestinal tract where it can replicate in lymphoid cells of the Peyer's patches in the lower gut. Replication also occurs in the intestinal epithelium.

FIGURE 29-3 ▶

Pathogenesis of Poliovirus. *It is noteworthy that most infections of nonimmune human beings result in an inapparent infection (90%) or a mild febrile respiratory illness with or without gastroenteritis (9%). Central nervous system disease occurs in only 1% of infected persons. IgA = immunoglobulin A; IgG = immunoglobulin G.*

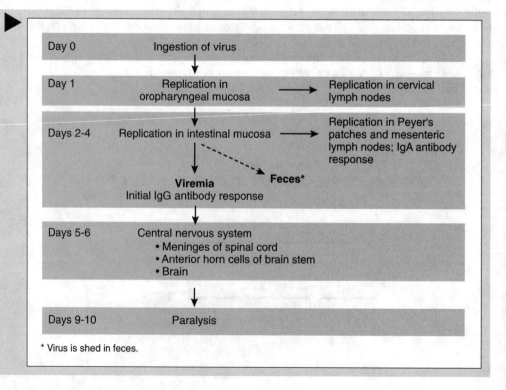

Day 0	Ingestion of virus	
Day 1	Replication in oropharyngeal mucosa	→ Replication in cervical lymph nodes
Days 2-4	Replication in intestinal mucosa	→ Replication in Peyer's patches and mesenteric lymph nodes; IgA antibody response
	Viremia Initial IgG antibody response ⤑ Feces*	
Days 5-6	Central nervous system • Meninges of spinal cord • Anterior horn cells of brain stem • Brain	
Days 9-10	Paralysis	

* Virus is shed in feces.

It is important to recognize that more than 90% of these infections are inapparent in nonimmune people. In about 10% of infections, the individual experiences the symptoms of a mild common cold, a relatively moderate gastroenteritis, or both. Because of damage to the intestinal lining, a viremia results. In 99% of infections in nonimmune people, the antibody response prevents polioviruses from gaining access to the spinal column or brain and no neurologic disease occurs. However, in 1%–2% of these infections, poliovirus particles cross the blood–brain barrier either by (1) growth in, and damage to, blood vessel cells or by (2) replication and spread via nerve fibers directly to the central nervous system (CNS). Cells may be infected in the spinal column, in the meninges and the anterior horn (aseptic meningitis). Virus penetration into the brain results in encephalitis, with virus growth confined largely to the extracerebral areas. Paralysis of autonomic functions including respiration may ensue. One of the most important features of poliomyelitis is the acute flaccid paralysis that afflicts infected individuals with CNS involvement. Because the spinal column and brain can be infected concurrently, severe cases of poliomyelitis take the form of a meningoencephalitis. It is noteworthy that many of the coxsackieviruses, echoviruses, and other enteroviruses cause a poliomyelitis-like illness.

Diagnosis

The presumptive diagnosis of poliomyelitis is based on clinical examination and epidemiologic factors. However, because other enteroviruses cause clinically similar diseases, it is not possible to diagnose poliomyelitis solely by its clinical presentation. Confirmation can be obtained by (1) isolating the virus (usually from the CNS or feces) from the diseased patient or by (2) testing acute and convalescent blood samples for a significant increase (> 4-fold) in antipoliovirus antibodies to one or more of the three serotypes, using virus neutralization or other serotype-specific tests.

Prevention and Treatment

There is no effective chemotherapy for enterovirus infection. Current prevention relies on two approaches. The first involves adequate sanitation practices, including the proper treatment of sewage and the availability of drinking water that is uncontaminated by poliovirus. The second is vaccination, using either an injected, enhanced, chemically inactivated poliovirus vaccine (EIPV) or an orally administered, live attenuated vaccine (OPV). Both virus formulations contain all three serotypes of poliovirus that are associated with the disease. The advantages and disadvantages of the EIPV and the OPV are summarized in Table 29-5. Since the development of the oral vaccine the incidence of polio has dropped to fewer than 10 cases (all vaccine related) annually within the United States.

IPV, developed by Professors Jonas Salk and Julius Youngner, was licensed in 1955 for use in the United States. This vaccine is administered by intramuscular injection and is commonly referred to as the Salk vaccine. OPV, developed by Professor Albert Sabin and generally referred to as the Sabin vaccine, was licensed in 1963 for use in the United States. OPV, generally accepted as the most protective of the two polio vaccines, carries a small risk for causing polio.

TABLE 29-5 ▶
Advantages (+) and Disadvantages (−) of Poliovirus Vaccines

Property	Live Virus	Killed Virus
Immunogenicity	+	+
Induction of IgA antibody in gut	+	−
Lifelong immunity	+	+[a]
Herd immunity	+	−
Safety (reversion to virulence)	−	+[b]
Ease of administration	+	−
Stability of product	+	−
Likelihood of contamination	+[c]	+[d]
Cost of production	+	−

[a] Requires booster shots at later times.
[b] Only the killed virus vaccine is recommended for older adults and immunocompromised individuals.
[c] Virus is made in human cells.
[d] Virus is prepared in monkey cells; future preparations may be made in human cells.

Polio Vaccine Controversy. In the last two decades the live attenuated vaccine itself has been identified as causing paralytic polio in a small number of children who received the vaccine and in a few adults who had close contact with recently vaccinated children. The risk of contracting polio this way is exceedingly low. This risk is greatest among people who have immunodeficiencies resulting from AIDS, cancer, or other diseases that make it hard for the body to fight infection. To prevent these rare but recurring instances of vaccine-associated poliomyelitis, the United States Public Health Service recommended in early 1997 the initial inoculation of young children (3 months old) with two sequential doses of EIPV vaccine followed by administration of OPV (see Table 29-2). The logic behind this is that vaccinees will benefit from the immune induction afforded by the EIPV without the risk of infection. Upon inducing an effective immune response, the vaccinees will be much better suited to receive the OPV and enjoy the benefits of long-range protection without risk. For nonimmune adults or immunocompromised individuals, only the EIPV should be administered because of the increased risk of disease from the live virus oral vaccine.

Although the modern EIPV does not appear to cause adverse reactions, at this time some public health authorities still recommend the OPV because it is more cost effective. The reasons for this are that it does not require repeated booster immunizations to maintain a high level of immunity, it is easier to administer than the injectable vaccine, and OPV spreads from vaccinees to unvaccinated individuals, helping to distribute immunity to the population at large.

ILLUSTRATIVE PATHOGEN: Varicella-zoster virus

Biologic Characteristics

Approximately 15% of the United States population suffers from herpes zoster (shingles) sometime during their life.

Varicella-zoster virus (VZV), a member of the Herpesviridae family, causes varicella (chickenpox) in children and herpes zoster (shingles) in adults. Like other herpesviruses, the VZV particle is composed of an enveloped icosahedral nucleocapsid enclosing a dsDNA genome. Similarly, VZV possesses the capacity to cause latent infections (see Chapter 3) and can specifically infect and become quiescent in regional sensory nerve ganglia. In most cases, the virus never reactivates. However, should reactivation occur, the virus replicates, migrates to the area of the skin enervated by that ganglion (dermatome), infects epithelial cells, and causes an outbreak of vesicular lesions (shingles).

Reservoir and Transmission

The only known reservoir for VZV is human beings. Transmission from person to person is the result of direct contact with infectious material from lesions by droplets, aerosols, or secretions from the respiratory tract. Clinical varicella can also result from intrauterine infection of the fetus. Congenital varicella syndrome is the consequence of prenatal infection in women infected during pregnancy. It is characterized by low birth weight, scarring of the newborn's skin, and a variety of birth anomalies including microencephaly, limb hypoplasia, and cataracts. Infection of pregnant women within 1 week of delivery is particularly dangerous because approximately 25% of these infants experience a severe case of chickenpox that is associated with a significant mortality rate. The contagiousness of varicella is of particular concern to hospitals (nosocomial infections) and other institutions, where patient isolation and special care procedures must be implemented should an outbreak occur. For example, a nonimmune child exposed to infectious material from an adult patient with shingles may contract chickenpox.

Virulence Factors

The capacity of herpesviruses to cause latent infections was described in Chapter 9. However, the viral genes responsible for herpesvirus latency and other aspects of herpesvirus pathology remain a mystery. What is known is that once VZV (and other herpesviruses) become latent, a restricted set of viral, non-messenger RNA molecules (referred to as lat [latent] RNAs) are synthesized in the nucleus from the unintegrated, plasmid-like viral genome. In this state no virus-encoded proteins are expressed; therefore, the infected cell is invisible to the immune system. The precise role of the lat RNAs in controlling latency remains obscure.

Pathogenesis

VZV is contracted via the respiratory tract, typically by inhalation of infectious secretions. VZV pathogenesis (chickenpox) proceeds by the virus gaining access to, and infecting cells of, the oropharyngeal mucosa, conjunctiva, or other sites in the upper respiratory tract. During this time, virus replication eventually leads to a viremia and infection of cells of the reticuloendothelial system. Despite an immune response, an overwhelming secondary viremia ensues, allowing VZV to spread to the skin where the characteristic cutaneous vesicles appear. The incubation period between exposure and outbreak of clinical chickenpox averages about 2 weeks. Over the third week or so, these lesions eventually dry, crust, and heal; however, the lesions are usually itchy and, if scratched or opened, they are susceptible to secondary infections by purulent bacteria such as staphylococci. If infected, the lesions may become pus filled (pustules) with subsequent scarring. Chickenpox is a common childhood disease that almost always resolves without serious sequelae. Despite this fact, in the United States about 40 children per year die from complications arising from chickenpox, including bacterial infections of the lungs (pneumonia) or brain (encephalitis). In addition, immunocompromised patients who contract VZV are more prone to develop potentially fatal viral pneumonia or encephalitis.

Herpes zoster (shingles) is the direct consequence of a VZV infection that may reactivate up to 40 or more years after the original viral infection. During latency, VZV is harbored in sensory ganglia such as the thoracic, geniculate, or trigeminal ganglia. Upon activation, presumably resulting from a deterioration of cellular immunity to VZV, the virus begins to grow. Newly synthesized virions travel antidromically down the sensory nerve to its endings and deposit in the skin. Before skin lesions appear, the patient usually experiences an acute neuralgia in the area where lesions will develop. Eventually, there is an eruption of vesicular lesions, usually confined to a particular dermatome. The role of a viremia in shingles remains controversial. It is noteworthy that the introduction of immunosuppression for a variety of medical reasons has markedly increased the rate of shingles.

Diagnosis

Chickenpox and shingles are diagnosed by their clinical manifestations, although the early neuralgia in shingles in the absence of lesions can be misleading. Once the clusters of lesions develop, diagnosis is usually straightforward. Although not routine, recovery of VZV from varicella lesions and the ability of VZV to cause a recognizably unique cytopathic effect in human cell cultures can be used to confirm the diagnosis. Identification of the virus can be accomplished using direct immunofluorescent antibody staining of the cultured infected cells. The two most common tests used to detect anti-VZV antibodies in patient sera are the indirect fluorescent antibody and ELISA tests, both of which are highly sensitive and specific. Other tests, such as radioimmunoassay procedures, are of equal reliability but require instrumentation and reagents that often are not available in the diagnostic virology laboratory.

Prevention and Treatment

VZV vaccine (e.g., Varivax) was first licensed in the United States in 1995 after extensive testing in Europe (1984), Japan (1986), and Korea (1988). It is an attenuated live virus vaccine intended for children 12–18 months of age; it is recommended for all children under 13 years of age. Recent evidence suggests that effective immunity is maintained for 20 years but the need for booster doses in adults requires ongoing evaluation. Adequate immunity is particularly important in the elderly to protect against shingles. However, the extent to which the widespread use of Varivax will impact the epidemiology of shingles remains to be determined. For immunocompromised individuals or persons exposed to chickenpox, passive immunization with varicella-zoster immune globulin (VZIG) is recommended.

Several antiherpesvirus drugs can be used to treat exposed individuals or infected immunocompromised persons. Acyclovir and famcyclovir (see Chapter 4) can ameliorate disease severity and mortality if given within 24 hours of development of the exanthem (rash). However, this is not a typical means of managing varicella disease.

Chickenpox Vaccine Controversy. The recently introduced live attenuated vaccine for the prevention of chickenpox is a double-edged sword. Infants often contract this disease from their older siblings or from their day care partners without demonstrating significant symptoms. The question becomes whether or not a reliable history of chickenpox can be established. If the parents suspect that the child has had chickenpox or are convinced that in the near future the child may contract this disease, they may deny or delay vaccination. It has been argued that because of this we may be lowering herd immunity (as described in the overview) and may in fact see an epidemic of chickenpox in our youth in the not so distant future. A second controversy about this vaccination is whether the administration of an attenuated vaccine affords the same level of immunity, over time, as infection by the natural virus. The concern is that a generation after this vaccine has gained acceptance, there may be an increased number of shingles cases because of waning immunity. One solution would be to require booster vaccination of adults.

RESOLUTION OF CLINICAL CASE

The patient was suffering from pertussis (whooping cough), which is generally associated with children but has been occurring with increased frequency in adults. If a vaccinated individual has an appropriately high immune response to this bacterial pathogen, they are generally immune to disease. However, if they have not been exposed to this pathogen since childhood vaccinations, their vaccine-induced immunity is lowered and they become susceptible to pertussis. This explains why the individual in this case contracted this disease. The initial symptoms of the catharral stage of pertussis infection are indistinguishable from other bacterial and viral infections. Because of this, it is impossible to know whether to place the patient on antiviral or antibacterial therapies. However, the clinical history and the patient's symptoms suggested that he was in the paroxysmal stage of a pertussis infection. The fact that *B. pertussis* could not be isolated from this patient on a cough plate is not surprising because these organisms are difficult to isolate late in the course of pertussis.

REVIEW QUESTIONS

Directions: For each of the following questions, choose the **one best** answer.

1. Which one of the following statements is most accurate about current strategies for creating vaccines against infectious diseases?

   (A) Live attenuated vaccines generally require yearly administration to an individual to establish an effective immune response

   (B) Toxoiding is used to convert an active toxin into an inactive toxin that is safe to use as a vaccine

   (C) Subunit bacterial or viral vaccines generally require a single administration to an individual to establish an effective immune response

   (D) Vaccination with a live attenuated virus or bacterium has proven to be ineffective in protecting individuals against infectious diseases

   (E) Inactivated whole-cell viral or bacterial vaccines generally establish a protective immune response on a single administration because large quantities of this material can be used to immunize an individual without concern for infection or toxic side effects

2. A 3-year-old child, whose parents elected not to comply with the current childhood immunization recommendations, presents at the emergency room with a distinctive rapid series of coughs and a slight fever. The parents report that the child demonstrated signs of an upper respiratory tract infection 2 weeks ago and that these symptoms cleared, except for the persistent cough. The parents became concerned when they observed the child experiencing a convulsion after a coughing episode. Which one of the following infectious agents is the most likely cause of this child's symptoms?

   (A) *Haemophilus influenzae*

   (B) *Neisseria meningitidis*

   (C) *Escherichia coli*

   (D) *Bordetella pertussis*

   (E) Varicella-zoster virus

3. Which one of the following statements is most accurate about vaccination for the protection against disease caused by poliovirus?

   (A) There is no effective vaccine for the prevention of polio

   (B) There are no health risks associated with receiving the live attenuated oral polio vaccine

   (C) When given as a single immunization, the inactivated polio vaccine is more effective at establishing a protective immune response than is the live attenuated oral polio vaccine

   (D) When given as a single immunization, the live attenuated oral polio vaccine is more effective at establishing a protective immune response than is the inactivated polio vaccine

   (E) Polio has been virtually eradicated within the developed world; therefore, there is no longer any need to vaccinate individuals against this disease

4. Which one of the following statements is correct about the current formulation of the varicella vaccine?

    (A) This vaccine is an inactivated whole virus that needs to be given only once to provide a protective immune response

    (B) This vaccine has proven to be protective against shingles, an adult form of chickenpox

    (C) Currently, this vaccine is administered to all children in the United States

    (D) This vaccine is part of the diphtheria, tetanus, and pertussis (DTP) vaccine

    (E) This vaccine has been shown to be effective in preventing chickenpox in young children but remains controversial because data are lacking as to its effectiveness in providing long-lasting immunity into adulthood

5. A small number of serious adverse effects associated with the diphtheria, tetanus, and pertussis (DTP) vaccine have been linked to the inactivated whole-cell pertussis component of this vaccine. This has led to the diphtheria, tetanus, and acellular pertussis (DTaP) reformulation of this vaccine. Which one of the following statements is most accurate about the reformulation of DTP vaccine?

    (A) The DTP vaccine was never proven to be protective against pertussis and has always been associated with significant side effects

    (B) The inclusion of the live attenuated pertussis component (aP) of DTaP has made this vaccine much safer to administer

    (C) The inclusion of the subunit pertussis component (aP) of DTaP has made this vaccine much safer to administer

    (D) DTP is an effective vaccine but is much more costly to produce than the current DTaP

    (E) Proper vaccination with the DTP vaccine, which in the past was given 3 times to infants within their first year, induces lifelong immunity against diphtheria, tetanus, and pertussis. The DTaP reformulation of the DTP vaccine uses a single immunization to achieve the same level of protection

ANSWERS AND EXPLANATIONS

1. **The answer is B.** Option B is correct because it is true that toxins that have been detoxified can make effective vaccines (e.g., tetanus and diphtheria vaccines). Option A is incorrect because live attenuated vaccines generally have the advantage of being given only a few times in a person's life. Option C is incorrect because subunit vaccines, like inactivated whole bacterial or viral vaccines, require multiple booster immunizations to establish an effective immune response (e.g., see the DTP immunization schedule described in Table 29-2). Option D is incorrect because live vaccines for both viral (e.g., polio, rabies, measles, mumps) and bacterial (e.g., tuberculosis) diseases are in general use. Option E is incorrect because inactivated whole bacterial or viral vaccines require multiple booster immunizations to establish an effective immune response and because products such as endotoxin can cause significant adverse side effects.

2. The answer is D. *B. pertussis* is the most likely cause of this child's symptoms since (1) the child may not have been immunized against this disease, (2) the child has a history consistent with the catarrhal stage of pertussis, and (3) the child is now experiencing symptoms (convulsions, characteristic cough, slight fever) that are consistent with the paroxysmal stage of pertussis. Option A is incorrect because while *H. influenzae* causes respiratory tract symptoms, it generally does not result in this characteristic cough. Option B is incorrect because *N. meningitidis* is not even considered to cause respiratory tract symptoms. Option C is incorrect because the characteristic cough is not associated with respiratory symptoms caused by *E. coli*. Option E is incorrect because varicella-zoster virus is associated with a characteristic rash.

3. The answer is D. In general, live attenuated vaccines such as the oral polio vaccine need be administered only a few times for an individual to achieve protection. If given as a single immunization, the live attenuated vaccine will be much more effective than the inactivated vaccine. Option A is incorrect because both the inactivated and the live attenuated oral polio vaccines are very effective at preventing this disease. Option B is incorrect because there have been a handful of polio cases linked to the live attenuated oral polio vaccine. Option C is incorrect because, in general, inactivated vaccines have to be given at multiple intervals to establish a protective immune response. Option E is incorrect because while polio has been controlled through vaccination, it has not been eradicated within the developed world and is still present in developing countries.

4. The answer is E. The effectiveness of varicella vaccine in providing long-lasting immunity into adulthood remains controversial. It is also controversial because many parents choose not to have their children vaccinated because they believe their children have been exposed to chickenpox. Option A is incorrect because the varicella vaccine is a live attenuated (not an inactivated) vaccine. What *is* true about this option is that this vaccine needs to be given only once to obtain a protective immune response. Option B is incorrect because this is a recently introduced vaccine, and data for the prevention of shingles, the adult form of chickenpox, have yet to be obtained. Option C is incorrect because this vaccine is not administered to all children within the United States. This is because of the perception by many parents that their children have been exposed to chickenpox, that chickenpox is a relatively harmless disease, and that this vaccine may not be as effective as the wild-type virus in providing lifelong immunity. Option D is incorrect because the DTP vaccine formulations include components to protect against diphtheria, tetanus, and pertussis.

5. The answer is C. The inclusion of the subunit pertussis component (aP) of the DTaP has made this vaccine much safer to administer while maintaining the effectiveness of this vaccine against pertussis. Option A is incorrect because the DTP vaccine is both safe and effective. While minor side effects are associated with the administration of this vaccine, the benefits of DTP vaccination far outweigh the consequent risk for contracting diphtheria, tetanus, and pertussis if not vaccinated. Option B is incorrect because "aP" does not refer to a live attenuated pertussis component but to an acellular pertussis component that consists of purified proteins that play significant roles during pertussis infection. However, it is true that inclusion of these purified components has made this a much safer vaccine. Option D is incorrect because the cost associated with a subunit vaccine is higher than that associated with a whole-cell vaccine preparation. Option E is incorrect because the current DTaP vaccine has to be administered on the same schedule as the DTP vaccine (see Table 29-2).

Diagnostic Medical Microbiology

INTRODUCTION

Diagnostic medical microbiology encompasses the detection and identification of bacterial, fungal, parasitic, and viral pathogens from patient specimens. The environment is full of both nonpathogenic and potentially pathogenic microorganisms, yet the vast majority of these microorganisms are not associated with infection. So how does one determine which of these microbes is causing disease? The answer to this rhetorical question is that dedicated medical microbiology laboratories identify the offending microorganism from the many microorganisms associated with the human body. The purpose of this appendix is to give a brief introduction to how a microbiology laboratory goes about identifying a microbial pathogen in the context of two specific disease states, pneumonia and urinary tract infection (UTI). For the sake of brevity, this discussion is confined to the isolation of pathogenic bacteria from relevant biologic specimens.

Classifying Microorganisms

Bacteria are broadly classified according to their Gram-staining characteristics and morphology. Within each of these categories, successive subdivisions are made according to various metabolic or phenotypic activities, such as growth in the absence or presence of a defined nutrient (e.g., oxygen, sugars, amino acids) or inhibitor (e.g., bile, colistin, vancomycin), motility, lysis of red blood cells, and many others. The system is "hierarchical" in that certain activities are given greater weight than others. The reasons for this are partly historical and partly practical; they involve, among others, a historical understanding of bacterial metabolism and the ease of carrying out the specific test. Since morphologic criteria were developed long before metabolic and phenotypic assays were understood, fundamental classifications of bacteria tend to be more artificial than evolutionary. More recently, genetic criteria (e.g., having a particular G + C content, the presence of a particular gene, or the similarity of ribosomal RNA sequences) have been useful in identifying microorganisms and in defining new microbial pathogens. In sum, the classification of microorganisms is dynamic and somewhat imprecise, but an important area of study in discerning the significance of an organism in the infectious process.

Choosing the Appropriate Specimen

An important first step in this process is choosing and obtaining an appropriate specimen that is enriched for the pathogenic microorganism. This relies largely on clinical symptomology. For example, if a patient is complaining of pulmonary symptoms, specimens such as sputums from the lung would be analyzed. If the patient is complaining of pain in the kidneys, urine would be obtained for study, and so forth. Upon obtaining the appropriate specimen, they are processed for their microbial content in one of three general ways—(1) by microscopically observing the specimen after staining; (2) by isolating the pathogenic microorganism in pure culture; and (3) by identifying the pathogenic microorganisms using biochemical, genetic, immunologic, or serologic methods.

METHODS OF IDENTIFICATION

Staining and Microscopic Observation

Appropriate staining of clinical samples or isolated microorganisms (see below) is arguably one of the most important tools for the immediate diagnosis of an infectious agent. The hallmark method for staining bacteria is the Gram stain (see Chapter 1). This staining is described in Table A1-1 and serves to discriminate gram-positive (purple to red-staining) from gram-negative (pink-staining) bacteria. In addition, microscopic examination reveals information pertaining to size (e.g., small or large), shape (e.g., bacillus or coccus), and cellular organization (e.g., occurring in chains, clusters, or pairs). This information is extremely important for identifying a particular bacterial pathogen within a clinical specimen.

TABLE A1-1 ▶

Gram Stain Procedure

1. With a sterile loop, place up to 3 drops of broth culture on a clean slide.
2. Spread the drop to form a *thin* film.
3. Allow to air dry.
4. *Fix organisms to slide by passing three times through a flame. Do not get slide too hot!
5. *Flood the slide with crystal violet for 30–60 sec.
6. Rinse with tap water.
7. *Cover with Gram's iodine and allow to set for 30–60 sec.
8. Rinse with tap water.
9. *Decolorize with alcohol.
10. *Rinse with tap water.
11. *Counterstain with safranin for 30 sec.
12. Rinse with tap water.
13. Blot dry and examine under an oil immersion lens.

Note. *Indicates basic steps of the Gram stain.

Isolation

With the exception of obligate intracellular pathogens, the spirochetes, and some species of *Mycobacterium*, most pathogenically important bacteria can be isolated on agar media.

Isolation on Nonselective Agar Media. Since many bacteria may be found in a specimen, it would be expected that several types of bacteria could be cultivated from a given clinical sample. For the general cultivation of most bacteria, media rich in metabolic nutrients is provided. These media generally include agar (acting as a semisolid support), a carbon source (e.g., glucose), and a degraded source of cellular material (e.g., peptone). Because of their relatively undefined composition, these types of media are referred to as complex media. Blood and chocolate agar are two common complex and nonselective media (Table A1-2).

Isolation on Selective Agar Media. Because of the sheer number of microorganisms that typically reside at the site of sampling, a complex array of organisms will likely be associated with these specimens (most of which would grow on nonselective agar). For this reason, selective media are used to eliminate large numbers of irrelevant bacteria from mixed cultures. The basis for selective media is the incorporation of an inhibitory agent that specifically selects against the growth of irrelevant bacteria. Examples of such agents are sodium azide, bile salts, colistin, and nalidixic acid. MacConkey and Columbia CNA agars are two common complex and selective media utilized in a bacteriology laboratory to isolate Enterobacteriaceae and gram-positive organisms, respectively (Table A1-3).

Streaking for Isolation on Selective and Nonselective Media. Obtaining bacteria in pure form is an important aspect of medical microbiology. This is typically done by isolating single colonies to which the microbiologist can readily ascribe observed properties to a

- *Sodium azide selects gram-positive organisms over gram-negative organisms.*
- *Bile salts (sodium deoxycholate and related species) select gram-negative enteric organisms over gram-negative mucosal and gram-positive pathogens.*
- *Colistin and nalidixic acid inhibit growth of many gram-negative pathogens.*

Blood agar

Trypticase-soy agar (trypsin-treated soy bean extract)	100 mL
Blood, defibrinated	4 mL

Prepare trypticase-soy agar. After autoclaving, bring to 45°C and add 4.0 mL of defibrinated sheep blood for each 100 mL of trypticase-soy agar; mix gently but well. Pour plates.

Blood agar is a rich medium used for the cultivation of fastidious microbes. It also is a differential medium used to determine the hemolytic phenotypes of organisms.

Chocolate agar

Pancreatic casein digest	7.5 g
Peptone (peptic animal tissue digest)	7.5 g
Cornstarch	1.0 g
Dipotassium phosphate	4.0 g
Monopotassium phosphate	1.0 g
Sodium chloride	5.0 g
Agar	10.0 g
Distilled water	1.0 g

Prepare sterile base. Add 5%–10% defibrinated blood and heat at 80°C for 15 min. Allow to cool and pour plates.

Chocolate agar is a rich medium used for the isolation of fastidious microbes. It is of particular importance for the isolation of *Haemophilus influenzae*.

TABLE A1-2
Composition of Some Common Nonselective Bacteriologic Media

MacConkey agar

Mixed peptones	20.0 g
Neutral red	30 mg
Lactose	10.0 g
Crystal violet	1 mg
Bile salts	1.5 g
Sodium chloride	5.0 g
Agar	13.5 g

Bring to 1 L in dH_2O and autoclave.

Mechanism of selection: MacConkey agar uses bile salts and crystal violet to suppress gram-positive and gram-negative mucosal pathogens while allowing gram-negative enteric bacteria to grow. Lactose-fermenting organisms form colonies that are visibly pink to reddish. Such organisms include *Escherichia coli*, *Enterobacter* spp., and *Klebsiella* spp. Bacteria unable to utilize lactose form colorless or transparent colonies; such bacteria include *Salmonella* spp., *Shigella* spp., *Proteus* spp., and *Yersinia* spp.

Columbia CNA agar (CNA)

Polypeptide peptone	10.0 g
Biosate peptone	10.0 g
Myosate peptone	3.0 g
Cornstarch	1.0 g
Sodium chloride	5.0 g
Agar	13.5 g

Prepare sterile base by the addition of water to 1 L. After autoclaving, bring to 45°C and add 40 mL of defibrinated sheep blood, 50 mg colistin, and 50 mg nalidixic acid. Mix gently but well and pour plates.

Mechanism of selection: CNA agar selects against gram-negative organisms by incorporating colistin and nalidixic acid in the agar.

TABLE A1-3
Composition of Some Common Selective Bacteriologic Media

single organism type. Consider the nature of a bacterial colony—in principle it originates from a single bacterial cell deposited on the agar surface, which has expanded by binary fission into a macroscopic colony, visible to the naked eye. So, how many bacteria comprise a colony growing on the surface of an agar plate? It takes as many as 1×10^6 bacteria to be seen as a single colony. Practically, with replication rates (such as *Escherichia coli*) of some 20 min per generation, it requires overnight incubation of most cultures in order to see a single colony. This can be exploited for the isolation of pure bacterial clones from a complex bacterial sample. Technically, however it requires both appropriate sterile precautions and a technique that appropriately dilutes the bacteria so that they occupy an isolated section of a plate. To accomplish this the procedure for streaking for isolation is generally employed (Figure A1-1).

FIGURE A1-1 ▶
Streaking a Bacterial Culture for Isolated Colonies

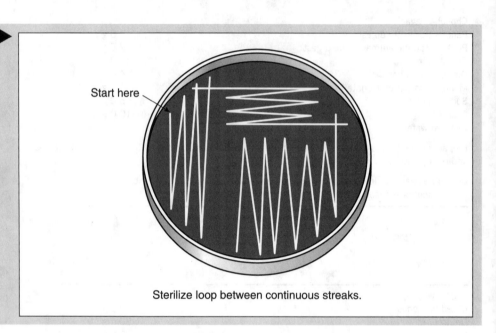

Sterilize loop between continuous streaks.

Biochemical, Genetic, Immunologic, and Serologic Methods

Upon isolating a bacterium isolated in pure culture, a variety of methods are used for its identification. Biochemical methods employ the ability of a bacterium to react with a chemical in a specific way. For example, the catalase reaction is a biochemical reaction that differentiates streptococci from staphylococci. Genetic methods such as quantitative polymerase chain reaction or DNA hybridization are commonly used to detect a specific organism. Immunologic methods involve using a specific antibody to detect the presence of an antigen on a target organism. These assays often use the format of enzyme-linked immunoassays (ELISAs). Serology measures the levels of preformed antibody in a patient's serum for their reactivity to purified antigens. For example, the test for human immunodeficiency virus type 1 (HIV-1) currently screens patient sera using an ELISA in which a specific HIV-1 protein has been incorporated. A positive ELISA requires confirmation by a more specific Western blot, a technique that separates proteins based on their size and then analyzes whether antibodies within the patient serum sample can recognize them.

EXAMPLES OF LABORATORY DIAGNOSIS

To illustrate the principles of diagnosis, two specific examples—laboratory diagnoses of pneumonia and urinary tract infections—are described.

Diagnosis of Pneumonia

When physical signs (e.g., cough, chest pain, etc.), radiographic findings, and case history suggest that a patient's illness may be pneumonia, the laboratory can play an important role in confirming this diagnosis. Traditionally, the first step in laboratory confirmation of pneumonia involves collecting a sputum sample. Sputum samples must be collected carefully to avoid heavy contamination by normal flora of the upper respiratory tract and to ensure that the microorganism(s) present in the lower respiratory tract are obtained. Therefore, it is essential that sputum be collected from a deep cough. Preferably, this collection is performed early in the morning, when overnight secretions are most likely to contain concentrated amounts of pathogens. In some cases (e.g., when there is little sputum, or when routine sputum collection has been uninformative), other collection techniques (e.g., transtracheal aspiration, bronchoscopy, broncheoalveolar lavage) are used to obtain specimens.

Once a suitable specimen has been obtained, it is usually first examined microscopically. The presence of elevated levels of neutrophils in a sputum sample is usually indicative of a bacterial infection. On the other hand, the presence of large numbers of squamous epithelial cells indicates that the sample has been heavily contaminated with normal flora of the nasopharynx and may be unreliable for determining what microorganisms are present in the lower respiratory tract. When a sputum sample contains elevated neutrophil levels, Gram stain of the biologic specimen may provide tentative information regarding the causative bacterium (e.g., the presence of large numbers of gram-positive diplococci in a sputum sample containing high levels of neutrophils would suggest the involvement of *Streptococcus pneumoniae*). When bacterial organisms are not found upon a microscopic evaluation of sputum, it must be kept in mind that several bacterial pathogens cause pneumonia (e.g., *Mycoplasma pneumoniae*, *Legionella pneumophila*) and that these organisms do not Gram stain. Further, if tuberculosis is considered a possibility, acid-fast staining of sputum should also be performed.

To confirm suspicions provided by microscopic examination of sputum from patients with suspected bacterial pneumonia isolation is usually essential. Specimens are typically cultured on several media, including blood agar plates, MacConkey agar, and chocolate agar. Depending on the results obtained from these cultures, further tests (e.g., determining optochin sensitivity if *S. pneumoniae* is suspected) can be performed to precisely identify the causative bacterial pathogen. Similar approaches can be used to identify fungal causes of pneumonia. Recovery of dimorphic fungi from sputum samples is usually informative, but several positive cultures of ubiquitous fungi such as *Aspergillus* must be obtained before these findings can be considered informative. If the patient produces limited sputum, this may indicate a viral pneumonia. Specimens can be cultured on tissue culture cells and/or subjected to serologic tests (e.g., specific ELISAs) to attempt to identify the responsible virus.

Diagnosis of Urinary Tract Infections

Urinary tract infections (UTIs) represent the most common genitourinary disease in children and adults. Critical to the diagnosis of UTI is a bacterial culture showing a significant number of bacteria, fungi, or virus particles. This is generally performed using quantitative culture on selective and nonselective agar. Bladder urine is normally sterile, but during the act of voiding, the urine can be contaminated from the anterior urethra, vagina, or surrounding structures. Thus, bacteriuria (i.e., bacteria growing within the urine) is defined as the presence in voided urine of pathogenic organisms in quantities that exceed those commonly caused by contamination. This usually means a culture of voided urine containing >100,000 colony-forming units (cfu) per mL. In general, if a single voiding shows 10^5 cfu/mL, there is an 80% chance of clinical disease. If a sample contains <10^4 cfu/mL, there is a very low probability that the patient has UTI. Because bacteriuria is used as evidence of UTI, methods of collection, transport, and subsequent handling of the urine specimen can significantly affect the culture results. Methods other than quantitative laboratory culture can be used to demonstrate bacteriuria. For example, examination of fresh uncentrifuged urine for bacteria can be used. A finding of even one bacterium per high-power field corresponds to 10^5 bacteria per mL and thus strongly suggests UTI. A high concentration of protein and a low glucose content may also be indicative of a UTI.

Escherichia coli is the most common organism causing UTI, accounting for >80% of first infections and 75% of recurrences. Only a small number of the known *E. coli* serotypes cause two-thirds of all *E. coli* UTIs. Other gram-negative organisms, such as *Klebsiella*, *Enterobacter*, *Proteus*, and *Pseudomonas*, are frequently seen in complicated or recurrent infections, and they account for about 10% to 15% of UTIs. Therefore, MacConkey agar is often used for their isolation. Although they are frequently considered contaminants, staphylococci have been responsible for UTIs as have *Clostridium perfringens*; *Bacteroides* and *Fusobacterium* spp. are usually found with obstruction and urinary stasis. Because of this culture on nonselective agar, anaerobic culture must also be considered. In addition, *Mycobacterium tuberculosis* and various fungi and yeasts are occasional causes of UTIs.

Control of Pathogens by Sterilization, Pasteurization, and Disinfection

Sterilization, pasteurization, and disinfection are three important processes used to protect humans from the many potentially pathogenic microorganisms that are ubiquitous in our environment.

Sterilization completely kills or removes (e.g., by filtration) all microorganisms from a particular material. For example, many medical instruments and supplies (including all surgical instruments) are routinely sterilized to prevent the introduction of microorganisms into the body during medical procedures. Commonly used sterilization techniques and their applications are listed below.

TABLE A2-1
Commonly Used Sterilization Methods

Technique	Example of Application
Autoclaving (moist heat)	Surgical dressings and instruments
Dry heat	Glassware
Ionizing radiation	Single-use disposable equipment (e.g., plastic syringes)
Ultraviolet light	Air sterilization at critical hospital sites
Ethylene oxide	Fragile, heat-sensitive instruments
Filtration	Heat-sensitive pharmaceuticals, air (e.g., some operating rooms)

Pasteurization is the process whereby materials (usually liquids) are heated to temperatures between approximately 55°–75°C in order to kill important pathogens; however, pasteurized materials are not necessarily sterile; for instance, bacterial spores may remain viable in pasteurized material. Pasteurization is particularly useful for heat-sensitive materials that cannot be acceptably sterilized. For example, sterilization of large quantities of milk is difficult to achieve without unacceptable loss of flavor, but pasteurized milk is free of important pathogens and retains its flavor.

Disinfection results in the killing of many, but not all, pathogens. Disinfection is usually achieved using chemical agents called disinfectants. It is important to appreciate that not all disinfectants work equally well against all pathogens; for example, mycobacteria (due to their waxy coat), bacterial spores, and some viruses are relatively resistant to many disinfectants. An *antiseptic* is a disinfectant that can safely be applied to surfaces of the human body to reduce numbers of microbial pathogens. Some commonly used disinfectants and antiseptics are listed in Table A2-2.

TABLE A2-2 ▶

Examples of Commonly Used Disinfectants and Antiseptics

Agent	Example	Uses
Phenols	Hexachlorophene, chlorhexidine	Environmental decontamination, mouthwashes, sore throat remedies, skin antiseptic
Halogens	Iodine, chlorine	Skin antiseptic, decontamination of glassware or other materials contaminated with difficult to kill pathogens (e.g., viruses, bacterial spores); water treatment
Alcohols	Ethanol (70%–90%), isopropyl alcohol (90%–95%)	Skin antiseptic
Surfactants	Quaternary ammonium compounds (e.g., benzalkonium chloride)	Skin antiseptic, general disinfectant
Aldehydes	Formaldehyde, glutaraldehyde	Effective sterilization of medical instruments

Table: Review of Medically Important Pathogens

This table (which begins on the following page) serves several purposes: (1) it provides a taxonomic organization of medically important microbial pathogens for those who prefer the traditional approach rather than a principles-oriented approach; (2) it presents information about some microbial pathogens not covered in the text; and (3) it provides a source for quick information about microbial pathogens, the disease(s) they cause, their notable characteristics, their reservoir and transmission, their virulence factors, and their vaccine status. A list of abbreviations used in the table is presented below for your convenience.

ARD	acute respiratory disease
BCG	the bacille Calmette-Guérin strain of mycobacteria that is used as a live, attenuated vaccine
CAMP test	a pattern of growth on specialized media
CF	cystic fibrosis
CFA	colonization factor of adherence
CID	cytomegalic inclusion disease
CMV	cytomegalovirus
CT	cholera toxin
DGI	disseminated gonococcal infection
DTH	delayed-type hypersensitivity
EBV	Epstein-Barr virus
FHA	filamentous hemagglutinin
gp120	major surface glycoprotein of HIV-1 virion
HA	hemagglutinin
HBsAg	hepatitis B surface antigen
HHV	human herpes virus
HSV	herpes simplex virus
JC	Jakob-Creutzfeldt disease
KOH	potassium hydroxide
LT	heat-labile enterotoxin
MHC	major histocompatibility complex
Mip	macrophage infectivity potentiator
NA	neuraminidase
NSP4	a rotaviral nonstructural protein
OSPs	outer surface proteins
PCP	*Pneumocystis carinii* pneumonia
PID	pelvic inflammatory disease
SSPE	subacute sclerosing panencephalitis
STa	heat-stable enterotoxin
STD	sexually transmitted disease
Stx	shiga toxin
TAT	trans-activator of transcription
TCP	toxin coregulated pili
TSST	toxic shock syndrome toxin
UTI	urinary tract infection
VZV	varicella-zoster virus
Yops	*Yersinia* outer membrane proteins

Pathogen	Disease(s)	Notable Characteristics	Reservoir/ Transmission	Virulence Factors	Vaccine Status
BACTERIA					
Gram-negative cocci					
Moraxella catarrhalis	Sinusitis; otitis; bronchitis; pneumonia	Considered normal flora	Humans/spread by aerosols	Endotoxin; most produce β-lactamase	None indicated
Neisseria gonorrhoeae	Urethritis; salpingitis; pharyngitis; PID; DGI; arthritis	Diplococci; oxidase-positive; does not ferment maltose	Humans; 5% males and 30% females are asymptomatic/spread by sexual contact	Pili; afimbrial adhesins; endotoxin; antigenic variation; IgA protease; natural transformation; transferrin-binding proteins; some produce β-lactamase	Indicated, not available
Neisseria meningitidis	Septicemia; meningitis	Diplococci; oxidase-positive; ferments maltose	Humans; maintained in population by asymptomatic carrier state/spread through inhalation; rarely causes disease	Weakly immunogenic capsule; endotoxin; pili; afimbrial adhesins; IgA1 protease; natural transformation; transferrin-binding proteins	Indicated, available for most common serogroups (A, C, Y, and W-135), except serogroup B
Gram-negative coccobacilli					
Bartonella	Emerging pathogen causing cat-scratch fever in immuno-competent individuals and bacillary angiomatosis (in immunocompromised individuals)	Pleomorphic rods; fastidious growth requirements (requires blood for growth)	Animals; associated with oral flora of cats/spread by the bite or scratch of an animal	Endotoxin	None indicated
Bordetella pertussis	Whooping cough	Small; encapsulated; pleomorphic rod; grows on Bordet-Gengou medium	Humans/spread through inhalation	Endotoxin; FHA; pertussis toxin; adenylate cyclase; tracheal cytotoxin	Indicated; "P" component of the DPT vaccine; vaccine very effective and in broad use; now an acellular version (D$_a$PT)
Campylobacter intestinalis (also known as *C. fetus*)	Infrequent pathogen causing enterocolitis in children; bacteremia can ensue	Motile; small; comma-shaped rods; oxidase-positive; urease-negative; microaerophilic	Domestic animals (cows, chickens, dogs)/spread by ingestion of contaminated food products	Endotoxin; probably involves inflammation from invasion (an enterotoxin may play a role)	None indicated
Campylobacter jejuni	Enterocolitis in adults and children; can cause bacteremia; major cause of diarrhea in the U.S.	Motile; small; comma-shaped rods; oxidase-positive; urease-negative; microaerophilic; grows at either 25°C or 42°C	Domestic animals (cows, chickens, dogs)/spread by ingestion of contaminated food products	Endotoxin; disease suspected to be associated with yet undefined enterotoxin	None indicated

Organism	Disease	Characteristics	Epidemiology/Transmission	Virulence Factors	Vaccine
Francisella tularensis	Tularemia; infrequent zoonotic infection	Small; pleomorphic rod	Enzootic (i.e., endemic to animals)/spread to humans by arthropod transmission; human-to-human spread does not occur	Endotoxin; mode of entry into host profoundly influences disease manifestations	None indicated
Haemophilus aegyptius	Infrequent pathogen causing Brazilian purpuric fever	Small; coccobacilli; fastidious growth requirements	Humans/transmission pattern poorly understood	Endotoxin	None indicated
Haemophilus ducreyi	Chancroid, an infrequent STD	Small; coccobacilli; fastidious growth requirements	Sexually transmitted	Endotoxin	None indicated
Haemophilus influenzae	Meningitis; epiglottitis; sinusitis; otitis media	Small; coccobacilli; fastidious growth requirements on chocolate agar in order to supply NAD (factor X) and heme (factor V) for growth	Human nasopharynx/transmission occurs between humans	Weakly immunogenic capsule; pili; afimbrial adhesins; IgA1 protease; natural transformation; transferrin-binding proteins; endotoxin	Indicated, Hib vaccine, a protein-carbohydrate conjugate administered to infants
Helicobacter pylori	Gastritis; peptic ulcers; cancer	Small; motile; comma-shaped rods; oxidase-positive; urease-positive; microaerophilic	Human stomach/clustering of disease within families suggests transmission between humans	Urease production may result in mutagenic free radical generation, giving rise to tissue toxicity or the generation of carcinoma; endotoxin	Indicated, not available
Kingella kingae	Opportunistic infection causing infrequent bacterial vaginitis	Rod; fastidious	Human pharnyx, vaginal flora/human-to-human transmission	Endotoxin	None indicated
Bacteroides spp.	Opportunistic anaerobic infections including sepsis, peritonitis, abscesses	Anaerobic; non-spore-forming; *B. fragilis* is the most common species associated with disease	Endogenous to humans; predominant organism in the human colon; also found in vaginal tract and oral cavity/not considered communicable	Polysaccharide capsule; endotoxin; a few strains produce exotoxins; commonly antibiotic resistant	None indicated
Fusobacterium spp.	Opportunistic mixed anaerobic infections; also isolated from pulmonary, intra-abdominal, and pelvic abscesses	Anaerobic; display characteristic "cigar-shaped" morphology	Endogenous human flora of mouth, intestine, and vagina/not considered communicable	Endotoxin	None indicated
Porphyromonas spp.	Opportunistic infection causing gingivitis and dental abscesses	Anaerobic; non-spore-forming rod	Endogenous human flora of the mouth and vagina/not considered communicable	Endotoxin	None indicated
Prevotella melaninogenicus (formerly *Bacteroides melaninogenicus*)	Opportunistic infection associated with oral, pharyngeal, and pulmonary abscesses	Anaerobic; non-spore-forming rod	Endogenous human flora of the mouth and vagina/not considered communicable	Endotoxin	None indicated

Pathogen	Disease(s)	Notable Characteristics	Reservoir/ Transmission	Virulence Factors	Vaccine Status
Citrobacter spp.	Opportunistic infection associated with bacterial sepsis in immunocompromised individuals	Oxidase-negative rod; member of the Enterobacteriaceae, related to *Salmonella* spp.	Endogenous to human colon and the environment/ transmission pattern poorly understood	Endotoxin	None indicated
Enterobacter spp.	Opportunistic, nosocomially acquired lung and urinary tract infections	Lactose-fermenting; oxidase-negative rod; member of the Enterobacteriaceae, related to *Serratia* and *Klebsiella* spp.	Endogenous to human colon; the environment/ transmission pattern poorly understood	Endotoxin; highly resistant to antimicrobials	None indicated

Escherichia coli	Gastrointestinal illness; UTI; sepsis; meningitis	Lactose-fermenting; oxidase-negative rod; member of the Enterobacteriaceae; disease depends on virulence factors associated with each disease isolate	Endogenous to human colon; the environment/ transmission pattern depends on the isolate	Depend on the isolate, including
				• endotoxin
				• adhesins
				  CFA
				  intimin
				• type 3 secretion systems
				• toxins
				  STa
				  LT
				  Stx
				  hemolysin
				• capsules
				  K1
				• siderophores
				  enterobactin
				  enterochelin
				  aerobactin
					Indicated under certain circumstance—traveler's diarrhea

Klebsiella pneumoniae	Opportunistic, nosocomially acquired lung and urinary tract infections	Lactose-fermenting; oxidase-negative rod; member of the Enterobacteriaceae, related to *Serratia* and *Enterobacter* spp.	Human colon; in soil and water/transmission patterns poorly understood	Endotoxin; capsule	None indicated
Morganella morganii	Opportunistic infection associated with UTI and pneumonia	Non-lactose-fermenting; motile; oxidase-negative; urease-positive rod; member of the Enterobacteriaceae, closely related to *Proteus* spp. Some demonstrate "swarming" morphology when grown on blood agar	Human colon; in soil and water/transmission patterns poorly understood	Endotoxin; flagella	None indicated

Proteus mirabilis	Opportunistic infection causing UTI and pneumonia	Non-lactose-fermenting; motile; oxidase-negative; urease-positive rod; member of the Enterobacteriaceae, closely related to *Proteus* spp. Some demonstrate "swarming" morphology when grown on blood agar	Human colon; in soil and water/transmission patterns poorly understood	Endotoxin; flagella	None indicated
Proteus vulgaris	Opportunistic infection causing UTI and pneumonia	Non-lactose-fermenting; motile; oxidase-negative; urease-positive rod; member of the Enterobacteriaceae, closely related to *Proteus* spp. Some demonstrate "swarming" morphology when grown on blood agar	Human colon; in soil and water/transmission patterns poorly understood	Endotoxin; flagella	None indicated
Providencia spp.	Opportunistic infection causing UTI and pneumonia	Non-lactose-fermenting; motile; oxidase-negative; urease-positive rod; member of the Enterobacteriaceae, closely related to *Proteus* spp. Some demonstrate "swarming" morphology when grown on blood agar	Human colon; in soil and water/transmission patterns poorly understood	Endotoxin; flagella	None indicated
Salmonella spp.	Gastroenteritis; septicemia; typhoid fever	Motile; non-lactose-fermenting; oxidase-negative rod; pathogenic member of the Enterobacteriaceae	Fecally contaminated foods; some species (i.e., non-typhoid salmonella) have zoonotic reservoir; *S. typhi* have only a human reservoir/spread by personal contact with food followed by ingestion	Requires a large innoculum; dependent on ability to invade cells; Vi antigen (a capsule) important for typhoid fever; endotoxin	Indicated, live attenuated vaccine in development
Serratia marcescens	Opportunistic, nosocomially acquired lung and urinary tract infections; also eye infections	Lactose-fermenting; oxidase-negative rod; member of the Enterobacteriaceae, closely related to *Klebsiella* and *Enterobacter* spp.	Human colon; the environment/transmission patterns poorly understood	Endotoxin	None indicated

Pathogen	Disease(s)	Notable Characteristics	Reservoir/ Transmission	Virulence Factors	Vaccine Status
Shigella spp.	Gastrointestinal disease associated with bloody diarrhea and occasional vomiting	Non-motile; non-lactose-fermenting; oxidase-negative rod; pathogenic member of the Enterobacteriaceae	Common food-borne illness; humans the only reservoir/spread by fecal-oral transmission	Requires few organisms; some strains produce Stx; endotoxin	Indicated, not available
Yersinia enterocolitica	Enterocolitis; mesenteric adenitis	Oxidase-negative; non-lactose-fermenting; oval rod; grows better at 25°C than at 37°C; pathogenic member of the Enterobacteriaceae	Enzootic/transmitted to humans through ingestion of food contaminated by excretia of domestic animals (e.g., dogs, cats, cattle)	Invasins—Inv and Ail; Yops; iron acquisition; endotoxin	None indicated
Yersinia pseudo-tuberculosis	Enterocolitis; mesenteric adenitis	Oxidase-negative; non-lactose-fermenting; oval rod; grows better at 25°C and at 37°C; pathogenic member of the Enterobacteriaceae	Enzootic/transmitted to humans through ingestion of food contaminated by excretia of domestic animals (e.g., dogs, cats, cattle)	Invasins—Inv and Ail; Yops; iron acquisition; endotoxin	None indicated
Yersinia pestis	Bubonic plague; pneumonic plague	Oxidase-negative; non-lactose-fermenting; rod; exhibits bipolar staining; pathogenic member of the Enterobacteriaceae	Enzootic, exists in wild rodents/gains access to humans through flea bite	Capsule; endotoxin; F-1 envelope antigen; exotoxin; V antigen; W antigen; iron acquisition	None indicated
Aeromonas hydrophila	Wound infections; diarrhea; sepsis	Motile; oxidase-positive; hemolytic rod	Found in water and contaminated foods/ transmitted via ingestion	Pili; aerolysin; endotoxin	None indicated
Pasteurella multocida	Wound infections; cellulitis	Small rod	Found in mouths of many domestic animals/ transmitted via animal bites or scratches	Capsule; endotoxin	None indicated
Vibrio cholerae	Cholera	Comma-shaped rod; oxidase positive	Human colon; in water/ transmitted via ingestion	TCP; endotoxin	Indicated, currently under development
Pseudomonas spp.	Sepsis; pneumonia; UTIs; wound infections (burns); eye infections; associated with repeated lung infections in CF patients	Motile; oxidase-positive; grows on MacConkey agar; non-lactose-fermenting; many isolates produce pigment; characteristic fruity aroma	Found in water and soil; 10% of individuals carry *P. aeruginosa* in their colon	Exotoxin A; exotoxin S; pili; elastase; alginate (in cystic fibrosis strains); endotoxin	None indicated

Organism	Disease	Characteristics	Reservoir/Transmission	Toxins/Virulence factors	Prevention
Burkholderia cepacia (formerly *Pseudomonas cepacia*)	Opportunistic pathogen associated with repeated lung infections in CF patients	Non-lactose-fermenting	Found in water, soil, and on plants/transmitted upon exposure to the environment	Endotoxin; highly antibiotic resistant	None indicated
Legionella spp.	Legionellosis, which typically presents as a pneumonia	Small; slow growing; fastidious growth requirements	Found in water supplies and to a lesser extent in soil/transmitted upon exposure to contaminated reservoirs	Cytotoxin; endotoxin; extracellular proteases; Mip; penicillin resistance	None indicated
Gram-positive rods					
Bacillus cereus	Food poisoning (both emetic and diarrheal forms); eye infections; opportunistic infections due to use of medical devices; intravenous drug use	Large rods; grow aerobically and anaerobically; form heat-resistant endospores; motile; hemolytic	Ubiquitous in soil, plants, etc./transmitted by contaminated foods, through wounds, dirty needles, etc.	Heat-labile diarrheal enterotoxin; heat-stable emetic toxin	None indicated
Bacillus anthracis	Anthrax has three forms, all can lead to generalized sepsis and death if bacteria enter the blood: • inhalation anthrax (also known as "wool-sorters disease") • cutaneous anthrax • gastrointestinal anthrax	Large rods; grow best aerobically; form heat-resistant endospores; chains of cells visible microscopically; nonmotile; nonhemolytic	Contaminated animal products (e.g., wool or meat) and soils/inhalation anthrax via breathing in spores; cutaneous anthrax via implantation of spores in a wound (forming a sore called an eschar); gastrointestinal anthrax via ingestion of meat contaminated with spores or cells; biowarfare potential	Polypeptide capsule; tripartite toxin consisting of protective antigen (binding component), edema toxin (increases cAMP levels), and lethal toxin (kills mammalian cells)	Vaccine available for high-risk individuals (e.g., veterinarians, soldiers)
Clostridium botulinum	Food-borne botulism; infant botulism; wound botulism	Grows anaerobically; forms endospores	Soils and some foods/can cause intoxication by ingestion of preformed toxin (food-borne botulism) or in vivo toxin production (wound and infant botulism)	Botulinum neurotoxin causes flaccid paralysis	Vaccine available for research workers and other high-risk individuals
Clostridium difficile	Pseudomembranous colitis; antibiotic-associated diarrhea	Grows anaerobically; forms endospores	Nosocomial environment (e.g., hospital rooms)/acquired by inhalation of spores	Toxins A and B (these toxins have potent proinflammatory properties)	None indicated
Clostridium perfringens	Gas gangrene; wound infections; food poisoning; antibiotic-associated diarrhea; necrotizing enteritis	Grows anaerobically; forms endospores; double zone of hemolysis	Soils; animal and human feces; sewage/transmitted via ingestion or through wounds	Produces many toxins, significantly: • α-toxin (associated with gas gangrene and wound infections) • enterotoxin (associated with common food poisoning)	None indicated

Pathogen	Disease(s)	Notable Characteristics	Reservoir/ Transmission	Virulence Factors	Vaccine Status
Other histotoxic Clostridia (C. histolyticum, C. novyi, etc.)	Gas gangrene; wound infections	Grows anaerobically; forms endospores	Soils; sewage; feces/ transmitted by ingestion or through wounds	Produces many toxins	None indicated
Clostridium tetani	Tetanus	Grows anaerobically; forms endospores	Soils/spores contaminate wounds and germinate if redox potential drops	Tetanus toxin causes spastic paralysis	Tetanus toxoid; the "T" component of the DPT vaccine
Corynebacterium diphtheriae	Diphtheria	Small; pleomorphic (club-shaped); arranged in palisades or "Chinese letters"; grows best aerobically; nonhemolytic	Human reservoir/spread by inhalation	Diphtheria toxin causes necrosis and inflammation	Diphtheria toxoid; the "D" component of the DPT vaccine
Listeria monocytogenes	Listeriosis (meningitis and bacteremia)	Short rod; motile; hemolytic; can grow at refrigeration temperatures; facultative anaerobe	Zoonotic reservoir/ foodborne spread (often in dairy products)	Listeriolysin O; other phospholipases; internalin	None indicated
Propionibacterium spp.	Contributes to acne (sometimes causes opportunistic infections)	Anaerobic; short rod	Normal skin flora/not communicable	No notable virulence factors described	None indicated
Erysipelothrix rhusiopathiae	Erysipeloid (a painful skin infection)	Short rod	Zoonotic reservoir; decaying organic matter/transmitted by exposure to the environment	No notable virulence factors described	None indicated
Nocardia spp., especially N. asteroides	Nocardiosis (an opportunistic disseminated illness that often begins with a respiratory focus)	Slow growing; aerobic; forms branching filaments; shows partial "acid fastness"	Soil; decaying vegetation/ transmitted by inhalation or implantation into cuts	No notable virulence factors described	None indicated
Actinomyces spp., especially A. israelii	Actinomycosis (a swelling, typically of the cervicofacial region); can result in abscess formation; can (rarely) disseminate	Branching filaments; sulfur granules; non-acid-fast; anaerobic; slow growing	Soil; mouth/transmitted by trauma (e.g., dental work) to tissue	No notable virulence factors described	None indicated

Gram-positive cocci

Organism	Diseases/infections	Characteristics	Reservoir/transmission	Virulence factors	Vaccine
Staphylococcus aureus	Furuncles and carbuncles (boils and abscesses); impetigo; deep lesions (e.g., osteomyelitis); wound infections; toxic shock syndrome; staphylococcal food poisoning	Grape-like clusters; nonmotile; facultative anaerobes; very hardy; coagulase-positive; catalase-positive; may or may not be hemolytic	Nares of many healthy people; on body surface; in human environment (sometimes food)/transmitted through wounds, ulcers, breaks in skin, and by ingestion	Protein A; capsule; TSST; α-toxin; enterotoxins; coagulase; DNAse; hyaluronidase	None indicated
Coagulase-negative staphylococci, e.g., *S. epidermidis, S. saprophyticus*	Nosocomial infections	Grape-like clusters; facultative anaerobes; coagulase-negative; catalase-positive	Endogenous flora of skin and nares/enters through wounds via medical devices (e.g., catheters)	Some form a polysaccharide slime layer	None indicated
Streptococcus pyogenes	Pharyngitis; impetigo; wound infections; toxic shock syndrome; infection leads to sequelae such as rheumatic fever and glomerulonephritis	Belong to Lancefield group A; often occur in chains; catalase-negative; β-hemolytic; facultative anaerobes	Endogenous human throat or skin flora/transmitted by aerosols from person to person	Streptolysin O; pyrogenic exotoxins; hyaluronic acid capsule; M proteins; lipoteichoic acid; protein G	Indicated, currently under development
Streptococcus agalactiae	Neonatal sepsis; meningitis	Belong to Lancefield group B; form short chains or diplococci; β-hemolytic; facultative anaerobes; catalase-negative; CAMP-test positive	Endogenous to human vagina or respiratory tract/transmitted from mother to infant during birth	Capsule; C5a peptidase	Indicated, capsular vaccine under development
Streptococcus pneumoniae	Pneumococcal pneumonia; meningitis; most common in young, old, and immuno-compromised	Lancet (bullet)-shaped; catalase-negative; facultative anaerobes; α-hemolytic; autolytic; optochin-sensitive; bile-soluble	Endogenous flora of human throat and nares/spread by aerosols	Capsule; pneumolysin	Indicated; capsular vaccine available for use in the elderly and immunocompromised; capsular conjugate vaccine under development for use in infants
Viridans streptococci	Opportunistic cause of subacute bacterial endocarditis	α-Hemolytic; bile-insoluble; optochin-resistant; facultative anaerobes	Endogenous flora of human throat and nares/transmission patterns are poorly defined	No notable virulence factors described	None indicated
Enterococci, especially *Enterococcus faecalis*	Opportunistic cause of urinary tract and endocardial infections; bacteremia	Lancefield group D antigen; catalase-negative; facultative anaerobes	Endogenous flora of human intestinal tract/transmission patterns are poorly defined	Very antibiotic resistant	None indicated

Pathogen	Disease(s)	Notable Characteristics	Reservoir/ Transmission	Virulence Factors	Vaccine Status
Peptococcus spp. and Peptostreptococcus spp.	Opportunistic cause of abscesses	Anaerobe; catalase-negative	Endogenous flora of the human skin, intestine, and vagina/ transmission patterns poorly defined	No notable virulence factors described	None indicated
Bacteria that do not Gram stain					
Treponemes					
Treponema pallidum Borrelia burgdorferi Leptospira interogans	Syphilis Lyme disease Leptospirosis	Thin; corkscrew-shaped; periplasmic flagella; difficult or impossible to culture; typically observed by dark field microscopy	• T. pallidum is an obligate human pathogen/sexually transmitted • B. burgdorferi is a zoonotic disease/ transmitted by tick bites • L. interrogans is a foodborne disease/ transmitted by ingestion	OSPs; other virulence factors are not well described	Indicated for Lyme disease, not for syphilis or leptospirosis
Mycoplasma	Broncho-pneumonia; genital and interuterine disease	Small; lack a cell wall; require sterols for growth	Humans; animals; the environment/ transmitted by sexual contact & by inhalation	M. pneumoniae produces catalase, which reduces ciliary clearance	None indicated
Chlamydia trachomatis	Nongonococcal urethritis; lymphogranuloma; pneumonia; neonatal conjunctivitis	Small; obligate intracellular bacteria; exist in two forms—elementary body and reticulate body	Obligate human pathogens that cause disease on genito-urinary mucosa, in lung, or on conjunctiva/ spread by sexual or person-to-person contact; spread to infants within the birth canal	Not well defined	Indicated, not available
Rickettsiae	Rocky Mountain spotted fever; scrub typhus; Q fever	Small; obligate intracellular rods	Zoonoses with rodents as a reservoir/transmitted by arthropod vectors	Energy parasite; ability to escape the phagosome	Available for Rocky Mountain spotted fever but not indicated because of infrequency of disease
Mycobacterium spp.	Primary and secondary tuberculosis; tuberculoid and lepromatous leprosy	Acid fast; thin rods; M. tuberculosis grows extremely slow in culture; M. leprae cannot grow in culture	Obligate human pathogens/M. tuberculosis spread by inhalation; M. leprae spread by close contact	Ability to cause chronic inflammation as a consequence of persistence in macrophages; causes the release of specific cytokines	BCG live vaccine of arguable efficacy

VIRUSES

DNA viruses

Virus	Disease	Structure/Genome	Host/Transmission	Pathogenesis	Vaccine
Herpesviruses	Oral, genital lesions (HSV-1, HSV-2); chickenpox, varicella-zoster (VZV); infectious mononucleosis (EBV, CMV); CID (CMV); roseola (HHV-6); Kaposi's sarcoma (HHV-8)	dsDNA genome; icosahedral capsid; enveloped	Humans/spread by intimate contact or sexual intercourse	Capacity to cause latent infections; viral proteins that regulate MHC antigen presentation	Indicated, live attenuated chickenpox vaccine in use
Hepadnaviruses	Hepatitis B; hepatitis D	Partially circular dsDNA genome; icosahedral capsid; enveloped	Humans/spread by intimate contact, sexual intercourse, contaminated blood products	Overproduction of excess HBsAg acts as a decoy, binding antiviral antibodies	Indicated, hepatitis B subunit (HBsAg) vaccine in use
Adenoviruses	Upper & lower respiratory disease; ARD	Linear dsDNA genome; icosahedral capsid; nonenveloped	Humans/spread by respiratory aerosols or fecal-oral route	Early proteins E1A/E1B block cell-cycle regulation and cause apoptosis; MHC class I antigen presentation blocked	Not indicated for broad use; live adenovirus serotypes 4 & 7 vaccine for military personnel only
Papovaviruses Papillomavirus JC virus	Papillomatosis Progressive multifocal leukoencephalopathy	Circular dsDNA genome; icosahedral capsid; nonenveloped	Humans and animals/spread by parenteral (germline) inoculation or sexual intercourse	Capacity to persist by integrating into host chromosome; capacity to cause tumors	None available
Parvoviruses B19 virus	Blood dysplasias	Linear ssDNA (+ or −) genome; icosahedral capsid; nonenveloped	Humans/spread by parenteral (germline) inoculation	Capacity to persist by integrating into host chromosome	None available
Poxviruses	Smallpox	Linear dsDNA genome; asymmetrical core containing many enzymes; enveloped	Humans/spread by intimate contact	Virus encodes a variety of homologs that mimic or counteract host immunoreactive molecules	Smallpox vaccine using live attenuated vaccinia virus; not currently in use due to absence of smallpox

RNA viruses

Virus	Disease	Structure/Genome	Host/Transmission	Pathogenesis	Vaccine
Picornaviruses Enteroviruses Rhinoviruses Hepatitis A	Polio Common cold Hepatitis A	Linear ssRNA[+] genome; icosahedral capsid; nonenveloped	Humans/spread by fecal-oral route or respiratory aerosols	Viral proteases cleave cellular factors involved in transcription and translation of host mRNA	Indicated; killed and live poliovirus vaccines in broad use; killed hepatitis A vaccine available
Togaviruses Rubella virus	German measles	Linear ssRNA[+] genome; icosahedral capsid; enveloped	Humans/spread by close contact	Unknown	Indicated, live attenuated rubella virus vaccine in broad use
Flaviviruses Dengue Yellow fever Hepatitis C virus Hepatitis G virus	Hemorrhagic fever Hemorrhagic fever Hepatitis Hepatitis	Linear ssRNA[+] genome; icosahedral capsid; enveloped	Birds; monkeys in the case of yellow fever/ spread by respiratory aerosols or parenteral inoculation	Unknown	Not indicated; live, attenuated, yellow fever virus vaccine available
Coronaviruses	Common cold	Linear ssRNA[+] genome; helical capsid; enveloped	Humans/spread by respiratory aerosols and fomites	S glycoprotein causes vacuolization and spindling of host cell	Indicated, not available

Pathogen	Disease(s)	Notable Characteristics	Reservoir/ Transmission	Virulence Factors	Vaccine Status
Caliciviruses Hepatitis E virus Norwalk virus	Acute GI illness in adults Acute GI illness in adults	Linear ssRNA[+] genome; icosahedral capsid; nonenveloped	Humans/spread by fecal-oral route or fomites	Unknown	Not indicated
Filoviruses Ebola virus	Severe hemorrhagic fevers	Linear ssRNA[−] genome; helical capsid; enveloped	Unknown reservoir/spread by contact with contaminated body fluids	Unknown	Indicated, none available
Rhabdoviruses Rabiesvirus	Rabies	Linear ssRNA[−] genome; helical capsid; enveloped; bullet-shaped virion	Rodents; bats/spread by animal bite and possibly by inhalation of bat feces	Envelope proteins disrupt cytoskeleton; tropism for CNS	Indicated, inactivated virus vaccine available
Paramyxoviruses Respiratory syncytial virus Human para-myxoviruses Morbillivirus	Upper & lower respiratory infections Mumps Measles	Linear ssRNA[−] nonsegmented genome; helical capsid; enveloped	Humans/spread by respiratory aerosols, fomites, and direct contact	Host range determined by the virus envelope glycoproteins; mumps M protein (SSPE)	Indicated, live, attenuated vaccines against measles and mumps in broad use
Orthomyxoviruses Influenzavirus A Influenzavirus B	Influenza Influenza	Linear ssRNA[−] genome (8 segments); helical capsid; enveloped	Humans; aquatic birds; swine/spread by respiratory aerosols	Mutability of viral envelope proteins HA and NA permits escape from previous immune responses	Indicated viral subunit (HA & NA) vaccine; effectiveness short-lived due to changes in HA and NA; requires yearly injections
Bunyaviruses Hantaviruses	Encephalomyelitis; systemic hemorrhagic-like fevers	Linear ssRNA[− or +] genome (3 segments); helical capsid; enveloped	Birds; rodents/inhalation or insect bites	Envelope glycoproteins	Indicated, not available
Arenaviruses	Hemorrhagic fevers	Linear ssRNA[+] genome (2 segments); helical capsid; enveloped	Rodents/spread by aerosols of rodent feces	Unknown	Not available
Reoviruses Rotaviruses	GI disease in children	Linear dsRNA genome (10–12 segments); icosahedral capsid; nonenveloped	Humans/spread by fecal-oral route	NSP4 may exert entertoxin-like activity affecting calcium homeostasis	Indicated, recently recommended as part of childhood vaccination regimen
Retroviruses Oncoviruses Lentiviruses	Adult T-cell leukemia AIDS	Linear diploid ssRNA[+] genome; icosahedral capsid; enveloped; reverse transcriptase	Humans/spread by parenteral inoculation and unprotected sexual activities	Infidelity of reverse transcription and functionality of mutant envelope proteins permits creation of quasispecies; TAT regulatory protein stimulates immunomodulatory host proteins; gp120 affects calcium homeostasis	Indicated, none available

EUKARYOTIC PATHOGENS
Cutaneous and subcutaneous mycoses

Epidermophyton, Trichophyton, and *Microsporum* spp.	Dermatophytoses	Infect superficial keratinized structures (e.g., ringworm, jock-itch, athlete's foot); scrapings of skin or nail placed in 10% KOH show microscopic hyphae	Humans and animals/spread by direct contact from human to human. *Microsporum* spp. is transmitted by animals (e.g., dogs, cats)	Not well defined	None indicated
Sporothrix schenckii	"Rose gardener's" disease (a.k.a., sporotrichosis)	Subcutaneous dimorphic fungi; round or cigar-shaped budding yeast observed microscopically in tissue specimens	Environment/spread by the subcutaneous introduction of organisms into skin, such as by the prick of a rose thorn	Not well defined	None indicated

Systemic mycoses

Coccidioides immitis	coccidioidomycosis (a.k.a., San Joachim Valley fever or desert rheumatism)	Dimorphic fungus that exists as a mold in soil, but as a yeast in tissue; spherules filled with yeast endospores are seen in tissues examined microbiologically; skin tests with fungal extract result in a DTH response	Endemic to soils of arid regions of southwestern U.S. and Latin America/inhalation is the major mode of transmission	Not well defined	None indicated
Histoplasma capsulatum	Histoplasmosis is mostly a disease of the immunocompromised but also is associated with immuno-competent hosts that demonstrate repeated exposure to bird or bat droppings	Dimorphic fungus existing as a mold in soil, but as a yeast in tissue; oval yeasts found within macrophages derived from tissues or bone marrow aspirates	Endemic to soils of the Ohio and Mississippi River valleys—particularly those containing large concentrations of bird or bat droppings/spread by inhalation	Capsule	None indicated
Blastomyces dermatidis	Blastomycosis, a granulomatous disease typically confined to the respiratory tract	Dimorphic fungus existing as a mold in soil, but as a yeast in tissue; examination of tissues demonstrates thick-walled yeast cells with broad-based buds	Endemic to North and Central American soils/spread by inhalation	Not well defined	None indicated

Pathogen	Disease(s)	Notable Characteristics	Reservoir/ Transmission	Virulence Factors	Vaccine Status
Opportunitic mycoses					
Candida spp.	Causative agent of thrush, vaginitis, chronic mucocutaneous-candidiasis	Budding yeast with pseudohyphae are seen microscopically; not dimorphic; oval yeast with a single bud	Endogenous to human oral and vaginal flora/ not considered communicable	Not well defined	None indicated
Aspergillus spp.	Aspergillosis within the immunocompromised host	Microscopic examination of infected tissue demonstrates molds with septate, branching hyphae; not dimorphic, exist as molds only	Widely distributed in nature/spread to humans by aerosols	Not well defined	None indicated
Protozoa					
Plasmodium spp.	Malaria	Systemic protozoa	Humans/spread by the bite of a female anopheline mosquito	Ability to multiply intracellularly	Indicated, none available
Toxoplasma gondii	Toxoplasmosis, manifested as mononucleosis in relatively healthy individuals; congenital disease if transmitted in utero; encephalitis in the immunocom-promised	Tissue protozoa	Infected cats and other animals/spread by inhalation of fecal material	Ability to persist within a zoonotic host	None indicated
Pneumocystis carinii	PCP occurring in immunocompromised individuals	Atypical fungus	Infected humans and animals/acquired by inhalation of airborne fomites	Ability to persist within humans and animals	None indicated
Trypanosoma spp. *T. cruzi* *T. brucei*	Trypanosomiasis Chagas' disease African sleeping sickness	Systemic protozoa	Infected humans and animals/transmitted via insect bite	Antigenic variation; resistance to human complement components	Indicated, none available
Giardia lamblia	Giardiasis, a watery diarrhea; may cause malabsorption	Intestinal protozoa	Infected humans, animals, and waters/ acquired by ingestion	Ability to persist within the environment	None indicated
Entamoeba histolytica	Amebiasis	Intestinal protozoa	Infected humans/spread via ingestion of cysts	Ability to adhere to human intestinal mucosa; ability to cause asymptomatic infection	None indicated
Cryptosporidium parvum	Cryptosporidiosis, a watery diarrhea commonly occurring in AIDS patients	Intestinal protozoa	Animal reservoir or infected humans/ spread by fecal-oral transmission	Ability to persist within the environment	None indicated
Trichomonas vaginalis	Vaginosis	Vaginal protozoa	Common inhabitant of human vagina/ transmitted via sexual intercourse	Ability to persist within the vagina	None indicated

INDEX

NOTE: An "f" after a page number denotes a figure; a "t" after a page number denotes a table.

α-Hemolysin (Hly), 195

Abscess, 33, 33t

ACE. *See* Toxin(s), accessory cholera enterotoxin

N-Acetylglucosamine (GlcNAc), 12, 12f, 15, 66, 66f, 68f

N-Acetylmuramic acid (MurNAc), 12, 12f, 15, 66–67, 66f, 68f

Acquired immunodeficiency syndrome (AIDS), 403–410. *See also* Human immunodeficiency virus

  case of, 403–404, 410

  criteria for diagnosis of, 410t

  and cryptosporidiosis, 114

  epidemic, magnitude of, 1, 404

  and susceptibility to sepsis, 331–332

Actinomyces genus, 32t

Acute respiratory disease (ARD), 126

Acyclovir (Acv), 72, 72t, 73f, 153

Adenosine triphosphate (ATP), 30

Adenoviruses, 46f, 47t, 49t, 50, 125–126

Adenylate cyclase system, 313t, 316–317, 316f, 439f

Adherence, 99, 123, 190–192

Adhesins

  and antigenic variation among various pathogens, 267t

  associated with urinary tract infections, 199

  as basis for microbial adherence, 123, 191–192, 191f

  colonization factor of adherence (CFA) adhesins, 195–196, 350t, 354

  as virulence factors of

    Bordetella pertussis, 438–439, 439f

    Escherichia coli, 195–196, 196t, 199

    Helicobacter pylori, 228

    Neisseria gonorrhoeae, 270

    Streptococcus pneumoniae, 288. *See also* Fimbrial adhesins *and* Nonfimbrial (afimbrial) adhesins

Aerobes, 30

Aerotolerants, 30

Agar media, 452–454, 453t

AgrC and AgrA, 300

AIDS. *See* Acquired immunodeficiency syndrome

Alanine aminotransferase (ALT), 111

Amantadine, 72t, 73, 73f

Aminoglycosides, 65t, 69

Ammonium (NH$_4$+), produced by *Helicobacter pylori*, 228

Amphotericin B, 71, 79, 421

Ampicillin, 82, 184

Anaerobic

  bacteria. *See* Bacteria, anaerobic

  cellulitis, 34t, 36

  infections

    clostridial, 33–34, 34t

    nonclostridial, 32–33, 33t

Anthrax, 38–39, 137t. *See also Bacillus anthracis and* Toxin(s), anthrax

Antibacterial therapy, 63–70

Antibiotics. *See also specific antibiotics*

  cell wall inhibitor type, 65–68, 65t, 66f, 83, 84t

  definition of, 62

  effects of on normal flora, 182–186

  β-lactam

    efficacy of against

      Haemophilus influenzae, 130

      Legionella pneumophila, 237–239

      Staphylococcus aureus, 302

      Streptococcus pneumoniae, 289

    hydrolysis of by resistant bacteria, 85

    mechanism of action of, 66f, 67, 68f

    structure of, 67f

  mechanisms of action of, 65–70

  membrane inhibitor type, 65t, 68–69, 84t

  metabolism inhibitor type, 65t, 70, 84t

  nucleic acid inhibitor type, 65t, 69, 84t

  principles of use of, 62–63

  protein inhibitor type, 65t, 69–70, 84t

  resistance to, 2, 62, 81–92, 291t

Antibodies, 235, 337, 408

Antigen(s)

  K, H, and O, 17, 18, 194

  T (T-Ag), 50

  translocon, 209

  V and W, 142–143

  virulence (Vi), 370

Antigenic variation, 265–277, 270f

Antimicrobial

  peptides, 366

  therapy, 61–77. *See also* Resistance, antimicrobial

Antiseptics, commonly used, 458t

Antiviral therapy, 71–75

  via blockade of viral

    genome replication, 72

    protein processing, 74

  during early stages of infection, 73

  via inhibition of reverse transcriptase of HIV, 74

  using natural products, 74–75

Apoptosis, 308

ARD. *See* Acute respiratory disease

Arenaviruses, 47t, 52

Ascariasis, 23t

Ascaris lumbricoides, 23t

Aseptic transfer, 29

Aspartate aminotransferase (AST), 111

Aspergillosis, 422

Aspergillus spp., 21t, 332, 419t, 422

Aspiration, 124
Autolysin, 288
Azidothymidine (AZT)
    mechanism of action of, 9, 71–72, 72t
    resistance to, 84
    structure of, 73f
    in treatment of HIV, 409
Azoles, 65t, 71

B cells, 108, 330t
Bacillus ("rod") morphology, 14f
Bacillus anthracis, 38–39
    anthrax toxin produced by, 298t, 313t
    capsule of, 64, 282t, 283
    macrophages killed by, 318
    transmission of, 38, 137t
Bacillus cereus, 98t, 103, 105t, 117, 313t
Bacillus megaterium, 15f
Bacillus spp., classification of, 5t
Bacitracin, 65t, 66f, 68, 79
Bactec method, 338
Bacteremia, 128t, 289
Bacteria, 9–20, 27–41, 460–468. See also
            Pathogens, prokaryotic
    anaerobic, 31, 31t, 32t, 181t
    anatomy of, and basis for Gram stain, 15–19
    antigenic variation by, 267, 268f
    arrangements of, 14f
    capsules of, 13–14, 64
    cell wall of, 12–13, 12f, 66f
    chain growth of, 66–67
    chromosomal rearrangement in, 11, 11t
    common
        biology of, 10–11
        structures of, 12–14, 13f
    cross-linking of, 66, 68f
    cytoplasm of, 63, 64f
    cytoplasmic membrane of, 12, 13f, 64, 64f
    distinguishing characteristics of, vs. other pathogen
            types, 8, 8t
    diversity of, antigenic and phenotypic, 9–10, 11t
    DNA of, inhibition of synthesis of, 69
    envelope of
        components of, 12–13, 64, 64f
        gram-negative, 16–18
        gram-positive, 15–16, 15f
    exotoxins of. See Exotoxins
    fastidious, 33
    genetic exchange between, 10–11
    gram-negative vs. gram-positive, 13, 13f
    growth of, 27–41
        anaerobic, 31–34
        in vivo, and physiology of, 29–30
        measurement of, 28–29, 29f
    haploid chromosomes in, 10
    morphologies of, 14f
    phage transfer by, 11, 11t
    protein expression in, 11
    ribosomes in, 11
    RNA of, inhibition of synthesis of, 69
    sizes of, 8, 9f
    somatic mutations of, 11, 11t
    structural differences among, 14
    structure of, 10, 10f, 12–13, 13f
    therapy for. See Antibacterial therapy
    transduction by, 11, 11t
    in tumorigenesis, 394–395

    virulence of. See Virulence, bacterial
Bactericidal vs. bacteriostatic agents, 62
Bacteriocins, 143, 182
Bacteriuria, 92, 455
Bacteroides fragilis, 34–35, 181, 181t
Bacteroides spp., 31t, 32t, 181t
Bacteroides-like spp., 34–35, 43
Bartonella henselae, 337t
BCG. See Vaccine(s), bacille Calmette-Guérin
Benzylpenicillin, 83
Bethesda system, 398, 398t
Bile, 107
Binary fission, 10
Biofilm, 89
Blastomyces dermatitidis, 5t, 21t, 419t
Blastomycosis, 420
Blood agar, composition of, 453t
Bloodborne infections. See Infection(s), bloodborne
Bordetella pertussis, 437–441
    adenylate cyclase secreted by, 298t
    adhesion by, 123
    biologic characteristics of, 438
    classification of, 5t
    filamentous hemagglutinin expressed by, 192
    oxygen requirements of, 30
    pathogenesis of, 439–440
    prevention and treatment of, 440–441
    receptor interactions of, 191t
    reservoir and transmission of, 98t, 438
    respiratory invasiveness of, 121t
    toxins produced by, 313t
    two-component regulatory system of, 365t
    virulence factors of, 438–439
Borrelia burgdorferi, 19–20, 98t, 137t, 146–149,
            432t
Borrelia spp., 5t, 146, 146t
Botulinum toxin. See Toxin(s), botulinum
Botulism
    antitoxin, 322
    case of, 311–312, 322–323
    diagnosis of, 322
    foodborne, 4, 103–104, 320–322
    general features of, 105t, 320–322
    infant, 320–322
    wound, 320, 322
Bovine papillomavirus, 46f
Braun's lipoprotein, 13f, 18
Bronchiolitis, 124f
Bronchitis, 124f, 125t
Brucellosis, 137t
Bubonic plague. See Plague
Bullous lesions, 301
Bundle-forming pili (BFP), 196t, 197, 197f
Bunyaviruses, 47t, 52, 140
Burkholderia cepacia, 88

E-Cadherin, 235t
Calcium, dependence of Yersinia pestis on, 141–142
Caliciviruses, 47t, 52, 54f, 111
Campylobacter fetus, 111
Campylobacter jejuni, 101–102, 105t, 111–112,
            115, 117
Campylobacter spp., 5t, 30, 228
Cancer, association of with infectious disease, 377–
            378
Candida albicans
    antigenic variation by, 267t

Candida albicans (*Continued*)
  candidiasis caused by, 421–422
  classification of, 5t
  with other fungal pathogens, 21t
  opportunism of, as function of CD4+ count, 417f
  with other causes of STDs, 155t
Candida spp., 419t
Candidiasis, 421–422
CAP. *See* Pneumonia, community-acquired
Capsids, 46, 46f, 48, 48f
Capsules, microbial, 281–291
  appearance of, 283f
  cellular location of, 282–283
  chemical composition of, 282t, 283–284, 283t
  table of, 282t
  as virulence factors, 284–286, 285f, 286f, 356
Carbapenems, 67f
Carrier state, 253, 381
Catalase, 31
Catheterization, 414–415, 415t
Cefotaxime, 82
Ceftriaxone, 120, 131, 332
Cefuroxime, 290
Cell-mediated immune (CMI) responses, 309
Cell wall(s), of bacteria, 12–13, 13f
Cephalosporins, 65t, 66f, 67f, 184
Cercariae, 341, 341f
Cervical intraepithelial neoplasia (CIN), 398, 398t
Cestodes. *See* Tapeworms
Chancroid, 155t
Chickenpox, 444–446
Chitin, 8t, 20, 418
Chlamydia psittaci, 137t, 151
Chlamydia spp., 5, 99, 157, 206t
Chlamydia trachomatis, 155t, 156–158
  biologic characteristics of, 156–157
  diagnosis of, 158
  elementary bodies (EBs) of, 157, 166
  and Gram stain, 158
  life cycle of, 157f
  pathogenesis of, 157–158
  persistence of, 380t
  prevention and treatment of, 158
  reservoir and transmission of, 157
  serovars of, 156t
Chloramphenicol, 65t
Chocolate agar, 127, 453t
Cholangitis, ascending, 91
Cholecystitis, 81
Cholera. *See Vibrio cholerae and* Toxin(s), cholera
Chromosomes, haploid vs. diploid, 10
Cidofovir (Cdv), 72t
Cilia, 225
Classification of microorganisms, 451
Clavulanate, 28
Clavulanic acid, 67
Clindamycin, 65t, 179–180, 183–184
Clonal proliferation, 10
Clostridia, histotoxic, 34t, 36–37
Clostridium barati, 320
Clostridium botulinum
  biologic characteristics of, 105t, 320. *See also*
        Botulism *and* Toxin(s), botulinum
  diagnosis of, 322
  pathogenesis of, 321–322
  prevention and treatment of, 322
  reservoir and transmission of, 104, 320–321

  toxins of, 313t
  virulence factors of, 321
Clostridium butyricum, 320
Clostridium difficile
  antibiotic-associated colitis caused by, 70, 179–
        180, 182, 186
  biologic characteristics of, 182
  colitis induced by, appearance of, 185f
  diagnosis of, 184
  pathogenesis of, 183–184
  prevention and treatment of, 184–186
  reservoir and transmission of, 182–183
  toxins A and B of, 313t, 316
  virulence factors of, 183, 183f, 188, 354t
Clostridium histolyticum, 36
Clostridium novyi, 36
Clostridium perfringens
  enterotoxins produced by, 298t
  features of, 34t, 36–37, 38, 105t
  toxins produced by, 298t, 313t, 316
  two-component regulatory systems of, 365t
Clostridium septicum, 36
Clostridium spp., 5t, 31t, 32t, 98t
Clostridium tetani
  characteristics of, 39–40
  clostridial disease caused by, 34t
  oxygen requirements of, 30
  toxin production by, 313t. *See also* Toxin(s), tetanus
  vaccine for, 432t, 434, 436t
Coagulase, 299
Coagulation system, 330–331
Cocci arrangement of bacteria, 14f
Coccidioides immitis
  classification of, 5t
  with other fungal pathogens, 21t
  general features of, 419t, 420
  opportunism of, as function of CD4+ count, 417f
  with other opportunistic pathogens, 122t
  with other pathogens causing granulomatous
        disease, 337t
Coccidioidomycosis, 420–421
Coccobacillus morphology, 14f
Coccus morphology, 14f
Cold, common, 206
Colon, normal flora of. *See* Flora, gastrointestinal
Colonization
  factor antigens (CFAs), 108, 195–196, 350t
  factors of *Vibrio cholerae*, 356
  by microbial pathogens, 97–99, 189–201
  of stomach by *Helicobacter pylori*, 227–230
Columbia CNA agar, 453t
Commensal organism, defined, 2
Community-acquired infection, 83, 290–291
Complement system, 330, 334, 416
Conjugation, 11, 11t, 86, 86f
Conjunctivitis, 124f, 156
Contingency loci, 268, 268f
Coronaviruses
  electron micrograph of, 46f
  limitation of to respiratory epithelium, 207
  with other pathogens infecting respiratory tract, 125t
  receptors of, 49t, 52
  RNA virus features of, 47t, 52
Corynebacterium diphtheriae, 352–354
  adherence by, 123
  arrangements of, 352f
  case of, 349–350, 358–359

Corynebacterium diphtheriae (*Continued*)
  classification of, 5t, 352
  invasiveness of, 121t
  lysogenic infection of with β-phage, 351, 351f
  toxin produced by. *See* Toxin(s), diphtheria
  vaccine for, 432t, 434, 436t
Crackles, 403
Crepitus, 28
Cross-talk, 207
Croup, 124f
Cryptococcus neoformans
  capsule of, 282–283, 282t, 283f
  cryptococcosis caused by, 422
  extracellular classification of, 5t
  invasiveness of, 121t, 122t
  morphology of, 21t
  opportunism of, as function of CD4+ count, 417f
  treatment of, 79
Cryptosporidiosis, 105–106, 114–115
Cryptosporidium parvum, 106, 114–115
Cryptosporidium spp., 5t, 106t, 417f
Cyclic adenosine monophosphate (cAMP), 316–317,
    316f
Cycloserine, 67
Cystic fibrosis, 89
Cystitis, 155t, 200–201
Cytokines, 317, 329, 329f
Cytomegalovirus (CMV). *See* Human cytomegalovirus
Cytoplasmic membrane. *See* Bacteria, cytoplasmic
    membrane of
Cytosol
  presence of in major microbial pathogens, 8t
  in structure of bacteria, 10f
Cytotoxin, 196t, 197, 199–200, 228, 313t

Dane particles, 169
Decay accelerating factor (DAF), 342
Defenses of body, overcoming, 223–230
Dermatophytoses, 419t
Diagnostic medical microbiology, 451–456
Diaminopimelic acid (DAP), 13
Diarrhea. *See also* Dysentery
  associated with
    antibiotics, 179–180, 184, 186
    Campylobacter jejuni, 101–102, 115, 117
    clostridial diseases, 34t
    Clostridium difficile, 182–186
    common waterborne pathogens, 106t
    Escherichia coli, 193t, 196–198
    rotaviruses, 109–110
    Salmonella spp., 193t
    Shigella spp., 193t, 205–206, 215
    Vibrio cholerae, 4
  enterohemorrhagic, 137t
Didanosine, 72t
Diplococci arrangement of bacteria, 14f
Diploid chromosomes, 10
Diseases, infectious
  acquired by
    ingestion, 101–115
    inhalation, 119–131, 121t
  as cause of death in U.S., 1
  introduction to, 1–5
  nature and medical importance of, 1–2
  transmission of. *See* Transmission of infectious
    diseases
Disinfection (disinfectants), 457, 458t

Disseminated
  gonococcal infection (DGI), 269f, 270
  intravascular coagulation (DIC), 331
DNA
  conjugation of, 11, 11t, 86–87, 86f
  diversity of in bacterial pathogens, 10–11, 11t
  in major microbial pathogens, 8t
  positive- and negative-polarity, 48
  proviral, 53
  slipped-strand synthesis of, 267
  transduction of, 11, 11t, 86, 86f
  transformation of, 85–86, 86f
  viruses. *See* Viruses, DNA
DPT vaccine. *See* Vaccine(s), diphtheria-pertussis-
    tetanus
Dysentery, 193t, 214
Dyspnea, 290

Ear infection, 7
Ectopic pregnancy, 156
Edema, 41
Effector molecules of *Salmonella* spp., 369–370
Elastase, 298
Elementary bodies (EBs), 157, 166
Elephantiasis, 23, 23t
Encephalitis, 160, 443
Endocytosis, pathogen-directed, 207, 235, 235t, 314f
Endospores, 37–38
Endotoxic shock, 17, 328
Endotoxin(s). *See* Lipopolysaccharide
Energy theft, 30
Entamoeba histolytica, 23, 23t, 106t
Enterobacter cloacae, 82
Enterobacter spp., principal diseases caused by, 194t
Enterobacteriaceae, 192–194, 193t, 194t, 199, 368
Enterochelin, 196t
Enterococcus faecalis, 82, 87, 89–90, 256, 256t,
    257f
Enterotoxin(s)
  five B subunit:one A subunit (5B:1A) family of, 315,
    315f
  heat-labile (LT), 196t, 313t, 315, 350t
  heat-stable (STa), 196t, 313t, 315–316, 350t
  producers and actions of, 313t
  staphylococcal
    A, 350t
    six serotypes of, 300, 313t
  as virulence factor of
    Clostridium difficile, 34t, 35
    enterotoxigenic *Eschrichia coli*, 196t
    Salmonella spp., 370
Enterovirus(es), 106t, 441
Enzyme-linked immunoassays (ELISAs), 446, 454
Enzymes, and immune evasion, 297–298, 300
Epidermophyton spp., 21t, 418
Epiglottitis, 124f, 125t, 128t
Episomal transfer, 11, 11t
Epithelial surfaces, invasion of by pathogens, 205–
    215, 206t, 207t
Epstein-Barr virus (EBV), 49t, 173, 380t, 395
Erythema
  chronicum migrans rash, 148f
  nodosum, 420
Erythromycin, 65t, 70, 290, 431
Escherichia coli, 194–201
  adherence by, 190, 191
  biologic characteristics of, 194

Escherichia coli (Continued)
  capsule of, 282t, 283
  classification of, 5t, 30
  enteroaggregative (EAEC), 196t, 197
  enterohemorrhagic (EHEC), 196t, 197–198, 350t
  enteroinvasive (EIEC), 196t, 197
  enteropathogenic (EPEC), 192, 196t, 197, 354t
  enterotoxigenic (ETEC), 103, 196–197, 196t, 315–316, 350, 350t
  gram-negative response of, 16
  growth of, 28
  as normal GI flora, 108, 181t
  O4:H5, 199–201
  O157:H7, 103, 105t, 194t, 197–198, 312
  pathogenesis of, 196
  reservoir and transmission of, 194–195
  serotypes of, 194, 194t, 204
  shiga toxin produced by. *See* Toxin(s), shiga
  sites of entry of, 137t
  tests for differentiating, 193t
  toxins produced by, 313t, 314
  and triple sugar iron slants, 193, 193t
  urinary tract infection by, 70, 181, 189–190, 198–201, 203, 456
  uropathogenic, 191t, 354t
  virulence factors of, 195
Eubacteria, 9
Eukaryotes. *See* Pathogens, eukaryotic
Excystation, 114
Exfoliatin, 300, 313t
Exotoxin(s), 307–308, 311–322
  A, produced by *Pseudomonas aeruginosa*, 314
  that induce pathologic immune responses, 318, 318f, 319f
  molecular action of, 312–320
  protein synthesis-inhibiting, 312–314

F-1 antigen, 142
Factor H, 258
Facultative aerobes, 30
Famciclovir, 72t, 73f
Fecal-oral route. *See* Transmission of infectious diseases, fecal-oral route of
Fermentation, 30
Ferric uptake repressor (fur), 364
Fibronectin, 259f
Filamentous hemagglutinin (FHA), 192, 438, 439f
Filoviruses, 47t
Fimbrial adhesins, 191–192, 195–196, 267t
Flagella
  protozoal, 22, 23t
  of *Helicobacter pylori*, 228
  of *Salmonella* spp., 370, 370f
  of typical bacteria, 10f, 13–14, 13f, 64, 64f
Flagellates, 23t
Flagellin, 370, 370f
Flaviviruses, 47t, 52
Flora, normal human, 108, 179–186
  gastrointestinal, 31t, 44, 108, 180–182, 181t
  mucosal, 3, 180, 181t
Flucytosine, 65t, 71
Flukes, 23, 23t
Fluorochrome stains, 341
Folate-synthesis inhibitors, 70
Food poisoning, 37, 104, 105t, 301, 369
Foodborne route. *See* Transmission of infectious diseases, foodborne route of

Forssman antigens, 16
Foscarnet, 72t, 73f
Francisella tularensis, 98t, 137t, 138
Fungi, 417–422. *See also* Mycoses
  distinguishing characteristics of, 8, 8t, 20–22, 21f, 21t
  facultative intracellular vs. extracellular, 5t
  summary table of, 419t
  therapy of, 71
  toxins produced by, 308
Fur. *See* Ferric uptake repressor
Fusiform morphology, 14f, 15
Fusobacterium, 32t

Ganciclovir, 72, 72t, 73f
Gardnerella vaginalis, 155t, 226
Gas gangrene. *See* Myonecrosis
Gas production, in nonclostridial anaerobic infection, 33
Gastrointestinal
  -associated lymphoid tissue (GALT), 102–103, 108
  flora. *See* Flora, gastrointestinal
  tract, defenses of, 107–108, 226
Genes. *See also* DNA *and* RNA
  conversion of, 266–268, 268f
  factors influencing expression of, 208–209
  housekeeping, 14
  plasticity of, 266
  rearrangement (recombination) of, 266–268, 268f
  retroviral, expression of, 55f
  virulence, 14
Gentamicin, 69, 82, 91
Germination, bacterial, 38
Giardia lamblia, 5t, 22, 23t, 106, 106t, 112–113, 113f
GlcNAc. *See* N-Acetylglucosamine
Glomerulonephritis, 261–262
Glucan, 8t, 20
Glycerol, 16
Glycocalyx, 13
Gonococcus. *See* Neisseria gonorrhoeae
Gonorrhea. *See* Neisseria gonorrhoeae
Gram-negative anaerobic bacteria, 32t
  cell envelopes, 16–18, 17f
Gram-positive anaerobic bacteria, 32t
  cell envelopes, 15–16, 15f
Gram stain, 12–20
  basis of, 15–18, 15f, 16f, 17f
  importance of, 14–15
  steps of, 452t
Granulocyte abnormalities, 416
Granuloma, 337, 337f
Griffith experiment, 284, 285f
Griseofulvin, 71
Growth curve(s), 29, 29f, 43f, 44
Guanosine, 73f

Haemophilus ducreyi, 129, 155t
Haemophilus influenzae, 127–130
  biologic characteristics of, 127
  bronchitis and, 125f
  diagnosis of, 129–130
  gram-negativity of, 18
  invasive disease, 129
  invasiveness of, 121t
  meningitis caused by, 119–120, 130–131
  mucosal disease, 129

Haemophilus influenzae (*Continued*)
    pathogenesis of, 128–129, 128f
    prevention and treatment of, 130
    reservoir and transmission of, 98t, 127
    treatment of with chloramphenicol, 69
    type b (Hib), 128f, 129, 130f, 132, 282t, 432t
    vaccine for, 432t, 434–435, 436t
    virulence factors of, 127–128
Haemophilus spp., 5t, 127f
Hageman factor, 330–331, 330t
Hantavirus, 140–141, 152
    pulmonary syndrome, 137t
Haploid chromosomes, 10
Helicobacter pylori, 228–230
    case of, 223, 230
    survival strategies of in stomach, 107, 220, 227f
    and tumorigenesis, 393t, 394–395
Helicobacter spp., 5t, 30
Helminths, 8, 9f, 22–24, 23t
Hemolysins, 259, 300, 354t
Hemolytic
    patterns of streptococci, 256, 257f, 264
    uremic syndrome, 197–198
Hepadnaviruses, 47t, 53–56, 56f, 168
Hepatitis A virus (HAV), 103–104, 105t, 106t, 110–
        111
Hepatitis B virus (HBV), 168–171
    chronic active (CAH), 168, 170f
    core antigen (HBcAg) and surface antigen (HBsAg),
        167, 169, 169f
    forms of, 169f
    HBeAg antigens, 170f, 171
    and liver dysfunction, 155t
    persistent chronic (PCH), 168, 170f, 380t
    serology of, 170f, 171t
    in tumorigenesis, 395
    vaccine for, 432t, 434, 436t
Hepatitis C virus (HCV), 395
Herpes simplex virus (HSV), 159–163
    atypical, opportunism of, 417f
    case of, 153–154, 163
    diagnosis of, 162–163, 166
    infection, primary vs. recurrent, 160
    latency of, 159, 160f
    life cycle of, 159–160, 159f
    lytic and latent infection by, 51f
    pathogenesis of, 161–162
    persistence of, 380t
    photomicrograph of, 46f
    reactivation of, 159, 160f
    receptors for, 49t
    serotypes of, 160
    virulence factors of, 161, 161t
Herpesviruses. *See also* Herpes simplex virus *and*
        Varicella-zoster virus
    characteristics of, 47t, 155t, 172–173
    replication of, 51–52, 51f
    therapy for, 9
Hib. *See Haemophilus influenzae* type b
Highly active anti-retroviral therapy (HAART), 409
Histoplasma capsulatum
    classification of, 5t
    with other fungal pathogens, 21t
    general features of, 137t, 419t, 421
    opportunism of, as function of CD4+ count, 417f
    with other pathogens causing granulomatous
        disease, 337t

Histoplasmosis, 137t, 421
Host
    defenses, deficits in, 415
    definitive vs. intermediate, 22
HPV. *See* Human papillomavirus
HTLV-1. *See* Human T-cell leukemia virus 1
Human cytomegalovirus (CMV), 172–175, 380t,
        417f
Human immunodeficiency virus (HIV), 406–410. *See
        also* Acquired immunodeficiency syndrome
    cultured, identification of, 454
    genes and proteins of, summarized, 406t
    pathogenesis of, 407–409, 408f
    persistence of, 380t
    prescription of AZT for, 9
    receptor interactions of, 49t, 191t
    reverse transcription of, 406–407, 407f
    schematic representation of, 405f
    and susceptibility to *Mycobacterium tuberculosis*,
        340
Human papillomavirus (HPV), 396–399
    with other causes of STDs, 155t
    infection and growth of in epidermal layers, 397f
    with other pathogens limited to epithelial cells, 206t
    persistence of, 380t
Human T-cell leukemia virus(es) [HTLV-1, -2], 395,
        405, 405t
HUS. *See* Hemolytic uremic syndrome
Hyaluronic acid, 282t, 284t, 293
    capsule of group A streptococci, 259, 264
Hyaluronidase activity of group A streptococci, 259
Hydrogen sulfide (H_2S), production of by
        Enterobacteriaceae, 193, 193f
Hydrolysis of cell wall, 15f, 26
β-Hydroxymyristic acid, 18
Hyperplasia, 50
Hyphae, 21, 21f, 21t
Hypogammaglobulinemia, 417

Iatrogenic immunosuppression, 172
Identification, methods of, 452–454
Idoxuridine, 73f
IFNs. *See* Interferons
IgA1 protease, 272
Immune complex formation, 336
Immunity
    cell-mediated, abnormalities in, 417
    herd, 427, 443t
    innate and specific, 219–220
Immunization, 139, 427–429, 436t. *See also*
        Vaccine(s)
Immunoglobulin A (IgA), 108, 121
    protease, 123, 133, 254, 288
Immunoglobulin G (IgG), 296, 296f
Immunopathology
    pathogen-elicited, mechanisms of, 336–337
    in response to infection, 336
Immunosuppression
    and opportunistic infection, 414–415
    types of, 415–417, 415t
    viral, 172
Impetigo, 300–301
Infection(s)
    bloodborne, 168–171, 211t
    of compromised hosts, 122, 122t
    defined, 97–98, 102–103
    host's inability to clear, 377–378

Infection(s) (*Continued*)
  immunopathology in response to, 336
  vs. intoxication, 4, 102
  lysogenic vs. lytic, 351, 351f
  of noncompromised hosts, 122–123, 123t
  opportunistic, 181, 413–424
  persistent, 197
  point source, 197
  transplant-associated, 171–175
Infectious diseases. *See* Diseases, infectious
Infiltrates, lobar vs. patchy, 76
Inflammatory response(s)
  immunopathologic consequences of, 335–343
  indirect host damage caused by, 308–309
  systemic, in sepsis, 328–329, 329f, 334
Influenzavirus
  antigenic variation by, 267t, 274–275, 279
  biologic characteristics of, 274–275
  diagnosis of, 276
  electron micrograph of, 46f
  limitation of to respiratory epithelium, 98t
  and noncompromised individuals, 123, 123t
  pathogenesis of, 276
  pneumonia, case of, 265–266, 277
  prevention and treatment of, 73, 276–277
  reassortment of, 57
  receptors for, 49t
  reservoir and transmission of, 98t, 275
  structure of, 275f
  vaccine for, 432t
  virulence factors of, 275–276
Interferons (IFNs), 74–75, 74t, 171
Interleukin, 328, 329f, 330t
Internalin(s), 235, 235t
Intestines
  invasion of by pathogens, 102–103, 208–211
  motility of, 107
  normal flora of. *See* Flora, gastrointestinal
Intoxication, 103–104
  vs. infection, 4, 102
Intracellular survival of pathogens, 234–236
Invasin(s), 208–209, 217, 235, 235t
Invasion by microbial pathogens, 99, 102–103, 234–236
Iridoviruses, 47t
Iron
  acquisition of by
    Escherichia coli, 195, 199
    Neisseria meningitidis, 254
  and bacterial growth, 29–30, 225
  dependence on of *Yersinia pestis*, 142
Isolation of bacteria on agar media, 452–454, 453t
Isoniazid, 65t, 70

Ketodeoxyoctalonate (KDO), 17f, 18
Klebsiella pneumoniae, 282t
Klebsiella spp., 5t, 193t, 194t
Koch's postulates, 2–3

β-Lactams. *See* Antibiotics, β-lactam
Lactobacillus spp., 181t, 226
Lactoferrin, 30, 224–225
Lamina propria, 371
Laryngitis, 124f
Latency, 159, 160f, 381
Legionella pneumophila, 237–239, 238f
Legionella spp., 5t

Leishmania spp., 5t, 23t
Lentiviruses, 405–406
Leprosy. *See Mycobacterium leprae*
Leptospira interrogans, 137t, 146t
Leptospirosis, 137t
Leukocidin, 300
Leukocyte count, and opportunistic infection, 416, 417f
Leukotrienes, 330t, 331
Lipid A, 17f, 18
Lipooligosaccharide (LOS)
  and gram-negative cell envelope, 17f, 18
  and immune evasion, 297
  produced by
    Neisseria gonorrhoeae, 271f, 271t, 272, 273f
    Neisseria meningitidis, 254
Lipopolysaccharide (LPS)
  and immune evasion, 297
  and inflammatory response, 329
  produced by
    Escherichia coli, 195, 196t
    Haemophilus influenzae type b, 127, 133
    Helicobacter pylori, 228
    Legionella pneumophila, 237
    Neisseria gonorrhoeae, 297
    Neisseria meningitidis, 254
    Salmonella spp., 369
    Shigella spp., 212
    Vibrio cholerae, 356
  in structure of gram-negative bacteria, 17–18, 17f, 26
Lipoteichoic acid (LTA), 16, 16f, 258, 259f
Listeria monocytogenes, 239–242
  acquisition and symptoms of, 103, 105t, 137t
  classification of, 5t
  compared to other pathogens, 249
  listeriolysin produced by, 313t
  parasite-directed endocytosis used by, 235t
  progression of infection by, 241f
Listeriosis, 137t
Low-grade squamous intraepithelial lesion (LSIL), 391
Lyme disease, 146–149
  case of, 135–136 , 149
  clinical manifestations of, 148t
  and Gram stain, 19–20
  means of spread of, 137t
  notable characteristics of, 146t
Lymphogranuloma venereum, 156t
Lysogeny, 351–352
Lysozyme, 15, 15f, 224, 232

M cells, 108, 208, 210f, 213–214, 213f
MacConkey agar, 198, 200, 204, 453t
Macrophage(s)
  alveolar, 238, 238f
  infectivity potentiator (Mip), 237, 238f
  journey of bacterium through, 236f
Malaria, 242, 242t
Malnutrition, 122
Mannan, 8t, 20
Measles virus, 49t, 206, 436t
Meningitis, caused by
  Escherichia coli K1, 252t
  Haemophilus influenzae, 119–120, 128t, 130–131
  Listeria monocytogenes, 241, 249
  Neisseria meningitidis, 252–256, 252t
Merozoites, 22

Mesenteric lymphadenitis, 208
Metronidazole, 28, 65t, 113, 185–186
Microaerophiles, 30
Microbial
  entry, colonization, and disease, 3–4
  flora, normal, 180–182, 181t
  growth in stomach, 227–228
  ligand–host cell receptor interactions, 191t
  pathogenesis, principles of, 3–5
  pathogens, 7–24. *See also specific pathogens*
  subversion of host defenses, 219–221
  toxins, 312
  virulence, genetics of, 347–348
Microscopy, 8, 9f
Microsporum spp., 21t, 418
Mip. *See* Macrophage infectivity potentiator
Miracidia, 341, 341f
Mitochondria, 8t
Molds, 21
Molecular mimicry, 220–221, 251–262, 252t, 272
Mollicutes, 20
Molluscum contagiosum, 155t
Monobactams, 67f
Monospot test, 414
Moraxella spp., 98t
Mouth, normal flora of, 31t, 181t
mRNA. *See* RNA, messenger
MRSA. *See Staphylococcus aureus*, methicillin-
      resistant
Mucinase, 228
Mucociliary escalator, 121
Mucopeptide, 12
Mucopurulent cervicitis, 156t
Mucus, 107
Multiplication of microbial pathogens, 99
Murein, 12, 16f
MurNAc. *See N*-Acetylmuramic acid
Mutation(s)
  frameshift, 267
  point, 56, 266–268, 268f, 275
Mycobacterium avium, 70, 417f
Mycobacterium bovis, 338, 432
Mycobacterium leprae, 385–387
  classification of, 5t
  Gram stain nonreactivity of, 19
  with other causes of granulomatous disease, 337t
  Koch's postulates and, 2
  persistence of, 380t
Mycobacterium spp., 5t, 19, 19f, 236t
Mycobacterium tuberculosis
  antibiotic resistance of, 63
  biologic characteristics of, 28, 338
  case of, 335–336, 343
  diagnosis of, 340
  Gram stain response of, 19, 19f
  granuloma formation with, 337f
  opportunism of, as function of CD4+ count, 416,
      417f
  with other opportunistic pathogens, 122t
  pathogenesis of, 339–340
  persistence of, 380t
  prevention and treatment of, 340–341, 345
  reservoir and transmission of, 338, 345
  rifampin effective against, 69
  vaccine for. *See* Vaccine(s), bacille Calmette-
      Guérin
  virulence factors of, 338–339

Mycoplasma hominis, 155t
Mycoplasma pneumoniae, 75–77, 76t, 121t,
      123t
Mycoplasma spp., 12, 20, 79
Mycoses
  classification of, 418
  cutaneous, 418–420
  opportunistic, 419t, 421–422
  subcutaneous, 420
  systemic, 419t, 420–421
Myonecrosis, 34t, 36–37, 41

Nafcillin, 296
Necrotizing enteritis, 37
Negri bodies, 139
Neisseria gonorrhoeae
  antibiotic resistance of, 85
  antigenic variation by, 267t
  biologic characteristics of, 269
  classification of, 5t
  diagnosis of, 273–274
  expression of LPS by, 18
  and gonorrhea, 155t, 269–274
  and Koch's postulates, 2
  pathogenesis of, 272–273, 273f
  pili of, antiphagocytic effects of, 297
  prevention and treatment of, 274
  properties of, 253t
  receptor interactions of, 191t
  reservoir and transmission of, 269–270, 269f
  virulence factors of, 270–272, 271t
Neisseria meningitidis
  biologic characteristics of, 252–253, 253t
  capsule of, 282t, 283
  classification of, 5t
  diagnosis of, 255
  immune response to, 220–221
  invasiveness of, 120, 121t
  LPS expression by, 18
  molecular mimicry by, 252–256, 252t
  pathogenesis of, 254–255
  prevention and treatment of, 255–256
  reservoir and transmission of, 253
  vaccine for, 432t, 435
  virulence factors of, 253–254
Neisseriaceae, properties of, 253t
Nematodes, 23t
Neuraminidase, 288, 432t
Neurotoxins. *See under* Toxin(s)
Neutrophilic pleocytosis, 130, 130f
Nevirapine, 72t
Nitric oxide (NO), 330t, 331, 339
Noncapsular surface factors, 296–297
Nonclostridial diseases. *See* Anaerobic infections,
      nonclostridial
Nonfimbrial (afimbrial) adhesins, 191–192, 195
Nongonococcal urethritis (NGU), 155t, 156, 156t
Norwalk and Norwalk-like viruses, 105t, 106t
Nosocomial infections, 83, 87, 91, 168, 199t
Nucleases, 260
Nucleocapsid(s), 46, 46f, 55
Nucleus, presence of in major microbial
      pathogens, 8t
Nystatin, 71

Obligate intracellular pathogens. *See* Pathogens,
      intracellular, obligate

Omeprazole, 230
Oncogene, viral, 50. *See also* Oncoviruses *and* Tumorigenesis
Oncoviruses, 405t
One-carbon transfer reactions, 70
Opportunistic infections. *See* Infections, opportunistic
Opsonins, 235
Orthomyxoviruses, 47t, 52, 274
Otitis media, 24, 124f, 125, 289
Oxygen
    and bacterial growth, 30
    sensitivity of strict anaerobes to, 31

PAI. *See* Pathogenicity islands
PAP. *See* Pili, P blood group antigen–associated
Papanicolaou (Pap) smear, 391, 398–399, 398t
Papillomaviruses, 396
Papovaviruses, 46f, 47t
Parainfluenza virus, 49t, 123t
Paralysis, 33t, 40, 40f, 321
Paramyxoviruses, 47t, 52
Parasites, 22–24
    distinguishing characteristics of, 8, 8t, 22
    malarial, 243, 243f
Parvoviruses, 46f, 47t, 49t
Pasteurella haemolytica, 98t
Pasteurella multocida, 137t
Pasteurellosis, 137t
Pasteurization, 457
Pathogenic
    cycle, 4, 97–99
    strategies, 3
Pathogenicity islands, 195, 209, 350, 354–355, 354t
Pathogens
    acquired by inhalation, 119–131
    bacterial. *See* Bacteria *and* Pathogens, prokaryotic
    bloodborne, 168–171, 211
    eukaryotic, 8, 8t, 10, 20–24, 471–472
        difficult-to-categorize, 24
        immune survival strategies of, 234–236
        protein expression in, 11
    extracellular, 8, 8t
        acquired by inhalation, 123
        vs. intracellular, 4–5, 5t
    Gram stain nonreactivity of, 19–20
    inhibition of by normal flora, 179–186
    intracellular
        acquired by inhalation, 124
        vs. extracellular, 4–5, 5t
        facultative, 4, 5t
        obligate, 4, 5t
    major divisions of, 8, 8t
    microbial, biology of, 7–24
    persistent, 380t
    postinvasion fates of, 211–212
    prokaryotic, 9–20. *See also* Bacteria
        defined, 8, 8t, 10, 10f
        growth of, 28–30
        immune survival strategies of, 234–236
        protein expression in, 11
        reproduction of, 10
        structural differences among, 14
    sizes of, 8, 9f
    table of, 459–472
    viral. *See* Viruses
Penciclovir TP, 72t, 73f

Penicillin(s)
    -binding proteins (PBPs), 83, 84t
    mechanism of action of, 65t, 66f
    resistance to of
        gonorrhea, 91, 272, 274
        pneumococci, 291t
    structure of, 67f
Pepsinogen 1, 267t
Peptidase, C5a, 259
Peptide, autoinducing, 367, 367f, 368f
Peptidoglycan
    in cell wall synthesis, 66
    as characteristic of bacteria, 8t
    in cross-linking of layers of bacterial cell wall, 67–69, 68f
    fragments, and inflammation, 300
    in mycobacteria, 19, 19f
    structure of, 12f
    in structure of gram-negative cell envelope, 16
Peptococcus genus, 32t
Peptostreptococcus genus, 32t
Periplasmic space, 13f, 18
Peroxidases, 31
Pertactin, 438
Pertussis. *See also Bordetella pertussis*
    case of, 431, 446
    signs and symptoms of, 437–438, 438t
    vaccine for, 435, 436t
Pesticin, 143
Petechiae, 255
Petri plates, 28
Peyer's patches, 108, 208, 442
PfEMP-1. *See Plasmodium falciparum* infected erythrocyte membrane protein 1
Phage
    β-, 351
    CTXφ, 355
    transfer, 11, 11t
Phagocytosis
    host-directed, 235, 236f, 236t
    inhibition of by capsules, 284–285, 284t
Pharyngitis, 61, 124f, 125t, 251–252, 260, 262
Pharynx, normal flora of, 31t, 181t
Phenotypic variation, 266–268
Picornaviruses, 46f, 47t, 52, 53f, 110, 441
Pilus (pili)
    of bacteria, 10f, 13f, 64, 64f
    bundle-forming (BFP), 196t, 197, 197f
    as colonization factor antigens (CFAs), 108, 195–196, 350t
    common, 10f, 64
    and microbial adherence by
        Escherichia coli spp., 195, 196t, 199, 252t, 253
        Neisseria gonorrhoeae, 270
        Neisseria meningitidis, 253–254, 439, 439f
        various bacteria, 191–192, 191t
    P blood group antigen–associated (PAP), 191t, 199, 225
    PilC and PilE components of, 270, 271f, 271t
    sex, 10f, 11, 64
    toxin-coregulated (TCP), of *Vibrio cholerae*, 356, 357f, 365t
    type 1, 191t, 196t, 199
    type 4, 191t
Pinta, 146t
Piperacillin, 82, 91

Pla protease, 143
Plague, 137t, 141–143, 142f, 193t
Plasmids, 86–87
　fertility/sex (F-factors), 86
　resistance (R-plasmids or R-factors), 11, 11t, 86–87, 93
　virulence, 86
Plasmodium falciparum, 22, 242–245, 242t, 244f, 267t
　infected erythrocyte membrane protein 1 (PfEMP-1), 244, 244f, 267t
Plasmodium malariae, 22, 242–245, 242t
Plasmodium ovale, 242t, 244
Plasmodium spp., 5t, 23t, 242–245, 242t
Plasmodium vivax, 242t, 244, 380t
Platelet-activating factor, 330t
Pleomorphic bacteria, 35
Pleuritic pain, 290
Pneumococcal surface protein A (PspA), 288
Pneumococcus. See Streptococcus pneumoniae
Pneumocystis carinii, 5t, 24, 70, 121–122, 417f
Pneumolysin, 288, 293
Pneumonia
　caused by Legionella pneumophila, 237–239, 249
　community-acquired (CAP), 290–291
　diagnosis of, 455
　with other diseases caused by Haemophilus influenzae, 128t
　infant, 156t
　mycoplasmal, 75–77, 76t
　pathogens associated with, 125t
　pneumococcal, 3–4, 76t, 288–289, 293
Pneumonic plague, 137t, 141–143
Point tenderness, 223
Poliovirus
　biologic characteristics of, 441–442
　neurovirulence of, 441f
　pathogenesis of, 442–443, 442f
　receptor for, 49t
　reservoir and transmission of, 442
　vaccination for, 436t, 444
　virulence factors of, 442
Polyenes, 65t, 71
Polymicrobic contamination, 32–33
Polymorphoneutrophils (PMNs), 271, 273f
Polymyxins, 65t, 68–69
Polypeptide capsule, 12
Polyribitolphosphate, 130, 130f
Polysaccharides, and immune evasion, 297. See also Lipopolysaccharide and Lipooligosaccharide
Porins, 13f, 17, 271f, 271t, 272
Porphyromonas genus, 34
Poxviruses, 47t, 52
Prevotella genus, 34
Prevotella spp., 31t
Prokaryotes. See Pathogens, prokaryotic
Protease inhibitors, 74, 74f, 409
Proteases. See specific proteases
Protein(s)
　A, 296–297, 296f, 299
　expression of in bacteria. See Bacteria, protein expression in
　G, 296–297, 296f
　Gi, 316–317, 316f
　glycoprotein gp120, 191–192
　Gs, 316, 316f

IcsA and IcsB, 212–214
Ipa (invasion plasmid antigen), 209, 210f, 212, 235t
M, 123, 258, 259f, 267t, 297, 309
Mxi-Spa, 209, 210f, 212–213, 217
opacity-associated (Opas), 271–272, 271f, 271t
outer membrane, of
　Neisseria meningitidis, 254
　Salmonella spp., 370
penicillin-binding (PBPs), 83, 84t
pneumococcal surface protein A (PspA), 288
PfEMP-1, 244, 244f, 267t
Rho, 183, 183f, 188
secreted, and immune evasion, 297–298
ToxR and ToxT, 357, 357f, 365t
transferrin-binding (Tbps), 271f, 272, 273f
viral nonstructural, 109
Yersinia outer (Yops), 142, 208, 350t
Proteinuria, 200
Proteolytic
　enzymes, 107
　nicking of toxins, 314f, 320
Proteus spp., 5t, 193t, 194t
Protoplasts, 15, 15f
Protozoa, 22–23, 23t, 243
Proviruses, 9
PRP. See Polyribitolphosphate
Pseudomembranous colitis, 184, 185f, 188
Pseudomonadaceae, morphology of, 88f
Pseudomonas aeruginosa
　elastase secreted by, 298
　exotoxin A secreted by, 11, 88, 313t, 314
　leukocidin secreted by, 298t
　quorum-sensing system of, 367, 367f
Pseudomonas cepacia, 88
Pseudomonas spp., 5t
Pseudomonas treatment of, 69, 82
Psittacosis, 137t
Purpura, 255
Pyelonephritis, 201
Pyoderma, 260
Pyogenic infection, 260, 299
Pyrogenic
　endotoxins, 300
　exotoxins, 259
Pyrogens, 195

Quellung reaction, 290
Quinolones, 65t, 69
Quorum-sensing systems, 366–368, 367f, 368f

R-plasmids. See Plasmids, resistance
Rabies and rabies virus, 137t, 138–139, 433
Rales, 61
Reactivation, 159, 160f, 381
Reagin, 385
Reassortment, 266–268
Rebound tenderness, 41
Receptor-mediated endocytosis, 48
Receptors, virus, 49t
Recombination, 56, 266–268
Redox potential, 31
Regulatory systems, two-component, 364–368
Reiter's syndrome, 156
Reovirus family, 47t, 53, 109
Resistance, antimicrobial, 81–92
　genetic basis of, 85–87

Resistance, antimicrobial (*Continued*)
  importance of, 82–83
  mechanisms of, 83–85, 84t
  prevention of spread of, 90–91
  of respiratory pathogens to phagocytes, 123
  to stomach acid, 107
  via
    alteration of antimicrobial site of action, 83–84
    bypass of targeted site of action, 8
    limiting access to site of action, 85
    modification of antimicrobial agent, 85
    overproduction of the target, 84
Respiration, 30
Respiratory syncytial virus (RSV), 123t
Respiratory tract, 124f
  host defenses of, 121–124
  infectious diseases of, 3–4, 124–125, 125t
Retrovirions, 55
Retroviruses, 47t, 53–56, 55f, 267t, 405t
Reverse transcriptase, 9, 74f, 406, 409
Rhabdoviruses, 47t, 52, 138
Rheumatic fever, 260–262, 261t
Rhinitis, 124f, 125t
Rhinoviruses, 49t, 121t, 123t, 125t, 207
Rhizopods, 23, 23t
Ribavirin (Rbv), 72t, 73f, 141
Ribosomes, 11
  presence of in major microbial pathogens, 8t
  30S and 50S ribosomal subunits, 69–70
Ribotol, 16
Rickettsia akari, 144t
Rickettsia prowazekii, 380t
Rickettsia ricketsii, 143–146
  cell-to-cell spread of, 145f
  compared to *Escherichia coli*, 144f
  Gram stain properties of, 19
  testing for, 151
  vectors of, 137t
Rickettsia typhi, 144t
Rifampin, 65t, 69
Rigor, 290
Rimantadine, 72t, 73, 73f
Ritonavir, 72t
RNA
  genomes, [+] and [−], 52–53
  in HIV-1 infection, 405–406, 407f
  in lentivirus infection, 405–406
  messenger (mRNA), and protein expression in
      prokaryotes, 11
  poliovirus genomic, influence of on neurovirulence,
      441f
  positive and negative polarity, 47t
  pre-genomic, 55, 56f
  viruses. *See* Viruses, RNA
Rocky Mountain spotted fever, 19, 137t, 144–146,
      151–152. *See also Ricketsia ricketsii*
Rose spots, 363
Rotaviruses, 106t, 109–110, 117, 312, 436t
Roundworms, 23–24, 23t

Sabouraud's agar, 418, 421
Salmonella spp., 368–371
  biologic characteristics of, 368
  classification of, 5t
  disruption of by streptomycin, 182
  invasion of intestinal epithelium by, 209–211,
      217

  nontyphoid, 105t, 137t, 368–369, 370–372
  pathogenesis of, 370–372
  pathogenicity island of, 354t
  prevention and treatment of, 372–373
  principal diseases caused by, 193t
  reservoirs and transmission of, 368–369
  tests for differentiating, 193t
  two-component regulatory system of, 365t, 366
  typhoid, 369, 371–372
  virulence factors of, 369–370
Salmonella typhi
  acquisition of, 103, 369
  capsule of, 282t
  case of, 363, 373
  persistence of, 380t
  vaccine for, 432t, 433
Salmonella typhimurium, 193t, 235t
Salmonellosis, 137t
Schistosoma spp., 341–343, 342t
  biology of, 24, 341
  geographic distribution of, 342t
  with other helminth pathogens, 23t
  life cycle of, 341f
  with other pathogens causing granulomatous
      disease, 337t
Schistosomiasis, 23, 23t
Sepsis, 327–332
  case of, 327, 332
  caused by *Pseudomonas aeruginosa*, 92
  host factors related to, 331–332
  management of, 332
  mediators of, 330t
  pathogenesis of, 328–331
  stages in progression of, 332t
Septicemia, 37
Serovariation, 156
Serratia marcescens, 98t
Serum glutamate pyruvate transaminase (SGPT), 111
Serum glutamic-oxaloacetic transaminase (SGOT), 111
Sexually transmitted diseases (STDs), 153–163. *See
      also specific STDs*
  major causes of, 155t
Shedding, 381
Shigella boydii, 212
Shigella dysenteriae, 99, 103, 212, 214, 313t
Shigella flexneri, 193t, 212, 235t
Shigella sonnei, 205–206, 212, 214–215
Shigella spp.
  acid resistance of, 227
  biologic characteristics of, 212
  classification of, 5t
  diagnosis of, 214–215
  as foodborne pathogens, 105t, 107
  invasion of intestinal epithelium by, 209, 210–211,
      210f, 213–214, 213f, 217
  pathogenesis of, 213–214, 213f
  prevention and treatment of, 215
  reservoir and transmission of, 212
  tests for differentiating, 193t
  transmission of, 104, 206t
  virulence factors of, 212–213
Shingles, 444–445
Shock, 309, 331
Sickle cell anemia, 331–332
Siderophores, 195
Sin Nombre virus, 140
Sinusitis, 124f, 289

Skin
    normal flora of, 31t, 181t
    as physical defense, 224
Spheroblasts, 15
Spirochetes, 14f, 19–20, 20f, 146t
Sporothrix schenckii, 21t, 419t, 420
Sporozoa, 23t
Sporulation, bacterial, 38
Spumaviruses, 405t
Staphylococcus aureus
    antibiotic resistance of, 84, 302
    biologic characteristics of, 299
    cases of, 295–296, 302, 305
    diagnosis of, 301
    as foodborne pathogen, 104, 105t
    leukocidin secreted by, 298t
    methicillin-resistant (MRSA), 302
    molecular mimicry by, 252t
    as normal flora, 181t, 299
    opportunistic infections by, 416
    pathogenesis of, 300–301
    prevention and treatment of, 302
    protein A, antiopsonic/antiphagocytic effects of,
        296–297, 296f
    reservoir and transmission of, 98t, 299
    toxins secreted by, 298t, 313t, 317f
    two-component regulatory system of, 365t, 367–
        368, 368f
    virulence factors of, 299
Staphylococcus epidermidis, 181, 181t, 416–417
Staphylococcus spp., 5t, 83
STDs. *See* Sexually transmitted diseases
Sterilization, control of pathogens by, 457
Stomach
    acidity of as antimicrobial defense, 220, 226–230
    microbial growth in, 227, 227f
Streaking of bacterial cultures, 453–454, 454f
Streptococci
    group A, 5t, 256–262, 257f, 261f, 284, 284t
    group B, 5t, 285, 286f
    pathogenic, table of, 256t
    viridans, 181t, 256t, 257f
Streptococcus agalacticae, 256, 256t, 257f
Streptococcus mutans, 191t
Streptococcus pneumoniae
    antibiotic resistance of, 291t
    appearance of, 287f
    biologic characteristics of, 286–287
    capsule of, 282t, 283–284, 283t, 285f, 287–288
    clinical syndromes associated with, 125t
    diagnosis of, 289–290
    erythrogenic toxins of, coding for, 350t
    hemolytic pattern of, 257f
    infection of compromised hosts by, 122, 122t
    pathogenesis of, 288–289
    pneumolysin secreted by, 313t
    prevention and treatment of, 290
    properties of, 256t
    receptor interactions of, 191t
    reservoir and transmission of, 3, 98t, 287
    sepsis caused by, 327, 332
    teichoic acids of, 16
    vaccine for, 432t, 435
    virulence factors of, 287–288
Streptococcus pyogenes
    antigenic variation by, 267t
    biologic characteristics of, 256t, 257–258, 257f

C5a peptidase secreted by, 298
capsule of, 282t
diagnosis of, 262
exotoxins secreted by, 313t
hemolytic pattern of, 257f
M protein of, and immune evasion by, 297
molecular mimicry by, 252t
pathogenesis of, 260–262
prevention and treatment of, 262
protein G of, antiopsonic/antiphagocytic effects of,
    296f, 297
pyrogenic exotoxins A and C produced by, 313t,
    318
receptor interactions of, 191t
reservoir and transmission of, 258
resistance of phagocytosis by, 123
with other respiratory pathogens, 123t, 125f
streptolysin O secreted by, 298t
toxic shock–like illness caused by, 301
virulence factors of, 258–260
Streptokinase, 260
Streptolysins O and S, 259–260
Streptomycin, 69
Strict anaerobes, 30, 31
Subclinical infection, 307
Sulbactam, 67
Sulfamethoxazole, 70
Sulfonamides, 62, 65t, 70, 70f
Superoxide dismutase, 31
Svedberg units, 11
Syncytium, 308
Syphilis. *See also Treponema pallidum*
    case of, 379–380, 387
    clinical stages of, 383t
    secondary, clinical manifestations of, 384t
    with other STDs, 155t
Systemic inflammatory response syndrome (SIRS),
    327–328, 328f

T cell(s)
    count
        opportunistic infection as function of, 416,
            417f
        in pathogenesis of HIV, 408, 408f
    in *Mycobacterium tuberculosis* infection, 337f,
        339–340
    in Peyer's patches, 108
    stimulation of by conventional antigens vs. by
        superantigenic toxins, 318, 318f, 319f
    with other TNF-α targets, 330t
Tachypnea, 290
Taenia spp., 23t
Tapeworms, 23–24, 23t
Taxonomy, 8, 459–472
TB. *See* Tuberculosis
TCP. *See* Pili, toxin-coregulated
Teichoic acid, 15–16, 15f, 16f, 300
Tenesmus, 184
Tetanus, 34t, 38–41, 44, 434, 436t. *See also
    Clostridium tetani and* Toxin(s), tetanus
Tetracyclines, 65t, 69
Tetrahydrofolate synthesis, 70, 70f, 80
Thymidine, 73f
Ticarcillin, 28, 82, 91
TNF-α. *See* Tumor necrosis factor-α
Tobramycin, 82
Togaviruses, 47t, 52, 54f

Toxic shock syndrome
    case of, 281–282, 302
    clinical criteria for defining, 303t
    toxin (TSST-1), 300–302, 313t, 318
Toxin(s).   See also Exotoxins and Intoxication
    α-, 34t, 313t, 317f, 365t
    θ, 365t
    A and B, 34t, 313t, 316, 354t
    accessory cholera enterotoxin (ACE), 354t, 356
    anaphylatoxins, 330
    anthrax, 298t, 318
    botulinum. See also Clostridium botulinum
        and clostridial disease, 34t
        and GI tract defenses, 108
        molecular action of, 319–320, 319f
        antitoxin, 322
    cholera, 315–316, 354t, 356–358, 365t
    damage to host by, 307–308
    diarrheal, 313t
    diphtheria
        gene for, carried by mobile genetic factor, 350t
        mechanism of action of, 312–314, 313t, 314f,
            353
        regulation of by iron, 351–352, 352f
    emetic, 313t
    P-fimbriae, 354t
    fungal, 308
    and immune evasion, 298, 298t
    membrane-active, 317, 317f
    neurotoxins, 319–320, 319f
    pertussis, 313t, 365t, 431, 439
    production, in vivo, 103
    progenitor, 321
    shiga (Stx)
        gene for, carried by mobile genetic factor,
            350t
        as in vivo toxin, 103
        mechanism of action of, 213, 313t, 314–315
        production of by Escherichia coli, 195, 196t,
            350t
    streptococcal erythrogenic, 350t
    superantigenic, 318, 318f, 319f
    tetanus, 312, 313t, 319–320, 319f, 350t
    zonula occludens (ZOT), 354t, 356
Toxogenic infection, 260
Toxoplasma gondii, 422–424
    case of, 413–414, 424
    opportunism of, as function of CD4+ count, 417f
    parasite-directed endocytosis by, 235t
    with other persistent pathogens, 380t
    with other protozoal pathogens, 23t
    transmission of, 137t, 423
Toxoplasmosis, 137t, 422–424
Tracheitis, 124f
Trachoma, 156t
Transduction, 11, 11t, 86, 86f
Transformation, genetic, 85–86, 86f, 284
Translational regulation, 267, 268f
Translocon, Mxi-Spa, 209, 210f, 217
Transmission of infectious diseases, 97–98, 98t
    fecal-oral route of, 104
    foodborne route of, 104, 105t
    waterborne route of, 105–106
Transplant-associated infection. See Infection(s),
            transplant-associated
Transposons, 87, 94
Trematodes, 23t

Treponema pallidum, 381–385
    Gram stain nonreactivity of, 19
    invasiveness of, 207t
    persistence of, 380t, 383
    with other spirochetes, 146t
    with other causes of STDs, 155t
Treponema spp., 5t, 146t
Treponemes. See Spirochetes
Trichinella spiralis, 23t, 105t
Trichinosis, 23t, 24
Trichomonas vaginalis, 23t, 155t
Trichophyton spp., 21t, 418
Trifluorothymidine, 73f
Trimethoprim, 65t, 70, 70f, 79
Triple sugar iron (TSI) slants, 193, 193t
Trophozoites, 22
Tropism
    of normal flora, 180
    viral, 48
Trypanosoma brucei, 5t, 23t, 268
Trypanosoma cruzi, 5t, 23t, 137t, 380t
Trypanosomes, African, 267t, 268
Trypanosomiasis, American, 137t
TSST-1. See Toxin(s), toxic shock syndrome toxin
Tuberculosis. See Mycobacterium tuberculosis
Tularemia, 137t
Tumor
    formation, mechanisms of, 393–394
    necrosis factor-α (TNF-α)
        cell targets of, 330t
        and mechanism of gonococcal disease, 273f
        as mediator of sepsis, 330t
        production of, 317, 328–329, 329f
        release of stimulated by TSST-1, 301
    terminology, 392t
Tumorigenesis, 391–397
    bacteria and viruses associated with, 393t
Turbidity, 28
Type III secretion systems of Salmonella spp., 369–
            370
Typhoid fever. See Salmonella spp., typhoid

Ulcers
    decubitus, 27
    peptic, 229
Uncomplicated gonococcal infection (UGI), 269f, 270
Ureaplasma urealyticum, 155t
Urease, 227–228, 227f, 229
Urinary tract infections (UTIs)
    diagnosis of, 455–456
    by Escherichia coli, 70, 181, 189–190, 198–201,
            203, 456
    treatment of, 70
Urogenital tract defenses, 225–226
Uterine infection, 37

Vaccine(s)
    administration of, 435–437, 436t
    bacille Calmette-Guérin (BCG), 341, 432–433,
            432t
    chemically inactivated, 433–434
    chickenpox, 433, 446
    composition of, 428–429
    conjugate, 435
    dead, 433–434, 433t
    diphtheria-pertussis-tetanus (DPT), 40, 354, 440–
            441

Vaccine(s) (*Continued*)
  killed whole pathogen, 429
  live
    attenuated, 429, 432–433, 433t
    vs. dead, advantages and disadvantages of, 433t
  measles-mumps-rubella (MMR), 436t, 437
  pertussis, 433, 449
  polio
    advantages and disadvantages of, 443t
  enhanced inactivated (EIPV). *See* Vaccine(s), Salk
    inactivated (IPV). *See* Vaccine(s), Salk
    oral (OPV). *See* Vaccine(s), Sabin
  principles of, 428
  Sabin, 432, 443–444
  Salk, 432t, 433, 443–444
  subunit, 429, 434–435
  table of, 432
  useful, properties of, 427–428
  varicella-zoster virus (VZV), 436t, 445
Vaccinologic therapy, 138
Vaccinology, principles of, 432–435
Vagina, normal flora of, 31t
Vaginosis, 155t
Vancomycin, 65t, 66f, 68, 185, 332
Variable surface glycoprotein (VSG), 267t
Variation, antigenic, 221
Varicella-zoster virus (VZV), 380t, 444–446
Veillonella genus, 32t
Venereal diseases. *See* Sexually transmitted diseases
Vibrio morphology, 14f, 15
Vibrio cholerae, 355–358
  and acidity of stomach, 107
  cholera toxin secreted by, 313t
  electrolyte solutions used to treat for, 358t
  and molecular Koch's postulates, 3
  pathogenic cycle of, 4, 106t
  pathogenicity island of, 354t
  receptor interactions of, 191t
  symptoms of, 116
  ToxR-regulated expression of virulence factors in, 357, 357f
  two-component regulatory system, 365t
  vaccine for, 432t
  virulence factors of, 356–357, 357f
Vibrio parahemolyticus, 105t, 137t
Vibriosis, 137t
Vidarabine (Vdb), 72t, 73f
Virions, 49–50, 53f
Virulence
  bacterial
    regulation of expression of, 363–373
    role of mobile genetic elements in, 349–359, 350t
  definition of, 2–3
  genes, 11, 364–368, 365f
  genetics of, 347–348

Virus(es). *See also* specific viruses
  antigenic variation by, 56–57, 59, 266, 267t
  capsids, 46, 46f, 48, 48f
  classification of, 9, 47t
  composition and architecture of, 45–46
  constituents of, synthesis and assembly of, 48–49
  cytopathic effects (CPEs) of on cells, 308
  direct fusion by, 48
  distinguishing characteristics of, 8, 8t, 46t, 59
  DNA, 47t, 48–52, 51f, 469
  enveloped vs. nonenveloped, 46, 46f, 51f
  fractionation of, 434
  genomes of, reassortment of, 57, 57f
  growth cycles of, 45–58
  oncogenesis by, 395, 395f
  particles, 46, 46f
  proteins of, 49
  receptors of, 49t
  release of, 49–50
  resistance of, 57, 59
  RNA, 47t, 48–49, 52–53, 53f, 54f, 266, 469–470
  sizes of, 8, 9f
  therapy of. *See* Antiviral therapy
  transmission of, 9
Vulvovaginitis, 155t
VZV. *See* Varicella-zoster virus

Warts, genital, 155t
Waterborne route. *See* Transmission of infectious diseases, waterborne route of
Weil-Felix test, 145, 151
Whooping cough. *See* Pertussis
Wuchereria bancrofti, 23t

Xenozoonosis, 138

Yaws, 146t
Yeasts, 8, 9f, 21, 21f, 21t
Yersinia enterocolitica, 105t, 141, 208
Yersinia outer proteins (Yops), 142, 208
Yersinia pestis, 137t, 141–143
Yersinia pseudotuberculosis, 137t, 141, 208, 235t
Yersinia spp.
  classification of, 5t
  invasion of intestinal epithelium by, 208–211, 217
  tests for differentiating, 193t
Yersiniosis, 137t

Zidovudine. *See* Azidothymidine (AZT)
Zoonotic
  diseases, 135–149
    general characteristics of, 136
    modes of entry of, 137, 137f
    transmission of, 136–137, 136f
  reservoir, 39, 136